Decision Making in
OPHTHALMOLOGY
An Algorithmic Approach

THIRD EDITION

Editor

Johan Zwaan MD PhD
Professor of Ophthalmology, Pediatrics, and Structural and Cellular Biology (Retired)
The University of Texas Health Science Center
San Antonio, Texas, USA

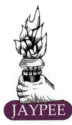

JAYPEE

JAYPEE BROTHERS MEDICAL PUBLISHERS (P) LTD

Philadelphia • New Delhi • London • Panama

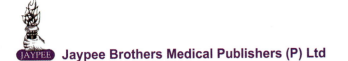

Jaypee Brothers Medical Publishers (P) Ltd

Headquarters

Jaypee Brothers Medical Publishers (P) Ltd
4838/24, Ansari Road, Daryaganj
New Delhi 110 002, India
Phone: +91-11-43574357
Fax: +91-11-43574314
Email: jaypee@jaypeebrothers.com

Overseas Offices

J.P. Medical Ltd
83, Victoria Street, London
SW1H 0HW (UK)
Phone: +44-2031708910
Fax: +02-03-0086180
Email: info@jpmedpub.com

Jaypee-Highlights.
Medical Publishers Inc
City of Knowledge, Bld. 237
Clayton, Panama City, Panama
Phone: +1 507-301-0496
Fax: +1 507-301-0499
Email: cservice@jphmedical.com

Jaypee Medical Inc.
The Bourse
111 South Independence Mall East
Suite 835, Philadelphia, PA 19106, USA
Phone: +1 267-519-9789
Email: jpmed.us@gmail.com

Jaypee Brothers
Medical Publishers (P) Ltd
17/1-B Babar Road, Block-B
Shaymali, Mohammadpur
Dhaka-1207, Bangladesh
Mobile: +08801912003485
Email: jaypeedhaka@gmail.com

Jaypee Brothers
Medical Publishers (P) Ltd
Shorakhute, Kathmandu
Nepal
Phone: +00977-9841528578
Email: jaypee.nepal@gmail.com

Website: www.jaypeebrothers.com
Website: www.jaypeedigital.com

Decision Making in Ophthalmology: An Algorithmic Approach

Third Edition: **2014**
ISBN: 978-93-5152-091-7
Printed at: Ajanta Offset & Packagings Ltd., New Delhi

Dedicated to

Three men have had a significant influence on my career in ophthalmology, as mentors and friends, and I wish to dedicate this book to three of them.

Dr Richard M Robb, then Chief of Pediatric Ophthalmology, Children's Hospital of Boston, MA, USA, exposed me to clinical ophthalmology and awakened my interest in the discipline. When I asked him for advice about a career in ophthalmology, he enthusiastically encouraged me to pursue it.

I knew Dr Robert D Reinecke, then Chair of the Department of Ophthalmology, Albany Medical Center, Albany, NY, USA, from my days as a member of one of the NIH Visual Sciences Study Sections. Hearing about my plans for an ophthalmology residency, he immediately invited me to join his department, eased my entry in many ways, and provided a great training program. I admired him particularly for his all-out support of the residents, his high ethical standards, and his terrific organizational talents.

At the end of my residency, Dr Claes H Dohlman, then Chief of the Department of Ophthalmology, Harvard Medical School, Boston, MA, USA, asked me to return to Boston, MA, USA, to the Massachusetts Eye and Ear Infirmary and later made me the Head of Pediatric Ophthalmology at the hospital. He obviously had more confidence in my capacities than I had myself, and I hope that I did not disappoint him.

All the three men have given me an example of what a dedicated ophthalmologist should be like.

Contributors

Gelareh Abedi MD
Assistant Professor
Department of Ophthalmology
The University of
Texas Health Science Center
San Antonio, Texas, USA

Ron A Adelman MD MPH MBA
Professor and Director of Retina Center
Department of Ophthalmology and
Visual Science
Yale University School of Medicine
New Haven, Connecticut, USA

Negin Agange MD
Resident, PGY-3
Department of Ophthalmology
The University of
Texas Health Science Center
San Antonio, Texas, USA

Kent L Anderson MD PhD
Associate Professor, Clinical
Department of Ophthalmology
The University of
Texas Health Science Center
San Antonio, Texas, USA

John Awad
Medical Student
The University of
Texas Health Science Center
Houston, Texas, USA

James E Bell MD
Resident
Department of Ophthalmology
Moran Eye Center
University of Utah
Salt Lake City, Utah, USA

Susan M Berry MD
Pediatric Ophthalmology
Alamo City Eye Physicians
San Antonio, Texas, USA

John W Boyle IV MD
Gulf South Eye Associates
Metairie, Louisiana, USA

John E Carter MD
Professor
Departments of Neurology and
Ophthalmology
The University of
Texas Health Science Center
San Antonio, Texas, USA

Timothy P Cleland MD MSE
Adjunct Associate Professor
Department of Ophthalmology
The University of
Texas Health Science Center
Retina Associates of South Texas, PA
San Antonio, Texas, USA

Steven R Cohen MD
Resident
Department of Ophthalmology
The University of
Texas Health Science Center
San Antonio, Texas, USA

Armand Daccache MD
Assistant Clinical Professor
Yale Eye Center
Danbury, Connecticut, USA

Lindsay T Davis MD
Department of Ophthalmology
The University of
Texas Health Science Center
San Antonio, Texas, USA

Christopher M DeBacker MD FACS
Assistant Professor
Department of Ophthalmology
The University of
Texas Health Science Center
San Antonio, Texas, USA

Manishi A Desai MD
Assistant Professor
Department of Ophthalmology
Boston University
Boston, Massachusetts, USA

Sonya Dhar MD
Adjunct Assistant Professor
Department of Ophthalmology and
Visual Science
John A Moran Eye Center
University of Utah
Salt Lake City, Utah
Clinical Instructor
Department of Ophthalmology
New York University
New York, New York, USA

Clinton Duncan MD
Resident
Department of Ophthalmology
The University of Texas
Health Science Center
San Antonio, Texas, USA

Ambar Faridi MD
Resident
Department of Ophthalmology
Oregon Health and Science University
Portland, Oregon, USA

Sandra M Fox OD
Assistant Professor, Clinical
Department of Ophthalmology
The University of
Texas Health Science Center
San Antonio, Texas, USA

Constance L Fry MD
Associate Professor
Department of Ophthalmology
The University of
Texas Health Science Center
San Antonio, Texas, USA

Kevin Gamett MD
Department of Ophthalmology
University of Virginia School of Medicine
Charlottesville, Virginia, USA

Mitchell J Goff MD
Rocky Mountain Retina Consultants
Salt Lake City, Utah, USA

Melanie P Gonzalez OD FAAO
Assistant Professor, Clinical
Department of Ophthalmology
The University of
Texas Health Science Center
San Antonio, Texas, USA

Mary Kelly Green MD
Adjunct Assistant Professor
Department of Ophthalmology
The University of
Texas Health Science Center
San Antonio, Texas, USA

Ankur Gupta
Medical Student
University of Virginia
School of Medicine
Charlottesville, Virginia, USA

Barrett G Haik MD FACS
Hamilton Professor
Department of Ophthalmology
The University of Tennessee Health
Science Center
Memphis, Tennessee, USA

Joseph M Harrison PhD
Associate Professor
Department of Ophthalmology
The University of
Texas Health Science Center
San Antonio, Texas, USA

Angela M Herro MD
Department of Ophthalmology
The University of
Texas Health Science Center
San Antonio, Texas, USA

Eric Hink MD
Assistant Professor
Department of Ophthalmology
University of Colorado
Aurora, Colorado, USA

David EE Holck MD FACS
Adjunct Associate Professor
Department of Ophthalmology
The University of
Texas Health Science Center
San Antonio, Texas, USA

Deeba Husain MD
Associate Professor
Department of Ophthalmology
Harvard Medical School
Boston, Massachusetts, USA

Maria Q Husain MD
Resident
Department of Ophthalmology
The University of
Texas Health Science Center
San Antonio, Texas, USA

Maria Stephanie R Jardeleza MD
Assistant Professor
Department of Ophthalmology
The University of
Texas Health Science
Center San Antonio, Texas, USA

Daniel A Johnson MD
Professor
Department of Ophthalmology
The University of
Texas Health Science Center
San Antonio, Texas, USA

Ekta Kakkar BS BA
Medical Student
Department of Ophthalmology
The University of
Texas Health Science Center
San Antonio, Texas, USA

Marilyn C Kincaid MD
Clinical Professor
Department of Ophthalmology and
Pathology
Saint Louis University
School of Medicine
St Louis, Missouri, USA

Nitya Kumar
Medical Student
Department of Ophthalmology
The University of
Texas Health Science Center
Houston, Texas, USA

Lorena Larez MD
Ophthalmologist
Wilmer Eye Institute
Johns Hopkins School of Medicine
Baltimore, Maryland, USA

Bailey L Lee MD
Houston Eye Associates
Houston, Texas, USA

Irene M Lee MD
Clinical Instructor
Department of Surgery
Division of Ophthalmology
The Warren Alpert
Medical School of Brown University
Providence, Rhode Island, USA

Gary L Legault MD
Cornea Fellow
Department of Ophthalmology
Duke University
Durham, North Carolina, USA

Alvaro PC Lupinacci MD PhD
Private Practice
Vinhedo, São Paulo, Brazil

Farhan F Malik MD
Department of Ophthalmology
Boston University School of Medicine
Boston, Massachusetts, USA

Lina Marouf MD
Adjunct Professor
Department of Ophthalmology
The University of Texas Health Science
Center at San Antonio
Retina Associates of South Texas, PA
San Antonio, Texas, USA

Mark L McDermott MD MBA CPE
Professor
Department of Ophthalmology
Wayne State University School of
Medicine
Detroit, Michigan, USA

J Kevin McKinney MD, MPH
Glaucoma Specialist
Eye Health Northwest
Portland, Oregon, USA

John Ryan McManus MD
Instructor
Department of Ophthalmology
University of Virginia
Charlottesville, Virginia, USA

James L Mims III MD
Clinical Professor
Department of Ophthalmology
The University of
Texas Health Science Center
San Antonio, Texas, USA

Amir Mohsenin MD PhD
Resident
Department of Ophthalmology and
Visual Science
Yale University School of Medicine
New Haven, Connecticut, USA

Reid A Mollman BS
Medical Student
University of Colorado School
of Medicine
Aurora, Colorado, USA

Jorge A Montes MD
Assistant Professor Clinical
Department of Ophthalmology
The University of
Texas Health Science Center
San Antonio, Texas, USA

Kundandeep S Nagi MD
Assistant Professor Clinical
Department of Ophthalmology
The University of
Texas Health Science Center
San Antonio, Texas, USA

Patricia C Nelson MD
Resident PGY-4
Department of Ophthalmology
San Antonio Military Medical Center
San Antonio, Texas, USA

Steven Ness MD
Assistant Professor
Department of Ophthalmology
Boston University School of Medicine
Boston, Massachusetts, USA

Peter A Netland MD PhD
Vernah Scott Moyston
Professor and Chair
Department of Ophthalmology
University of Virginia School of Medicine
Charlottesville, Virginia, USA

Anhtuan H Nguyen BS
Medical Student
Department of Ophthalmology
The University of
Texas Health Science Center
San Antonio, Texas, USA

Lilian Nguyen BA
Medical Student
Department of Ophthalmology
The University of
Texas Health Science Center
San Antonio, Texas, USA

Joshua Nunn
Medical Student
University of Virginia School of Medicine
Charlottesville, Virginia, USA

Lanny S Odin MD
Clinical Assistant Professor
Prairie Eye Center
Southern Illinois University
School of Medicine
Springfield, Illinois, USA

Mary A O'Hara MD
Professor
Departments of Ophthalmology
and Pediatrics
University of California, Davis
Sacramento, California, USA

Abbie S Ornelas BS
Medical Student
Department of Ophthalmology
The University of
Texas Health Science Center
San Antonio, Texas, USA

Sotiria Palioura MD PhD
Resident
Department of Ophthalmology
Massachusetts Eye and Ear Infirmary
Harvard Medical School
Boston, Massachusetts, USA

Thanos D Papakostas MD
Resident
Department of Ophthalmology
Massachusetts Eye and Ear Infirmary
Harvard Medical School
Boston, Massachusetts, USA

John M Parkinson MD
Private Practice
Durango, Colorado, USA

Aaron J Parnes MD
Eyecare Medical Group
Portland, Maine, USA

Mark Pennesi MD PhD
Assistant Professor
Department of Ophthalmology
Oregon Health and Science University
Portland, Oregon, USA

*Kenneth L Piest MD

Vasiliki Poulaki MD PhD
Associate Professor
Department of Ophthalmology
Boston University School of Medicine
Boston, Massachusetts, USA

Omar S Punjabi MD
Retina Staff Physician
Department of Ophthalmology
Charlotte Eye Ear Nose and Throat
Associates
Charlotte, North Carolina, USA

Ashvini K Reddy MD
Assistant Professor
Department of Ophthalmology
University of Virginia School of Medicine
Charlottesville, Virginia, USA

Juan E Rubio Jr MD
Retina Associates of South Texas, PA
San Antonio, Texas, USA

David K Scales MD
Clinical Professor
Department of Ophthalmology
The University of
Texas Health Science Center
San Antonio, Texas, USA

Brian P Schallenberg
Medical Student
School of Medicine
The University of
Texas Health Science Center
San Antonio, Texas, USA

Martha P Schatz MD
Assistant Professor Clinical
Department of Ophthalmology
The University of
Texas Health Science Center
San Antonio, Texas, USA

Frank W Scribbick MD
Professor, Clinical
Department of Ophthalmology
The University of
Texas Health Science Center
San Antonio, Texas, USA

Elizabeth Shane BS
Medical Student
The University of
Texas Health Science Center
Houston, Texas, USA

Olga A Shif MD
Resident
Department of Ophthalmology
The University of
Texas Health Science Center
San Antonio, Texas, USA

*Deceased

Dimitrios Sismanis MD
Fellow, Oculoplastics
San Antonio, Texas, USA

Scott D Smith MD MPH
Chairman, Eye Institute
Cleveland Clinic, Abu Dhabi
United Arab Emirates

Tomy Starck MD
Private Practice
Houston, Texas, USA

Kristin Story Held MD
Clinical Professor
Department of Ophthalmology
The University of
Texas Health Science Center
San Antonio, Texas, USA

Manju Subramanian MD
Associate Professor
Department of Ophthalmology
Boston University School of Medicine
Boston, Massachusetts, USA

WAJ van Heuven MD
Professor and Herbert F Mueller
Chair of Ophthalmology
The University of
Texas Health Science Center
San Antonio, Texas, USA

Lisa Vogel
Medical Student
School of Medicine
The University of
Texas Health Science Center
San Antonio, Texas, USA

Martha A Walton MD
Clinical Associate Professor
Department of Ophthalmology
The University of
Texas Health Science Center
San Antonio, Texas, USA

Nisha Warrier MD MPH
Chief Resident
Department of Ophthalmology
Boston University Medical Center
Boston, Massachusetts, USA

Roy Whitaker Jr MD
President
Eye Consultants of Greensboro, PA
Greensboro, North Carolina, USA

Ronald E Wise MD
Assistant Professor
Department of Ophthalmology
University of Colorado
Denver, Colorado, USA

John P Wooten BS
Medical Student
Department of Ophthalmology
The University of
Texas Health Science Center
San Antonio, Texas, USA

Elizabeth Yang MD
Resident
Department of Ophthalmology
Yale-New Haven Hospital
New Haven, Connecticut, USA

Richard W Yee MD
Private Practice
Houston, Texas, USA

Johan Zwaan MD PhD
Professor of Ophthalmology,
Pediatrics, and Structural and
Cellular Biology (Retired)
The University of
Texas Health Science Center
San Antonio, Texas, USA

Preface

Physicians approaching a patient or a clinical problem come to the right diagnosis or the most appropriate treatment by a process of selection and elimination of choices. Some of this takes place subliminally and the more experience the practitioner has, the quicker and more automatically the process becomes.

This is a book of algorithms or 'decision trees' which make the process of decision-making visible. Not everyone follows the same pathways of thinking, and you may find chapters in the book where you would have made different choices, but in most cases, you hopefully would have finished at the same end point(s).

To emphasize the central position of the 'decision trees' in the chapters, I have moved them to the front of the chapters, with the text amplifying points of the tree (marked by capital letters referring to paragraphs of the text) to follow.

Other changes from previous editions include the use of tables and graphs and inclusion of color illustrations. The 'trees' have partially been color-coded: surgical treatments are shown in red, pharmaceutical ones in green, and other treatments in blue.

In each chapter, the text is not meant to provide a complete review of a topic and the references mostly refer to the text in general, not to a specific paragraph. This is also true for the figures.

Within the framework of the book, the authors had a great deal of freedom in composing their chapters. For those readers who used the previous editions, you will notice that some chapters have stayed virtually the same, while others have been (almost) completely rewritten. All chapters have been reviewed.

I hope that this edition will be found equally useful to practitioners of eyecare at any level as the previous editions were.

Johan Zwaan

Acknowledgments

A book of this nature requires the cooperation of many different authors. I am grateful to all the contributors to the book, but some stand out, going well beyond the call of duty.

First, I wish to thank Dr WAJ van Heuven, retired Chair of the Department of Ophthalmology, University of Texas Health Science Center, San Antonio, Texas, USA. He was the one who started the Decision Making in Ophthalmology book (the first and second editions). I was quite honored, when he asked me to be a co-editor. He was very gracious in allowing me to start work on a third edition.

Dr Gelareh Abedi did not only contribute several chapters, but did so very fast. She was also very helpful in recommending other potential authors.

Dr Lina Marouf recruited several other authors, in addition to submitting her own chapters.

Dr Daniel A Johnson, Chair of Ophthalmology, University of Texas Health Science Center, San Antonio, Texas, USA, wrote several chapters and got his entire department to collaborate.

The staff of the Philadelphia office, USA, of Jaypee Brothers Medical Publishers (P) Ltd., bent over backwards to make the production of this manuscript pleasant, professional, and fast.

Contents

SECTION 1

General Ophthalmology

Visual Loss

WAJ van Heuven

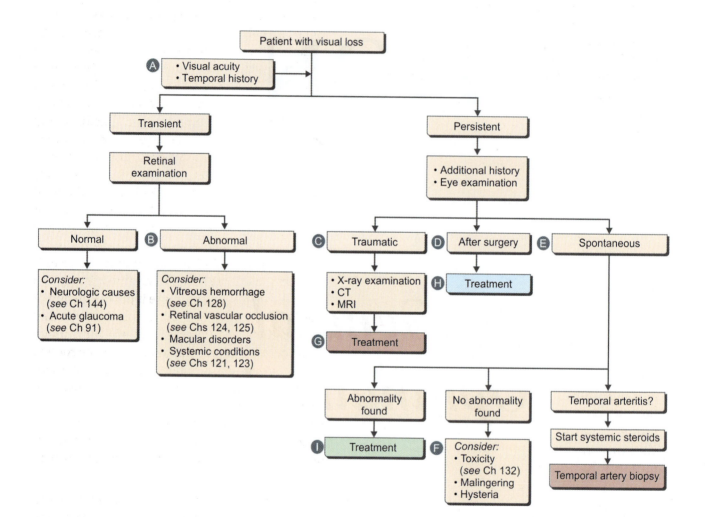

Vision is the most precious sense, so loss of vision is a serious complaint that requires immediate attention. Untreated and permanent, it changes the patient's life significantly, especially if it is bilateral.

A. If visual loss is spontaneous and without apparent cause (e.g. trauma), the persistence of sudden severe vision loss in one or both eyes may indicate retinal arterial occlusion, a medical emergency.

Thus rapid documentation of this condition (vision test, pupil and retina examination), done within 2 hours of the onset of symptoms, may allow early successful emergency treatment, which can consist of ocular massage, paracentesis of the cornea to decrease ocular pressure and increase perfusion, retrobulbar injection of vasodilators, and breathing of CO_2. There is evidence that, after 90 minutes of complete central occlusion of the retinal artery, the retina is permanently damaged and will not recover.

B. *Nontraumatic vitreous hemorrhage* is usually caused by vitreous detachment. The bleeding can originate from vitreous adhesions to vascular structures on the surface of the retina, such as normal disc vessels or neovascularization of any cause, and from retinal vessels when the retina tears. Small vitreous hemorrhages clear rapidly from the visual axis by gravity, so patients may not appreciate the potential danger. Perform a thorough retinal examination in all patients whose eyes have vitreous hemorrhage of any amount to rule out retinal tears and to confirm vitreous detachment. Treat symptomatic horseshoe-shaped retinal tears to prevent retinal detachment. *Vein occlusions* may produce macular edema, which may resolve in weeks or months. Central or branch occlusions of the retinal arterioles are usually embolic and may produce only temporary symptoms when the embolus moves downstream. Treatment is usually directed at making this happen by creating sudden vasodilation. Several *macular disorders* produce transient visual symptoms. Central serous choroidopathy almost resolves completely within 6 weeks to 6 months. Some presumed inflammatory conditions, such as idiopathic stellate neuro-retinopathy and acute multifocal punctate pigment epitheliopathy, resolve in a few weeks, as may hemorrhage in some macular degenerations (e.g. age-related or angioid streaks). When these clear, vision may be improved even though the underlying cause persists and will ultimately lead to permanent visual loss. Macular edema caused by a solar burn after eclipse watching or sun gazing often results in surprising recovery of vision. Severe and especially sudden systemic disorders, particularly those causing hypertension (e.g. idiopathic, eclampsial or severe metabolic imbalance such as acute renal failure), may cause temporary vision loss, usually from macular edema or secondary retinal detachment, until the primary condition is cured.

C. Blunt trauma to the head is less likely to cause visual loss than direct trauma to the eye and orbit, but has been known to cause brain injury, especially to the occipital cortex, and contrecoup optic nerve and retinal damage. If optic nerve contusion is suspected, consider high-dose systemic steroids. Direct trauma can take many forms. Blunt injury may cause visual loss by mechanisms ranging from severe lid edema to optic nerve avulsion and includes orbital fractures, ocular hemorrhages, cataracts and retinal damage. Pupillary examination to elicit an afferent pupillary defect (Marcus Gunn) is helpful in determining damage to the visual pathway. Echography is an easy, cheap and noninvasive way to rule out a pathologic condition. Computed tomography (CT) scan and magnetic resonance imaging (MRI) may be helpful, particularly in determining orbital fractures, and optic nerve and brain damage. In severe direct trauma, always suspect ocular perforation. Severe hypotony, chemosis and visual loss are especially suspicious. Echography, particularly standardized A-scan, can be helpful. A common ocular perforation is caused by a sliver of steel, usually magnetic, that enters the eye while the patient is hammering on a metal object. Because the sliver is small and thin, it perforates easily through a minute entry wound, which may make it difficult to find. A history of eye injury should thus include detailed questioning about the manner in which the injury occurred. Plain films of the orbit should be routine if any such injury is even remotely suspected. Sharp pointed objects (e.g. darts, pencils, nails) that cause eye injuries, even though they may seem to have perforated the eye anteriorly only, often leave double perforations. Echography can help rule this out. MRI should not be used if a metal foreign body is suspected.

D. After surgery, visual loss can occur from several obvious ocular complications (e.g. hyphema). However, after ocular or orbital surgery, orbital hemorrhage, optic nerve damage, ocular perforation and intravascular injection during retrobulbar anesthesia must be considered.

E. Spontaneous "idiopathic" persistent visual loss, when bilateral, most often results from nonocular disease. However, some patients insist that the loss was bilateral when, in fact, the event was unilateral, and the second eye had previously been blinded by another or similar disorder. All cases of visual loss should be considered eye emergencies until the examination indicates otherwise. Of special importance is the severe monocular visual loss in the elderly patient due to temporal (cranial) arteritis. An elevated sedimentation rate helps suggest the diagnosis, at which time systemic steroids should be given immediately to prevent involvement of the other eye. Biopsy of the temporal artery can confirm the diagnosis later, and results will still be abnormal for several days after steroid treatment has begun.

F. Toxic visual loss is often bilateral and may be caused by quinine or methyl alcohol poisoning. The latter, as well as the use of numerous illegal drugs may be difficult to glean from the patient's history unless specifically elicited.

G. Treatment for traumatic visual loss usually is surgical.

H. Postoperative visual loss may require various treatments, depending on the findings.

I. Depending on findings, patients may need steroids, antibiotics and other treatments.

BIBLIOGRAPHY

1. Augsburger JJ, Magargal LE. Visual prognosis following treatment of acute central retinal artery obstruction. Br J Ophthalmol. 1980;64:913-7.
2. Deutsch TA, Feller DB. Paton and Goldberg's Management of Ocular Injuries, 2nd Edition. Philadelphia: WB Saunders; 1985.
3. Hayreh SS, Kolder HE, Weingeist TA. Central retinal artery occlusion and retinal tolerance time. Ophthalmology. 1980;87:75-8.
4. Spoor TC, Hartel WC, Lensink DB, et al. Treatment of traumatic optic neuropathy with corticosteroids. Am J Ophthalmol. 1990;110:665-9.

Transient Visual Loss

2

John E Carter, Susan M Berry, Martha P Schatz

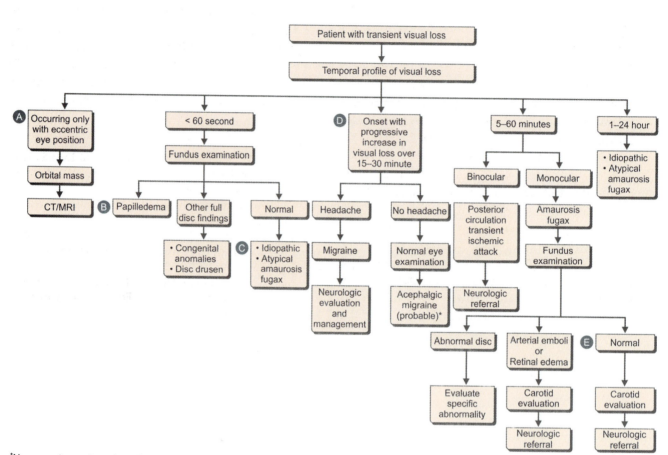

*New onset symptoms in patients older than 40 years and without a previous history of migraine should prompt a neurologic evaluation.

The two important factors in the approach to the patient with transient loss of vision are: (1) the temporal profile of the event and (2) the fundus examination.

A. Patients who experience visual loss when they look to one side usually have an intraorbital mass that compresses or stretches the optic nerve as it moves with rotation of the eye. The examination may be normal, or there may be evidence of a mild optic neuropathy in the form of an afferent pupil defect, color desaturation or disc edema.

B. Transient obscurations of vision occur in 50% of patients with papilledema secondary to intracranial hypertension. Vision is obscured or lost, usually in one eye, for seconds. Common descriptions include "sparkly lights, distortion, waterfalls or droplets" in the center field. This often occurs with change in body position from supine to erect. Any condition resulting in tightly packed nerve fibers as they enter the disc to form the optic nerve may produce such symptoms.

C. Most patients who experience amaurosis fugax have episodes lasting minutes. Very brief or very prolonged episodes of transient visual loss may be caused by carotid atherosclerotic disease, but the likelihood of carotid occlusive lesions is much smaller. Other factors that identify the patient as having increased risk for cardiovascular disease, including age, hypertension, coronary artery disease, peripheral vascular disease and family history, must be taken into consideration.

D. The presence of a small area of visual loss or a mild disturbance of vision that progressively increases over 15 minutes or more is highly characteristic of migraine. The patient need not have a headache for this diagnosis to be made. Most patients have some abnormal visual symptoms associated with the episodes, most commonly fortification spectra around an area of scotoma or distortions within the area of visual disturbance resembling heat waves or water running down a glass. Similar abnormal visual disturbances, often accompanied by headache, may occur with cerebral lesions, such as arteriovenous malformations or meningiomas, but they do not have the characteristic buildup and resolution. Instead, these structural lesions produce symptoms that steadily increase in duration and frequency until they are present daily throughout much of the day.

E. Patients may experience transient monocular visual loss at any age. If the fundus examination is normal, the most helpful indicator of carotid occlusive disease is age. Patients younger than 40 years of age are unlikely to have carotid disease in the absence of other risk factors. Most cases in these patients are idiopathic, although transient visual loss may occur in association with migraine, Raynaud's phenomenon, diseases causing increased viscosity of the blood, and from cardiogenic embolism.

BIBLIOGRAPHY

1. Burde RM, Savino PJ, Trobe JD. Clinical Decisions in Neuro-ophthalmology, 2nd Edition. St Louis, Missouri: Mosby-Year Book; 1992.
2. Glaser J. Neuro-ophthalmology, 2nd Edition. Philadelphia: Lippincott; 1990.
3. Lee AG, Brazis PW. Clinical Pathways in Neuro-ophthalmology: An Evidence-based Approach. New York: Thieme; 1998.
4. Miller NR, Newman NJ. Walsh and Hoyt's Clinical Neuro-ophthalmology, 6th Edition. Philadelphia: Lippincott Williams & Wilkins; 2005.

Distorted Vision

WAJ van Heuven

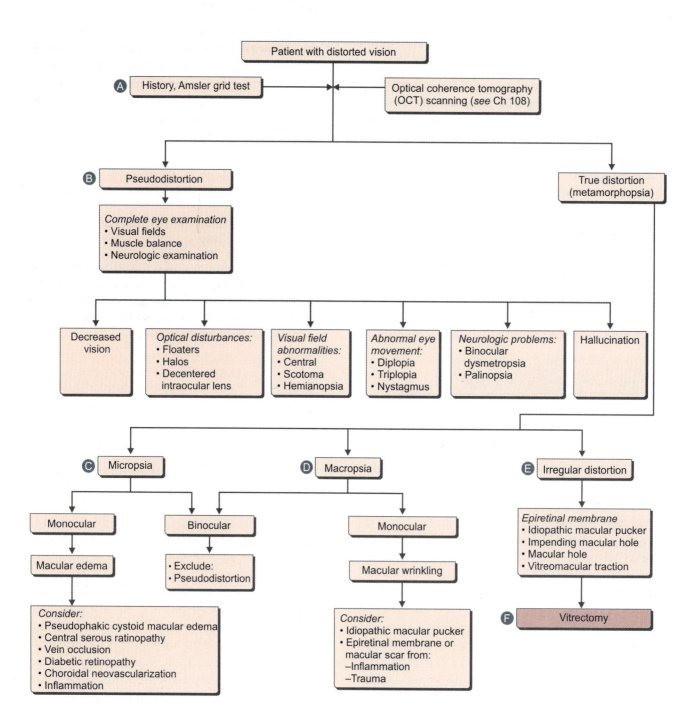

3

Distorted vision, or irregularities of lines and figures in the central visual field, is called *metamorphopsia.* Micropsia and macropsia, the two forms of dysmetropsia (seeing abnormal size), are forms of metamorphopsia in which objects appear smaller or larger than they really are.

A. Take a careful history because patients complaining of distorted vision are often nonspecific in describing symptoms. They also often do not know whether the distortion is monocular or binocular, or whether it is associated with other symptoms. Testing for distortion, one eye at a time, is easily done using the Amsler grid, which tests the central 20° of vision at reading distance. Optical coherence tomography (OCT) can yield significant information (Chapter 108).

B. Some patients use the word *distortion* to describe the perception of blur caused by acquired decreased vision or central scotoma in one eye. Monocular visual acuity and Amsler grid testing elicit these causes. Occasionally, large vitreous floaters, usually from vitreous detachment, may interfere with vision, especially at close range, and mimic monocular distortion. Halos around lights, with or without blurring of vision, may indicate glaucoma. Diplopia or triplopia, whether monocular or binocular, must be investigated initially with a careful examination of muscle balance. Acquired nystagmus requires a thorough neurologic evaluation. Binocular dysmetropsia, although usually retinal in origin, may be cerebral. Cerebral micropsia is more common than macropsia. It may be associated with other neurologic conditions such as migraine, epilepsy, hysteria, schizophrenia, drug intoxication and focal lesions. These symptoms may be difficult to differentiate from hallucinations. *Palinopsia,* a term meaning visual perseveration, which is the persistence of visual perception after the object has been removed, also requires neurologic evaluation. Visual hallucinations occur from a variety of causes, most of which are not ocular. They represent complex integrative processes and often have little value in topical diagnosis. However, formed hallucinations are often the result of temporal lobe involvement, and unformed ones suggest involvement of the occipital lobe. Many hallucinations are associated with cerebral tumors, although they can be caused by cerebral injury or infection. A complete neurologic evaluation is indicated because different forms of epilepsy, visual field defects and other neurologic findings may help localize the cause.

C. Micropsia from ocular causes, so-called peripheral metamorphopsia, is often monocular. If binocular, just like binocular macropsia, central metamorphopsia (i.e. resulting from cerebral causes) must be ruled out. True ocular micropsia is caused by an abnormal separation of the rods and cones, usually in the macular region, which causes fewer retinal receptors to be stimulated by an object than would normally be stimulated by that object. Therefore, the brain receives and perceives the object to be smaller. Conditions that separate the retinal receptors, such as stretching or edema of the retina, cause micropsia.

D. True peripheral or retinal macropsia, in contrast to micropsia, is caused by the retinal photoreceptors being closer together than normal. Thus more retinal receptors are stimulated by an object than would normally be stimulated by that object, which causing the brain to receive and perceive that the object is larger than actual. Conditions causing shrinkage of the retina, such as retinal scars, are the most common cause of macropsia. If a retinal condition, such as inflammation or trauma, initially causes edema and later causes scarring, macropsia may follow micropsia.

E. Irregular metamorphopsia can result from any condition that causes an irregular distortion of the retina, so the photoreceptors are no longer evenly spaced. Patients perceive straight lines to be crooked and, if the condition involves the fovea, may also have blurred vision. Any condition that causes scarring of the retina or shifting of the retina because of traction may cause metamorphopsia. Patients with impending macular holes or small full-thickness macular holes may also have complaints of metamorphopsia. Like the vitreomacular traction syndrome, these may not be obvious unless one performs careful contact lens biomicroscopy.

F. Pars plana vitrectomy and membrane stripping can improve vision and distortion in patients with epiretinal membranes and vitreomacular traction syndrome. Macular holes can be closed with improved vision after vitrectomy and fluid-gas exchange. Because of the high rate of spontaneous resolution of impending macular holes, these are generally observed unless a full-thickness hole develops.

BIBLIOGRAPHY

1. Gass JDM. Macular dysfunction caused by vitreous and vitreoretinal interface abnormalities. Stereoscopic Atlas of Macular Diseases: Diagnosis and Treatment, 4th Edition. St Louis: Mosby; 1997.
2. Miller NR. Walsh and Hoyt's Clinical Neuro-ophthalmology, 5th Edition. Baltimore: Williams & Wilkins; 1998.

Poor Color Vision

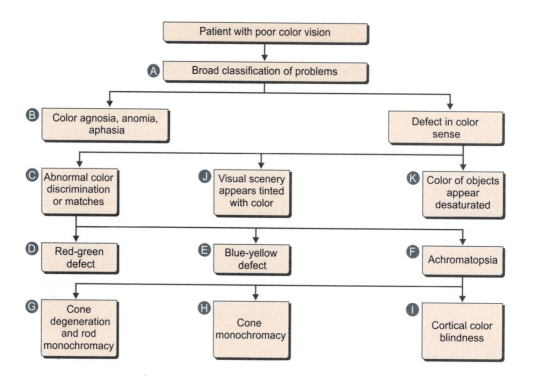

Joseph M Harrison

4

The evaluation of color vision complaints is important primarily because poor color vision may be an early sign of acquired disease or may help differentiate among alternative diagnoses. Occasionally, color vision evaluation is needed in the certification of personnel for occupations that require chromatic discrimination.

A. Color vision problems can be broadly classified as those affecting high-level mental functions involving colors but not the color sense *per se* and those primarily affecting the color sense. Problems affecting the color sense are manifested by poor color discrimination, abnormal mixtures of primary colors required to match a standard light, disturbances in the color appearance of objects or the like. Problems affecting high-level mental functions involve the name of colors of familiar objects, the categorization of different colors, topographical memory linked with colors, the attachment of emotion with colors, and so forth.

B. Brain disorders can produce difficulties associated with colors (e.g. color agnosia, anomia, aphasia) without affecting the color sense. Many of the problems are associated with the language aspect of colors but it is perhaps worth mentioning that visual-verbal or verbal-visual dissociations (i.e. the inability to name the color of shown objects or to correctly point to color named objects) are not adequate evidence of such problems. Additional information required includes whether color discrimination is normal or whether there is an evidence of nonvisual (e.g. verbal-verbal) dissociations, such as the inability to name the color of a named fruit (e.g. banana, apple). Consider neurologic referral.

C. A patient has a defect in the color sense if he or she fails the pseudoisochromatic plates test (e.g. American Optical Hardy-Rand-Rittler, Ishihara, Dvorine, Tokyo Medical College), color arrangement tests (e.g. Farnsworth D-15 and 100-hue, Lanthony desaturated panel, Sahlgren saturation test), or color matching tests (e.g. the Nagel, the Neitz, and the Pickford-Nicolson anomaloscopes). Based on the portion of the visible spectrum in which the performance deficits occur, the color vision defects can be further classified as 'red-green' (i.e. middle and long wavelength spectrum), 'blue' or 'blue-yellow' (i.e. short wavelength spectrum), or nonspecific (i.e. the entire spectrum).

D. In the general population, most people with red-green color vision defects have a congenital, stationary, X-linked recessively inherited trait. This trait, present in about 8% of men and 0.42% of women, is generally not considered as a health-related problem but the color vision defect may be important to the patient because it cannot be corrected and may affect early success in school or his or her career plans (e.g. in transportation, military, law enforcement professions). The diagnosis of the inherited color vision trait is supported by a history of a stationary red-green color defect from a young age, the absence of other significant ocular or visual defects (e.g. having good visual acuity), or a family history of color vision problems consistent with X-linked recessive inheritance. Rayleigh matches (the red and green color mixture that appears perceptually identical to a spectral yellow field) provide the definitive data for classifying red-green defects into anomalous trichromacy (i.e. protanomaly and deuteranomaly) or dichromacy (i.e. protanopia and deuteranopia). The Rayleigh matches are made using an anomaloscope. In the absence of evidence that the red-green defect is stationary, X-linked recessive, and so on, consider the possibility that a red-green defect is secondary to an acquired disorder. The loss of red-green discrimination as

demonstrated by pseudoisochromatic plates or color arrangement tests suggests involvement of the central 5° of visual field but contrary to early clinical correlations, seldom provides information about whether the lesion lies in the optic nerve versus outer retina. However, abnormalities in the Rayleigh matches strongly indicate either a photoreceptor or prereceptoral disturbance.

E. Patients with a 'blue' or 'blue-yellow' defect typically confuse blues and greens or yellows and violet. Because cases of stationary, inherited, blue-yellow defects are so rarely reported, one would assume, until proven otherwise, that a patient with a blue-yellow defect probably has an acquired problem. The visual pathway for the blue cone signals is thought to be more vulnerable to diseases and ocular insults than the pathway for red or green cone signals. So, a blue-yellow defect may be an indication of early stage disease. In addition to neuronal lesions, a blue-yellow defect may originate from aging changes in the lens of the eye.

F. Nonspecific color vision defects (i. e. significant discrimination losses throughout the entire light spectrum) occur in several distinct clinical entities, all of which fall into the broad classification of 'achromatopsia'.

G. When nonspecific color discrimination losses are accompanied with normal night vision but poor visual acuity, the cone-mediated vision may be selectively compromised. Progressive cone degeneration and congenital, autosomal recessively inherited, rod monochromacy are among likely diagnoses. Both disorders are associated with poor day-vision function (e.g. visual acuity of 20/200 or worse) and little, if any color vision. Rod monochromats also have photophobia and nystagmus, which tend to diminish with age. There is also a rare, X-linked recessive incomplete ('blue-cone') achromatopsia with similar clinical symptoms except for residual blue-yellow color vision and visual acuity as good as 20/60.

H. When nonspecific color discrimination losses are accompanied with normal visual acuity and a history of the disorder from early age, consider cone monochromacy. Cone monochromacy is believed to be a defect of the visual pathway in which chromatic information is not transmitted to the brain despite the presence of cone photoreceptors.

I. When nonspecific color discrimination losses occur after head trauma or vascular cerebral disorder, a probable diagnosis is cortical color blindness. This condition is distinguished from other abnormalities associated with cerebral lesions, such as color agnosia, anomia, or aphasia, in that cortical color blindness involves a loss of the color sense. In the classic cases of cortical color blindness, visual acuity was spared but the achromatopsia was accompanied by ancillary symptoms such as visual field defects (particularly in the upper quadrant), inability to recognize faces (prosopagnosia), inability to spatially navigate in familiar surroundings (topographical disorientation), or inability to recognize objects (object agnosia).

J. Another clue of an abnormality involving the color sense is the disturbance in color appearance of objects, for example, the patient may report that portions of the visual scenery or the entire visual scenery in one or both eyes appears 'tinted' purple, green, blue, red, or yellow (chromatopsia). Depending on the color of the tint, the problem can be classified as erythropsia (red), xanthopsia (yellow), cyanopsia (blue), or chloropsia (green). Chromatopsia almost always suggests an acquired visual defect. It is a symptom reported in association with retinal side effects from drugs and toxic agents. Drugs of particular clinical significance include cardiac glycosides such as digoxin and digitoxin, antimalarial agents such as quinine and chloroquine, and psychotherapeutic drugs such as thioridazine. Chromatopsia may arise optically when substances such as blood or fluorescein collect in front of the retina and alter the wavelength composition of light reaching the photoreceptors. Chromatopsia is also experienced after exposure to high illumination for long periods.

K. Patients may report that the color of an object appears pale, washed-out, or desaturated, another clue of a disturbance of the color sense. Such subjective descriptions are particularly credible when the problem occurs in one eye, and the patient is able to appreciate the difference seen by the better eye. The report of color desaturation suggests a loss in the color sense with relatively greater preservation of the luminance sense. Some clinicians believe that the desaturation in the color of red objects is a sensitive indicator of significant macular or optic nerve disease.

▌BIBLIOGRAPHY

1. Grusser OJ, Landis T. The world turns grey: Achromatopsia, colour agnosia and other impairments of colour vision caused by cerebral lesion. In: Visual Agnosia and Other Disturbances of Visual Perception and Cognition. Boca Raton: CRC Press; 1991.
2. Krastel H, Moreland JD. Colour vision deficiencies in ophthalmic diseases. In: Inherited and Acquired Colour Vision Deficiencies. Boca Raton: CRC Press; 1991.
3. Miller NR. Walsh and Hoyt's Clinical Neuro-ophthalmology, 5th Edition. Baltimore: Williams & Wilkins; 1998.
4. Pokorny J, Smith VC, Verriest G, Pinckers AJLG. Congenital and Acquired Color Vision Defects. New York: Grune & Stratton; 1979.
5. Report of Working Group 41 (Committee on Vision). Procedures for Testing Color Vision. Washington, DC: National Academy Press; 1981.

Poor Night Vision

Joseph M Harrison

5

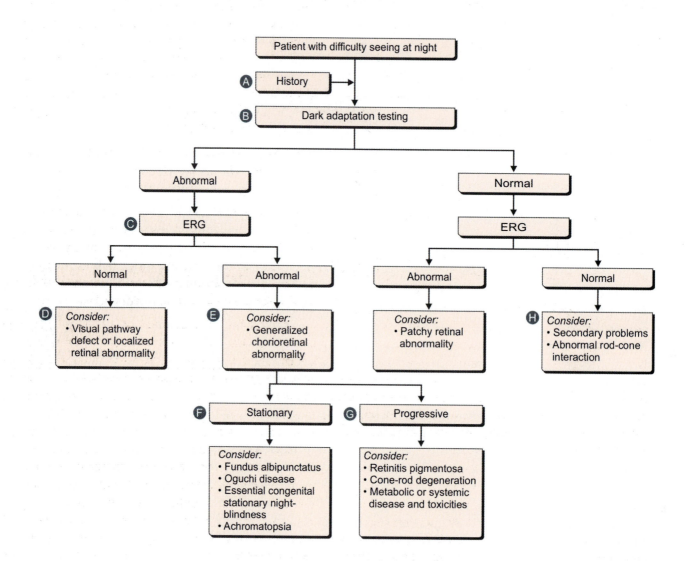

A. The patient history for night vision problems is notoriously unreliable. Even in the cases of very reduced dark-adapted sensitivity, decreased night vision is often not the patient's complaint. Many complaints of vision problems at night are related to depressed cone rather than rod sensitivity because sufficiently dim ambient illumination is rarely encountered in developed countries.

B. Dark adaptation is classically tested with a Goldmann-Weekers adaptometer. The pupil is dilated and the full visual field of the eye is light adapted for 7 minutes to about 2,000 lumens/m²

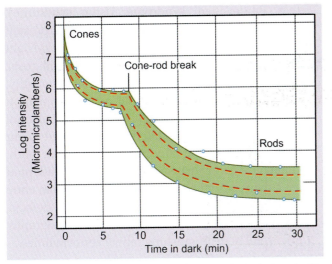

Fig. 5.1: The dark adaptation curve. The area between the dashed curves includes 80% of the data from 110 normal observers. The upper and lower lines represent the upper and lower extremes from this sample. (Adapted from Hecht S, Mandelbaum J. JAMA 1939;112:1911. Copyright 1939. American Medical Association).

illumination of the interior of the partial sphere serving as a projection perimeter. The adapting light is turned off, and the test light, 11° in diameter and flashing two times per second, appears in an area centered at 15° from a dim red central fixation spot. At frequent intervals, the luminance of the test light is decreased and increased manually to bracket the value that is just visible to the patient determined by feedback between the patient and the examiner. The dark adaptation curve shows the logarithm of the threshold test light luminance as a function of time in the dark after light adaptation (Fig. 5.1). The time of the inflection in the curve separating the cone and rod branches, and the threshold in the cone and rod branches are compared with normal values. Long and short wavelength test lights can be used to determine relative cone and rod contributions, and the position of the fixation light can be varied to test other parts of the visual field.

Recently, automated commercial dark adaptometry instruments have become available. Some of these instruments test threshold automatically by criterion-free two alternative forced choice psychophysical techniques. In addition, powerful new analysis techniques based on a cellular model for regeneration of rhodopsin yield more specific information about the pathophysiology involving the visual cycle in photoreceptors and the retinal pigment epithelium. The new instruments and analytical techniques have renewed the interest in measuring dark-adapted sensitivity, particularly in hereditary retinal degenerative disease.

C. The electroretinogram (ERG) is the bioelectrical response of the retina produced with flashes of light or other temporal patterns of changing visible stimuli. The usual clinical ERG is a mass response arising from the entire retina and can be used to determine rod versus cone and inner versus outer retinal involvement in disease, as well as the lateral extent of involvement.

D. Localized areas of abnormal retina are usually visible on fundus examination as chorioretinal lesions or pigmentary changes.

E. Chorioretinal abnormality is used to encompass a wide variety of disorders. An important distinction to make is the progressive versus stationary nature of the disease. The progressive or stationary nature of the disease is determined by history but the ERG helps in the diagnosis of type of disorder.

F. Fundus findings are an important component of fundus albipunctatus and Oguchi disease. Both cone and rod adaptation are delayed in fundus albipunctatus, which is associated with slower cone and rod photopigment kinetics. Only rod system adaptation is delayed in Oguchi disease. Delayed cone-rod break times are also seen in dysfunctions of the retinal pigment epithelium, such as fundus flavimaculatus and dominant drusen. Fundus findings are subtle, if present, in essential congenital stationary night blindness, which can also be distinguished from the two other stationary night-blind disorders (fundus albipunctatus and Oguchi disease), which have improved rod sensitivity with prolonged dark adaptation (> 180 minutes). Some stationary diseases affect only cone function. In complete achromatopsia or rod monochromatism, there is reduced visual acuity and no cone ERG or cone branch during dark adaptation but normal rod threshold.

G. Retinitis pigmentosa (RP) and cone-rod degeneration are the two major primary progressive photoreceptor dystrophies associated with decreased night vision. A distinction between the two is that the elevation of the final rod threshold in cone-rod degeneration is usually less than hundred-fold and in rod-cone degeneration is more than hundred-fold. Also, in cone-rod degeneration, color vision is affected more than expected on the basis of visual acuity, and photophobia is the more common complaint. Most or all patients with RP have prolonged implicit times of the cone ERG. The ERG is absent by standard recording techniques in about 70% of patients. The ERG and dark adaptation can be completely normal in central cone dystrophy, which may be detectable only by changes in the fundus, visual acuity, color vision, and/or multifocal ERG. In some cone degenerations, the cone branch of dark adaptation and the cone ERG are absent with a normal rod threshold and ERG. There are also hereditary forms of choroidal atrophy such as choroideremia and choroidal sclerosis, which cause a secondary photoreceptor dystrophy and result in poor night vision early in the disease. Avitaminosis is not a common dietary problem in developed countries but may occur secondary to other conditions such as malabsorption syndromes and gut resection. It can also occur in liver and pancreas diseases and cystic fibrosis and in disorders causing urinary excretion of vitamins. Conditions leading to zinc deficiencies (e.g. alcoholic cirrhosis, chronic pancreatitis) are associated with night vision problems. In addition, a variety of systemic diseases are associated with retinal degenerations affecting night vision: lipid abnormalities (e.g. Bassen-Kornzweig syndrome, or abetalipoproteinemia) resulting in low plasma levels of vitamins A and E, ceroid lipofuscinosis, mucopolysaccharidoses, metabolic disorders such as Refsum disease (elevated serum phytanic acid) and gyrate atrophy (elevated plasma ornithine), degenerative myopia and neurologic disease (e.g. Bardet-Biedl syndrome, Usher syndrome). Some forms of occult cancer can also present initially with symptoms of night-vision loss. Night vision can be reduced in the later stages of siderosis. Vascular occlusive disease and diabetic retinopathy, luetic retinopathy, panretinal photocoagulation and phenothiazine, chloroquine, and ethyl alcohol toxicity are also associated with reduced night vision in either the cone or rod branch or both. Glaucoma can cause small losses of dark-adapted sensitivity, which are greater for the rod than cone branch in areas outside of visual field defects. Fundus examination and fluorescein angiography are useful in distinguishing retinal abnormalities.

H. Secondary problems include glare from media opacities; night myopia, which is an inappropriate midpoint of accommodation under dark conditions; and miosis from age or drugs. Some patients also show an exaggerated depression of cone sensitivity during the rod branch of dark adaptation detectable with a flickering red stimulus. These patients complain of problems driving at night.

BIBLIOGRAPHY

1. Arden CB, Hogg CR. Rod-cone interactions and analysis of retinal disease. Br J Ophthalmol. 1985;69:404-15.
2. Krill AE. Hereditary Retinal and Choroidal Diseases, Vol I, Evaluation. Philadelphia: Harper and Row; 1972: 189-26.
3. Lamb TD, Pugh Jr EN. Phototransduction, dark adaptation, and rhodopsin regeneration. Invest Ophthalmol Vis Sci. 2006;47:5138-52.
4. Liebowitz HW, Owens DA. Night-time driving accidents and selective visual degradation. Science. 1977;197: 422-3.
5. Massof RW, Finkelstein D. Two forms of autosomal dominant primary retinitis pigmentosa. Doc Ophthalmol. 1981;51:289-346.
6. Roman AJ, Schwartz SB, Aleman TS, et al. Quantifying rod photoreceptor-mediated vision in retinal degenerations: dark-adapted thresholds as outcome measures. Experimental Eye Res. 2005;80:259-72.

Isolated Diplopia

6

Susan M Berry, John E Carter, Martha P Schatz

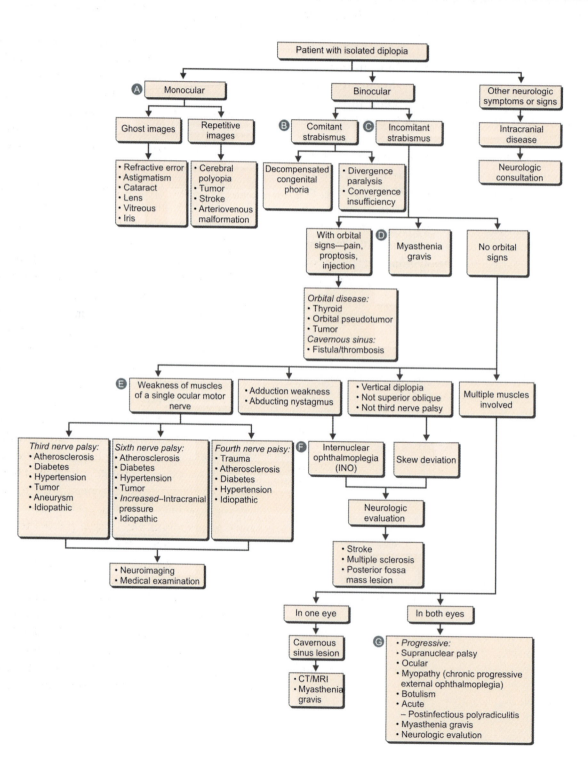

Diplopia most often occurs as an isolated symptom. The presence of other neurologic symptoms indicates more extensive neurologic disease and merits referral for a neurologic evaluation.

A. Monocular diplopia is most commonly caused by some refractive disturbance, including astigmatism or some opacity in the ocular media. The patient may not have realized that there is diplopia when using an eye individually, in which case testing of each eye individually by the clinician may save the patient from an extensive evaluation. Cerebral lesions, usually in the posterior hemisphere, may produce polyopia, but polyopia is usually distinct from the distortion or ghost image seen with ocular disturbances. Patients with cerebral polyopia often see multiple images. This is enhanced when the object is moving; a car passing by may look like a procession of cars. Other visual disturbances, including perseveration of an image in the visual environment (palinopsia) or visual hallucinations, often accompany cerebral polyopia. A homonymous visual field defect is often associated with these phenomena.

B. A truly comitant strabismus is often benign and may be caused by decompensated congenital phoria (this does not apply to any form of childhood strabismus or diplopia, which must be fully evaluated in a separate context). Convergence insufficiency type exodeviation is often treated conservatively unless there are other neurologic concerns. Divergence insufficiency esodeviation must be evaluated for restrictive or paralytic causes to include bilateral sixth nerve paresis, thyroid orbitopathy and myasthenia gravis.

C. An incomitant strabismus must be classified as neural, myoneural junction, myopathic or restrictive. Orbital processes causing a restrictive strabismus are usually obvious from the presence of proptosis, pain, hyperemia and abnormal forced ductions. Computed tomography (CT) or magnetic resonance imaging (MRI) of the orbits is indicated. Cavernous sinus fistula or thrombosis may mimic orbital disease because of the proptosis and chemosis.

D. The history makes the diagnosis of myasthenia gravis. Ptosis and/or diplopia that varies from hour to hour, day to day, and week to week; that is usually present late in the day or that resolves for a period after a nap is often myasthenia gravis. A Tensilon (edrophonium) test is helpful, if positive but in patients with small deviations or with absent symptoms in the office, myasthenia may be difficult to diagnose. Laboratory evaluation for acetylcholine receptor antibodies and electromyography are diagnostic, if positive. If ptosis is present, then an ice-pack test may be helpful. A trial of Mestinon (pyridostigmine) for 1–2 weeks may serve as a diagnostic tool as well. Neurologic evaluation is indicated in all patients in whom the diagnosis of myasthenia gravis is being entertained.

E. The evaluation of diplopia caused by injury to any of the individual ocular motor nerves is specific to the nerve and the history. If the nerve fascicles are involved within the brainstem, the patient is expected to have additional neurologic symptoms or signs. The differential diagnosis for the cause of peripheral third, fourth and sixth cranial nerve palsies is similar, but the diagnosis of most concern varies with the particular nerve. The third nerve may be injured by an aneurysm of the posterior communicating artery; surgery before the aneurysm ruptures may be lifesaving. Aneurysmal third nerve palsies involve the pupil in 96% of cases, but the pupil is rarely involved with microvascular etiologies associated with diabetes and hypertension. A pupil-sparing complete (all muscles served by the third nerve affected) third nerve palsy is rarely aneurysmal in origin. MRI and MR angiography/CT angiography are indicated in pupil-involving third nerve palsies to rule out aneurysm. Catheter angiography is also done in select cases, but noninvasive angiography can be done as an initial study. The diagnosis of most concern in the patient with a sixth nerve palsy is neoplasm. Because of its long course along the base of the skull, the sixth nerve is often involved by dural metastases or by nasopharyngeal malignancies eroding through the bone. MRI with contrast demonstrates most such lesions. Benign isolated ocular motor nerve palsies should resolve within 3 months, and pain associated with their onset should resolve within 1–2 weeks. Failure to recover indicates the need for more thorough evaluation and repeat imaging studies.

F. Diplopia associated with an internuclear ophthalmoplegia (INO) or with skew deviation indicates intrinsic brainstem disease and requires a neurologic evaluation. Skew deviation is diagnosed when the patient complains of an acquired vertical diplopia that is not caused by orbital disease or myasthenia and that on examination cannot be attributed to a dysfunction of the third or fourth nerve. The vertical strabismus may be comitant or incomitant.

G. Although patients with progressive supranuclear palsy, chronic progressive external ophthalmoplegia (CPEO), and Fisher's variant of acute postinfectious polyradiculitis (ataxia, ophthalmoplegia, and depressed reflexes) have strabismus, many do not complain of diplopia. These entities are characterized by weakness in most extraocular muscles in both eyes. Progressive supranuclear palsy usually has additional abnormalities in the form of involuntary eye movements such as square wave jerks and neurologic signs of parkinsonism.

BIBLIOGRAPHY

1. Burde RM, Savino PJ, Trobe D. Clinical Decisions in Neuro-ophthalmology, 2nd Edition. St Louis: Mosby; 1992. pp 224-88.
2. Glaser JS. Neuro-ophthalmology, 2nd Edition. Philadelphia: Lippincott; 1990.
3. Miller NR, Newman NJ. Walsh and Hoyt's Clinical Neuro-ophthalmology, 6th Edition. Baltimore: Williams & Wilkins; 2005.

Photophobia

7

Johan Zwaan

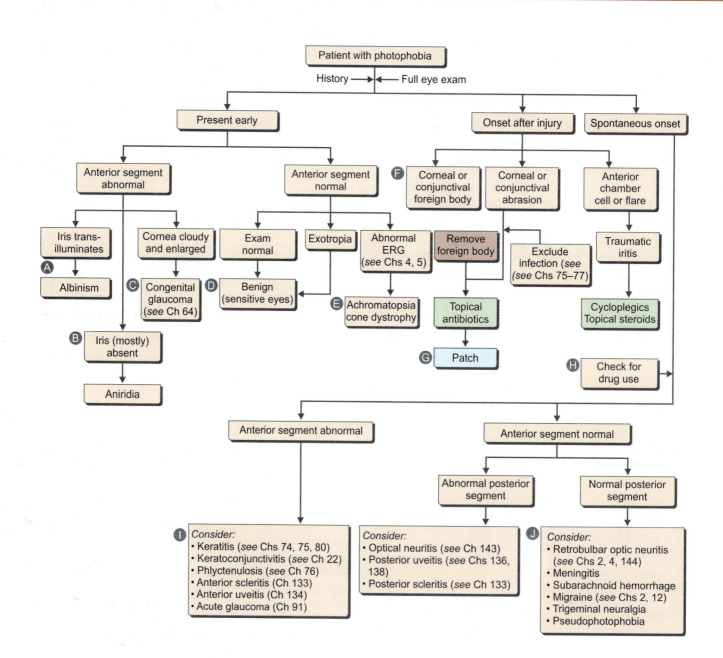

Photophobia is a fairly common patient complaint. It may not indicate a serious problem, but it can and therefore a thorough eye examination is necessary. The history may give significant clues regarding possible underlying pathology. Particularly, the time and manner of onset offers an idea about the cause of the photophobia.

A. In addition to transillumination of the iris, both oculo-cutaneous albinism (which is inherited in an autosomal recessive pattern) and ocular albinism (which is X-linked recessive) have a number of other findings in common. Nystagmus, foveal hypoplasia, a hypopigmented retina and lack of stereopsis are seen in both.

B. A (partial) congenital absence of the iris is a consequence of aniridia, due to autosomal dominant inheritance or to a deletion of chromosome 11p13. In the latter, which is sporadic, there is a risk for Wilms tumor, genitourinary abnormalities and mental retardation (WAGR or Miller syndrome). Both types share foveal hypoplasia and nystagmus with albinism.

C. An enlarged cloudy cornea almost certainly indicates congenital glaucoma. These kids often are so photophobic that they stay kneeled down in their crib with their head buried in the pillow or coverings. Because of this, they are not infrequently considered to be developmentally delayed (Chapter 64). Urgent treatment is indicated.

D. Children often complain of photophobia, while the eye examination is completely normal. In most cases, all that is needed is reassurance of the parents and patients. A sub-group consists of children with (intermittent) exotropia. These patients often are photophobic and tend to close one or both eyes when they step outside into bright sunlight.

E. The classification of cone photoreceptor functional abnormalities is becoming increasingly complicated and more variations are recognized all the time, based on electrophysiology, i.e. electroretinography (ERG), visual evoked response (VER), and dark adaptometry, and on genetic analysis. Cone-rod degenerations complicate the picture even more. Detailed descriptions are beyond the scope of this book.

F. One type of quite painful severe keratitis/abrasion is caused by ultraviolet (UV) exposure (snow blindness; welder's eye).

G. The use of a patch after a traumatic abrasion is somewhat controversial. It makes the eye more comfortable, but some evidence indicates that it delays healing.

H. A number of medications may produce photophobia. Among them are anticonvulsants (mephenytoin, methsuximide, paramethadione, trimethadione, valproic acid), antineoplastic agents (cytarabine, fludarabine, procarbazine, vindesine), topical eye medications (belladonna type products, dexamethasone, vidarabine) as well as clofibrate, oral retinoids, ketoconazole, phenothiazines and others.

I. Any type of inflammatory condition of the cornea produces photophobia due to irritation of the corneal nerves. The cornea has one of the highest concentrations of sensory nerves in the body. It may be tempting to prescribe topical anesthetics, but they only give very temporary relief and delay healing.

J. Occasionally, malingering may be accompanied by a complaint of photophobia.

BIBLIOGRAPHY

1. Carden S, Boissy RE, Schoettker PJ, et al. Albinism: modern molecular diagnosis. Brit J Ophthalmol. 1998;82:189-95.
2. Deeb SS, Motulsky AG. Disorders of color vision. In: Traboulsi EI, (Ed). Genetic Diseases of the Eye, 2nd Edition. New York: Oxford University Press; 2012. pp. 448-66.
3. Drummond PD. A quantitative assessment of photophobia in migraine and tension headache. Headache. 1986;26:465-9.
4. Hazin R, Abuzetun JY, Daoud YJ, et al. Ocular complications of cancer therapy: a primer for the ophthalmologist treating cancer patients. Curr Opin Ophthalmol. 2009;20:308-17.
5. Traboulsi EI. Cone dysfunction syndromes, cone dystrophies, and cone-rod degenerations. In: Traboulsi EI, (Ed). Genetic Diseases of the Eye, 2nd Edition. New York: Oxford University Press; 2012. pp. 410-20.

Flashes and Floaters

WAJ van Heuven

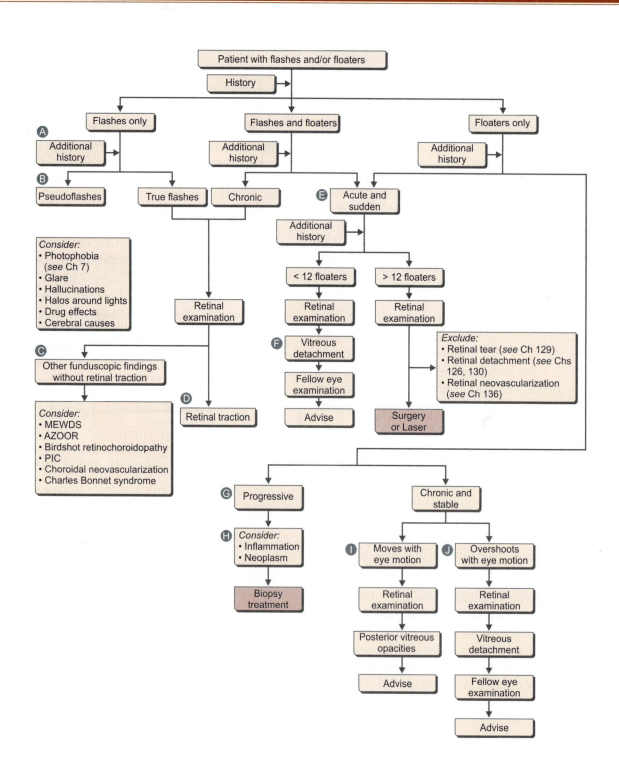

A common chief complaint, particularly in adults, is "seeing flashes or floaters". These symptoms usually stem from ocular sources. The flashes of light indicate mechanical stimulation of the retina and are best seen in the dark or with the closed eyes when the flashes do not compete with ambient light. When the retina is mechanically stimulated, a message is transmitted to the brain, which the brain presumes to be light because the stimulus originated in the retina. Firm massage of the globe can produce such retinal stimulation with resultant flashes. Floaters, which are usually caused by opacities in the ocular media that cause shadows to be cast on the retina, are best seen in bright light or against a bright background. Floaters caused by opacities near the retina appear small and distinct, whereas those farther forward are larger and blurrier. Floaters move with eye movement, and, depending on the tissue in which they are embedded, either follow the eye movements precisely, overshoot the eye movements, or move with gravity.

A. A history is important to determine whether flashes are true entoptic flashes or pseudoflashes. True flashes are better seen in the dark and are usually vertical and temporal. Some patients complain of the flashes only at night.

B. When flashes occur mostly in or around bright lights, the patient may really be complaining of glare, halos or photophobia. Glare is usually caused by media opacities, varying from cataracts to intraocular lenses to contact lenses or dirty and scratched spectacles. Although halos can be caused by any opacities in the ocular media, a common cause is corneal edema from increased intraocular pressure. In fact, when eliciting a history of glaucoma, ask for the symptom of halo or rainbow vision. Many drugs that affect the corneal epithelium can also produce halos. Photophobia, abnormal intolerance to bright light, may be caused by glare. However, photophobia in children, in whom media opacities are less common, warrants consideration of congenital disorders such as cone dystrophy, albinism, or achromatopsia. Numerous systemic drugs can also cause photophobia. Hysteria and malingering are also more common than generally appreciated. As with all entoptic phenomena, cerebral causes such as migraine headaches and their variants must be considered, and a careful history and neurologic examination may be indicated (Chapter 12).

C. In addition to vitreoretinal traction, other retinal pathologic conditions can also lead to symptoms of photopsia. These include inflammatory disorders such as multiple evanescent white dot syndrome (MEWDS), acute zonal occult outer retinopathy (AZOOR), birdshot retinochoroidopathy, and punctate inner choroidopathy (PIC). Also patients with decreased central vision from choroidal neovascularization can have symptoms of flashing lights or even formed hallucinations (Charles Bonnet syndrome).

D. True flashes, with or without floaters, indicate retinal stimulation, which is most often caused by traction on the retina. The most common form of retinal traction is vitreous traction, in which the vitreous gel, at a point of firm vitreoretinal adhesion, pulls the retina forward. This problem can be caused by congenital abnormalities, such as congenital retinal traction tufts and congenital meridional folds at the ora serrata. Vitreous traction can also be acquired when the vitreous gel, which tends to liquefy with increasing age, collapses forward and produces sudden traction on the retina at the posterior edge of the vitreous base. Vitreous traction can also occur in 'secondary' vitreous detachment, in which a slow shrinkage of the vitreous gel, caused by inflammation or chronic vascular leakage, causes slow progressive traction on those retinal structures to which the vitreous is firmly attached, such as the disk, major retinal vessels, and areas of abnormal retinal vascular lesions, such as neovascularization and vascular tumors (von Hippel). Retinal traction can also occur tangentially to the retina from preretinal fibrosis, which occurs in spontaneous idiopathic macular pucker and in proliferative vitreoretinopathy. The latter most often results from proliferation of retinal pigment epithelial cells, which have migrated through a retinal hole into the vitreous cavity and settled on the retina. Intraretinal traction can also occur after chorioretinal injuries with resultant scars, which shrink with time. A complete retinal examination, using indirect ophthalmoscopy and scleral depression, usually permits diagnosis of the source of flashes and floaters caused by retinal traction.

E. Acute and sudden symptoms of flashes and floaters usually indicate vitreous detachment. Patients may call the office for an appointment, and the determination of whether the patient should be seen immediately must often be made during the telephone conversation. Thus, it is wise, particularly in a retina practice, to instruct the secretaries to ask, whether the floaters are fewer or more than a dozen. If the floaters are few, it is often safe to assume that a benign vitreous detachment has occurred, in which the floaters represent the opacities on the posterior vitreous surface, where the vitreous was previously attached to the disk. If the floaters are numerous, particularly if they are described as a 'cloud', 'spider web', or 'curtain', assume that there has been a vitreous hemorrhage, which may mean that there is now a retinal tear. Other common causes of vitreous hemorrhage are vitreous detachment without retinal tear, in which the hemorrhage originates at the disk, and vitreous traction on neovascularization of the retina as a result of diabetic retinopathy, retinal vein occlusion, or other ischemic retinopathies. Ocular trauma can also produce vitreous hemorrhage.

F. Acute, or rhegmatogenous, vitreous detachment is a sudden collapse of the vitreous gel caused by a sudden outpouring of central liquefied vitreous through one of the posterior holes in the vitreous cortex overlying the disk and macula. The vitreous gel usually retracts forward with the central liquefied vitreous moving through the posterior vitreous hole into the space between the vitreous surface and the retina. The separation of vitreous from the retina stops anteriorly at the posterior edge of the vitreous base, which represents the strongest adhesion between vitreous and retina. The sudden cessation of the vitreous detachment at the vitreous base creates traction on the retina at that location and may tear the retina. When that occurs, there is usually bleeding, causing many floaters. If no retinal tear occurs, the floaters represent small pieces of glial tissue on the posterior surface of the vitreous, where it separated from the optic disk. Always

examine the fellow eye for vitreous detachment. If it is not present, advise the patient that symptoms of floaters in the fellow eye should again prompt a visit to the ophthalmologist.

G. Progressively worsening floaters, although they could represent rebleeding from neovascularization of the retina, often indicate uveitis, particularly peripheral uveitis (pars planitis). Also consider reticulum cell sarcoma (Chapter 135).

H. If the vitreous appears liquefied or is detached, vitreous biopsy can be done easily with a needle through the pars plana. If the vitreous is solid and not detached, it is safer to do a partial vitrectomy to avoid causing vitreous traction on the retina during the biopsy. Specimens should be cultured and stained for cytologic examination. Fungi may need special stains (e.g. silver).

I. Vitreous floaters that are chronic and stable and *move* precisely with eye movement are common, particularly in myopic patients. They represent opacities in the posterior vitreous near the retina and are of no clinical significance. They may remain constant for decades.

J. Vitreous opacities that overshoot (i.e. *move* more than the eye movement and then return to the visual axis) indicate vitreous opacities on the posterior surface of a detached vitreous gel. No matter how long the symptoms have been present, examine the fellow eye for vitreous detachment. If it is not present, advise the patient of the significance of new floaters in the fellow eye.

BIBLIOGRAPHY

1. Brown GC, Murphy RP. Visual symptoms associated with choroidal neovascularization: Photopsias and the Charles Bonnet syndrome. Arch Ophthalmol. 1992;110:1251-6.
2. Eisner G. Biomicroscopy of the Peripheral Fundus. New York: Springer-Verlag; 1973.
3. Gass JDM. Acute zonal occult outer retinopathy. J Clin NeuroOphthalmol. 1993;13:79-97.
4. Jampol LM, Sieving PA, Pugh D, et al. Multiple evanescent white dot syndrome. I. Clinical findings. Arch Ophthalmol. 1984;102:671-4.
5. Schepens CL. Retinal Detachment and Allied Diseases. Philadelphia: WB Saunders; 1983.

Acquired Increasing Myopia

9

Johan Zwaan

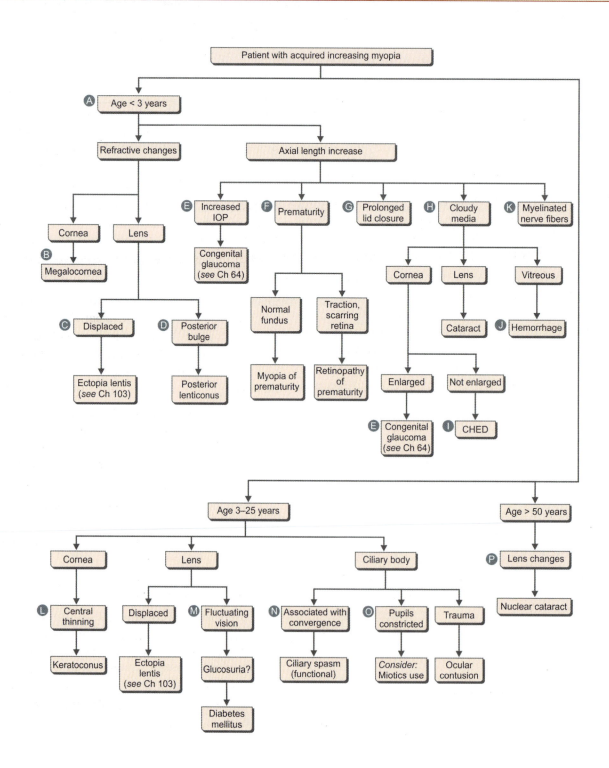

Four factors determine the ocular refractive state: (1) the optical power of the cornea, (2) the optical power of the lens, (3) the distance between these two, (i.e. anterior chamber depth) and (4) axial length. Accommodation for near vision and scleral resistance versus intraocular pressure (IOP) plays a role in the genesis of myopia, and both genetic and environmental influences are suspected.

Myopia is the most common ocular anomaly seen in developed countries. Most affected individuals have so-called simple myopia. In the United States, 15–25% of the population have or will have this type of myopia. In most people, the refractive error becomes manifest between the ages of 6 and 13 years and worsens, becoming reasonably stable around the age of 17. A much smaller group, almost all college students, becomes myopic in early adulthood.

Second, a large group of syndromes and inherited diseases are commonly associated with myopia. Examples are Marfan, Ehlers-Danlos, Stickler, Down, fetal alcohol syndromes and retinitis pigmentosa. The diagnosis of these diseases obviously does not depend on the finding of myopia.

In the third group of patients, myopia is a major presenting sign. These are discussed in this chapter. It is useful to divide these patients by age and to consider the anatomic structures involved in the genesis of myopia [i.e. cornea, lens, ciliary body (muscle) and vitreous size (axial length)].

A. Up to the age of 3 years, corneal power and lens power are adjusted to correlate with different increases of axial length. The result is that more than 95% of eyes end up with a refraction close to emmetropia (between (+) 4.00 and (−) 4.00 diopters of refractive error). The regulatory factors involved are only poorly understood.

B. Megalocornea is associated with myopia because the cornea is steeper than normal. It is inherited, and all three patterns of Mendelian inheritance have been reported. It is usually an isolated condition but can be associated with juvenile glaucoma or ectopia lentis.

C. Ectopia lentis can cause significant myopia as a result of tilting of the lens. In some types (Marfan syndrome, autosomal recessive ectopia lentis et pupillae), the axial length is also increased.

Fluctuation of the refraction is common, related to shifts in lens position, and the patient may indeed go all the way from high myopia to high hyperopia if the lens dislocates completely and disappears out of the visual axis.

D. Posterior lentiglobus is an axial deformation of the posterior aspect of the lens. It results in high myopia through the center of the lens, although the periphery can be emmetropic.

E. An enlarging corneal diameter and an axial length increasing beyond the expected normal growth in an infant should alert one to the possible presence of congenital glaucoma, even in the absence of clearly abnormal IOP. Other signs usually present are an enlarging optic cup and corneal edema.

F. Even mild cicatricial retinopathy of prematurity, expressed as retinal pigmentation and dragging of retinal vessels and macula, is almost always associated with myopia. It is less well known that prematurity *per se* is a risk factor for the development of severe myopia.

G. Both animal experiments and findings in patients with capillary hemangiomas, severe ptosis, plexiform neurofibroma or patching have demonstrated that in addition to causing severe amblyopia, prolonged eyelid closure may cause myopia as a result of an increase in axial eye length.

H. A severely blurred image on the fovea during infancy not only is amblyogenic but can also cause myopia. Typical causes are a cloudy cornea resulting from birth trauma, a cataract or a vitreous hemorrhage.

I. Congenital hereditary endothelial dystrophy (CHED), an autosomal recessive disease leading to diffuse corneal clouding, is always associated with myopia. It is differentiated from congenital glaucoma because the IOP is normal or close to normal, the cornea is greatly thickened, and its diameter does not increase.

J. A vitreous hemorrhage related to birth can cause high myopia. It is often not recognized because retinal examinations are not done routinely on all newborns. Because of the dense structure of the infant vitreous, such a hemorrhage clears only slowly and its amblyogenic influence may be present for months.

K. A syndrome has been reported in which monocular presence of significant myelination of retinal nerve fibers is combined with high myopia, fairly intractable amblyopia and strabismus. The pathogenesis is not understood.

L. Inability to obtain a clear endpoint on retinoscopy should lead to slit lamp examination. Central thinning of the cornea and irregular mires and rings seen with keratometry, keratoscopy or corneal topographical determinations confirm the presence of keratoconus, which usually manifests itself at puberty.

M. Fluctuating distance vision is often the presenting sign for previously undiagnosed diabetes. The fluctuations are presumably caused by changes in lens hydration, related to the variations in osmotic effects of swings in blood glucose. Ask patients about other signs and symptoms such as weight loss, polydipsia and polyuria. A simple dipstick test can confirm glucosuria, which should lead to immediate referral to the internist or endocrinologist.

N. Episodes of blurred and double vision, associated with headaches or eye pain, may be caused by a spasm of the near reflex. Examination should reveal convergence of the eyes and miosis during the attacks. The problem is most often seen in female adolescents and is self-limited, although it may recur for several years. The attacks can be incapacitating and may last several hours. Although underlying abnormalities are rare and the problem is almost always functional, neurologic and neuro-ophthalmologic examinations are recommended. Treatment consists of cycloplegics and binocular glasses, although paradoxically, miotics have also been used with success, presumably by reducing the central drive.

O. Pilocarpine is notorious for inducing disturbing, if transient, myopia in young people. Other miotics, such as echothiophate and isoflurophate, which sometimes used to be prescribed for esotropia therapy, can also cause myopia. Many drugs may occasionally lead to myopia, presumably because of induced edema of the ciliary body. In cases of unexplained recently acquired myopia, it is worthwhile to question the patient about medication use.

P. In elderly patients, gradually increasing myopia is almost always the result of lens changes. These changes may be subtle but eventually it becomes clear that a nuclear cataract is developing.

BIBLIOGRAPHY

1. Curtin BJ. The Myopias: Basic Science and Clinical Management. Philadelphia: Harper and Row; 1985.
2. Dagi LR, Chrousos GA, Cogan DG. Spasm of the near reflex associated with organic disease. Am J Ophthalmol. 1987;103:582-5.
3. Goldberg MF. Clinical manifestations of ectopia lentis et pupillae in 16 patients. Ophthalmology. 1988;95:1080-7.
4. Rosner M, Belkin M. Intelligence, education, and myopia in males. Arch Ophthalmol. 1987;105:1508-11.
5. Straatsma BR, Foos RY, Heckenlively JR, et al. Myelinated retinal nerve fibers. Am J Ophthalmol. 1981;91:25-38.
6. Weale RA. Corneal shape and astigmatism: with a note on myopia. Br J Ophthalmol. 1988;72:696-9.
7. Working Group on Myopia Prevalence and Progression. Myopia: Prevalence and Progression. Washington DC: National Academy Press; 1989.

Acquired Hyperopia

Johan Zwaan

10

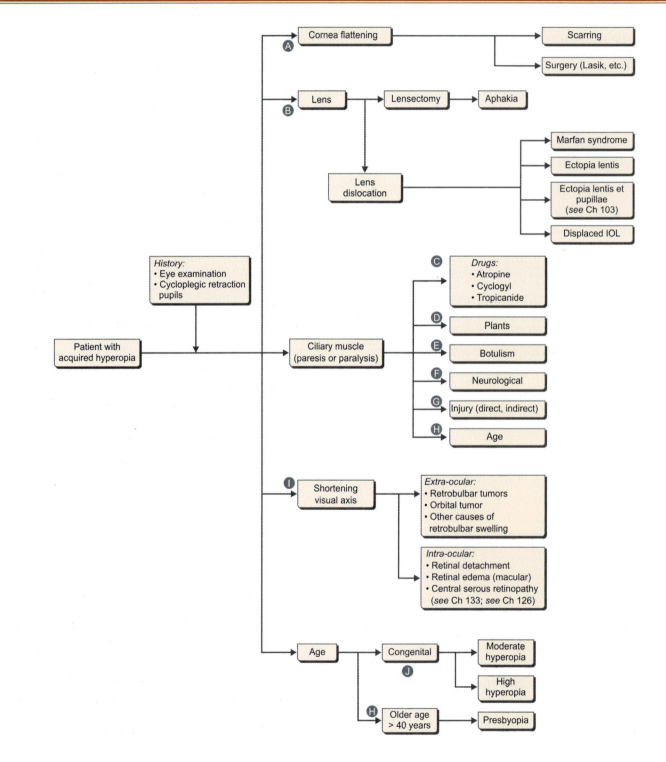

Hyperopia is an optical condition in which an object seen at a distance of 6 meters or more (optical infinity) is projected behind the retina. The focusing mechanisms of the eye need to converge the light so that the image falls on the retina. This is necessary, because the hyperopic eye is smaller and shorter than an emmetropic or a myopic eye, which have a longer axial length. In these two, the projected image falls on the retina or even in front of it. From front to back several parts of the eye are responsible for projecting the image on the retina, which is essential for sharp vision. The curvature of the cornea is the major factor in focusing the acquired image.

Next, as the name indicates the lens provides the fine focusing, which is partially controlled by the contractions of the ciliary muscle, which influences the curvature of the lens, and further by the elasticity of the lens tissue. Finally, the axial length can be modified by intraocular or extraocular conditions shortening the axial length.

A. Scarring of the cornea by injury can flatten the curvature of the cornea, changing the refraction of the eye away from myopia. Refractive surgery uses the same principle of flattening the cornea through selective thinning.

B. The absence of the lens from the visual axis, congenitally as in Hallerman-Streiff syndrome, surgically by lensectomy, displacement of the lens from the visual axis (usually upward in Marfan syndrome and down in ectopia lentis), or the displacement of an implanted intraocular lens, all have the same principal effect: a significant part of the accommodation mechanism is missing, resulting in high hyperopia.

C. Several drugs are used clinically to paralyze the ciliary muscle, to aid with refraction, for amblyopia treatment, or to increase comfort for a uveitis patient. Occasionally a parent will call in a panic, because she has rubbed her own eye after instilling drops in her child's eye with resulting ciliary paralysis and blurred vision.

D. In the same way, kids playing outside, or gardeners may be in touch with a plant with a high alkaloid content (Bella Donna, Thorn Apple) causing dilation.

E. Botulinum, either used for cosmesis, or ingested by food poisoning, can also cause pupillary dilation and paralysis of the ciliary muscle.

F. Lesions of the parasympathetic nuclei in the midbrain, as seen with a pineal tumor, with a complete third nerve palsy or encephalitis, may cause pupillary dilation and ciliary paralysis, increasing hyperopia.

G. If the eye is hit, particularly with a ball, it is not unusual for the pupil to be dilated and the vision blurry. Often this is temporary, but not always.

H. As people grow older their accommodation power gradually decreases. This is mostly due to the lens losing its elasticity, but weakening of the ciliary muscle also may play a role. Thus, around age 40 years, most of us require reading glasses to compensate for this presbyopia.

I. Axial length can be shortened when the retina moves forward. This may happen when the retina slowly becomes edematous or develops central serous retinopathy. Alternatively, the wall of the eye may be indented by a retrobulbar process.

J. A majority of children (75%) is born with hyperopia. In most the refractive error is modest and, with growth of the eye, will gradually diminish. Some kids have high hyperopia (5–6 diopters and beyond), which may not get much less. All hyperopic children need to be checked for amblyopia and esotropia, especially the ones with high hyperopia.

BIBLIOGRAPHY

1. Attebo K, Ivers RQ, Mitchell P. Refractive errors in an older population. Ophthalmology. 1999;106:1066-72.
2. Fraunfelter FT. Drug-Induced Ocular Side Effects and Drug Interactions, 3rd Edition. Philadelphia, PA: Lea and Febiger; 1989.
3. Gordon RA, Dontzis PB. Refractive development of the human eye. Arch Ophthalmol. 1986;103:785-9.
4. Katz J, Tielsch JM, Sommer A. Prevalence and risk factors for refractive errors in an adult inner city population. Invest Ophthalmol Vis Sci. 1997;38:334-50.
5. Mutti DO, Zadnik K, Egashira E, et al. The effect of cycloplegia on measurement of the ocular components. Invest Ophthalmol Vis Sci. 1994;35:515-27.

11

Low Vision

Sandra M Fox, Melanie P Gonzalez

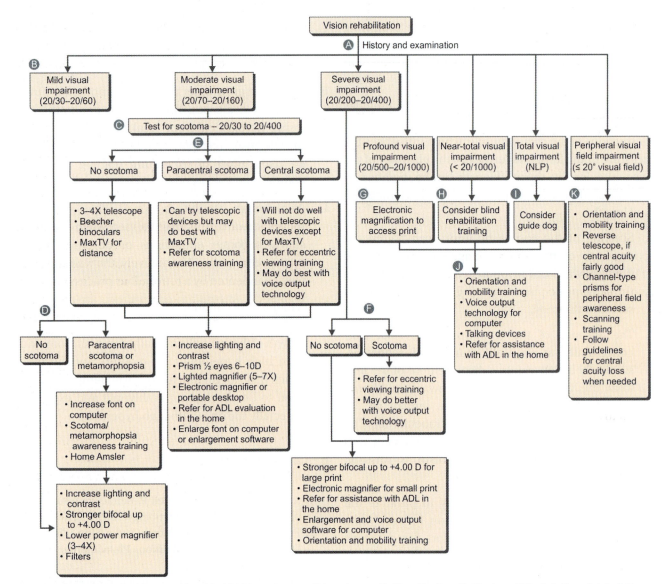

Abbreviations: NLP: No light perception; MaxTV: Binocular magnifying glasses; X: Magnification; D: Diopters; ADL: Activities of daily living

The goal of vision rehabilitation is to improve patients' functional vision in order to keep their independence, continue with activities of daily living (ADLs) and improve quality of life. The term functional vision is defined as the ability to accomplish a task that requires vision. When a patient experiences functional loss due to their vision, they are considered visually impaired. Patients experience functional deficits at different levels of visual acuity loss. A patient with low vision is defined as someone whose visual acuity cannot be enhanced with traditional spectacles, medical or surgical treatment. The estimated number of patients in the United States, older than 45 years, with visual impairment is 13.5 million. The majority of these patients are 65 years and older. The population of Americans older than 65 years was 40.3 million in 2010 and is projected to double by the year 2050. Therefore, the number of patients with visual impairment will continue to increase. The three most common causes of visual impairment are age-related macular degeneration, glaucoma, and diabetic retinopathy. The constant aim to successfully manage a patient's ocular disease may overshadow the proper attention needed to improve a patient's functional vision. It is important to recognize when a patient is experiencing visual deficits, thus a timely referral can be made for vision rehabilitation. When a patient can no longer answer "yes" to any of the following simple questions: "Can you see well enough to read?", "Can you see well enough to watch television?" and "Can you see well enough to perform your daily activities?"; then referral to a vision rehabilitation specialist is essential.

A. Complete patient assessment includes a thorough functional history and visual function measurement. Functional history is approached similarly as medical history. It is important to understand the patient's functional deficits and how these deficits correlate to the patient's ocular and medical history. A patient's ocular history can help determine the types of visual deficits a patient may experience. For example, a patient with an ocular history of retinitis pigmentosa may express difficulty navigating in unfamiliar areas. A patient with a significant medical history of arthritis may report difficulty reading with a hand-held magnifier. A thorough functional history should include task analysis. This analysis will define which tasks the patient has trouble performing; therefore, we can determine a plan to rehabilitate such tasks. It is essential to ask specific questions regarding near tasks, which include reading, writing, and ability to read and administer medications (e.g. insulin dependent diabetic patients). Intermediate tasks that visually impaired patients have a difficulty in performing include cooking, shopping, working with hobbies, shaving or working on the computer. It is also important to identify distance tasks that need improvement, such as watching television, independent travel, and especially driving. The functional history is the foundation to identify the goals and plan for vision rehabilitation.

B. It is imperative to accurately measure a patient's best-corrected visual acuity (BCVA) in order to monitor disease progression, determine their level of visual impairment, and provide proper vision rehabilitation. Most patients qualify for vision services through state agencies, if their vision is 20/70 or less. Legal blindness is defined as visual acuity of 20/200 or worse in the patient's better eye or a peripheral visual field of 20° or worse in the better eye. Distance visual acuity is commonly tested using the Feinbloom chart in low vision examinations. This chart can test a greater range of visual acuity compared to the Snellen chart. The ability to move the chart from its initial distance of 10 feet to a closer distance of 5 feet doubles the range of acuity. Near visual acuity is tested both monocularly and binocularly. Single letter charts are used to test monocular acuity while paragraph acuity charts are used to test binocular acuity. This dual acuity testing informs the examiner of the patient's potential acuity as well as how they function with their vision, especially in reading. In most low vision examinations, careful trial-frame refraction is the best way to determine the patient's BCVA. Trial-frame refraction offers many advantages. One of the main advantages is that the patient is able to look through a wider lens and therefore able to eccentrically fixate or in cases of nystagmus a null point can be maintained. An important benefit of trial-frame refraction is the ability to make large increment lens changes and Jackson cross cylinders are available in higher powers. It is also easier to check near visual acuity at a more natural position in the trial-frame as well as use telescopes over the lenses to test distance acuity. Trial frame refraction is performed in the same manner as subjective refraction. A clinical pearl for refraction is to show the patient the new manifest refraction versus their habitual correction. It is important for the patient to notice an improvement in vision before writing a new spectacle prescription.

C. It is important to evaluate for metamorphopsia and/or scotomas since these findings affect a patient's visual impairment and their performance with optical and nonoptical devices. Central visual field testing can be achieved with Amsler grid, central visual field test, and/or macular perimetry. Amsler grid is used to measure the central 20° of the visual field monocularly. It is helpful in diagnosing metamorphopsia and absolute scotomas; however, it is insufficient for detecting small and relative scotomas. Amsler grid will also fail to detect a scotoma, if the patient experiences perceptual completion. The California Fletcher central visual field test also measures the function of the central 20° of vision. This test is performed using a central tangent on white paper and three laser pointers of varying size and brightness, which allows for more sensitivity to evaluate for relative scotomas. A scotoma is plotted on the central tangent based on the patient's responses when they are unable to view the stimulus. The central tangent can be performed monocularly or binocularly. Macular perimetry which utilizes a scanning laser ophthalmoscope allows an examiner to visualize the specific area of the retina that is being tested with each stimulus. This apparatus maps the visual field defect with the exact retinal location. The precision of this diagnostic tool is especially valuable in eccentric viewing training and monitoring of disease progression.

D. *Mild visual impairment (20/30–20/60):* Most visually impaired patients will benefit from increased lighting and contrast because they allow for better detail resolution. Both of these will enhance a patient's ability to use optical aids as well as increase overall function. Tinted-lens filters can facilitate improved contrast sensitivity. A stronger bifocal up to +4.00 diopters (D) will improve near

vision. When prescribing higher Add powers, make sure to educate the patient on a closer near working distance, based on the new focal point. Low power 3–4X magnifiers will enhance small print and facilitate continuous text reading as magnifiers allow a greater working distance. For patients with paracentral scotomas or metamorphopsia, increasing contrast and/or enlarging the font on the computer are simple adjustments that will aid in computer tasks. It is also important for these patients to be referred for scotoma and/or metamorphopsia awareness training to improve overall visual function.

E. *Moderate visual impairment (20/70–20/160):* Patients with moderate visual impairment may benefit from high-plus prismatic glasses for near vision. These glasses have base-in prism that is ground-in to the spectacles so the patient can function binocularly. The advantage of spectacles over magnifiers is that they have a wider field of view and allow the patient to use their hands. These patients perform well with 5–7X illuminated magnifiers. They will also benefit from enlarging the font on the computer. Closed-circuit television (CCTV) systems or electronic magnification systems utilize a video camera that is attached to a monitor or even a television screen to display images. These electronic devices can enlarge the images and/or increase contrast and brightness based on the patient's preference for enhanced function. It is essential for these patients to have an ADL evaluation in their home in order to make modifications to the daily tasks they find challenging as well as to ensure they are able to function safely in their home and environment. Patients who have moderate visual impairment without any scotomas can enhance their distance vision with a 3–4X telescope, which is useful for intermittent distance spotting. Beecher binoculars are advantageous for continuous distance viewing such as at sporting events. MaxTV binocular glasses have about 2X magnification and are worn like eyeglasses for better distance vision. These MaxTV glasses are especially helpful for watching television and movies. Patients with paracentral scotomas can try a telescopic device for distance vision, but they may do best with MaxTV glasses. Patients with paracentral or central scotomas should be referred for eccentric viewing training. This training is imperative for patients to be able to develop tracking and scanning skills, and utilize optical devices in order to boost visual function especially in areas of reading. Voice output technology is valuable for visually impaired patients with central scotomas. The American Academy of Ophthalmology's (AAO) SmartSight patient handout can be presented to the patient at this time. It offers essential tips for making the most of the patient's remaining vision and provides information about services in the community.

F.   *Severe visual impairment (20/200–20/400):* A patient with severe visual impairment in their better eye is considered legally blind. Since some charts, like the Feinbloom, can test a wider range of acuity, it is important to know that a patient who cannot read any letters on the 20/100 line with their better eye is considered legally blind. A stronger bifocal up to +4.00 D can be prescribed if it allows the patient to see large print. These patients will require electronic magnification to be able to see small print. Assistance with ADLs in the home is necessary. Computer enlargement software and voice output technology becomes very useful for patients with severe visual impairment. At this stage of visual impairment, referral for orientation and mobility (O&M) training should be initiated.

G.   *Profound visual impairment (20/500–20/1,000):* Most patients with this level of vision loss will need electronic magnification to access print. Leisure reading is usually not possible since the print must be enlarged to such an extent that it is just too laborious, but a CCTV will allow the person with profound visual impairment to read medication bottles and sort their mail. Enlargement software is available for the computer and several have the option to use voice output as well. A referral to an assistive technology specialist is warranted to determine what technology will be necessary for the patient to remain independent.

H.   *Near-total visual impairment (< 20/1,000):* Patients with this level of vision loss will need to learn to use their other senses rather than vision. Blind rehabilitation training will teach visual substitution skills using tactile aids, such as raised dots for marking and braille as well as auditory aids, such as talking books, talking watches and even voice output technology. Braille may be indicated for young patients whereas, voice output technology may be more beneficial for older patients.

I.   *Total visual impairment (No light perception):* Total visual loss will require blind rehabilitation training. Many states have residential training facilities for those with new vision loss to learn the skills necessary to function independently. A guide dog can instill confidence for many people with total vision loss.

J.   All patients with profound visual impairment or worse will benefit from a referral to an O&M specialist. The O&M specialist will teach the person with profound vision loss how to use a blind cane as well as how to navigate within the community, including how to use other transportation options such as public transportation. Voice output technology is now available for the computer, tablets and smart phones as well as many other devices for daily living such as talking watches, microwaves, etc. Occupational therapists and vision rehabilitation specialists can assist the person with profound visual impairment to remain independent by teaching them strategies for managing their finances, medication management and meal preparation.

K.   *Peripheral visual field impairment:* Patients with visual field constriction present a special challenge because mobility is significantly affected. A referral to an O&M specialist is warranted. If the central vision is better than 20/40, a 2X reverse telescope may be beneficial. If a handheld telescope helps the patient ambulate more efficiently, a reverse telescope can be placed in a spectacle. If the central vision is worse than 20/40, base-out hemiprisms placed on the lateral aspect of both lenses can allow the patient to make smaller scanning movements. This technique can also benefit patients with hemianopsia as a result or acquired brain injury. Training in the use of the prism as well as scanning training will increase the level of success. If the patient has central acuity loss as well, magnification can be utilized up to a point. Too much magnification can make it more difficult because the letters may be too large for the patient's field of vision.

According to the AAO's Preferred Practice Pattern concerning vision rehabilitation, all ophthalmologists are encouraged to recommend vision rehabilitation as a continuum of their care and to provide information about rehabilitation resources for patients with vision loss. The AAO's SmartSight model of vision rehabilitation (*www.aao.org/smartsight*) asks all ophthalmologists to 'recognize and respond'—'recognize' the impact of even modest uncorrectable partial vision loss and 'respond' by assuring the patient that much can be offered with rehabilitation and when available, a referral for multidisciplinary rehabilitation should be considered.

The goal of vision rehabilitation is to teach the individual with vision loss how to safely and independently perform daily tasks with reduced visual function and this often requires a multidisciplinary approach. The multidisciplinary approach includes an evaluation by an ophthalmologist or optometrist who specializes in low vision and rehabilitative training that may include the services of a certified low vision therapist, occupational therapist that specializes in low vision or vocational rehabilitation specialist, as well as an assistive technology specialist and/or an O&M specialist. Psychosocial support services may include a referral to a psychiatrist, psychologist and/or support group. The low vision ophthalmologist or optometrist may also refer the visually impaired patient to a nonprofit or state agency or the Veterans Administration where additional support services such as employment assistance, help with ADLs in the home, assistance in purchasing low vision devices and participation in comprehensive residential rehabilitation training may be available for patients who qualify. Comorbidities are common in this patient population so referrals to other allied health disciplines, such as physical therapy, speech therapy and audiology, may also be warranted. Pediatric low vision services, while similar to adult services, are aimed at ensuring proper child development and academic success. A detailed approach to pediatric low vision services can be found in Appendix 5 of the Preferred Practice Pattern Vision Rehabilitation: Vision Rehabilitation for Children. Since loss of vision affects all areas of daily life, utilizing a multidisciplinary vision rehabilitation service can substantially improve quality of life and must be considered for all patients with functional vision loss.

BIBLIOGRAPHY

1. American Academy of Ophthalmology. Chapter 9: Vision Rehabilitation. Basic and Clinical Science Course. San Francisco, CA: American Academy of Ophthalmology; 2011. pp. 283-307.
2. American Academy of Ophthalmology Vision Rehabilitation Committee (2013) Preferred Practice Pattern® Guidelines. Vision Rehabilitation.[online] Available from *www.aao.org/ppp*.[Accessed May 2013]
3. Faye, Eleanor E, Darren LA, et al. The Lighthouse Ophthalmology Resident Training Manual: A New Look at Low Vision Care. New York: Lighthouse International; 2000.

Headache

Johan Zwaan

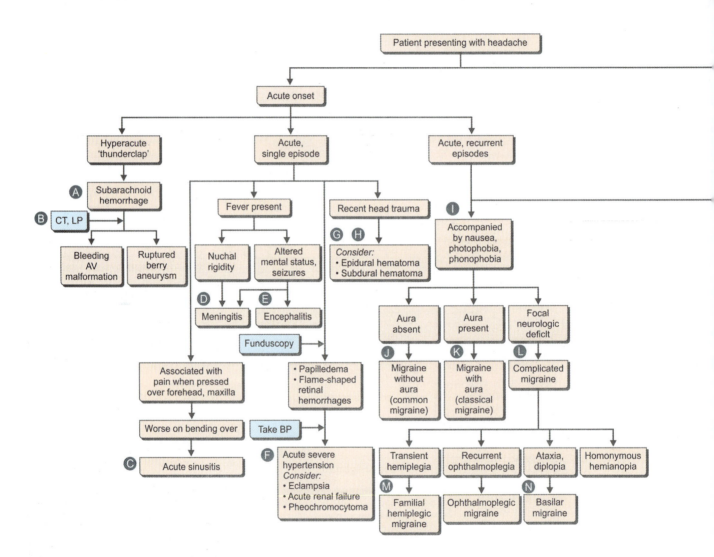

12

INTRODUCTION

One of the most common reasons for referral of a patient to the ophthalmologist is the complaint of headache, even though an ocular cause for headache is uncommon. Eye findings may be important and sometimes essential in the diagnosis of the type of headache. Muscular or tension headaches are by far the most common, followed by migraines and sinusitis. Other causes for headaches are much less common.

The diagnosis of headaches relies to a large extent on the history, which should be taken in great detail. Of particular importance are the length of the headache symptoms, its frequency and duration, location, associated symptoms, such as nausea, exacerbating and relieving features, possible triggers, and family history. The results of various examinations are useful for specific types of headaches but are generally less informative than the history. However, because patients

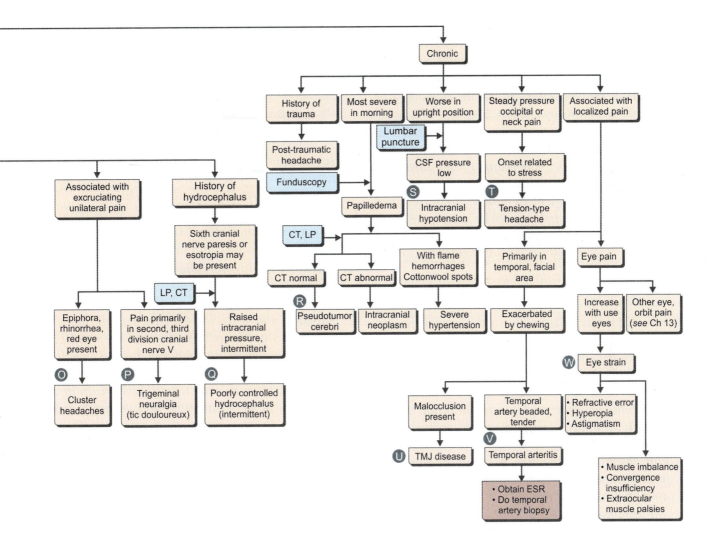

present in the belief that their headache is caused by an eye problem, a full eye examination is necessary.

In some headaches (e.g. subarachnoid hemorrhage, temporal arteritis, bacterial meningitis), a rapid and accurate diagnosis is essential to avoid permanent harm to the patient.

A. Patients report that the headache caused by a subarachnoid hemorrhage is the worst pain they have ever experienced. The pain reaches maximum intensity in a few minutes or less ('thunderclap'). A milder forewarning 'sentinel' headache may occur before the severe attack. In a few patients the headache is less severe and less acute. The diagnosis is missed in up to 25% of patients, half of whom will have bleeding again within 2 weeks, with an increased mortality rate.

B. An early computed tomography (CT) scan done within 72 hours is highly diagnostic with a sensitivity of up to 95%. If the CT is normal, a lumbar puncture (LP) will show blood in the cerebrospinal fluid (CSF) and, starting a few hours after the onset, xanthochromia. To avoid possible brain herniation, an LP should not be done if the CT is abnormal. If CT is unavailable, performing an LP is controversial.

C. Chronic sinusitis is rarely the cause of a headache. Acute sinusitis, associated with an upper respiratory tract infection or sometimes a severe allergy, gives a dull, constant ache, which increases when the patient bends over. Pressing on the area over the paranasal sinuses is uncomfortable. The diagnosis is confirmed by X-ray film or CT scan.

D. Most patients with headache and fever have an acute systemic illness and the headache will resolve when the temperature comes down. In meningitis, the headache increases in severity over hours to days. It often radiates to the neck and back and is somewhat relieved by lying flat. Altered consciousness and vomiting are common. Nuchal rigidity is highly typical. An LP is essential for the diagnosis.

E. Acute encephalitis overlaps in its symptoms with meningitis because the meninges are usually involved in any inflammation of the brain. However, an altered state of consciousness and mental status, seizures and focal neurologic signs are more severe than in meningitis.

F. The role of chronic hypertension in the causation of headache is controversial. Most authors now believe that it is not a factor. Acute, severe (diastolic pressure > 130 mm Hg) hypertension, on the other hand, can cause headache and is common when the blood pressure elevation is acute. Papilledema and retinopathy may be present.

G. An epidural hematoma is the result of arterial bleeding after a temporal or parietal skull fracture. Patients usually lose consciousness immediately after the trauma. They then regain it and a headache begins to develop. The headache increases over a few hours, and vomiting, seizures and focal signs occur. Loss of consciousness and often death follow. This typical scenario is not always followed, and some patients never regain consciousness after the trauma.

H. Subdural hematomas are caused by rupture of the bridging veins of dura and arachnoid. Trauma is the most common cause. In the acute form most patients are comatose after the injury. In subacute and chronic cases, minor trauma is common, but in one-third of patients such a history is absent. Older patients, epileptics, alcoholics and patients with coagulation disorders are prone to subdural hematomas developing. The headache is severe and may last days to weeks. Tapping on the head increases the pain.

I. Headache is never the only symptom of a migraine. In fact, migraine can be present without a headache. To be classified as migraineurs, patients should have at least five attacks lasting 4–72 hours. The headache should have two or more of the following characteristics: unilateral, throbbing, moderate to severe, and aggravated by movement. It should be accompanied by at least one of the following three: nausea, photophobia or phonophobia.

J. The term common migraine has been replaced by migraine without aura. Migraine without aura is considerably more common than that with aura.

K. Patients with migraine with aura, previously called classical migraine, often have a prodromal stage of fluid retention, changes in energy level and appetite, and a decrease in mental alertness as much as a day before the onset of the headache. The aura occurs within 1 hour before the headache and starts with scintillating scotomata consisting of jagged, often colored lines, which begin in the periphery of the visual field and gradually move centrally. Quadrantanopsia or hemianopsia may develop. Other sensory auras, such as paresthesias, are uncommon. The aura resolves in less than 60 minutes. Rarely, the deficits become permanent because of cerebral infarction. The headache follows the aura or occasionally coincides with it.

L. In complicated migraine, the headache is accompanied by focal neurologic deficits such as hemiplegia. Loss of consciousness may occur. The neurologic dysfunctions tend to outlast the headache.

M. A positive family history is common in migraine patients. Familial hemiplegic migraine shows autosomal dominant inheritance and a responsible gene has been localized on chromosome 19p13.1.

It encodes a protein subunit of one of the cellular calcium channels.

N. Basilar migraine is rare. The headache is preceded or accompanied by bilateral occipital lobe dysfunction (visual field abnormalities), brainstem abnormalities (diplopia) and/or cerebellar dysfunction (dysarthria and ataxia). Other cranial nerve signs may be present. This syndrome is usually seen in children. It is thought to result from disturbed blood flow in the vertebrobasilar arterial system.

O. Cluster headaches are uncommon and affect primarily adult men. The pain is severe and lasts only a few minutes. Attacks are frequent during a period of days to weeks and then disappear for prolonged periods, only to recur later. Alcohol is a known trigger. The conjunctiva is injected on the affected side and the nose is congested. A mild Homer syndrome may be present. The cause is unknown.

P. The attacks of trigeminal neuralgia last only very briefly but are very painful. They occur within the distribution of the second and third division of the trigeminal nerve and are repeated at a high frequency, often for weeks on end. Touching of the face or lips will trigger the attack. In most patients no cause is found. The condition can be so disabling that some patients become suicidal.

Q. Acute hydrocephalus, as seen when a ventriculo-peritoneal shunt malfunctions, or when a tumor, such as the subependymal astrocytomas of tuberous sclerosis, blocks the CSF flow, produces severe headache. Papilledema and later optic atrophy are usually the result. Other visual disturbances include cranial sixth nerve palsies and even concomitant esotropia.

R. In pseudotumor cerebri, papilledema is usually the sign leading to the diagnosis. The headache is initially relatively mild and may be present for weeks before the diagnosis is made. A CT scan is normal, but the ventricles may appear smaller than average. Intracranial pressure is elevated. Visual disturbances are frequent (i.e. cranial sixth nerve palsies with resulting diplopia, slightly blurred vision enlarged blind spots and constricted peripheral visual fields).

S. Intracranial hypotension (pressure < 90 mm H_2O) may be caused by a CSF leak, usually after an LP is performed. A traumatic dura tear or an avulsed nerve root and systemic dehydration may also lower the CSF pressure.

T. Tension-type headaches, previously called muscular contraction or tension headaches, are the most common headaches. They cause a steady pressure-like pain that may last for days. The headache is precipitated or exacerbated by stress. The patient has no nausea, photophobia or aura. The headache is generalized with frequent occipital or neck pain.

U. Temporomandibular joint disease, usually malo-cclusion, may lead to preauricular pain associated with chewing. Most patients develop facial pain and headache.

V. Temporal arteritis or giant cell arteritis needs to be diagnosed and treated promptly to avoid severe visual loss. This disease strikes older people and is diagnosed by the tenderness of the temporal artery, elevated sedimentation rate and temporal artery biopsy. The patient often has a history of malaise, anorexia, mild fever and aches, and anemia. In half of the patients this granulomatous arteritis is associated with polymyalgia rheumatica. If the disease is suspected, start treatment with high-dose steroids immediately, even before the results of the biopsy are known, to prevent progression of visual deficits. Once ischemic optic neuropathy has started, it may progress with startling rapidity.

W. Although 'eye strain' is a popular explanation by the lay public for all types of headaches, particularly tension-type, this opinion is usually wrong. If the headache is related to a refractive error or muscle imbalance, it will be absent in the morning and appear and then increase with use of the eyes.

BIBLIOGRAPHY

1. Frishberg BM. The utility of neuroimaging in the evaluation of headache in patients with normal neurological examinations. Neurology. 1994;44:1191-7.
2. Goadsby PJ, Olesen J. Diagnosis and management of migraine. BMJ. 1996;312(7041):1279-83.
3. Rasmussen BK. Epidemiology of headache. Cephalalgia. 1995;15:45-8.
4. Weir B. Headaches from aneurysms. Cephalalgia. 1994; 14:79-87.
5. Ziegler DK, Schwertfeger TL, Murrow RW. Headache. Clin Neurol. 1996;2:1-56.

Eye Pain

13

Tomy Starck, Lorena Larez

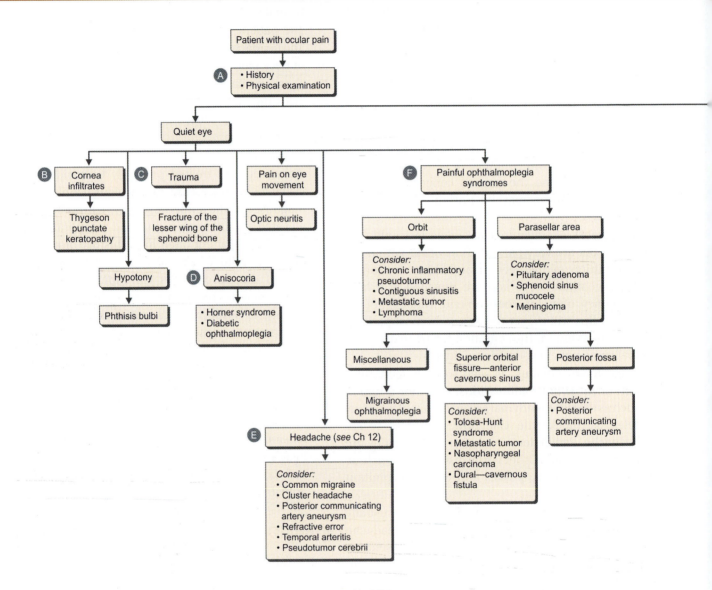

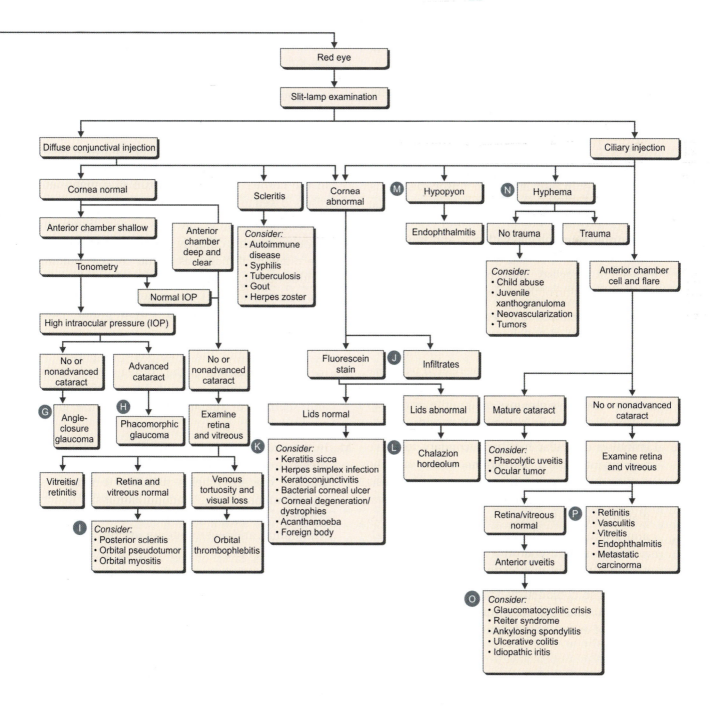

Red eye

Slit-lamp examination

Diffuse conjunctival injection

Ciliary injection

Cornea normal

Scleritis

Cornea abnormal

M Hypopyon

N Hyphema

Anterior chamber shallow

Anterior chamber deep and clear

Consider:
• Autoimmune disease
• Syphilis
• Tuberculosis
• Gout
• Herpes zoster

Endophthalmitis

No trauma

Trauma

Tonometry

Consider:
• Child abuse
• Juvenile xanthogranuloma
• Neovascularization
• Tumors

Anterior chamber cell and flare

Normal IOP

High intraocular pressure (IOP)

No or nonadvanced cataract

Advanced cataract

No or nonadvanced cataract

Fluorescein stain

J Infiltrates

G Angle-closure glaucoma

H Phacomorphic glaucoma

Examine retina and vitreous

Lids normal

Lids abnormal

Mature cataract

No or nonadvanced cataract

K

Vitreitis/retinitis

Retina and vitreous normal

Venous tortuosity and visual loss

Consider:
• Keratitis sicca
• Herpes simplex infection
• Keratoconjunctivitis
• Bacterial corneal ulcer
• Corneal degeneration/dystrophies
• Acanthamoeba
• Foreign body

L Chalazion hordeolum

Consider:
• Phacolytic uveitis
• Ocular tumor

Examine retina and vitreous

I *Consider:*
• Posterior scleritis
• Orbital pseudotumor
• Orbital myositis

Orbital thrombophlebitis

Retina/vitreous normal

P • Retinitis
• Vasculitis
• Vitreitis
• Endophthalmitis
• Metastatic carcinorma

Anterior uveitis

O *Consider:*
• Glaucomatocyclitic crisis
• Reiter syndrome
• Ankylosing spondylitis
• Ulcerative colitis
• Idiopathic iritis

A. The diagnosis of ocular pain covers a broad-spectrum of ophthalmic and nonophthalmic entities and may be a sign of a serious underlying disease process. A thorough clinical history, including detailed review of systems, adds to the complete physical examination.

B. Ocular pain without redness most likely does not involve the ocular surface, with the exception of Thygeson punctate keratopathy. Multiple small corneal epithelial and subepithelial areas of staining with flourescein dye usually highlight the diagnosis. Hypotony secondary to end-stage ocular diseases (phthisis bulbi) may be accompanied by chronic dull pain.

C. Patients with orbital pain and a history of trauma may reveal old orbital wall fractures on computed tomography (CT) scan, especially of the lesser wing of the sphenoid.

D. Horner syndrome should be considered in patients with ocular pain associated with anisocoria, ptosis, and anhidrosis. Although unlikely, microvascular causes, such as diabetes mellitus, may occasionally induce ophthalmoplegias with pain and anisocoria. Pain, with or without visual loss on ocular movement, suggests optic neuritis and requires careful evaluation of the visual pathways.

E. Headache is believed to be a common symptom of refractive errors, although in reality the association is uncommon. Several migraine syndromes may also prove to be causes of ocular-related pain (*See* Chapter 12). Systemic debilitating symptoms, such as loss of weight, loss of appetite, and scalp tenderness, may indicate temporal arteritis.

F. Limitation of ocular motility secondary to nerve involvement, called *ophthalmoplegia,* may be associated with pain. The differential diagnosis should include migraine syndromes, orbital inflammatory disease, contiguous sinusitis, tumors of the parasellar area, and superior orbital-cavernous sinus syndrome caused by vascular anomalies, tumors, or infection.

G. Pain, diffuse conjunctival injection, hazy cornea, high intraocular pressure, mid-dilated pupil, the absence of an advanced cataract, and iris bombé make the diagnosis of simple angle-closure glaucoma. Gonioscopy confirms the diagnosis.

H. In the case of an advanced cataract combined with the findings in Section G, phacomorphic glaucoma is the diagnosis, and immediate lens extraction is indicated.

I. After a thorough ocular examination that reveals only a red eye with severe pain, but no obvious ocular disease, further studies are indicated, including orbital ultrasonography, CT, or magnetic resonance imaging (MRI). Also consider posterior scleritis, orbital myositis, or pseudotumor.

J. Painful infiltrates of the cornea (with and without epithelial defects) can be a diagnostic dilemma. An infective corneal ulcer must be differentiated from a sterile ulcer by scraping the lesion for Gram stain and cultures. Bacterial, fungal, and viral ulcers with infiltrates must be treated specifically. Sterile corneal infiltrates are caused by immune responses in the cornea to a specific toxin or antigen and respond well to steroids.

K. Fluorescein staining of the cornea is usually associated with a diffusely red eye and some pain. The differential diagnosis of the corneal staining includes corneal abrasion, foreign body, keratitis sicca, herpes simplex keratitis, keratoconjunctivitis, corneal ulcers, corneal dystrophies, and degenerations.

L. Lid abnormalities that may cause exposure or mechanical abrasion of the cornea are trichiasis, ectropion, entropion, lagophthalmos, lid coloboma, and scarring of the lids that leaves the globe exposed.

M. In the red eye with pain and ciliary injection, the presence of a hypopyon (layer of white cells in the anterior chamber) helps narrow the diagnosis. Considerations are endophthalmitis, Behçet syndrome, malignancy (retinoblastoma, leukemia, lymphoma), and severe anterior uveitis.

N. Hyphema (a layer of red cells in the anterior chamber) after trauma makes the diagnosis in a painful red eye simple. In contrast, spontaneous hyphema, especially in children, should raise suspicion of juvenile xanthogranuloma (JXG) or child abuse. In adults, consider neovascularization and tumors.

O. If thorough examination reveals only anterior inflammation uveitis, the differential diagnosis is human leukocyte antigen (HLA)-B27-positive disease (Reiter syndrome, ankylosing spondylitis, inflammatory bowel disease, psoriasis), Behçet syndrome, or idiopathic iritis, the last one being the most common.

P. The painful red eye with anterior chamber inflammation may also exhibit posterior chamber inflammation in the form of vitritis, retinitis, vasculitis, or infective endophthalmitis. Consider life-threatening systemic diseases, such as syphilis, tuberculosis, sarcoidosis, and acquired immunodeficiency syndrome.

▌BIBLIOGRAPHY

1. Albert D, Jakobiec F. Atlas of Clinical Ophthalmology. Philadelphia: Saunders; 1996.
2. Basic and Clinical Science Course. Sections 3, 4, and 7. San Francisco: American Academy of Ophthalmology; 2013.
3. Cullom D, Chang B. The Wills Eye Manual Office and Emergency Room Diagnosis and Treatment of Eye Disease. Philadelphia: Lippincott; 1993.
4. Duane T, Jaeger E. Clinical Ophthalmology, 2nd Volume. Philadelphia: Lippincott; 1988.
5. Tomsak RL. Handbook of Treatment in Neuro-ophthalmology. Missouri: Butterworth-Heinemann; 1997.

Red Eye

Tomy Starck, Lorena Larez

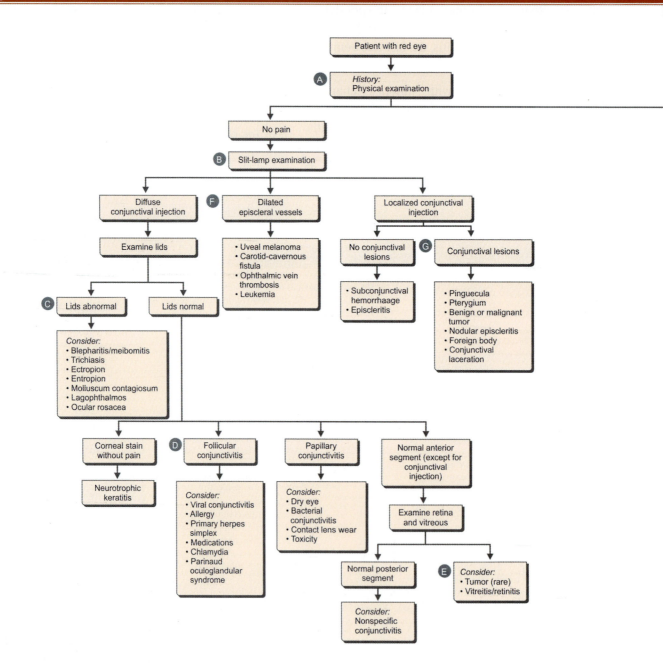

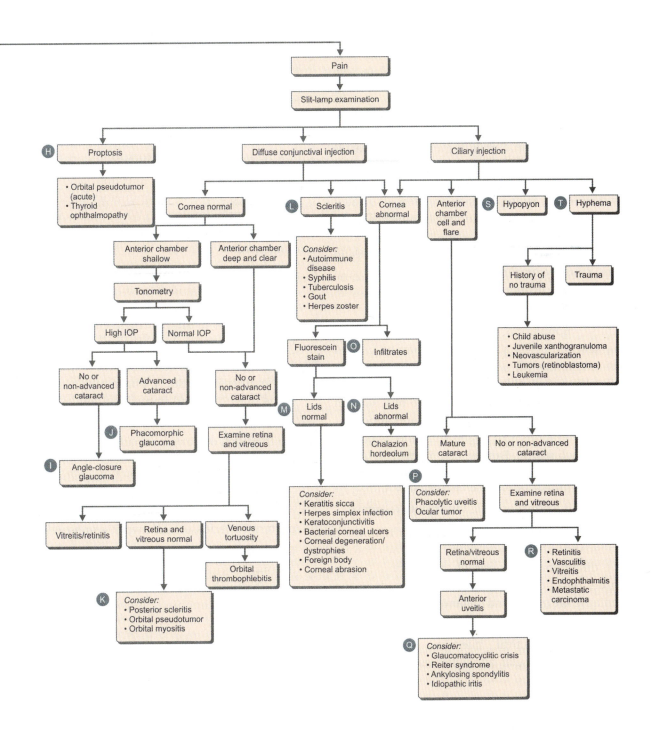

14

Pain

Slit-lamp examination

H — Proptosis

Diffuse conjunctival injection

Ciliary injection

• Orbital pseudotumor (acute)
• Thyroid ophthalmopathy

Cornea normal

L — Scleritis

Cornea abnormal

Anterior chamber cell and flare

S — Hypopyon

T — Hyphema

Anterior chamber shallow

Anterior chamber deep and clear

Consider:
• Autoimmune disease
• Syphilis
• Tuberculosis
• Gout
• Herpes zoster

History of no trauma

Trauma

Tonometry

High IOP

Normal IOP

• Child abuse
• Juvenile xanthogranuloma
• Neovascularization
• Tumors (retinoblastoma)
• Leukemia

No or non-advanced cataract

Advanced cataract

No or non-advanced cataract

Fluorescein stain

O — Infiltrates

J — Phacomorphic glaucoma

Examine retina and vitreous

M — Lids normal

N — Lids abnormal

Mature cataract

No or non-advanced cataract

I — Angle-closure glaucoma

Chalazion hordeolum

P — *Consider:*
Phacolytic uveitis
Ocular tumor

Examine retina and vitreous

Vitreitis/retinitis

Retina and vitreous normal

Venous tortuosity

Retina/vitreous normal

R — • Retinitis
• Vasculitis
• Vitreitis
• Endophthalmitis
• Metastatic carcinoma

Orbital thrombophlebitis

Consider:
• Keratitis sicca
• Herpes simplex infection
• Keratoconjunctivitis
• Bacterial corneal ulcers
• Corneal degeneration/ dystrophies
• Foreign body
• Corneal abrasion

Anterior uveitis

K — *Consider:*
• Posterior scleritis
• Orbital pseudotumor
• Orbital myositis

Q — *Consider:*
• Glaucomatocyclitic crisis
• Reiter syndrome
• Ankylosing spondylitis
• Idiopathic iritis

The differential diagnosis of the red eye encompasses a wide range of ophthalmic conditions, many of which are discussed in detail in other chapters.

A. One of the more helpful differentiating symptoms of the red eye, obtained from the history and physical examination, is pain. In general, the nonpainful red eye denotes a less serious, nonvision-threatening cause. A painful red eye is often a more serious problem.

B. Slit lamp examination, by which more than 90% of the red eye can be diagnosed, is most helpful. However, more than one disease process may be taking place, so perform a complete eye examination.

C. A nonpainful red eye with diffuse conjunctival injection may be caused by abnormalities of the lids. Debris and bacterial growth found in blepharitis and meibomitis can spill over into the conjunctiva. Ocular rosacea, a skin disease involving facial erythema and telangiectasias, is often associated with dysfunction of the meibomian glands. Trichiasis (ingrowth of eyelashes) may cause mechanical irritation. Malpositions of the eyelid may cause exposure. Molluscum contagiosum lesions on the lid margin usually result in a follicular conjunctivitis.

D. Diffuse nonpainful conjunctival injection in the absence of lid abnormalities may be caused by conjunctivitis. The distinctions between follicular and papillary conjunctivitis are helpful to determine treatment. Follicles are best seen in the inferior conjunctival cul-de-sac and appear as smooth elevations with vessels surrounding but not within each follicle. Papillae can be small or 'giant' and present a mosaic-like pattern. Each papilla has a central fibrovascular core. Papillary conjunctival injection is a nonspecific inflammatory response.

E. Rarely, a nonpainful diffuse red eye harbors a malignancy of the ciliary body, retina or choroid. The differential diagnosis of the tumor depends on the patient's age. Retinoblastoma leads in the pediatric age group, and melanoma leads in adults.

F. Generalized dilated episcleral vessels, with or without conjunctival injection, should raise suspicion of vascular anomalies such as carotid-cavernous fistula or low-grade flow dural-carotid shunts. Focal dilated episcleral vessels may signal an underlying intraocular malignancy (sentinel vessels).

G. Nonpainful focal lesions of the conjunctiva may become irritated and inflamed. Pinguecula and pterygium are easily diagnosed. Atypical inflamed lesions may need to be excised to rule out malignancy. Localized nonpainful 'redness' of the conjunctiva usually represents episcleritis, which includes episcleral vascular injection, or a subconjunctival hemorrhage, which is a localized collection of blood beneath the conjunctiva with normal conjunctival vessels. Both conditions are benign, but occasionally, the first may require the use of topical nonsteroidal drugs. Recurrent subconjunctival hemorrhage without trauma warrants a hematologic workup.

H. Proptosis, conjunctival injection, and pain are highly suggestive of inflammatory orbital disease (orbital pseudotumor). When pain is absent, consider thyroid ophthalmopathy in the differential diagnosis.

I. Pain, diffuse conjunctival injection, high intraocular pressure (IOP), mid-dilated pupil, the absence of an advanced cataract, and iris bombé make the diagnosis of simple angle-closure glaucoma. Gonioscopy confirms the diagnosis.

J. In the case of an advanced cataract combined with the findings in Section I, phacomorphic glaucoma is the diagnosis, and immediate lens extraction is indicated.

K. If a thorough ocular examination reveals only a red eye with severe pain but no obvious ocular disease, further studies are indicated, including orbital ultrasonography, computed tomography (CT), or magnetic resonance imaging (MRI). Consider posterior scleritis, orbital myositis, or pseudotumor.

L. Pain, diffuse conjunctival injection and scleral edema (scleritis) require a systemic workup based on a thorough review of systems to rule out both generalized immune diseases and infectious causes.

M. Fluorescein staining of the cornea is usually associated with a diffuse red eye and some pain.

The differential diagnosis of the corneal staining includes corneal abrasion, foreign body, keratitis sicca, herpes simplex keratitis, keratoconjunctivitis, corneal ulcers, corneal dystrophies and degenerations.

N. Lid abnormalities that may cause exposure or mechanical abrasion of the cornea are trichiasis, ectropion, entropion, lagophthalmos and scarring of the lids that leaves the globe exposed.

O. Painful infiltrates of the cornea (with and without epithelial defects) can be a diagnostic dilemma. An infective corneal ulcer must be differentiated from a sterile ulcer by scraping the lesion for Gram stain and cultures. Bacterial, fungal and viral ulcers with infiltrates must be treated specifically. Sterile corneal infiltrates are caused by immune responses in the cornea to a specific toxin or antigen and usually respond well to steroids.

P. With ciliary injection, anterior chamber cell and flare, and hypermature cataract, phacolytic uveitis (and possibly glaucoma) is the diagnosis. Diagnostic echography should be done to rule out a hidden malignancy of the posterior segment.

Q. If a thorough examination reveals only anterior inflammation, the differential diagnosis is HLA-B27-positive disease (Reiter syndrome, ankylosing spondylitis, inflammatory bowel disease, psoriasis), Behçet syndrome, or idiopathic iritis, the last one being the most common.

R. The painful red eye with anterior chamber inflammation may also exhibit posterior chamber inflammation in the form of vitreitis, retinitis, vasculitis, or infective endophthalmitis. Consider life-threatening systemic diseases, such as syphilis, tuberculosis, sarcoidosis and AIDS.

S. In the red eye with pain and ciliary injection, the presence of a hypopyon (layer of white cells in the anterior chamber) helps narrow the diagnosis. Considerations are endophthalmitis, Behçet syndrome, malignancy (retinoblastoma, leukemia, lymphoma), and severe anterior uveitis.

T. Hyphema (a layer of red cell in the anterior chamber) after trauma makes the diagnosis of a painful red eye simple. In contrast, spontaneous hyphema, especially in children, should raise suspicion of juvenile xanthogranuloma (JXG) or child abuse. In adults, consider neovascularization and tumors.

BIBLIOGRAPHY

1. Albert D, Jacobiec F. Atlas of Clinical Ophthalmology. Philadelphia: Saunders; 1996.
2. Basic and Clinical Science Course, sections 3, 4, and 7. San Francisco: American Academy of Ophthalmology; 2013.
3. Cullom D, Chang B. Wills Eye Hospital: Office and Emergency Room Diagnosis and Treatment of Eye Disease. Philadelphia: Lippincott; 1993.
4. Duane T, Jaeger E. Clinical Ophthalmology, Vol 2. Philadelphia: Lippincott; 1988.
5. Hampton F. Ocular Differential Diagnosis. Baltimore: Williams & Wilkins; 1997.
6. Newell FW. Ophthalmology: Principles and Concepts. St Louis: Mosby; 1992.

Itchy Eye

Kristin Story Held

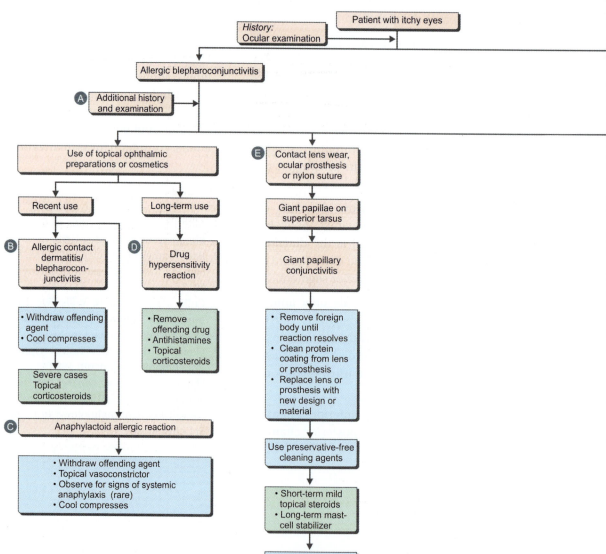

Patient with itchy eyes

History:
Ocular examination

Allergic blepharoconjunctivitis

Ⓐ Additional history and examination

Use of topical ophthalmic preparations or cosmetics

Recent use

Long-term use

Ⓑ Allergic contact dermatitis/ blepharocon-junctivitis

Ⓓ Drug hypersensitivity reaction

• Withdraw offending agent
• Cool compresses

• Remove offending drug
• Antihistamines
• Topical corticosteroids

Severe cases Topical corticosteroids

Ⓒ Anaphylactoid allergic reaction

• Withdraw offending agent
• Topical vasoconstrictor
• Observe for signs of systemic anaphylaxis (rare)
• Cool compresses

Ⓔ Contact lens wear, ocular prosthesis or nylon suture

Giant papillae on superior tarsus

Giant papillary conjunctivitis

• Remove foreign body until reaction resolves
• Clean protein coating from lens or prosthesis
• Replace lens or prosthesis with new design or material

Use preservative-free cleaning agents

• Short-term mild topical steroids
• Long-term mast-cell stabilizer

Discontinue contact lens wear if above measures fail

15

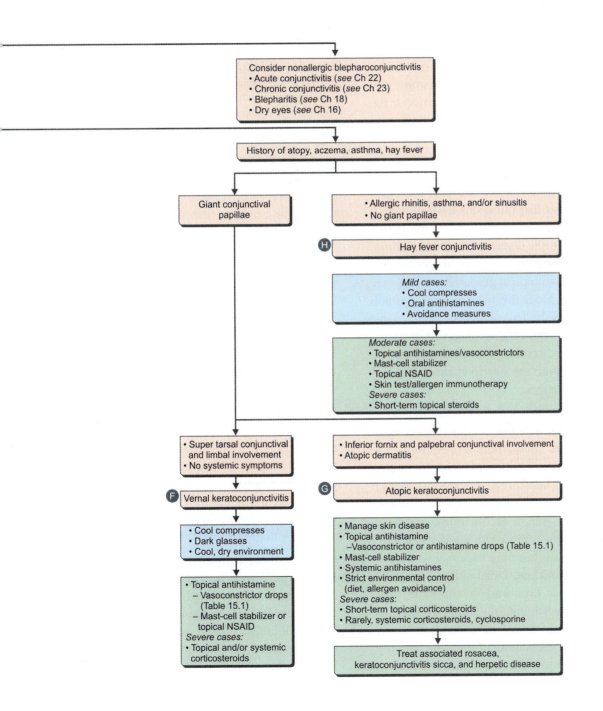

Consider nonallergic blepharoconjunctivitis
• Acute conjunctivitis (*see* Ch 22)
• Chronic conjunctivitis (*see* Ch 23)
• Blepharitis (*see* Ch 18)
• Dry eyes (*see* Ch 16)

History of atopy, aczema, asthma, hay fever

Giant conjunctival papillae

• Allergic rhinitis, asthma, and/or sinusitis
• No giant papillae

H Hay fever conjunctivitis

Mild cases:
• Cool compresses
• Oral antihistamines
• Avoidance measures

Moderate cases:
• Topical antihistamines/vasoconstrictors
• Mast-cell stabilizer
• Topical NSAID
• Skin test/allergen immunotherapy
Severe cases:
• Short-term topical steroids

• Super tarsal conjunctival and limbal involvement
• No systemic symptoms

• Inferior fornix and palpebral conjunctival involvement
• Atopic dermatitis

F Vernal keratoconjunctivitis

G Atopic keratoconjunctivitis

• Cool compresses
• Dark glasses
• Cool, dry environment

• Manage skin disease
• Topical antihistamine
  −Vasoconstrictor or antihistamine drops (Table 15.1)
• Mast-cell stabilizer
• Systemic antihistamines
• Strict environmental control
  (diet, allergen avoidance)
Severe cases:
• Short-term topical corticosteroids
• Rarely, systemic corticosteroids, cyclosporine

• Topical antihistamine
  − Vasoconstrictor drops
    (Table 15.1)
  − Mast-cell stabilizer or
    topical NSAID
Severe cases:
• Topical and/or systemic
  corticosteroids

Treat associated rosacea,
keratoconjunctivitis sicca, and herpetic disease

Itching is a common symptom of many ocular external diseases, including viral conjunctivitis, blepharitis, dry eye syndrome, and allergic blepharoconjunctivitis. It is just one of many other more significant symptoms in conjunctivitis, blepharitis and dry eye syndrome, but it is the primary and overwhelming complaint in allergic blepharoconjunctivitis. Intense itching is the most common and significant symptom of ocular allergic disease. Nonallergic causes can usually be ruled out after the initial history and physical examination.

A. After making the diagnosis of allergic blepharo-conjunctivitis, collect additional historical information. The types of allergic blepharoconjunctivitis include contact blepharoconjunctivitis, drug hypersensitivity reactions, giant papillary conjunctivitis, vernal keratoconjunctivitis, atopic keratoconjunctivitis and hay fever conjunctivitis. Elucidation of the patient's history and the clinical setting in which the itchy eye developed will lead to a highly accurate diagnosis. Key questions must be asked of every patient: What is the primary symptom? Is there a history of atopic disease, hay fever, asthma or eczema? Has there been exposure to specific environmental agents or topical preparations (e.g. eye drops, cosmetics)? Does the patient wear contact lenses or has he or she had ocular surgery? Associated signs include red eyes, swollen lids, tearing, rhinorrhea, stringy discharge, chemosis and papillary hypertrophy. Evert the lids to evaluate the superior tarsal conjunctiva.

B. Allergic contact blepharoconjunctivitis develops acutely, usually within 48 hours after contact with the offending agent. The patient is reexposed to a topical ophthalmic preparation to which he or she has been previously sensitized. A delayed (type IV) T-lymphocyte-mediated hypersensitivity reaction occurs. Neomycin sulfate is the most common offending ocular preparation. Other agents include antazoline phosphate, atropine sulfate, idoxuridine thimerosal, chlorhexidine, facial soaps, perfumes and cosmetics. The eyes and surrounding skin become acutely erythematous and edematous and intense itching develops, accompanied by a characteristic eczematoid dermatitis of the eyelid skin. Symptoms resolve upon removal of

Table 15.1: Allergy drops

Over-the-counter
- Naphazoline hydrochloride/pheniramine maleate eye drops (Ocuhist, Opcon-A, Naphcon-A)
- Naphazoline hydrochloride/antazoline phosphate eye drops (Vasocon-A)

By prescription
H1 antihistamines
- Levocabastine hydrochloride ophthalmic suspension (Livostin)

H1 antihistamines plus mast-cell stabilizer
- Olopatadine hydrochloride ophthalmic solution (Patanol, Pataday)

Mast-cell stabilizer
- Cromolyn sodium ophthalmic solution (Crolom, Opticrom)

Mast-cell stabilizer plus eosinophil suppressor
- Lodoxamide tromethamine ophthalmic solution (Alomide)

Nonsteroidal anti-inflammatory drugs
- Ketorolac tromethamine ophthalmic solution (Acular)

Steroids
- Loteprednol etabonate ophthalmic suspension (Alrex 0.2%, Lotemax 0.5%)
- Rimexolone ophthalmic suspension (Vexol) Fluorometholone (FML, Fluor-Op, Eflone, Flarex)

the causative agent. Supportive measures provide symptomatic relief.

C. Anaphylactoid reactions to topical preparations are rapid in onset and characterized by lid edema and conjunctival erythema and chemosis. Anaphylactoid reactions are type I (IgE-mediated) hypersensitivity reactions. These rarely occur, but the main offending agents are topical penicillin, sulfacetamide, bacitracin and topical anesthetics.

D. Long-term use of topical preparations, such as gentamicin, idoxuridine, pilocarpine, and echothiophate iodide, may result in a cytotoxic (type II) reaction. Their action is slow to develop and often follows use of a drug for weeks, months or even years. A conjunctival follicular response is usually present, and significant conjunctival scarring can develop.

E. Giant papillary conjunctivitis occurs in otherwise healthy persons who wear contact lenses or an ocular prosthesis, or who have monofilament nylon or another foreign body on the ocular surface. No history of atopic disease is associated. Eversion of the upper lid reveals the characteristic giant papillae. Definitive treatment is removal of the foreign body.

F. Vernal keratoconjunctivitis typically occurs in young males in the second decade of life. Symptoms peak in the spring and fall. The condition is worse in warm climates. Ocular symptoms are severe, but there are no associated systemic symptoms. There is a patient or family history of atopic disease. The classic sign is papillary hypertrophy of the superior tarsal conjunctiva and limbus. Trantas dots and shield ulcers may be seen. Abundant eosinophils and free eosinophilic granules are seen on conjunctival scrapings. No granules and fewer eosinophils are seen with atopic and hay fever keratoconjunctivitis. Because vernal keratoconjunctivitis tends to be self-limited, the goal of treatment is palliation.

G. Atopic dermatitis is familial and begins in childhood. From 10-20% of the population is atopic, and 25–40% of these patients have ocular involvement, which usually appears in the teens. The eye signs are accompanied by characteristic skin lesions on the face, trunk and flexor surfaces of the arms and legs. Atopic dermatitis is neither seasonal nor exacerbated by warm climates. Atopic keratoconjunctivitis is characterized by recurrent inflammation of the lids and conjunctiva. The inferior fornix and palpebral conjunctiva are predominately involved. Serious potentially blinding consequences may occur in relation to the corneal complications. One must take great care to recognize and treat associated acne rosacea, herpetic disease and keratitis sicca. Systemic antihistamines and strict environmental controls are important in successful management.

H. Hay fever conjunctivitis is characterized by hyperemic chemotic, baggy conjunctiva accompanied by allergic rhinitis, mild asthma, and/or sinusitis. Many allergens may cause this reaction. If pollens are the cause, the symptoms may vary with season and geographic location. If molds, house dust, or dander is the allergen, no seasonal variation exists. Conjunctival scrapings stained with Giemsa stain show eosinophils. The mainstay of treatment is removing the offending agent; treatment is otherwise supportive.

BIBLIOGRAPHY

1. Colby K, Dohlman C. Vernal keratoconjunctivitis. In: Jakobiec FA, Adamis AP, Pineda RA, (Eds). International Ophthalmology Clinics: Noninfectious Inflammatory Disorders of the Eye and Adnexa. Boston: Little, Brown and Company; 1996. 36:15-20.
2. Friedlaender MH. Management of ocular allergy. Ann Allerg Asthma lmmunol. 1995;75:212-24.
3. Power WJ, Tugai-Tutkun I, Foster CS. Long-term follow-up of patients with atopic keratoconjunctivitis. Ophthalmology. 1998;105:637-42.
4. Titi MJ. A critical look at ocular allergy drugs. Am Fain Physician. 1996;53:2637-42.

Dry Eye

Kristin Story Held

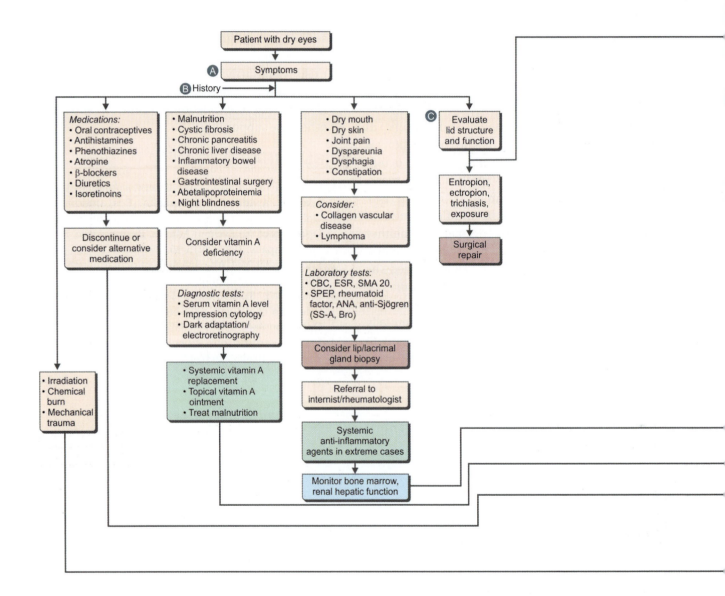

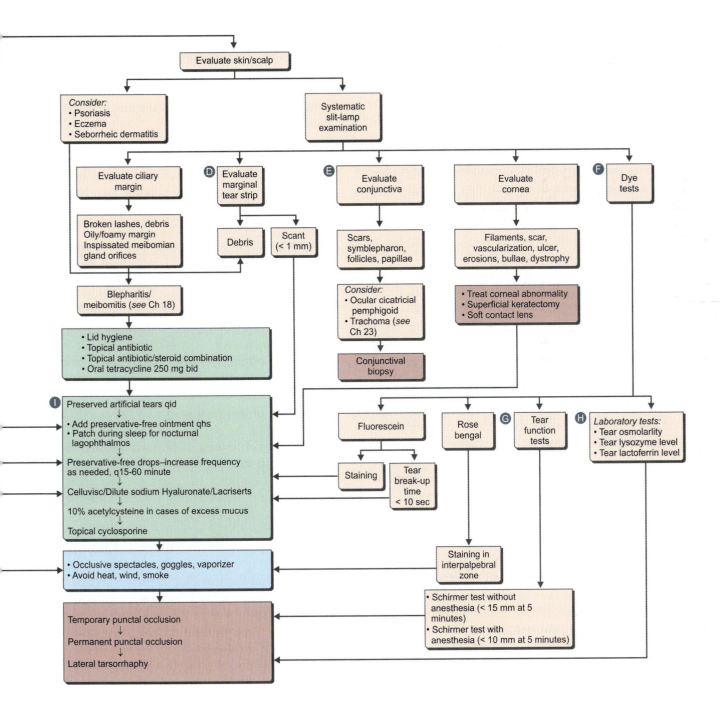

Evaluate skin/scalp

Consider:
• Psoriasis
• Eczema
• Seborrheic dermatitis

Systematic slit-lamp examination

Evaluate ciliary margin

D Evaluate marginal tear strip

E Evaluate conjunctiva

Evaluate cornea

F Dye tests

Broken lashes, debris
Oily/foamy margin
Inspissated meibomian gland orifices

Debris

Scant (< 1 mm)

Scars, symblepharon, follicles, papillae

Filaments, scar, vascularization, ulcer, erosions, bullae, dystrophy

Blepharitis/meibomitis (*see* Ch 18)

Consider:
• Ocular cicatricial pemphigoid
• Trachoma (*see* Ch 23)

• Treat corneal abnormality
• Superficial keratectomy
• Soft contact lens

• Lid hygiene
• Topical antibiotic
• Topical antibiotic/steroid combination
• Oral tetracycline 250 mg bid

Conjunctival biopsy

I Preserved artificial tears qid
↓
• Add preservative-free ointment qhs
• Patch during sleep for nocturnal lagophthalmos
↓
Preservative-free drops–increase frequency as needed, q15-60 minute
↓
Celluvisc/Dilute sodium Hyaluronate/Lacriserts
↓
10% acetylcysteine in cases of excess mucus
↓
Topical cyclosporine

Fluorescein

Rose bengal

G Tear function tests

H *Laboratory tests:*
• Tear osmolarlity
• Tear lysozyme level
• Tear lactoferrin level

Staining

Tear break-up time < 10 sec

• Occlusive spectacles, goggles, vaporizer
• Avoid heat, wind, smoke

Staining in interpalpebral zone

Temporary punctal occlusion
↓
Permanent punctal occlusion
↓
Lateral tarsorrhaphy

• Schirmer test without anesthesia (< 15 mm at 5 minutes)
• Schirmer test with anesthesia (< 10 mm at 5 minutes)

Dry eye affects millions of people worldwide, and it is a common problem leading patients to the ophthalmologist's office. There are many causes of dry eye, which results ultimately from abnormalities of the tear film and/or ocular surface. The tear film is composed of three layers: (1) the outermost lipid layer, derived from the meibomian glands; (2) the largest layer, the aqueous layer, derived from the main and accessory lacrimal glands; and (3) the mucin layer, derived from the goblet cells. Abnormalities of the meibomian glands, lacrimal glands or conjunctiva, which contains the goblet cells, obviously result in a defective tear film mechanism, as does any abnormality of the ocular surface (i.e. the cornea, eyelids, conjunctiva). An accurate diagnosis is important in determining appropriate treatment and resolving patients' complaints. A thorough history and physical examination are essential in making a proper diagnosis. Laboratory evaluation and histologic studies provide further information supporting the diagnosis.

A. The symptoms are variable and range from burning and foreign body sensation to severe pain and irritation out of proportion to clinical signs. Symptoms are often exacerbated by smoke, wind or prolonged use of the eyes. Paradoxical tearing may be present. One may complain of ropy mucus, vision that fluctuates with blinking and photophobia.

B. The patient history may often disclose the cause of the dry eye. Most types of dry eye are more common in women, and postmenopausal women are more likely to have aqueous tear deficiencies than premenopausal women. Many commonly prescribed medications, systemic and topical, can affect the tear film and should be eliminated when possible. Ask about specific systemic complaints that might suggest an underlying systemic disorder associated with dry eyes, particularly the autoimmune collagen vascular disorders and lymphoma. Dry eyes have been associated with certain dermatologic diseases as well. Congenital conditions associated with lacrimal hyposecretion include lacrimal gland hypoplasia, familial dysautonomia and multiple endocrine neoplasia. Acquired conditions include rheumatoid arthritis, systemic lupus erythematosus, polyarteritis nodosa, lymphoma, thrombocytopenic purpura, hypergammaglobulinemia, Hashimoto thyroiditis, sarcoidosis, graft-versus-host disease and viral dacryoadenitis. Conjunctival or lip biopsy may be useful in diagnosing Sjögren syndrome.

Irradiation, chemical burns or mechanical trauma to the lacrimal gland produce hyposecretion as well. A history of factors leading to vitamin A deficiency must be elicited because this is a common cause of dry eye worldwide, and rapid improvement in the ocular surface abnormalities occurs with systemic vitamin A therapy.

C. Perform a thorough evaluation of the lid structure and function, including observation of the blink mechanism and Bell phenomenon. Lid abnormalities such as ectropion, entropion, trichiasis and margin irregularity must be detected so that surgical repair can be undertaken. Rule out nocturnal lagophthalmos, Bell palsy and thyroid disease. Assess the integrity of the fifth and seventh cranial nerves.

D. The inferior marginal tear strip is observed initially. Normally, the height of the tear meniscus should be at least 1 mm and convex. A small, scanty tear strip suggests deficient tear volume. Debris in the tear film may indicate an inadequate tear volume in addition to blepharitis.

E. The conjunctival examination may indicate the underlying cause of the dry eyes such as ocular cicatricial pemphigoid, trachoma, chemical burn or Stevens-Johnson syndrome. Conjunctival biopsy is useful in the diagnosis of ocular pemphigoid. Severe cases may require systemic and topical immunosuppressive therapy. Conjunctival impression cytologic examination may be useful in evaluating the epithelium for squamous metaplasia and the presence of goblet cells.

F. Proper use of dye tests is of ultimate importance in diagnosing the dry eye. A fluorescein strip is moistened with a drop of preservative-free saline solution and gently touched to the inferior tear meniscus. The amount of fluorescence is an indirect measure of the aqueous tear volume. Observe the cornea for areas of punctate stain. Fluorescein stains areas that are devoid of epithelium as the water-soluble dye penetrates into the underlying corneal stroma. The tear breakup time, which indicates the stability of the tear film, is then recorded. It is the time between a blink and the appearance of a corneal dry spot. Normally it should be greater than 10 seconds. Tear breakup time is often abnormal (<10 seconds) in all types of dry eye conditions. The tear breakup time may help in assessing the efficacy of treatment; that is, a positive therapeutic effect would be indicated by an increased tear breakup time. If corneal drying repeatedly appears in the same area, suspect and treat a localized corneal abnormality. Rose bengal is a vital dye that stains devitalized epithelial cells rather than areas of actual epithelial cell loss. It is common to see rose bengal staining in the interpalpebral zone of exposure in keratoconjunctivitis sicca. Rose bengal stains this region in many cases in which fluorescein would show no defect.

G. Schirmer test is performed to measure tear secretion. Place a standardized strip (Whatman's 41 filter paper, 5 mm wide) in the lateral third of the lower eyelid for 5 minutes. The test is first performed without anesthesia to indicate the reflex or maximum amount of lacrimal gland secretion. Wetting of less than 15 mm at 5 minutes is abnormal. When performed after the instillation of topical anesthesia, the test measures the minimum or basal tear secretion. The normal value is greater than 10 mm at 5 minutes.

H. The tear film osmolality, lysozyme level and lactoferrin level are three laboratory tests that measure lacrimal gland function and may be useful in diagnosing dry eye. Tear film osmolality is increased (>312 mOsm/kg) in patients with keratoconjunctivitis sicca, whereas lysozyme and lactoferrin levels are decreased in tears of patients with decreased lacrimal gland secretion. Kits are available to perform these tests.

I. After establishing the diagnosis of dry eye by a thorough patient history and complete systematic clinical examination, initiate treatment in a logical, stepwise fashion. First, address the underlying cause of the dry eye. Lid abnormalities may be surgically corrected, blepharitis and meibomitis are treated, and associated inflammation is controlled. Refer patients with underlying systemic conditions for further medical consultation, and control the associated inflammation and immune processes by local and systemic immunosuppression as needed. Next, address localized conjunctival and corneal abnormalities. Modify systemic medications. The mainstay of dry eye treatment is artificial tear replacement. Treatment with preserved artificial tears with strict adherence to a schedule of at least four times daily is used on a conscientious basis in mild cases. Lubricating ointment may be added at bedtime. Patching with the lubrication may be helpful if nocturnal lagophthalmos is present. Niteye, a "dry eye bandage", is now available in the form of a plastic eye shield that acts as a moisture chamber for use when resting. Once the need for artificial tears exceeds four times daily, preservative-free drops must be used and, in some cases, may be used every 15–60 minutes. Celluvisc (carboxymethylcellulose sodium 1% lubricant), Ocucoat PF (hydroxypropyl methylcellulose), and sodium hyaluronate (dilute Healon) may afford decreased frequency of administration because of their increased viscosity. Lacriserts, sustained-release tear inserts, are available but difficult for many patients to insert. Patients should decrease external factors that increase the evaporation of the tear film or exacerbate symptoms. In cases of excess mucous strands, 10% acetylcysteine may be effective. As a rule, wearing soft contact lenses should be avoided, particularly if the tear breakup time is less than 10 seconds; however, on a short-term basis they may be useful in resolving persistent epithelial defects or filamentary keratopathy. If symptoms and signs of ocular surface injury persist, perform temporary punctal occlusion using absorbable collagen plugs or nonabsorbable silicone plugs. If occlusion of all four puncta affords clinical improvement and the patient tolerates this well, proceed with permanent punctal occlusion using thermal cautery, laser or radiodiathermy. In severe cases, refractory to all preceding measures, perform lateral tarsorrhaphy. Consider topical cyclosporine in severe cases. Patient reassurance is extremely important. The efficacy of therapy may be assessed by following the tear breakup time and the staining pattern with rose bengal, but the most important gauge is the patient's symptoms.

▌BIBLIOGRAPHY

1. Arffa RC. Grayson's Diseases of the Cornea, 4th Edition. St Louis: Mosby; 1997. p. 355.
2. deLuise VP. Management of dry eyes. In: Focal points: Clinical modules for ophthalmologists. San Francisco: American Academy of Ophthalmology; 1985.
3. Nelson ID. Dry eye syndrome-Current diagnosis and management. In: Schachat AP (Ed). Current Practice in Ophthalmology. St Louis: Mosby; 1992. p. 49.
4. Smolin G, Friedlaender M (Eds). International Ophthalmology Clinics: Dry eye, Vol 34(1). Boston: Little, Brown and company; 1994.

17

Epiphora

Kenneth L Piest*, Martha A Walton

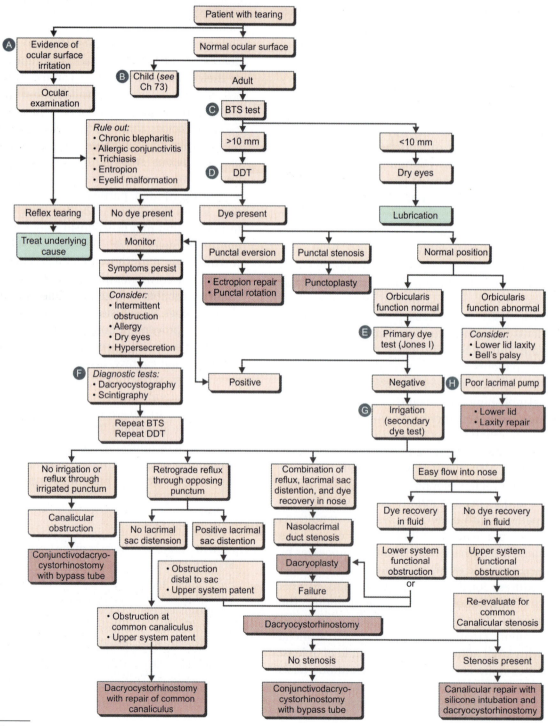

A. Tearing may result from reflex lacrimation, which may be caused by ocular surface irritation. It can also result from other entities that stimulate the ophthalmic division of the fifth cranial nerve, as in iritis or glaucoma.

B. Congenital nasolacrimal duct obstruction is a common disorder, occurring in up to 10% of newborns.

C. The basal tear secretion (BTS) is assessed by anesthetizing the conjunctiva and ocular surface with a topical agent and then measuring tear production. If the BTS is low, the quantity of tears required to keep the cornea moist is insufficient. This condition stimulates the reflex arc of the fifth and seventh cranial nerves, producing excessive reflex secretion. The lacrimal drainage system cannot handle the sporadic increase in volume, and overflow tearing (pseudoepiphora) occurs. Topical ocular lubrication is required to prevent stimulation of the reflex arc.

D. Dye disappearance testing (DDT) is one of the most useful tests of lacrimal outflow. A moistened fluorescein strip or 2% solution is placed in the conjunctival fornices. Clearance of the dye over 5 minutes is observed. Retention of dye after this period is abnormal and suggests obstruction. Further testing is necessary to determine the condition responsible for the obstruction.

E. The primary dye test Jones I, like the DDT, is a functional test investigating lacrimal outflow under normal physiologic conditions. However, it gives an abnormal result in approximately one-third of normal patients and is often performed improperly. The test consists of attempting to recover fluorescein dye from the inferior meatus by passing a cotton-tipped wire probe beneath the inferior turbinate. A wire is used because of the close approximation of the turbinate to the wall of the nose. A cotton-tip applicator is too large to enter this space. Attempts at dye recovery are also often accompanied by anesthetizing and shrinking of the mucosa to provide comfort and better visualization. This procedure may mask the true pathologic condition in patients in whom hypertrophy and impaction of the turbinate are compressing the opening of the nasolacrimal duct.

F. In selected patients, diagnostic testing may provide additional information. Scintigraphy can be used to evaluate the physiologic flow of tears, and therefore is a functional test. Structural information can be provided by dacryocystography. Newer digital subtraction imaging can provide detailed images and is useful when a mass, diverticulum or stenosis is suspected.

G. The secondary dye test (irrigation) is performed after an abnormal DDT and a primary dye test. It differentiates partial from complete obstructions and provides an estimate of the site of the block. Clear saline solution is used. If irrigation fails to transmit fluid into the nose, a total obstruction is present. If irrigation produces dye-containing fluid from the nose, dye was able to enter the lacrimal sac under physiologic conditions but could not pass down the duct.

H. A pump mechanism is responsible for the excretion of tears. A normal-functioning orbicularis muscle is a prerequisite. With eyelid closure, the heads of the pretarsal orbicularis compress the ampulla and shorten the canaliculi, while the preseptal fibers expand the sac. This action creates negative pressure and draws fluid into the sac from the ampulla and canaliculi. When the eye opens, the muscles relax. The resilience of the lacrimal sac fascia collapses the sac and forces tears from the sac into the duct. Disorders that affect this pumping mechanism, such as seventh cranial nerve palsy or lower lid laxity, can produce tearing.

BIBLIOGRAPHY

1. Bueger DG, Schaefer AJ, Campbell CB, et al. Acquired lacrimal disorders. In: Smith BC, Della Rocca RC, Nesi FA, Lisman RD (Eds). Ophthalmic Plastic and Reconstructive Surgery. St Louis: Mosby; 1988. p. 661.
2. Katowitz JA, Kropp TM. Congenital abnormalities of the lacrimal drainage system. In: Hornblass A (Ed). Oculoplastic, Orbital and Reconstructive Surgery, Vol 2. Baltimore: Williams & Wilkins; 1990. p. 1397.
3. Leone CR. The management of pediatric lacrimal problems. Ophthalmic Plast Reconstr Surg. 1989;1:34-9.
4. Patrinely JR, Anderson RL. A review of lacrimal drainage surgery. Ophthalmic Plast Reconstr Surg. 1986;2:97-102.

Blepharitis

Kristin Story Held

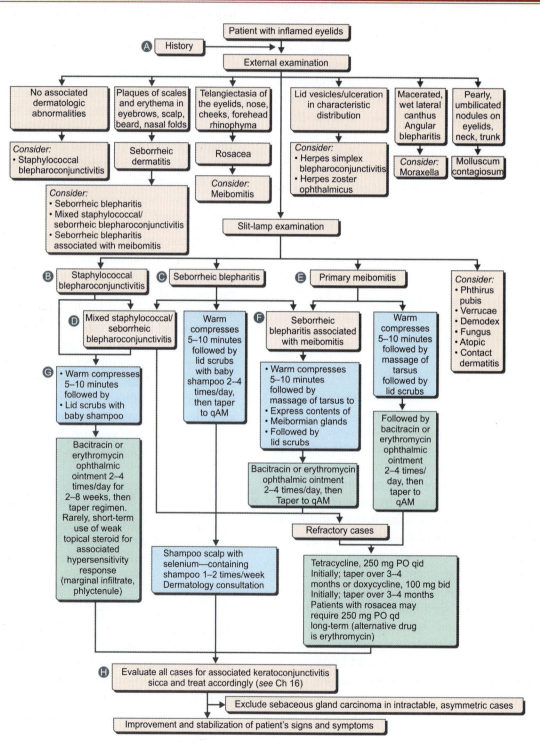

18

Blepharitis is chronic inflammation of the eyelids secondary to a broad spectrum of infectious and noninfectious causes. Patients with acne rosacea, seborrheic dermatitis, atopic disease, and Down syndrome have a greater than normal predisposition for blepharitis. Accurate diagnosis requires a complete patient history and thorough clinical examination. Once the appropriate diagnosis has been established, proper therapy can be implemented.

A. Patients often complain of burning, irritation, foreign body sensation, itching and mattering of the eyes particularly upon awakening. The course is usually chronic with varying degrees of waxing and waning. Associated dermatologic conditions may be present and helpful in establishing the diagnosis.

B. Staphylococcal blepharoconjunctivitis is by far the most common cause of infectious blepharitis and probably the most common chronic infection of the external eye. It occurs in a younger population (mean age, 42 years), and 80% of patients are female. The symptoms are generally shorter in duration, more severe, and maximally waxing and waning in nature. The classic clinical sign is the collarette. Other signs are poliosis, madarosis, misdirected lashes, erythema, ulcerated lid margins and hordeolum. Fifteen percent of patients exhibit bulbar and tarsal conjunctival changes. Recent studies have shown that a large percentage of lid cultures from these patients are positive for *Staphylococcus aureus* and *S. epidermidis.* A keratitis may develop secondary to the toxic effects of the organism. Punctate epithelial erosions develop over the inferior third of the cornea. Marginal catarrhal infiltrates may occur secondary to the bacterial antigen and host-antibody interaction, most often at the 8 to 10 and 2 to 4-o'clock positions. Secondary infections of these lesions may lead to an infectious corneal ulcer. Finally, phlyctenulosis may develop as a result of cell-mediated immunity (also consider tuberculosis). In most cases, the diagnosis is based on clinical evidence of infection, and cultures are not routinely done because most staphylococcal species are sensitive to bacitracin, erythromycin, and the aminoglycosides. Combination preparations (Polytrim, Maxitrol) are often effective. Cultures with sensitivity testing of the lid margins may be useful in patients, who have keratitis, marginal infiltrates, or phlyctenules or who have recalcitrant symptoms. The goal of treatment for staphylococcal blepharitis is to cure it. To achieve this goal, treatment must be implemented aggressively for a prolonged initial period before tapering of the regimen is begun. Of these patients, 50% have associated keratoconjunctivitis sicca, which must be treated concurrently.

C. Seborrheic blepharitis occurs in an older age group (mean age, 50 years). The course is more chronic with minimal waxing and waning of symptoms that last longer. The classic clinical sign is scurf, which is oily, greasy, debris on the lid margin. The lids are less inflamed than with staphylococcal blepharitis or meibomitis. Most patients have associated seborrheic dermatitis and may benefit by dermatologic consultation. Associated keratitis may be present. Many have concurrent keratoconjunctivitis sicca. The goal of treatment is to control and prevent complications. Topical antibiotics are unnecessary.

D. Patients may exhibit signs of both seborrheic and staphylococcal blepharoconjunctivitis. Most have underlying seborrheic dermatitis, and 35% have associated keratoconjunctivitis sicca. The course is that of chronic seborrheic blepharitis intermittently exacerbated by the staphylococcal component. Clinical findings include both collarettes on the lashes and oily, greasy crusting of the anterior eyelid. Almost all of these patients have positive lid cultures for *S. epidermidis,* and more than 80% are positive for *S. aureus.* Treatment is aimed at control of clinical signs and symptoms and requires a long-term commitment to compliance by the patient and diligent attention by the ophthalmologist.

E. Patients with primary meibomitis exhibit more inflammation than those with seborrheic blepharitis. The anterior lamellae are minimally involved with scurf; however, the meibomian glands are diffusely inflamed and inspissated with retained, thick secretions that are not easily expressed. These patients are predisposed to chalazia. Of patients, 63% have associated rosacea. Many have punctate epithelial erosions and stain with rose bengal in the interpalpebral zone. Systemic tetracycline is indicated; it is believed to alter the nature of the oily secretions (do not use in kids!). Omega-3 fatty acids per os helps thin meibomian secretions.

F. Patients, who have seborrheic blepharitis associated with meibomitis have more exacerbations than those with pure seborrheic blepharitis. They may complain of severe burning in the morning. The meibomian glands are engorged with retained secretions, and the tear film is foamy, especially laterally.

G. Successful treatment requires accurate diagnosis based on thorough patient history and clinical examination. Pure staphylococcal blepharoconj-unctivitis may be cured with aggressive long-term lid hygiene and topical antibiotics. The other types of blepharitis are difficult or impossible to eradicate. The goals of treatment are to improve the patient's symptoms and signs, stabilize the course with decreased exacerbations, prevent complications and preserve vision. This requires a great deal of commitment by the patient and the treating physician. The foundation of treatment is consistent lid hygiene that (1) removes eyelid debris and (2) restores normal flow of the meibomian secretions. Topical antibiotics are used in all patients except those with purely seborrheic blepharitis. Oral tetracycline is used in all patients with primary meibomitis, particularly in association with rosacea, and in refractory cases of seborrheic blepharitis associated with meibomitis. Initially, aggressive treatment is required and then tapered. Tetracyclin should not be prescribed to children. The morning is the most important time for lid hygiene because it targets organisms and debris that have accumulated overnight. Short courses of mild topical steroids may be used to treat staphylococcal hypersensitivity reactions. Furthermore, associated dermatologic conditions and underlying keratoconjunctivitis sicca must be managed.

H. Because up to 60% of patients with chronic blepharitis have concurrent keratoconjunctivitis sicca, all patients with blepharitis must be evaluated for dry eye and treated accordingly.

BIBLIOGRAPHY

1. Arffa RC. Grayson's Diseases of the Cornea, 4th Edition. St Louis: Mosby; 1997. p 339.
2. Brown DO, McCulley JP. Staphylococcal and mixed staphylococcal/seborrheic blepharoconjunctivitis. In: Fraunfelder FT, Roy FH, (Eds). Current Ocular Therapy, 3rd Edition. Philadelphia: WB Saunders; 1990. p 525.
3. Halsted M, McCulley JP. Seborrheic blepharitis. In: Fraunfelder FT, Roy FH, (Eds). Current Ocular Therapy, 3rd Edition. Philadelphia: WB Saunders; 1990. p 522.
4. McCulley JP. Meibomitis. In: Kaufman HE, Barron BA, McDonald MB, Waitman SR, (Eds). The Cornea. New York: Churchill Livingstone; 1988. p 125.

Nonpigmented Lesion of the Eyelid

19

Reid A Mollman, Eric Hink

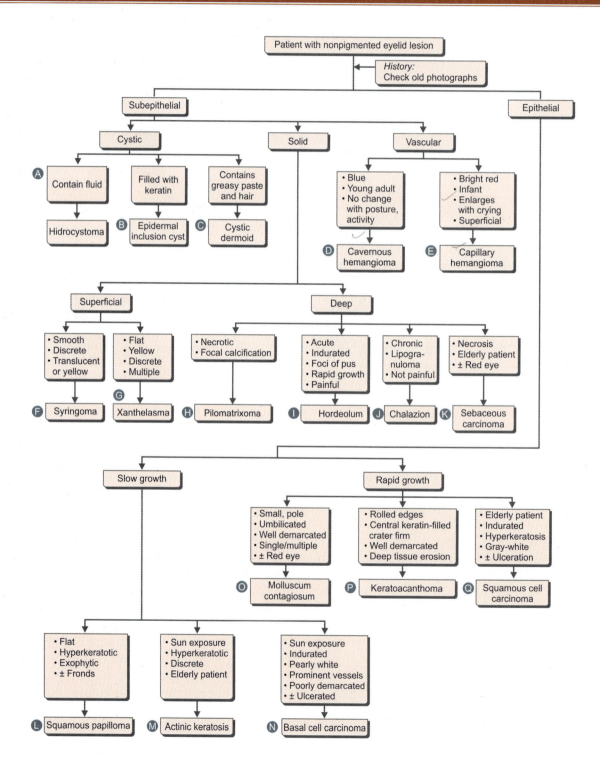

Patient with nonpigmented eyelid lesion

History: Check old photographs

Subepithelial

Epithelial

Cystic

Solid

Vascular

Ⓐ Contain fluid
→ Hidrocystoma

Filled with keratin
→ Ⓑ Epidermal inclusion cyst

Contains greasy paste and hair
→ Ⓒ Cystic dermoid

- Blue
- Young adult
- No change with posture, activity
→ Ⓓ Cavernous hemangioma

- Bright red
- Infant
- Enlarges with crying
- Superficial
→ Ⓔ Capillary hemangioma

Superficial

Deep

- Smooth
- Discrete
- Translucent or yellow
→ Ⓕ Syringoma

- Flat
- Yellow
- Discrete
- Multiple
→ Ⓖ Xanthelasma

- Necrotic
- Focal calcification
→ Ⓗ Pilomatrixoma

- Acute
- Indurated
- Foci of pus
- Rapid growth
- Painful
→ Ⓘ Hordeolum

- Chronic
- Lipogra-nuloma
- Not painful
→ Ⓙ Chalazion

- Necrosis
- Elderly patient
- ± Red eye
→ Ⓚ Sebaceous carcinoma

Slow growth

Rapid growth

- Small, pole
- Umbilicated
- Well demarcated
- Single/multiple
- ± Red eye
→ Ⓞ Molluscum contagiosum

- Rolled edges
- Central keratin-filled crater firm
- Well demarcated
- Deep tissue erosion
→ Ⓟ Keratoacanthoma

- Elderly patient
- Indurated
- Hyperkeratosis
- Gray-white
- ± Ulceration
→ Ⓠ Squamous cell carcinoma

- Flat
- Hyperkeratotic
- Exophytic
- ± Fronds
→ Ⓛ Squamous papilloma

- Sun exposure
- Hyperkeratotic
- Discrete
- Elderly patient
→ Ⓜ Actinic keratosis

- Sun exposure
- Indurated
- Pearly white
- Prominent vessels
- Poorly demarcated
- ± Ulcerated
→ Ⓝ Basal cell carcinoma

A. Hidrocystomas are benign cystic lesions that tend to originate on the lower eyelids and canthi, and are most common in adults aged between 30 years and 70 years. There are two types, eccrine and apocrine. Eccrine hidrocystomas are usually 1–6 mm and can be seen as a solitary nodule or in a cluster of nodules. Apocrine hidrocystomas are usually 3–15 mm, may be translucent or bluish, and are most commonly solitary nodules, but may be multiple. Treatment for both types is with surgical excision or marsupialization.

B. Epidermal inclusion cyst (also known as epidermoid cyst) is a benign, slow growing, firm cystic lesion that is filled with keratin. They can be caused by introduction of the epidermis into the dermal layer, such as in trauma or body piercing. Newborn infants commonly have multiple small epidermal inclusion cysts, which is referred to as milia. Large problematic cysts can be treated with surgical excision.

C. Cystic dermoids are benign lesions that contain skin appendages, such as hair shafts, differentiating them from epidermal inclusion cysts. They usually grow slowly and are located in the region of the lacrimal fossa, superotemporal to the globe. Occasionally, trauma results in cyst rupture, yielding an intense inflammatory response that mimics orbital cellulitis. When this diagnosis is suspected and excision contemplated, a CT scan may be necessary.

D. Cavernous hemangioma of the eyelid is a benign vascular proliferation that does not resolve spontaneously, in contrast to capillary hemangioma. They are typically blue in color, in contrast to capillary hemangiomas which are often red. There is typically no change in appearance of the lesion with posture or activity. Eyelid cavernous hemangiomas tend to be less well circumscribed than orbital cavernous hemangiomas. Steroid injections and laser therapy have been used in treatment.

E. Capillary hemangiomas or infantile hemangiomas are benign hamartomas. The lesion is typically bright red, and may enlarge with crying. They most often present as congenital lesions that enlarge in the first years of life, and then often regress slowly with spontaneous resolution in 70% of cases by age of 7 years. However, depending on location, they may cause amblyopia either by corneal distortion with resultant astigmatism or by eyelid ptosis with pupillary occlusion. Treatments include propranolol, steroid injection, radiotherapy, laser therapy, and surgery.

F. Syringoma is a benign tumor of the eccrine sweat glands which present as 1–3 mm firm, yellowish or skin colored nodules typically clustered on the lower eyelids. They are often misdiagnosed as xanthelasma due to their similarity in appearance. Treatment, when required, is with surgical excision.

G. Xanthelasma is plaque that can be found on the upper or lower eyelids. Hyperlipidemia is found in approximately 50% of individuals with xanthelasma, but xanthelasma can be found in individuals with normal cholesterol levels. Xanthelasma can be seen in up to 75% of older patients with familial hypercholesterolemia. There is an association with primary biliary cirrhosis. Treatment is with surgical excision, CO_2 laser, or topical 100% trichloroacetic acid, but recurrence is common.

H. The pilomatrixoma, also called *calcifying epithelioma of Malherbe,* is a benign lesion of hair-shaft origin. It tends to necrose and calcify at its center and may mimic an epidermal inclusion cyst. Treatment is total excision.

I. Hordeolum (commonly known as a stye) is a condition in which there is acute inflammation of the eyelid, which can result in the production of purulent exudate. The most commonly isolated pathogen is *Staphylococcus aureus*. There are two types, internal and external. Internal hordeolum is the result of an inflamed meibomian gland on the conjunctival side of the lid. External hordeolum is the result of inflammation at the lid margin near the hair follicles and apocrine sweat glands of Moll or sebaceous glands of Zeis. The lesions are often painful, but usually resolve in 7–10 days. Initial treatment consists of warm compresses. Antibiotics are occasionally prescribed, but the supporting evidence for their use is lacking. Unresolved hordeolum can progress to a chalazion.

J. Chalazion (also known as a meibomian gland lipogranuloma) is subacute or chronic inflammation of the eyelid which is typically nonpainful, as opposed to the painful acute inflammation of hordeolum. Additionally, chalazia are classically defined as the result of a blocked meibomian gland on the conjunctival side of the eyelid, and typically originate away from the lid margin. Chalazia are often associated with chronic blepharitis and rosacea. As with hordeolum, initial treatment consists of warm compresses and evidence for antibiotic usage is lacking. Occasionally, problematic chalazia are removed surgically with pathologic analysis to rule out malignancy, especially in recurrent or atypical cases. Steroid injection is occasionally used in combination with surgical excision.

K. Sebaceous carcinoma is an aggressive malignant tumor most commonly found in the elderly with high morbidity and mortality rates. It can mimic a chalazion and must be considered in the differential of recurrent chalazion, especially in the elderly. It can also mimic a unilateral blepharitis or conjunctivitis. The diagnosis should be suspected when the latter do not respond to topical medication. Tissue diagnosis and appropriate surgical intervention are mandatory under these circumstances.

L. Squamous papilloma, caused by the human papilloma virus, is the most common benign lesion of the eyelid. It is a hyperkeratotic, frond-like skin tag with central vascularity. Treatment with excision or cryotherapy is recommended.

M. Actinic keratosis (AK) is a premalignant skin lesion most commonly seen in the elderly with a history of sun exposure. AK is thought to be a precursor to squamous cell carcinoma (SCC) in 20% of cases. The lesions are typically in sun-exposed areas, dry, flat, and hyperkeratotic. Biopsy is recommended to confirm the diagnosis, followed by excision or cryotherapy.

N. Basal cell carcinomas (BCCs) are by far the most common malignant eyelid lesion, accounting for 85–90% of eyelid malignancy. They are associated with basal cell nevus syndrome (Gorlin-Goltz syndrome) and xeroderma pigmentosum. The classic lesions are indurated, firm and pearly in appearance, with prominent vessels. They grow slowly and almost never metastasize. Morbidity results from local extension. The most dangerous variant is morpheaform because the spread is subcutaneous, with accompanying fibrous proliferation that mimics scar tissue. The morpheaform variant is firm, plaque-like and ulcerated in appearance. Mohs surgery or frozen-section controlled excision may be necessary to ensure complete removal.

O. Molluscum contagiosum is a benign poxvirus infection that historically has been seen most commonly in children. However, up to 10–20% of patients with human immunodeficiency virus may develop these lesions. The lesions are small, pale, well demarcated with central umbilication. The lesions are typically diagnosed on appearance alone, with no biopsy necessary. Treatment includes surgical excision, cryotherapy, and desiccation.

P. Keratoacanthomas grow extremely rapidly and can attain a large size in weeks to months. They are firm and well demarcated with rolled edges and a keratin filled crater. They often regress spontaneously, but may erode surrounding tissues, including bone, with significant scarring and damage. Previously considered a benign entity, there is now controversy as to whether the lesions are benign or malignant. Most regress spontaneously, but they resemble SCC histologically, and there have been cases of invasive keratocanthoma with metastasis. This has caused most to treat it as a variant of SCC, with current recommendations being biopsy followed by complete surgical excision.

Q. Squamous cell carcinoma of the eyelid is a malignant lesion which is far less common than BCC (accounts for approximately 9% of malignant eyelid lesions), but faster growing and more likely to metastasize, although metastases are rare. The lesions are typically indurated, hyperkeratotic, ulcerated, and found in elderly individuals with a history of chronic sun exposure. Frozen-section control of surgical margins or Mohs surgery to ensure complete excision of the tumor is the current standard of practice. The prognosis is excellent if excision is complete.

▐ BIBLIOGRAPHY

1. Alfadley A, Al Aboud K, Tulba A, et al. Multiple eccrine hidrocystomas of the face. Int J Dermatol. 2001;40: 125-9.
2. Ben Simon GJ, Huang L, Nakra T, et al. Intralesional triamcinolone acetonide injection for primary and recurrent chalazia: is it really effective? Ophthalmology. 2005;112:913-7.
3. Cook BE, Bartley GB. Epidemiologic characteristics and clinical course of patients with malignant eyelid tumors in an incidence cohort in Olmsted County, Minnesota. Ophthalmology. 1999; 106:746-50.
4. Deans RM, Harris GJ, Kivlin JD. Surgical dissection of capillary hemangiomas. An alternative to intralesional corticosteroids. Arch Ophthalmol. 1992;110:1743-7.
5. Depot MJ, Jakobiec FA, Dodick JM, et al. Bilateral and extensive xanthelasma palpebrarum in a young man. Ophthalmology. 1984;91:522-7.
6. Kass LG, Hornblass A. Sebaceous carcinoma of the ocular adnexa. Surv Ophthalmol. 1989;33:477-90.
7. Lane CM, Ehrlich WW, Wright JE. Orbital dermoid cyst. Eye (Lond). 1987;1:504-11.
8. Reifler DM, Hornblass A. Squamous cell carcinoma of the eyelid. Surv Ophthalmol. 1986;30:349-65.
9. Robinson MR, Udell IJ, Garber PF, et al. Molluscum contagiasum of the eyelids in patients with acquired immune deficiency syndrome. Ophthalmology. 1992;99: 1745-7.
10. Scott KR, Kronish JW. Premalignant lesions and squamous cell carcinoma. In: Albert DM, Jakobiec FA (Eds). Principles and Practice of Ophthalmology: Clinical Practice, 3rd Volume. Philadelphia: WB Saunders; 1994. p.1733.
11. Vinger PF, Sachs BA. Ocular manifestations of hyperlipoproteinemia. Am J Ophthalmol. 1970;70:563-73.
12. Waugh MA. Molluscum contagiosum. Dermatol Clin. 1998; 16:839-41.

Pigmented Lesion of the Eyelid

20

Marilyn C Kincaid, Frank W Scribbick

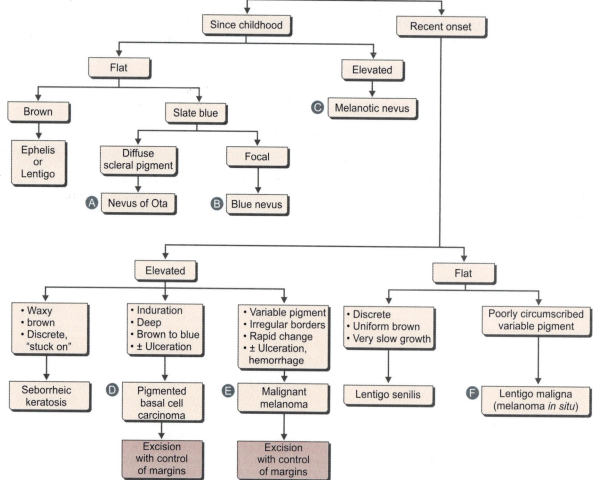
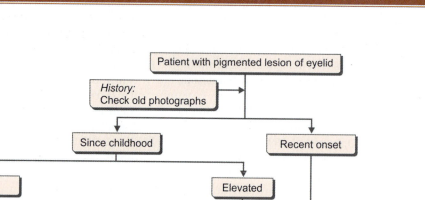

Patient with pigmented lesion of eyelid

History:
Check old photographs

Since childhood

Recent onset

Flat

Elevated

Brown

Slate blue

C Melanotic nevus

Ephelis or Lentigo

Diffuse scleral pigment

Focal

A Nevus of Ota

B Blue nevus

Elevated

Flat

- Waxy
- brown
- Discrete, "stuck on"

- Induration
- Deep
- Brown to blue
- ± Ulceration

- Variable pigment
- Irregular borders
- Rapid change
- ± Ulceration, hemorrhage

- Discrete
- Uniform brown
- Very slow growth

Poorly circumscribed variable pigment

Seborrheic keratosis

D Pigmented basal cell carcinoma

E Malignant melanoma

Lentigo senilis

F Lentigo maligna (melanoma *in situ*)

Excision with control of margins

Excision with control of margins

A. Nevus of Ota is characterized by a large blue nevus of the eyelid (see section B), scleral pigmentation, and increased numbers of uveal melanocytes. Though more common in Asian patients, affected Caucasian patients are at higher risk for developing uveal and intracranial melanoma and must be carefully evaluated.

B. A blue nevus results from proliferation of darkly pigmented, spindle-shaped melanocytic cells deep within the dermis. Diffraction of light waves by the skin fibroblasts results in a blue rather than a brown appearance (Tyndall effect). Blue nevi, like other melanocytic nevi, are benign and can be excised for cosmetic reasons.

C. Melanocytic nevi only rarely undergo malignant transformation. The chief reason for excision is cosmetic.

D. Pigmented basal-cell carcinomas (BCCs), which account for 10% of BCC, occur because benign melanocytes become passively entrapped in the proliferating mass of epithelial cells. Pigmentation in a BCC does not alter prognosis but may mislead the clinician into an incorrect diagnosis.

E. Malignant melanomas of the eyelid skin account for less than 1% of all eyelid malignancies. They can arise from a pre-existing nevus, from lentigo maligna (melanoma *in situ*), or apparently *de novo*. A new pigmented nodule demands prompt evaluation because the depth of invasion is strongly associated with the prognosis. The entire lesion is excised with frozen section control of the margins.

F. An older term for lentigo maligna is *Hutchinson's freckle*. Lentigo maligna is really melanoma *in situ*, a flat lesion composed of atypical melanocytes. Generally, they grow slowly, but development of nodules (the vertical growth phase) indicates invasive melanoma and demands prompt evaluation and excision.

BIBLIOGRAPHY

1. Garner A, Koornneef L, Levene A, et al. Malignant melanoma of the eyelid skin: Histopathology and behaviour. Br J Ophthalmol. 1985;69:180-6.
2. Grossniklaus HE, Mclean IW. Cutaneous melanoma of the eyelid: Clinicopathologic features. Ophthalmology. 1991;98:1867-73.
3. Hartmann LC, Oliver CF, Winkelman RK, et al. Blue nevus and nevus of Ota associated with dural melanoma. Cancer. 1989;64:182-6.

Lesion of the Conjunctiva

Marilyn C Kincaid, Frank W Scribbick

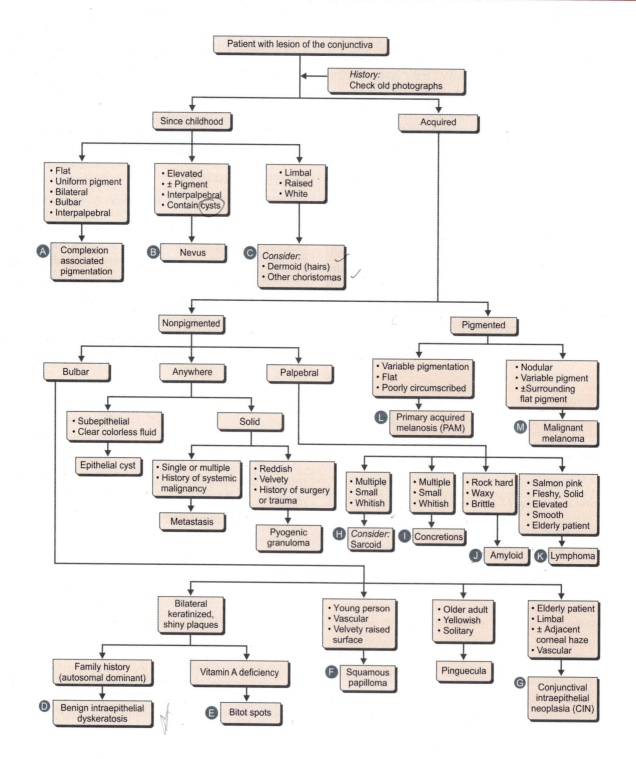

Conjunctival lesions are extremely common. A complete history and physical examination are mandatory. Often, excisional biopsy will also help establish the diagnosis.

A. Interpalpebral melanin deposition in the bulbar conjunctiva is extremely common in darker-skinned individuals and is also referred to as complexion associated pigmentation or racial melanosis. Regardless of the patients' degree of pigmentation, the presence of pigment on the palpebral conjunctiva or within the fornix is abnormal and should be biopsied. The combination of presence since childhood without subsequent change implies benign racial pigmentation.

B. Conjunctival nevi typically occur in the interpalpebral bulbar conjunctiva. They grow slowly but may become more prominent during puberty or young adulthood. Histologically, epithelial cysts are virtually always present, although they may be subtle clinically. Alternatively, they may be the predominant feature. Rarely, conjunctival nevi become malignant, necessitating regular follow-up examinations. Excision may be indicated for cosmesis. Pigmented caruncles are almost always nevi.

C. Solid dermoids contain hair shafts. Other types of epibulbar choristomas generally do not have hair but may have a variety of ectodermal or mesodermal elements. Excision must be approached with care because these lesions may extend into the interior of the eye. Also, epibulbar dermoids (usually bilateral) are features of Goldenhar syndrome, which may include renal and vertebral malformations, as well as preauricular skin tags.

D. Benign intraepithelial dyskeratosis is an uncommon autosomal dominant condition originally traced to a kindred in North Carolina, although more recent patients do not belong to this group. Despite a possibly worrisome clinical appearance, this lesion is not malignant.

E. Bitot's spots are areas of keratinization associated with vitamin A deficiency. In developed countries, vitamin A deficiency is rare except in individuals who have undergone extensive small bowel resection, for instance, for cystic fibrosis.

F. Squamous papillomas result from proliferation of conjunctival epithelium with associated fibrovascular stroma. They are usually found at the lid margin, caruncle, or limbus. Their occurrence in young individuals distinguishes them from the lesions of conjunctival intraepithelial neoplasia. In children and young adults, they are caused by human papilloma virus.

G. Conjunctival intraepithelial neoplasia ranges from mild dysplasia to frank carcinoma *in situ*. Even lesions that are histologically more benign can lead to invasive squamous cell carcinoma if not attended. Excisional biopsy with alcohol or cryotherapy to margins is recommended.

H. The conjunctival lesions of sarcoidosis, which represent discrete granulomas, are the ideal site for histologic confirmation of the diagnosis because there is virtually no morbidity of a biopsy at this site. However, the yield of blind biopsies is low.

I. Conjunctival concretions are white, subepithelial deposits on the palpebral conjunctiva. They are filled with an acellular, mucinous material that contain little or no calcium. They are rarely responsible for ocular surface symptoms and usually do not require removal.

J. Localized subconjunctival amyloid deposition is rare but distinctive. These often cause spontaneous subconjunctival hemorrhages. The deposits can be removed surgically, and generally do not recur.

K. The 'salmon patch' is virtually pathognomonic for conjunctival lymphoma. Evaluate the patient for more widespread local or systemic disease. Consider a biopsy of the salmon patch, with fresh tissue submitted for flow cytometric analysis.

L. Recently, acquired pigmentation to the conjunctiva in an adult Caucasian patient should be biopsied in order to rule out or in primary acquired melanosis (PAM) with or without atypia. Cases of PAM with atypia may also require treatment with alcohol or mitomycin C, patient referral to a specialist familiar with this condition and treatment.

M. Conjunctival malignant melanoma may arise from acquired melanosis, from a pre-existing nevus, or *de novo*, though most arise from PAM with atypia. Once the pigmented lesion in a patient with known PAM with atypia is elevated clinically, the presence of conjunctival melanoma must be assumed. Conjunctival melanoma will spread directly through the lymphatics; the pre-auricular and sub-mandibular lymph nodes require evaluation.

BIBLIOGRAPHY

1. Elsas FJ, Green WR. Epibulbar tumors in childhood. Am J Ophthalmol. 1975;79:1001-7.
2. Folberg R, Jakobiec FA, Bernardino VB, et al. Benign conjunctival melanocytic lesions: clinicopathologic features. Ophthalmology. 1989;96:436-61.
3. Grossniklaus HE, Green WR, Luckenbach M, et al. Conjunctival lesions in adults: A clinical and histopathologic review. Cornea. 1987;2:78-116.
4. Kiratli H, Shields CL, Shields JA, et al. Metastatic tumors to the conjunctiva: Report of 10 cases. Br J Ophthalmol. 1996;80:5-8.
5. Lee GA, Hirst LW. Ocular surface squamous neoplasia. Surv Ophthalmol. 1995;39:429-50.
6. Mansour AM, Barber JC, Reinecke RD, et al. Ocular choristomas. Surv Ophthalmol. 1989;33:339-58.
7. McDonnell, Carpenter JE, Jacobs P, et al. Conjunctival melanocytic lesions in children. Ophthalmology. 1989;96:986-93.

Acute Conjunctivitis

22

Kristin Story Held, Ronald E Wise

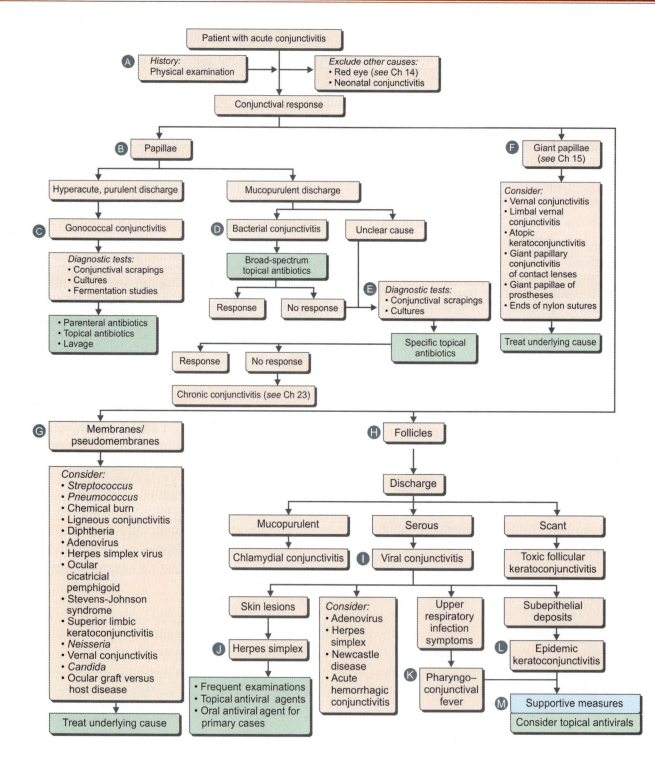

Conjunctivitis implies an inflammatory process of the conjunctival ocular surface. Certain characteristic clinical features may allow determination of an accurate clinical diagnosis (type of exudate, conjunctival response, preauricular adenopathy, and associated symptoms or signs).

A. Acute conjunctivitis is present for less than 4 weeks, is abrupt in onset, and is usually unilateral at first with involvement of the second eye occurring within 1 week. History should include the patient's age, allergies, medications, exposure to irritants, and ocular, genitourinary, and respiratory symptoms. A history of contagion is common. Patients often complain of red eye with watery, purulent or mucopurulent discharge, eyelids sticking on awakening, and burning foreign body sensation. Vision is usual normal, as are pupillary response, intraocular pressure, and funduscopic examination.

B. Inflammation of the conjunctiva can produce only a few clinical signs. A papillary response is non-specific, resulting from any type of inflammation. Papillae occur in the tarsal conjunctiva and contain a central vessel that branches on the surface in a spoke-like pattern readily evident on biomicroscopic examination. Numerous small papillae give the conjunctiva a red *velvety* appearance characteristic of bacterial conjunctivitis.

C. Hyperacute purulent conjunctivitis suggests infection with *Neisseria gonorrhoeae,* a highly virulent bacterium that can penetrate an intact corneal epithelium. There is rapid progression of a highly purulent conjunctivitis with lid edema, conjunctival hyperemia, and limbal chemosis to corneal perforation and blindness. This is the only bacterial conjunctivitis that commonly produces preauricular adenopathy. *N. meningitidis* is less common, but can produce septicemia and meningitis. Prompt laboratory evaluation and institution of specific treatment are mandatory. Smears for Gram and Giemsa stains should be taken from conjunctival scrapings rather than the exudate. Gram stain shows gram-negative intracellular diplococci in an overwhelming acute inflammatory response [polymorphonuclear lymphocytes (PMLs)]. Cultures are obtained on blood and chocolate agar (37°C, 10% CO_2). Carbohydrate fermentation studies should be obtained to differentiate *N. gonorrhoeae* from *N. meningitidis.* The patient with suspected gonococcal conjunctivitis is admitted for systemic parenteral full-dose antibiotics according to current recommendations of the Centers for Disease Control and Prevention. IV aqueous penicillin C, 10 million U per day for 5 days, is recommended for penicillin-sensitive gonorrhea. Ceftriaxone, 1 g IM daily for 5 days, is desirable for penicillinase producing strains and ease of administration. Tetracycline or erythromycin, 500 mg PO four times per day, is given for at least 1 week because of the high rate of associated chlamydial infections. Topical bacitracin may be administered, but is of secondary importance. The copious discharge should resolve within the first 24–48 hours, and the lid edema and hyperemia clear within 7–14 days.

D. Bacterial conjunctivitis is the most common type of infectious conjunctivitis. Historically, clinical diagnosis is made on the basis of a specific constellation of signs and symptoms; that is, the presence of a mucopurulent discharge, the absence of conjunctival follicles, and the absence of preauricular adenopathy. In adults the most common organisms isolated are *Streptococcus pneumoniae, Staphylococcus aureus,* and *Staphylococcus epidermidis.* In children the chief organisms are *Haemophilus influenzae, S. pneumoniae,* and *S. aureus. S. pneumoniae* is classically seen in cooler, temperate climates, whereas *H. aegyptius* is seen in warmer, southern climates. Bacterial conjunctivitis predominates *over* viral in the winter and spring. Most cases of bacterial conjunctivitis are self-limited, but appropriate antibiotics can shorten the course from 10–14 days to 1–3 days. Exceptions are *Moraxella lacunata* and *S. aureus,* which may result in chronic follicular conjunctivitis and chronic blepharoconjunctivitis, respectively. Initial treatment consists of broad-spectrum topical antibiotic solution or ointment (e.g. sulfacetamide drops or ointment four times daily, bacitracin ointment four times daily, or erythromycin ointment four times daily, for 5–10 days). Therapy is adjusted according to culture and sensitivity in refractory cases.

E. Because bacterial conjunctivitis is sufficiently identifiable on clinical grounds, self-limited and benign in nature, and highly responsive to empiric treatment, extensive laboratory evaluation is usually not needed. If the diagnosis is unclear or if the conjunctivitis is refractory to initial empiric treatment, perform a laboratory evaluation. Discontinue antibiotic treatment for 24 hours before obtaining specimens. Investigate all conjunctivitis in children. Obtain conjunctival scrapings for Gram and Giemsa stains. PMLs may be seen with Giemsa stain. Bacteria may be seen with Gram stain with a high level of specificity. Routine culture and sensitivity are obtained on blood and chocolate agar. Gram stain characteristics may allow presumptive diagnosis of the pathogen until culture and sensitivity results are available to guide selection of the specific topical antibiotics. Numerous preparations are available in the United States. Sulfacetamide covers *Staphylococcus*, *Pneumococcus*, *Haemophilus*, and *Moraxella* and, is inexpensive and relatively nontoxic. Agents containing neomycin are broad spectrum, but there is a high incidence of sensitivity to neomycin.

Chloramphenicol is broad spectrum and especially useful for *Haemophilus* and *Moraxella*, but a small risk of aplastic anemia exists, although no adverse systemic effects have been seen with short-term use. Aminoglycosides are broad spectrum, but are associated with a significant incidence of local hypersensitivity and toxicity. Furthermore, they are unreliable for *Pneumococcus* and other *Streptococcus* species and cause emergence of resistant strains. Fluoroquinolones are broad spectrum and highly effective and commonly used, but are more expensive. Topical therapy is preferred because it circumvents the toxic systemic side effects of many agents and allows the use of highly effective bactericidal agents, such as neomycin and bacitracin. Exceptions are *Neisseria*, *Chlamydia*, and *H. influenzae* type B in children (risk of septicemia, meningitis, orbital cellulitis and endogenous endophthalmitis), which require systemic treatment.

F. Giant papillae suggest a narrower differential diagnosis. They have a cobblestone appearance and are larger than 1 mm. They are more common in allergic and chronic conjunctivitis.

G. A pseudomembrane or membrane forms in certain inflammatory conditions as proteinaceous fluid and fibrin coagulate on the conjunctival surface. Pseudo-membranes are easily removed without bleeding. Membranes are more firmly adherent and bleed when stripped from the conjunctival surface.

H. The follicle is a focal lymphoid hyperplasia, which appears as a gray or white round structure with small vessels arising at its border and encircling it. A follicular response is a more specific clinical sign. Follicles are seen in most cases of viral conjunctivitis and all cases of chlamydial conjunctivitis except neonatal. Only trachoma produces a more severe follicular response in the upper tarsal conjunctiva than in the inferior fornix.

I. The clinical complex of a watery discharge, conjunctival follicles, and preauricular adenopathy suggests viral or chlamydial disease. Viral conjunctivitis occurs in all age groups. Epidemics are common. Adenoviruses are responsible for the most frequent epidemics in the United States. Viral conjunctivitis predominates over bacterial in the summer. As viral isolation techniques are expensive and of low yield, they are not routinely used. A morphologic diagnosis may be possible if the patient has associated corneal changes or systemic symptoms. However, if performed early in appropriately selected patients, viral isolation techniques may be helpful. The laboratory should be informed of a presumed diagnosis so that the appropriate cell line in which to inoculate the specimen may be selected. Cultures may also be taken from the pharynx and nares. Giemsa-stained conjunctival smears show predominantly lymphocytes or may show multinucleated giant cells. A Pap smear may show intranuclear inclusions. Immunofluorescent antibody techniques are available for diagnosing Herpes simplex, Herpes zoster, Adenovirus and *Chlamydia*. Lateral flow immunoassay testing is available to detect Adenovirus in tears.

J. Characteristic periorbital vesicles or pustules associated with a follicular, sometimes membranous, conjunctivitis and a palpable preauricular node are seen in primary herpes simplex blepharoconjunctivitis, which most often affects young children. The conjunctivitis caused by herpes simplex is self-limited, but may be followed by the classic dendritic keratitis; therefore topical antiviral agents for both the skin and eye are advocated. Trifluridine 1% solution, ganciclovir gel 0.15% or vidarabine 3% ointment are given five times daily for 7–10 days until the conjunctivitis has resolved. Topical acyclovir ointment or topical antibiotic ointment may be applied to the skin lesions. Cool compresses may provide symptomatic relief. Examine the patient every 2–3 days for the development of keratitis. Use oral acyclovir in primary cases of herpetic disease with corneal or eyelid involvement.

K. Pharyngoconjunctival fever is typically caused by Adenovirus with serotypes 3 and 7. The clinical complex of pharyngitis, fever, and follicular conjunctivitis help identify this diagnosis. Epidemics are often associated with public swimming pools in the summer.

L. Epidemic keratoconjunctivitis is caused by Adenovirus with serotypes 8 and 19. The clinical syndrome consists of preauricular lymphadenopathy, follicular conjunctivitis, pharyngitis, and characteristic subepithelial infiltrates that develop 5–12 days after the initial symptoms.

M. Viral conjunctivitis is usually self-limited and has a low morbidity rate, requiring no treatment. Antiviral agents, such as ganciclovir gel 0.15%, might be considered. Cold compresses provide symptomatic relief, as do artificial tears. Vasoconstricting antihistamine drops (naphazoline, pheniramine) may be given for itching. Inform the patient that the condition might worsen before it improves, and advise him or her to perform meticulous hand washing and to avoid direct contact with others. Health care personnel should refrain from direct patient contact for 14 days after the onset of symptoms.

BIBLIOGRAPHY

1. Arffa RC. Grayson's Diseases of the Cornea, 4th Edition. St Louis: Mosby, 1997. p. 107.
2. Dawson CR, Sheppard D. Follicular conjunctivitis. In: Tasman W, Jaeger EA (Eds). Duane's Clinical Ophthalmology, 4th Volume. Philadelphia: JB Lippincott Co; 1990.
3. Fitch CP, Rapoza PA, Owens S, et al. Epidemiology and diagnosis of acute conjunctivitis at an inner-city hospital. Ophthalmology. 1989;96:1215-20.
4. Friedlaender MH. A review of the causes and treatment of bacterial and allergic conjunctivitis. Clin Ther. 1995;17:800-10.
5. Mannis MJ. Bacterial conjunctivitis. In: Tasman W, Jaeger EA (Eds). Duane's Clinical Ophthalmology, 4th Volume. Philadelphia: JB Lippincott Co; 1990.
6. McDonnell PJ, Green WR. Conjunctivitis. In: Mandell GL, Douglas RG, Bennett JE (Eds). Principles and Practices of Infectious Diseases, 1st Volume, 3rd Edition. New York: Churchill Livingstone; 1990. pp. 975-82.

Chronic Conjunctivitis

23

Kristin Story Held

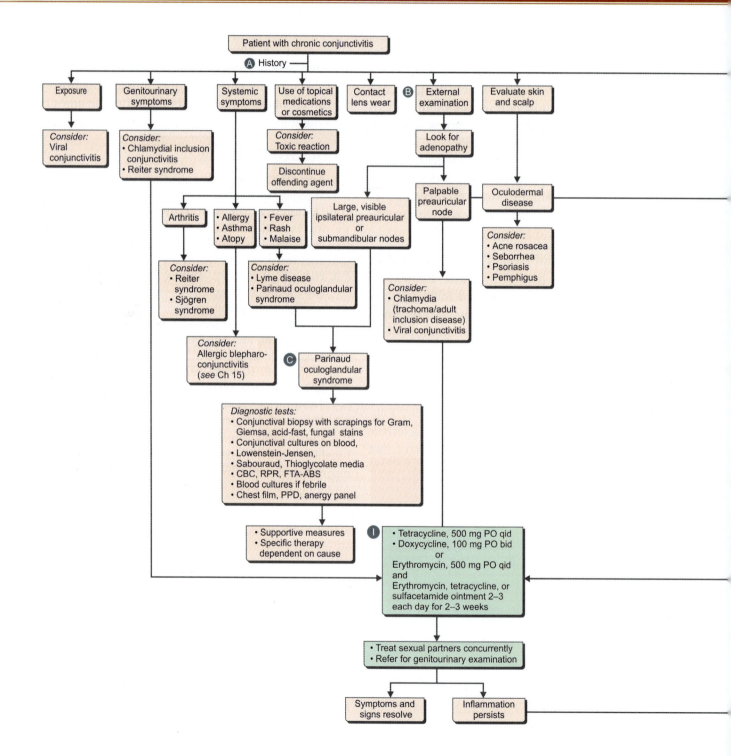

Patient with chronic conjunctivitis

Ⓐ History

Exposure

Consider:
Viral conjunctivitis

Genitourinary symptoms

Consider:
• Chlamydial inclusion conjunctivitis
• Reiter syndrome

Systemic symptoms

Use of topical medications or cosmetics

Consider:
Toxic reaction

Discontinue offending agent

Contact lens wear

Ⓑ **External examination**

Look for adenopathy

Evaluate skin and scalp

Palpable preauricular node

Oculodermal disease

Consider:
• Acne rosacea
• Seborrhea
• Psoriasis
• Pemphigus

Arthritis

• Allergy
• Asthma
• Atopy

• Fever
• Rash
• Malaise

Large, visible ipsilateral preauricular or submandibular nodes

Consider:
• Reiter syndrome
• Sjögren syndrome

Consider:
• Lyme disease
• Parinaud oculoglandular syndrome

Consider:
• Chlamydia (trachoma/adult inclusion disease)
• Viral conjunctivitis

Consider:
Allergic blepharoconjunctivitis (*see* Ch 15)

Ⓒ **Parinaud oculoglandular syndrome**

Diagnostic tests:
• Conjunctival biopsy with scrapings for Gram, Giemsa, acid-fast, fungal stains
• Conjunctival cultures on blood,
• Lowenstein-Jensen,
• Sabouraud, Thioglycolate media
• CBC, RPR, FTA-ABS
• Blood cultures if febrile
• Chest film, PPD, anergy panel

• Supportive measures
• Specific therapy dependent on cause

Ⓘ • Tetracycline, 500 mg PO qid
• Doxycycline, 100 mg PO bid
or
Erythromycin, 500 mg PO qid
and
Erythromycin, tetracycline, or sulfacetamide ointment 2–3 each day for 2–3 weeks

• Treat sexual partners concurrently
• Refer for genitourinary examination

Symptoms and signs resolve

Inflammation persists

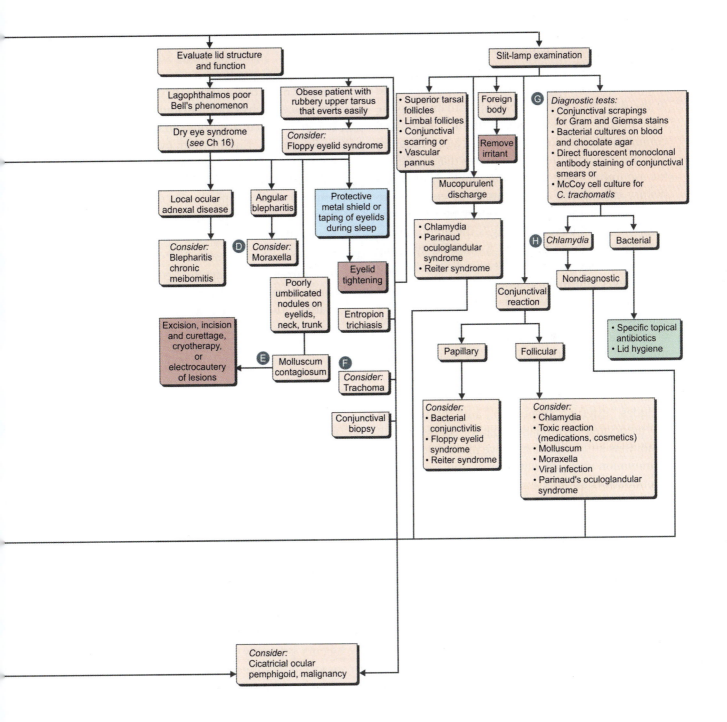

Evaluate lid structure and function

Lagophthalmos poor Bell's phenomenon

Dry eye syndrome (*see* Ch 16)

Obese patient with rubbery upper tarsus that everts easily

Consider: Floppy eyelid syndrome

Slit-lamp examination

• Superior tarsal follicles
• Limbal follicles
• Conjunctival scarring or
• Vascular pannus

Foreign body

Remove irritant

Ⓖ *Diagnostic tests:*
• Conjunctival scrapings for Gram and Giemsa stains
• Bacterial cultures on blood and chocolate agar
• Direct fluorescent monoclonal antibody staining of conjunctival smears or
• McCoy cell culture for *C. trachomatis*

Local ocular adnexal disease

Angular blepharitis

Protective metal shield or taping of eyelids during sleep

Consider: Blepharitis chronic meibomitis

Ⓓ *Consider:* Moraxella

Eyelid tightening

Mucopurulent discharge

Ⓗ *Chlamydia*

Bacterial

• Chlamydia
• Parinaud oculoglandular syndrome
• Reiter syndrome

Nondiagnostic

Poorly umbilicated nodules on eyelids, neck, trunk

Conjunctival reaction

• Specific topical antibiotics
• Lid hygiene

Excision, incision and curettage, cryotherapy, or electrocautery of lesions

Ⓔ Molluscum contagiosum

Entropion trichiasis

Ⓕ *Consider:* Trachoma

Papillary

Follicular

Conjunctival biopsy

Consider:
• Bacterial conjunctivitis
• Floppy eyelid syndrome
• Reiter syndrome

Consider:
• Chlamydia
• Toxic reaction (medications, cosmetics)
• Molluscum
• Moraxella
• Viral infection
• Parinaud's oculoglandular syndrome

Consider: Cicatricial ocular pemphigoid, malignancy

Chronic conjunctivitis is inflammation of the conjunctiva that persists greater than 2–4 weeks. There are many causes of chronic conjunctivitis, and effective treatment is available to alleviate the signs and symptoms of most types. Accurate identification of the specific cause of chronic conjunctivitis is the key to successful management. The symptoms are variable, and clinical signs may seem equally nonspecific. A systematic approach to the investigation of chronic conjunctivitis, including detailed history, thorough examination, and specific diagnostic tests, affords the most accurate diagnosis and treatment.

A. A detailed patient history provides important clues in the diagnosis of chronic conjunctivitis. Explore any history of exposure. Chronic adenoviral conjunctivitis is a clinical diagnosis, and laboratory tests are often of little help, although diagnostic kits for use in the clinic are now available. Likewise, a history of asthma, allergy, atopy or exposure to a specific allergen suggests one type of allergic blepharoconjunctivitis; itching is the predominant complaint in these patients. Associated systemic symptoms may suggest a specific diagnosis such as the fever and malaise associated with Parinaud oculoglandular conjunctivitis or the genitourinary symptoms associated with chlamydial disease. Finally, inquire about all topical preparations used, including cosmetics, contact lens solutions and contact lenses.

B. A thorough systemic examination is essential and includes external inspection and examination of associated lymphadenopathy, dermatologic conditions and local adnexal eye disease, including examination for lagophthalmos and poor Bell phenomenon. Slit lamp examination should evaluate the characteristics of the conjunctival reaction, discharge, presence of foreign bodies or irritants, adequacy of tearing, and presence of keratopathy.

C. Parinaud oculoglandular conjunctivitis is a syndrome characterized by a unilateral granulomatous lesion of the conjunctiva surrounded by follicles and large visible preauricular or submandibular lymph nodes on the same side. Fever, malaise and rash may be present. Several microorganisms may produce this syndrome, most commonly the bacillus of cat scratch fever.

More than two-thirds of these patients have been scratched by a cat 1–2 weeks before the onset of symptoms. Other common causes are tularemia, sporotrichosis, tuberculosis and other mycobacteria; syphilis; coccidioidomycosis; and less commonly, leukemia, lymphoma, mumps, mononucleosis, fungi, and sarcoidosis. Perform a diagnostic laboratory evaluation when the cause is unclear because treatment is directed at the specific causative agent.

D. *Moraxella lacunata,* large square gram-negative diplobacillus, produces a chronic angular blepharoconjunctivitis characterized by conjunctival injection and maceration of the inner and outer canthal angles. It can produce a chronic follicular conjunctivitis and keratitis. Culture and cytologic examination help establish this diagnosis. *M. lacunata* is readily cultured on blood and chocolate agar. *Moraxella* responds well to topical sulfacetamide, tetracycline, or erythromycin. Culture and sensitivity help guide treatment.

E. Molluscum contagiosum, a skin disease caused by a poxvirus, is characterized by multiple dome-shaped umbilicated nodules on the eyelid or lid margin. The virus causes a toxic reaction, which results in a chronic follicular conjunctivitis and keratitis that can progress to a trachoma-like picture. Recognition of the typical molluscum lesions, which may be inconspicuous or hidden by the lashes, is crucial. Treatment involves simple excision, incision and curettage, cryotherapy or electrocautery of the lesions.

F. *Chlamydia* is an extremely common cause of chronic eye infection, specifically trachoma, adult inclusion conjunctivitis, and neonatal inclusion conjunctivitis. Trachoma is the most common cause of preventable blindness or decreased vision in the world, affecting about 500 million people. It is a chronic follicular conjunctivitis that results in conjunctival and corneal scarring. The cicatricial phase of the disease causes conjunctival and lid deformation that ultimately leads to the blinding complications of corneal ulceration and opacification. Trachoma occurs primarily in the Third World countries in association with poverty and poor sanitation. The presence of two of the following signs suggests the diagnosis of trachoma: (1) lymphoid follicles on the upper tarsal conjunctiva, (2) typical conjunctival scarring, (3) vascular pannus, and (4) limbal follicles or their sequelae, Herbert pits. Cytologic examination of Giemsa-stained conjunctival smears to look for chlamydial inclusions is helpful. Direct fluorescent monoclonal antibody staining of conjunctival smears and McCoy cell culture for *C. trachomatis* are available as well.

G. Because many causes exist for chronic conjunc-tivitis, laboratory evaluation is required for diagnosis. Obtain conjunctival smears for cytologic evaluation with Gram and Giemsa stains. This is rapid and cost-effective Gram stain reveals bacterial pathogens, and Giemsa stain reveals cellular morphology. Bacterial infections are characterized by polymorphonuclear cells. Viral infections are characterized by lymphocytes. A mixed response is seen in chlamydial infection. Intraepithelial cytoplasmic inclusions are diagnostic of chlamydial infections; however, inclusions can be seen more readily in acute than in chronic chlamydial infection. Eosinophils suggest allergic eye disease. Cytologic examination may also reveal dysplasia or keratinization of the ocular surface. Bacterial culture is useful, particularly in partially treated or resistant cases. Cultures are taken after the patient has stopped taking antibiotics for 24–72 hours. Sensitivity results are particularly useful in guiding therapy. Blood and chocolate agar should be used. The rate of isolation in the chronic phase of an infection is often lower than during the acute phase, especially for viruses (e.g. adenovirus). Viral cultures are not particularly helpful in chronic conjunctivitis. McCoy cell culture is the standard for the laboratory-confirmed diagnosis of chlamydial conjunctivitis. Direct monoclonal antibody staining of conjunctival smears has been reported to have a sensitivity of 100%, specificity of 94%, and positive and negative predictive values of 94% and 100% respectively. However, the diagnostic tests are not perfect, and sexually active patients with follicular conjunctivitis should be considered to have chlamydial disease until proven otherwise. Therapeutic trials of tetracycline or erythromycin are important diagnostic and therapeutic steps in selected patients. In refractory cases, conjunctival biopsy is useful for detection of other potentially treatable causes, such as pemphigoid or malignancy (e.g. sebaceous gland carcinoma).

H. Chlamydial organisms are responsible for trachoma and adult inclusion conjunctivitis. Adult inclusion conjunctivitis usually occurs in sexually active adults, 15–30 years of age, who have acquired a new sexual partner within the past 2 months. It presents as an acute follicular conjunctivitis with mucopurulent discharge and has a chronic course. Keratitis may be a prominent feature later in the disease. Reiter syndrome has been reported in association with adult inclusion conjunctivitis. Nonspecific urethritis in men and chronic vaginal discharge in women are common. More than 4 million Americans acquire genital chlamydial infection each year, and 1 in 300 of these patients gets inclusion conjunctivitis. Treat all sexual partners simultaneously to prevent reinfection. Refer patients for evaluation of other venereal infections such as gonorrhea and syphilis.

I. *C. trachomatis* is the most common cause of chronic follicular conjunctivitis. Topical antibiotics are relatively ineffective. Adequate treatment requires systemic administration of tetracycline or doxycycline for 3 weeks. Tetracycline should not be administered to children less than 7 years of age or to pregnant or lactating women. In patients who are intolerant of tetracycline, use oral erythromycin. Administer erythromycin, tetracycline, or sulfacetamide ointment as an adjunct. Treat sexual partners concurrently and refer the patient for genitourinary examination.

BIBLIOGRAPHY

1. Dawson CR, Sheppard JD. Follicular conjunctivitis. In: Duane TD, (Ed.). Clinical Ophthalmology, Vol 4. Philadelphia: Harper & Row; 1990.
2. Huang MC, Dreyer E. Parinaud's oculoglandular conjunctivitis and cat-scratch disease. In: Jakobiec FA, Lucarelli MJ, (Eds). International Ophthalmology Clinics: Ocular Adnexal Infections. Boston: Little, Brown and Company. 1996;36:29.
3. Mannis MJ. Bacterial conjunctivitis. In: Duane TD, (Ed.). Clinical Ophthalmology, Vol 4. Philadelphia: Harper & Row; 1990.
4. Rapoza PA, Quinn TC, Terry AC, et al. A systematic approach to the diagnosis and treatment of chronic conjunctivitis. Am J Ophthalmol. 1990;109:138-42.

Subconjunctival Hemorrhage

24

Patricia C Nelson

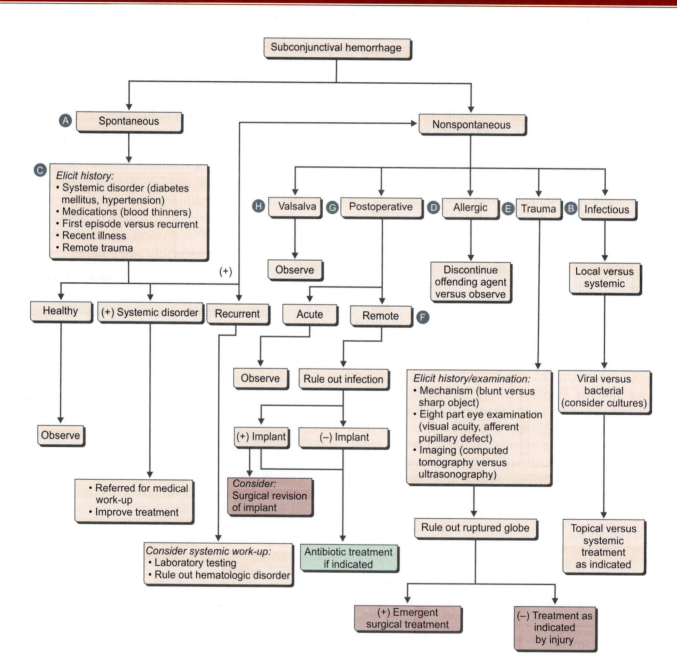

One of the most common ocular referrals is for a bright, 'blood red' looking eye; usually a subconjunctival hemorrhage. Often, this process is painless, and the patient themselves may be unaware until a friend or provider notes the finding. Despite the patient being otherwise asymptomatic, the appearance alone can cause much concern. While a simple subconjunctival hemorrhage, from a ruptured small blood vessel, requires no treatment, other concerning etiologies should be differentiated before educating the patient on spontaneous resolution. A differential would include etiologies such as infection (epidemic keratoconjunctivitis, acute hemorrhagic conjunctivitis), inflammation (uveitis, episcleritis, scleritis), vascular abnormalities, (diabetes mellitus, vessel fragility), trauma (laceration, ruptured globe), medications, postoperative and following Valsalva maneuvers.

Initial slit-lamp examination can help differentiate conjunctival hemorrhage from hyperemia, and also rule out intraocular inflammation, as well as identifying any palpebral conjunctival reaction. In a classic hemorrhage, the surrounding vessels are of a normal caliber and the hemorrhage is focal with diffusion over time as gravity comes into play. Over 2 weeks the hemorrhage resolves, like any other bruise, and may undergo color changes from red to yellow before complete resolution.

A. *Idiopathic/spontaneous*: Most common cause in a healthy adult. Often patient awakes with the finding. The incidence increases with age, capillary fragility, arteriosclerosis, and hypertension. In young patients without a history of trauma or infection, rule out systemic causes, specifically diabetes, vitamin C deficiency, hematologic or hepatic diseases, lupus erythematosus and parasites, particularly when the problem keeps on recurring.

B. *Infectious*: Some febrile systemic infections causing hemorrhage include viruses (adenovirus, enterovirus, influenza, smallpox, measles, yellow fever, sandfly fever), meningococcal septicemia, scarlet fever, typhoid fever, cholera, rickettsia (typhus) and parasites (malaria).

C. *Medications*: Not only 'blood thinners' but many other drugs and chemicals have been associated with hemorrhage, including aspirin, warfarin (Coumadin), clopidogrel (Plavix), dabigatran (Pradaxa), heparin, various antibiotics, contraceptives, steroids, alcohol, vitamins A and D, fish oil, ginseng, St John's wort and many other herbal supplements.

D. *Allergic reaction*: While some drugs and chemicals may cause hemorrhage directly, others cause ocular irritation, leading to eye rubbing, which produces a hemorrhage.

E. *Trauma*: Subconjunctival hemorrhage following direct or blunt ocular trauma should raise suspicion for an ocular perforation, often hidden by the blood. A globe rupture is an ocular emergency and requires timely surgical intervention. A globe perforation is unlikely and surgical globe exploration may not be necessary if the complete 8-part exam is normal, including vision, pupillary responses, intraocular pressure (IOP), slit lamp exam and a dilated exam with good view of the periphery. However, if there is hyphema or vitreous hemorrhage preventing complete visualization of the fundus, an ultrasound examination should be considered. Have a low threshold to consider globe exploration to rule out perforation if there is significant hemorrhagic chemosis present. Imaging, including computed tomography (CT) of the face and/or orbits, can show irregular globe contour, intraocular and retrobulbar air and hemorrhage, as well as intraocular foreign bodies and orbital fractures. Intraocular air or foreign bodies prove perforation. Poor prognostic signs following trauma are an afferent pupillary defect (APD), decreased presenting vision, and a retinal detachment. Clinically, very low IOP, deep or flat anterior chamber, peaked pupil, or positive Seidel testing all suggest perforations.

F. *Emboli*: Subconjunctival hemorrhage has been reported as a result of emboli from long bone fractures, chest compression, cardiac angiography, open-heart surgery, and other 'remote' operations.

G. *Postoperative*: Following ocular surgery, including refractive, periocular, and intraocular surgeries, it is considered a normal sequel to find blood under the conjunctiva. This finding is considered normal even if no conjunctival incision was made, as in transconjunctival cryotherapy. The conjunctival vessels are more fragile due to postoperative inflammation, thus bleeding may increase during the first few days following surgery. The postoperative hemorrhages would be expected to resolve within a few weeks of surgery. It is important to rule infectious etiologies, if hemorrhage occurs outside the immediate postoperative period, specifically with scleral buckle procedures.

H. *Valsalva*: With coughing, sneezing, or bearing down, subconjunctival hemorrhages can occur in any age group. They are seen more frequently in young, otherwise healthy, persons involved in heavy weight-lifting or pilots undergoing high magnitude G-force.

BIBLIOGRAPHY

1. Davis JR, Stepanek J, Fogarty JA. Fundamentals of Aerospace Medicine, 4th Edition. Philadelphia, PA: Lippincott Williams & Wilkins; 2008. p.92.
2. Fraunfelder FT. Drug Induced Ocular Side Effects and Drug Interactions, 3rd Edition. Philadelphia: Lea & Febiger; 1989.
3. Friberg TR, Weinreb RN. Ocular manifestations of gravity inversion. JAMA. 1985;253:1755-7.
4. Kubal, WS. Imaging of orbital trauma. Radiographics. 2008;28:1729-39.
5. Russell SR, Olson KR, Folk JC. Predictors of scleral rupture and the role of vitrectomy in severe ocular blunt trauma. Am Ophthalmol. 1988;105:253-7.
6. Unver YB, Kapran Z, Acar N, et al. Ocular trauma score in open globe injuries. J Trauma. 2009;66:1030-2.

Pigment Alterations of the Iris

25

Maria Q Husain

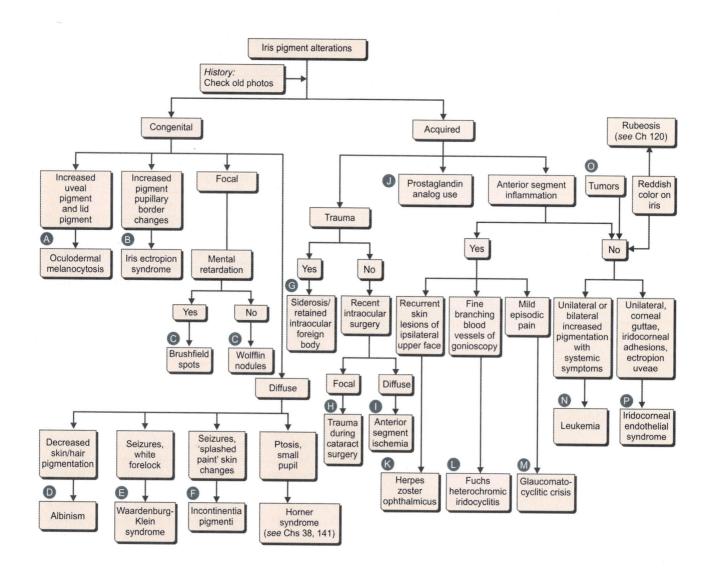

A. Oculodermal melanocytosis, or *Nevus of Ota*, is more common in Asian people. In patients with oculodermal melanocytosis, an almost thirtyfold increased risk of uveal, orbital and intracranial melanoma is present. Appropriate imaging studies should be ordered to monitor this. Patients with oculodermal melanocytosis risk development of glaucoma.

B. Congenital iris ectropion syndrome is associated with ectropion of the iris pigment epithelium, high iris insertion, dysgenesis of the drainage angle, glaucoma, and in many cases, ipsilateral ptosis. It may be a part of the spectrum of Axenfeld-Rieger syndrome.

C. Brushfield spots are often found in patients with Down syndrome (Trisomy 21). However, 24% of the population can have normal, similar looking colorations on the iris, and in this case, they are called Wolfflin nodules.

D. Oculocutaneous albinism is generally a straight-forward diagnosis and is inherited in an autosomal recessive fashion. However, patients with ocular albinism may have normal skin and hair and have X-linked inheritance. Both will have increased iris transillumination, foveal aplasia/hypoplasia, and decreased pigment in the posterior pole (Chapter 26).

E. Waardenburg-Klein syndrome includes iris hetero-chromia, lateral displacement of the medial canthi combined with dystopia of the lacrimal punctum, blepharophimosis, hypertrichosis of the medial part of the eyebrows, white forelock and deafness. It is mainly inherited by an autosomal dominant trait. The iris abnormalities can be complete, partial, or segmental and can be unilateral or bilateral.

F. Incontinentia pigmenti (Bloch-Sulzberger syndrome) has an X-linked dominant inheritance pattern, and nearly all cases are in females. Patients have a 'splashed paint' appearance on their skin with multiple small hyperpigmented macules. Systemic issues also include microcephaly, hydrocephalus, seizures, dental abnormalities and scoliosis. Aside from iris heterochromia, one-quarter to one-third of patients may have a proliferative retinal vasculopathy that is similar to retinopathy of prematurity in appearance.

G. Patients with intraocular foreign bodies may not present with the most compelling history. Suspicion should be heightened when the history involves an activity that could have resulted in a ferrous body in the eye. Removing the foreign body is imperative to prevent further deterioration of ocular function.

H. During intraocular surgery, if instrumentation chafes along the iris, atrophy may develop in the area. Alternatively, intraocular lens placement can cause iris chafing, which can lead to iris irritation, ocular inflammation and prostaglandin release. This can necessitate removal of the lens.

I. Anterior segment ischemia can occur when perfusion via the anterior ciliary arteries is interrupted during extraocular muscle surgery. It can also be seen after an episode of shock or other cause of hypoperfusion.

J. Prostaglandin analogs upregulate iridial melano-cytes and can cause darkening of irises. This effect is particularly prominent in patients with hazel or heterochromic eyes.

K. Herpes zoster ophthalmicus causes intraocular inflammation, which results in iris atrophy. If a patient has skin involvement at the tip of the nose (*Hutchinson sign*), there is a much greater likelihood of involvement of the eye as both areas are supplied by the nasociliary nerve.

L. Fuchs heterochromic iridocyclitis can result in iris depigmentation on the affected side, but if atrophy is severe, darkening can occur as a result of exposed iris pigment epithelium. The cornea can have fine stellate keratic precipitates. Secondary open angle glaucoma is a concern for these patients, and cataract surgery can be complicated by bleeding.

M. Glaucomatocyclitic crisis (*Posner-Schlossman*) presents with corneal edema and anterior uveitis resulting from elevated intraocular pressures. It occurs episodically and lasts hours to weeks. Pain is minimal, the angle usually stays open, and the iris can lighten on the affected side from atrophy. The prognosis is good, and visual fields usually remain full. Mild miotics can be used to treat this syndrome.

N. The initial manifestation of initial or returning leukemia may be darkening of unilateral or bilateral irides. The irides can return to their normal coloration after systemic treatment is administered.

O. Tumors of the iris can arise from the iris pigment epithelium in the fourth to sixth decade of life and are extremely rare. Iris metastases are exceedingly rare as well, and primary tumors are usually from the breast or lung. They usually appear as a solitary yellow-white or pink fleshy mass on the stromal surface. Approximately 2–5% of intraocular melanomas are primary iris melanomas, and they usually present in the fifth decade of life (Chapter 27).

P. Iridocorneal endothelial syndrome is a spectrum of disorders that are mainly characterized by iris changes, corneal edema and glaucoma. Essentially, endothelial cells morph into epithelial like cells and invade the angle and the surface of the iris. This syndrome occurs mainly in middle-aged females and is almost always unilateral.

BIBLIOGRAPHY

1. Catalano RA. Incontinentia pigmenti. Am J Ophthalmol. 1990;110:696-700.
2. Rennie IG. Don't it make my blue eyes brown: heterochromia and other iris abnormalities. Eye. 2012;26:29-50.
3. Stjernschantz JW, Albert DM, Hu DN, et al. Mechanism and clinical significance of prostaglandin-induced iris pigmentation. Surv Ophthalmol. 2002;47(Suppl 1): S162-75.
4. Velilla S, Dios E, Herreras JM, et al. Fuchs' heterochromic iridocyclitis: a review of 26 cases. Ocul Immunol Inflamm. 2001;9:169-75.
5. Wilson MC, Shields MB. A comparison of the clinical variations of the iridocorneal endothelial syndrome. Arch Ophthalmol. 1989;107:1465-68.
6. Wilson ME. Congenital iris ectropion and a new classification for anterior segment dysgenesis. J Pediatr Ophthalmol Strabismus. 1990;27:48-55.

Increased Transillumination of the Iris

Johan Zwaan

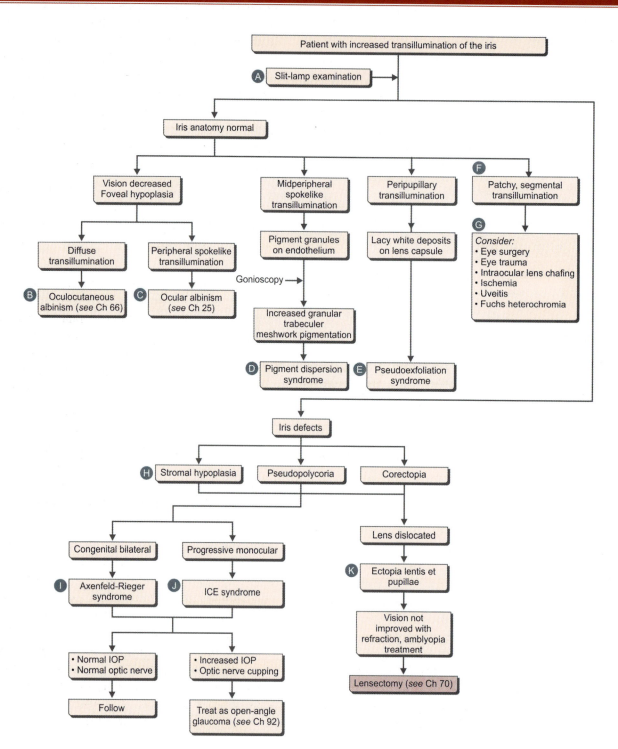

26

Transillumination of the iris indicates reduced melanin pigment in the double layer of pigmented iris epithelium that covers the posterior aspect of the iris. It may result from the absence or decrease of melanin within the cells, or there may be defects within the cell layers. The latter can be the result of congenital anomalies, trauma, or disease.

A. When there is a significant lack of pigment, the defects can be seen by transscleral transillumination with a bright light, such as a muscle light. In general, careful slit-lamp examination in a darkened room is essential to evaluate more subtle defects. In patients with dark irides the defects may be particularly difficult to see because pigment in the iris stroma blocks the light.

B. In oculocutaneous albinism the eyes, as well as the skin and hairs, show a significant lack of pigment. In tyrosinase-negative type 1 (OCA 1), melanin is completely missing. The lashes and hair are white, and transillumination of the iris is complete. Vision is significantly reduced because of foveal hypoplasia and lack of fundus pigment. Nystagmus is found. In tyrosinase-positive OCA 2, some pigment accumulates over time and the hair and lashes are yellowish. Vision is reduced less than in OCA 1. At least 10 different genetic types of OCA exist. Their discussion is beyond the scope of this chapter.

C. Patients with ocular albinism also have reduced vision, foveal hypoplasia, and nystagmus. Expression can be varied even within one family. Although skin changes are not obvious, electron microscopy has shown that abnormalities of pigmentation are present, primarily macromelanosomes. Four different types of ocular albinism exist.

D. Loss of pigment from the iris epithelium in pigment dispersion syndrome occurs primarily in a spoke like midperipheral pattern. It is caused by rubbing of the posterior leaflet of the iris epithelium against the lenticular zonules, associated with a concave iris plateau and a deep anterior chamber. It is found primarily in young adults with myopia and affects males more than females. The dislodged pigment granules are deposited in the trabecular meshwork and are visible with gonioscopy as a dense band of pigment. This may interfere with aqueous drainage and lead to glaucoma. Pigment also is deposited on the corneal endothelium in a vertical band, Krukenberg spindle, and on other anterior segment structures.

E. The deposition of flaky white material on the anterior surface of the lens is the hallmark of pseudoexfoliation. The material also may be found on the zonules, the drainage angle, the corneal endothelium, ciliary processes, and anterior vitreous face. Pigment accumulation in the-drainage angle is less pronounced than in pigment dispersion. The pigment is derived from the iris epithelium at the pupillary ruff as evidenced by scattered peripupillary transillumination defects. This pattern of pigment loss is not pathognomonic for pseudoexfoliation because it can also occur with aging.

F. Trauma, manipulation of the iris during surgery, and inflammation can lead to loss of pigment, usually in a patchy fashion. A careful history and slit-lamp examination will usually lead to the proper diagnosis.

G. Fuchs heterochromic iridocyclitis is a unilateral anterior uveitis that affects young adults. It manifests as progressive heterochromia; a painless decrease of vision may occur. The anterior chamber reaction is low grade with small keratic precipitates and no posterior synechiae. Cataracts may develop. Atrophy of the iris pigment epithelium is patchy.

H. Abnormal shapes of the pupil (dyscoria), corectopia, and holes in the iris (pseudopolycoria) can result from hypoplasia of the iris stroma. The hypoplasia may be congenital, as in Axenfeld-Rieger syndrome, or acquired, as in iridocorneal endothelial (ICE) syndrome. In both cases it can be progressive.

I. Axenfeld anomaly usually shows autosomal-dominant inheritance. It is characterized by posterior embryotoxon and bridges of iris tissue crossing the anterior chamber angle and inserting at Schwalbe line. It is often associated with glaucoma. This may be congenital or develop later, necessitating monitoring of the intraocular pressure (lOP) throughout life. In Rieger's anomaly the iris stroma is hypoplastic, in addition to the abnormalities found in Axenfeld anomaly. Both anomalies are termed syndromes if systemic abnormalities are present. Because both may be found within the same family, they are now considered variable manifestations of the same gene defect and the syndrome or anomaly is labeled Axenfeld-Rieger. The syndrome has been mapped to two different gene loci: 4q25 and 13q14. Autosomal-dominant iris hypoplasia and iridogoniodysgenesis with systemic features also map to the first locus.

J. ICE syndrome includes progressive essential iris atrophy, Chandler syndrome, and the iris-nevus, or Cogan-Reese, syndrome. It is almost always unilateral. Glaucoma is combined with corneal endothelial abnormalities, anterior synechiae, iris atrophy leading to pseudopolycoria, and iris nodules. The three subtypes show different degrees of these manifestations of the same disease.

K. Ectopia lentis et pupillae is an autosomal-recessive anomaly. The lens dislocation is in the opposite direction from the displacement of the pupil. The iris shows transillumination defects. Axial myopia is the rule.

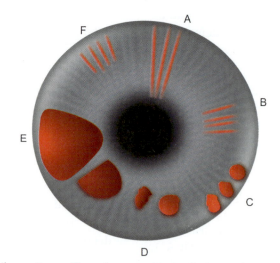

Fig. 26.1: Various iris transillumination patterns. There is some overlap between the patterns, but in general they are a good indication of the underlying pathology. (A) In oculocutaneous albinism (OCA) the entire iris tends to transilluminate; (B) Spoke like transillumination in the mid periphery is often seen in pigment dispersion syndrome; (C) Peripupillary transillumination is shown in pseudoexfoliation syndrome, but also occurs with aging; (D) Patchy dropout of pigment in a segmental fashion indicates possible eye trauma, sometimes surgical, and uveitis among others; (E) Large defects may happen in Axenfeld-Rieger syndrome associated with stromal hypoplasia; (F) In ocular albinism (OA) the transillumination often is less than in OCA, primarily with a peripheral spoke shaped pattern.

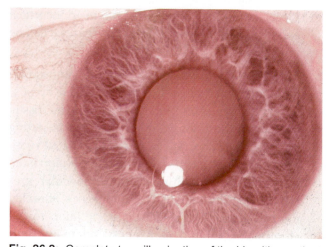

Fig. 26.2: Complete transillumination of the iris with a patient with oculocutaneous albinism type 1.

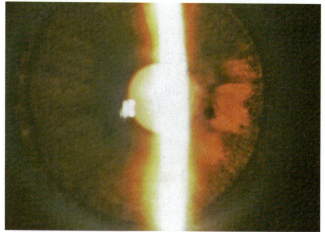

Fig. 26.3: Mid iris pigment defects after trauma.

BIBLIOGRAPHY

1. Brooks AMV, Gillies WE. The presentation and prognosis of glaucoma in pseudoexfoliation of the lens capsule. Ophthalmology 1988; 95:271-4.
2. Farrar SM, Shields MB, Miller KN, et al. Risk factors for the development and severity of glaucoma in the pigment dispersion syndrome. Am J Ophthalmol 1989;108:223-7.
3. Goldberg MF. Clinical manifestations of ectopia lentis et pupillae in 16 patients. Ophthalmology 1988; 95:1080-7.
4. Jones N. Fuchs' heterochromic uveitis: An update. Surv Ophthalmol 1993; 37:253-72.
5. King RA, Hearing Vj, Creel D, et al. Albinism. In: Scriver CR, Beaudet AL, Sly WS, Valle D, eds. The Metabolic and Molecular basis of Inherited Disease. New York: McGraw-Hill 1995: 4353-90.
6. Semina EV, Reiter R, Leysens NJ, et al. Cloning and characterization of a novel bicoid-related homeobox transcription factor, RIEG, involved in Rieger syndrome. Nature Genet 1996;14: 392-9.
7. Wilson MC, Shields MB. A comparison of the clinical variations of the iridocorneal endothelial syndrome. Arch Ophthalmol 1989; 107:1465-8.

27

Tumor of the Iris

Negin Agange, Johan Zwaan

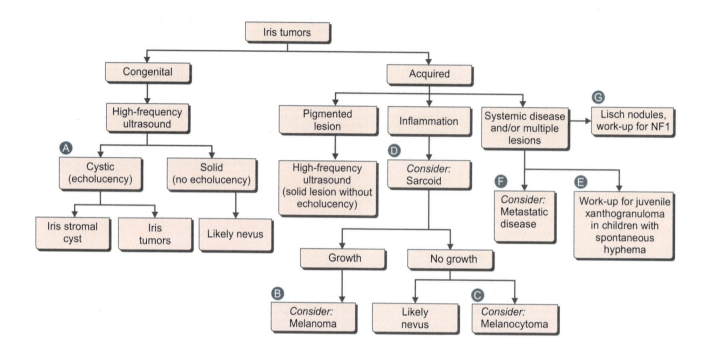

Recognition of iris tumors is important for early diagnosis and proper management of the lesions. Most pigmented iris tumors can be followed by clinical exam with photography or high-frequency ultrasound to establish a baseline for future comparisons. Iris tumors may also indicate systemic diseases like neurofibromatosis (NF1), sarcoidosis, juvenile xantho-granuloma (JXG), or metastatic disease. For most iris masses, observation alone is the initial treatment, and usually they do not require further treatment.

A. Cysts can be located in the iris stroma and are formed by a separation of pigmented epithelium. Iris cysts typically present as protrusion of the iris stroma anterior to the cyst. Gonioscopy can demonstrate focal anterior displacement of the iris stroma and is an important tool in evaluation of involvement of angle structures.

B. Though the majority of iris tumors are cysts or nevi, malignant melanomas can occur rarely as well. Most small iris melanomas can be surgically removed. Medium and large uveal melanomas are usually treated conservatively with local radiation plaque therapy, and generally, enucleation is restricted to those patients experiencing uncontrollable pain from secondary processes or failing local tumor control (Fig. 27.1).

C. A small iris melanocytoma on slit lamp exam is usually dark brown or black with a cobblestone appearance. It can be mistaken for a melanoma, but a melanocytoma is not likely to have intrinsic vascularity or to cause a sector cataract the way a melanoma could. One key difference on high-frequency ultrasound is that a melanocytoma has high reflectivity, unlike low reflectivity from an

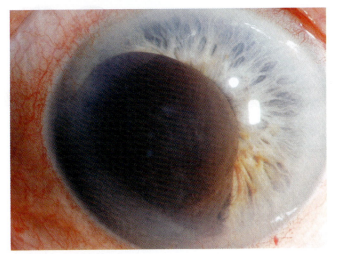

Fig. 27.1: Iris melanoma.
Courtesy: Dr Constance Fry.

iris melanoma. High-frequency ultrasound is also helpful in differentiating solid from cystic lesions on the iris. In such cases, the ultrasound provides a more objective way of measuring the size, depth, and location of iris tumors.

D. Sarcoidosis is a systemic granulomatous disease that can manifest with discrete vascular nodules on the iris. Nodules in the angle of the eye are referred to as Berlin nodules, when on the pupillary margin as Koeppe, and those in the periphery as Busacca nodules. When sarcoidosis is suspected, further testing is recommended with initial workup including angiotensin-converting enzyme and lysozyme blood testing, chest X-ray, and/or skin biopsy, if indicated.

E. JXG is a primarily pediatric dermatologic disorder that can be associated rarely with systemic manifestations in the eye. JXG typically presents with reddish brown skin papules or plaques commonly on the trunk, neck, and head. Ocular JXG can occur without skin lesions and can be associated with iris lesions, glaucoma, and spontaneous hyphema in children. No treatment is needed for skin lesions, and treatment for ocular JXG depends on associated eye complications.

F. Metastasis to the iris is relatively rare and often regresses when the underlying cancer is treated with systemic chemotherapy.

G. Lisch nodules associated with NF1 are elevated and often times pigmented hamartomas of the iris that are present in the majority of adult patients. Patients with NF1 tend to have bilateral Lisch nodules, and although these nodules carry no prognostic significance, earlier recognition will likely lead to earlier testing for the more dangerous neoplasms associated with NF1.

BIBLIOGRAPHY

1. Collaborative Ocular Melanoma Study Group. The COMS randomized trial of iodine 125 brachytherapy for choroidal melanoma: V. Twelve-year mortality rates and prognostic factors: COMS report No. 26. Arch Ophthalmol. 2006; 124:1664.
2. Shields CL, Kaliki S, Hutchinson A, et al. Iris nevus growth into melanoma: analysis of 1611 consecutive eyes. The ABCDEF guide. Ophthalmology. 2013; 120:766-72.
3. Venda Z, Walton D, Chen T. Glaucoma in juvenile xanthogranuloma. Semin Ophthalmol. 2006; 21:191-4.

Hyphema

28

John P Wooten, Kent L Anderson

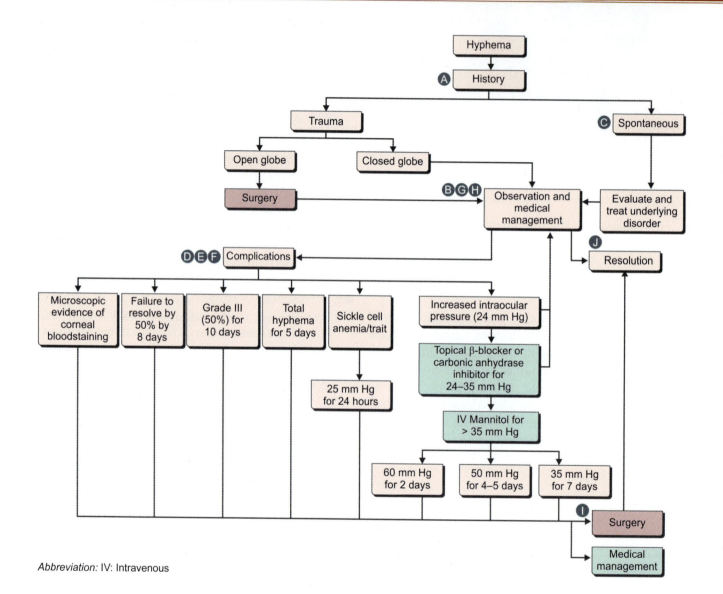

Abbreviation: IV: Intravenous

Hyphema, defined as blood in the anterior chamber of the eye, occurs most commonly as a complication of blunt or lacerating ocular injury. The anterior chamber, normally filled with clear aqueous humor secreted from the ciliary body, is bordered anteriorly by the cornea, posteriorly by the lens and iris, and circumferentially by the angle formed by the junction of the cornea and iris. Important angle structures include the anterior ciliary body, trabecular meshwork, and the canal of Schlemm. During direct blunt injury, there is rapid anterior-posterior compression of the globe, equatorial expansion and increased intraocular pressure. This may cause shearing of the blood vessels of the ciliary body and the iris root leading to hemorrhage into the anterior chamber of the eye. The tearing of the iris root and angle vasculature occurs as the iris and lens are displaced posteriorly. The most common site of bleeding is from the vessels of the anterior ciliary body; however, iris tears, iridodialysis, and cyclodialysis are possible. Hemorrhaging is usually limited due to platelet clot formation, vessel spasm and intraocular tamponade. Clot absorption occurs when fibrinolytic activity releases free red blood cells and fibrin degradation products, which are cleared from the anterior chamber via the trabecular meshwork and the canal of Schlemm. The vasculature within the iris also provides a small contribution to clearance of the clot. Bleeding from lacerating injury is due to direct injury to vessels. Postoperative hyphema is usually due to damaged uveal vessels or bleeding from granulation tissue. Hyphema can also be spontaneous or occur with minor trauma, which can be indicative of an underlying systemic disorder, intraocular tumor, or medication effect.

A. The first step in the evaluation of hyphema is obtaining a thorough history, including a history of present illness, medical and surgical history, medications, and prior eye injuries. Patients with hyphema commonly present with a history of trauma, decreased vision, and/or pain in the affected eye. Important conditions to remember when taking a history include sickle cell disease/trait, hematologic disorders, anticoagulation, and platelet inhibition since these processes can alter management and increase risk of complications. A complete eye examination including measurement of intraocular pressure and a dilated funduscopic examination must be done when evaluating a patient with hyphema. However, if trauma is the suspected cause, it is important to rule out an open globe with careful inspection and imaging before any manipulation of the eye since external pressure can lead to further expulsion of intraocular contents. Computed tomography of the orbit in fine (1.0–2.0 mm) axial and coronal cuts along with clinical reasoning is preferred in patients with a suspected open globe. Plain film and computed tomography may also reveal fractures, foreign bodies, cranial bleeds and retrobulbar hematomas. B-scan ultrasonography is also a useful tool in evaluating internal ocular anatomy and foreign bodies without exposure to radiation. Ultrasound provides a real-time view of the retina and vitreous

when a funduscopic examination is difficult. Even in the case of a suspected open globe, ocular ultrasound can be used carefully with excess gel applied to the eyelid as long as no contact is made between the probe and skin. Alternatively, ultrasound can be used after a globe repair. Until an open globe can be surgically repaired, an eye shield should be placed to prevent further manipulation and aggressive pain control and antiemetics should be administered to prevent increases in intraocular pressure from crying and vomiting.

B. Under slit-lamp examination, hyphema can be classified according to percentage of the anterior chamber filled with blood. Microhyphema is considered red blood cells visible under slit-lamp only. Most commonly, hyphemas are grade I, which is less than one-third of the anterior chamber filled with blood. Grade II is less than one half of the anterior chamber filled, grade III is greater than one half, but less than 100% filled, and grade IV is considered an anterior chamber completely filled with blood. Higher grade is associated with increased risk of secondary rebleeding, increased intraocular pressure and corneal bloodstaining. Hyphema grade, intraocular pressure and corneal bloodstaining should be evaluated daily, especially in the first 4 days following the onset of hyphema. Frequent documentation of the size of the hyphema is important in monitoring the clearance of blood from the anterior chamber, or it can indicate secondary hemorrhaging if fluid level is increased.

C. Trauma is the most common cause of hyphema; however, it can occur spontaneously or in concurrence with minor trauma. Spontaneous hyphema may occur in conditions such as rubeosis iridis (neovascularization of the iris associated with proliferative diabetic retinopathy, chronic retinal detachment, carotid artery stenosis, central retinal vein occlusion), juvenile xanthogranuloma, melanoma and leiomyosarcoma of the iris, iris vascular tufts (microhemangiomas), herpes zoster uveitis and fragile iris vasculature. In addition, hematologic disorders such as leukemia, hemophilia, von Willebrand disease, and thrombocytopenia may cause hyphema in the absence of trauma. Patients taking warfarin long-term for anticoagulation and medications that inhibit platelets are also at risk. In children without a history of trauma and a negative workup for underlying predisposing disorders, abuse must be considered. Spontaneous hyphema should be managed acutely; however, long-term management should be geared toward treating the underlying disease process.

D. Secondary hemorrhage is a common complication of hyphema as one fourth of grade I and the majority of grade III and IV hyphemas will result in secondary hemorrhage. These rebleeds usually occurs within a week of the initial injury and is typically more severe than the initial hyphema. It includes the above-mentioned risks with a worse prognosis. Patients with coagulopathies and hemoglobinopathies should be treated more aggressively as an increased risk of secondary hemorrhage has been reported. Additionally, platelet disorders and medications that inhibit platelet activity carry an increased risk of rebleed.

E. Elevated intraocular pressure (≥24 mm Hg), occurs in about one-third of patients. Debris such as erythrocytes, platelets, and fibrin degradation products may obstruct the trabecular meshwork decreasing fluid outflow and increasing pressure. Patients with sickle cell trait/disease are at increased risk for increased intraocular pressure. The hypoxic and relatively acidic environment within the anterior chamber promotes red blood cell sickling which leads to a higher likelihood of outflow obstruction. Elevated pressures for extended periods of time can cause irreversible damage to the optic nerve and anterior chamber structures causing secondary glaucoma.

F. Corneal bloodstaining is another complication of hyphema, occurring most commonly in association with grade III and IV hyphemas, secondary hemorrhage, and prolonged elevated intraocular pressure above 25 mm Hg. Prior or current corneal epithelial damage increases risk. Permanent vision loss is possible and staining can take as long as two years to resolve.

G. The main objectives in hyphema management are minimizing risk for secondary hemorrhage and secondary glaucoma. Hospital admission for treatment is based on clinical judgment and should be considered in higher risk patients with secondary hemorrhage, persistent increased intraocular pressure, grade II or higher hyphema, loss of vision, hematologic disorders, and for children and noncompliance. Patients with hyphema should be placed sitting at a 30° angle to allow the fluid level to settle inferiorly out of the visual axis, and to help increase clearance of the hyphema. A metal eye shield is typically used until resolution of the hyphema to prevent further injury and to help immobilize the eye. Some authors have argued against patching the eye closed due to increase in bacterial growth, so topical antibiotics may be appropriate. Bed rest with careful ambulation is important to prevent further injury. Video games should be avoided in patients with hyphema due to the increased eye movement that occurs; therefore, patients and/or parents of patients should be cautioned. However, watching television has not been shown to increase risk of complications. Sedation with benzodiazepines to help limit activity may be required in some patients.

H. Cycloplegics such as atropine are an important initial therapy for hyphema because they provide pain relief by decreasing ciliary spasm. Atropine, due to its mydriatic effects, may also facilitate healing by reducing stress on the vessels of the iris due to decreased pupil movement. It has not been shown that cycloplegics have a positive outcome on preventing secondary hemorrhage; however, they are still widely used with this in mind. Atropine, because of pupil dilation, also allows for a better posterior segment examination, which is important in evaluating trauma. In addition, atropine helps prevent the formation of posterior synechiae by keeping the pupil dilated. Atropine dosing for hyphema is one drop for children and up to three drops for adults of 1% atropine daily for up to 5 days. Topical corticosteroids have been shown to decrease intraocular inflammation and reduce the occurrence of secondary hemorrhage. Efficacy of systemic corticosteroids is uncertain; however, visual outcomes have been reported as similar to topical corticosteroids. Secondary hemorrhage can also be reduced with administration of topical and systemic antifibrinolytics. Aminocaproic acid (Amicar) is a lysine analog fibrinolytic that competitively inhibits conversion of plasminogen to plasmin, preventing clot lysis at the damaged blood vessel. Dosing is 50–100 mg/kg by mouth every four hours for 5 days, but not in excess of 30 g/day or one drop every four hours for 5 days. Aminocaproic acid should be used with caution in patients with large (grade III or IV) hyphemas as prolonged presence of a clot can increase intraocular pressure and increase risk of corneal bloodstaining. Intraocular pressures between 24 mm Hg and 35 mm Hg can be managed with topical β-blockers and carbonic anhydrase inhibitors. Acetazolamide should not be used in patients with sickle cell trait and disease because it lowers blood pH and promotes sickling of red blood cells, which further increases risk of outflow obstruction in a predisposed population. Patients with intraocular pressures above 35 mm Hg can be treated with systemic mannitol, which creates an osmotic gradient due to its impermeability to vessel membranes. Mannitol is given intravenously, and dosed at 1.5 mg/kg in 10% solution over 45 minutes twice daily for hyphema.

I. Surgical evacuation of the clot is indicated in patients with uncontrolled intraocular hypertension with a failed response to medical therapy. Suggested guidelines for surgical intervention are intraocular pressures greater than or equal to 60 mm Hg for 2 days, greater than or equal to 50 mm Hg for 4–5 days, and greater than or equal to 35 mm Hg for 7 days. Other suggested indications for surgery include hyphemas that are grade III or larger for more than 10 days duration, and microscopic evidence of early corneal bloodstaining. Patients with sickle cell anemia with pressures of at least 25 mm Hg for 24 hours or with pressures frequently spiking above 30 mm Hg require surgery. Persistent total hyphemas lasting more than 4 days or failure of anterior chamber volume to drop 50% by 8 days have also been suggested in the literature as indications for surgery.

J. Grade I hyphemas typically resolve within 5 days. Grades II, III, and IV are associated with increased risk of complications such as secondary hemorrhage, corneal bloodstaining, secondary glaucoma, elevated intraocular pressure with optic nerve atrophy, and vision loss. About three-fourths of all eyes with traumatic hyphema will return to a visual acuity of 20/50 or better; however, chances of returning to at least 20/50 decrease as grade increases. Follow-up care should include a 1-month gonioscopy examination to evaluate for potential bleeding sites and angle recession. A dilated retinal examination with scleral depression is also suggested at 1 month to exclude retinal damage.

BIBLIOGRAPHY

1. Blaivas M, Theodoro D, Sierzenski PR. A study of bedside ocular ultrasonography in the emergency department. Acad Emerg Med. 2002;9:791-9.
2. Brandt MT, Haug RH. Traumatic hyphema: A comprehensive review. J Oral Maxillofac Surg. 2001;59:1462-70.
3. Harlan JB Jr, Pieramici DJ. Evaluation of patients with ocular trauma. Ophthalmol Clin N Am. 2002;15:153-61.
4. Sankar PS, Chen TC, Grosskreutz CL, et al. Traumatic hyphema. Int Ophthalmol Clin. 2002;42:57-68.
5. Walton W, Von Hagen S, Grigorian R, et al. Management of traumatic hyphema. Surv Ophthalmol. 2002;47:297-334.

Hypopyon

29

Lilian Nguyen, Kent L Anderson

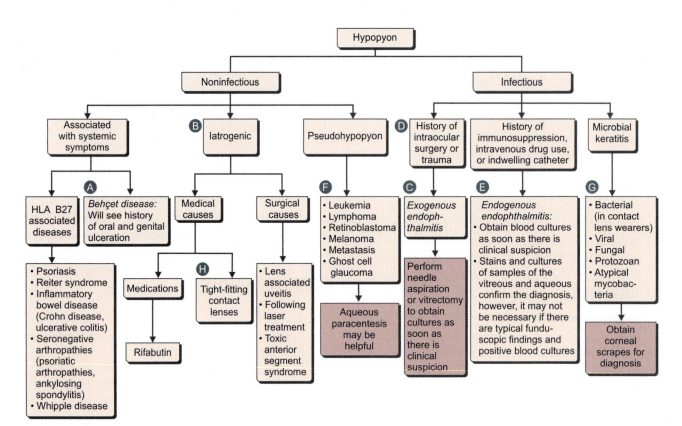

Abbreviation: HLA: Human Leucocyte Antigen

Hypopyon is the gravity-dependent layering of white blood cells in the anterior chamber. It is the continuum of uveitis, inflammation of the tissues of the eye seen as white blood cells dispersed throughout the anterior chamber. Hypopyon is a nonspecific reaction resulting from inflammation, infection, or malignancy, and also has an association with systemic disease. Obtaining a thorough history from the patient and performing a detailed examination of the eye is necessary to guide the differential diagnosis. When seen it is a useful clinical marker, as it tends to occur in specific conditions. Because the various underlying causes may have serious vision-threatening consequences requiring different management and treatment options, knowledge of the main causes of hypopyon is of utmost importance.

A. Hypopyon may be found in noninfectious diseases such as Behçet disease; a rare systemic disease affecting young adults 20–40 years of age. The common clinical feature is recurrent and painful mucocutaneous ulcers, however, the greatest morbidity and mortality occur with ocular disease as it may progress to blindness if left untreated. Ocular disease in Behçet disease includes bilateral and episodic pan-uveitis that may not completely resolve between episodes, hypopyon, retinal vasculitis and optic neuritis. Behçet disease is diagnosed on clinical grounds alone that rely on the recognition of ocular and systemic findings in a patient, commonly described as a triad of uveitis with oral and genital ulceration. The hypopyon usually resolves with topical corticosteroid treatment for several days; however, severe ocular disease with posterior segment involvement requires treatment with immunosuppressive agents such as infliximab, adalimumab or interferon-alpha.

B. There are iatrogenic causes of hypopyon as well. In a human immunodeficiency virus (HIV) positive patient, use of rifabutin—an agent used in the prophylaxis and treatment of *Mycobacterium avium* complex—may result in a sterile hypopyon. In this case, treatment with topical steroids leads to resolution within 24–48 hours. Other iatrogenic causes of hypopyon include surgical causes, in which case the first priority should be to exclude or treat infection. Sterile hypopyon may result from severe postoperative inflammation after intraocular surgery (toxic anterior segment syndrome) or as a reaction to retained lens fragments after cataract surgery (lens-associated uveitis). Definitive treatment is complete removal of lens remnants from the eye; however, postoperative inflammation should be treated with topical steroids. Hypopyon following laser treatment in either the anterior or the posterior segment has also been reported.

C. Hypopyon following cataract surgery is seen in exogenous endophthalmitis. The onset of symptoms—decreasing vision and pain—usually occurs within 1 week following cataract surgery. On physical examination, the lid may be swollen, the conjunctiva injected or edematous, a hypopyon is present, view of the retina is hazy, and slit-lamp examination reveals intraocular white blood cells and protein. Needle aspiration or vitrectomy to obtain cultures of the aqueous or vitreous should be done as soon as there is clinical suspicion. The endophthalmitis vitrectomy study (EVS) demonstrated the benefit of early intravitreal antibiotic injection and of vitrectomy if there is severe vision loss on presentation that fails to improve after 24–48 hours.

D. Chronic pseudophakic-related endophthalmitis is a rare complication of cataract surgery that may also present with hypopyon. This infection is characterized by low-grade intraocular inflammation that may last for months. Symptoms include decreased vision and mild eye pain. Slit-lamp examination reveals white blood cells in the anterior chamber and a characteristic white plaque in the posterior lens capsule, along with a hypopyon and white blood cells in the anterior vitreous. Diagnosis is based on clinical suspicion and confirmed by cultures of the aqueous or posterior lens capsule. As with acute postcataract endophthalmitis, treatment requires at least vitrectomy and intravitreal antibiotics. Removing the entire lens capsule and exchanging the intraocular lens for a new one may also be necessary. The EVS also showed the lack of benefit of systemic intravenous antibiotics in both acute and chronic cases.

E. Hypopyon is also seen in endogenous endophthalmitis, which results from seeding of the eye from the bloodstream. The most common cause is infection of a fungal species, but bacterial species may also be involved. In patients who present with eye pain, decreased vision and panuveitis, with risk factors—immunosuppression, intravenous drug use and an indwelling catheter—endogenous fungal endophthalmitis should be considered in the differential diagnosis. Findings in endogenous *Candida endophthalmitis* include fluffy white lesions in the choroid and retina, with overlying vitreous inflammation that has a clumped appearance, often described as 'fluff balls' or 'string of pearls'. Endogenous mold endophthalmitis often has a similar appearance. Blood cultures should be obtained from all patients with suspected endogenous endophthalmitis. Stains and cultures of samples of the vitreous and aqueous confirm the diagnosis. Obtaining intraocular samples for diagnosis may not be necessary if there are typical fundoscopic findings and positive blood cultures. Treatment may involve both systemic and local intravitreal antifungal therapy. Severe cases may require vitrectomy.

F. Malignancy may mimic hypopyon, as tumor cells may enter the anterior chamber and layer behind the cornea and is referred to as a pseudohypopyon. Retinoblastomas have a tendency to form pseudo-hypopyon because they are friable tumors that grow into and seed the vitreous, and then enter the anterior chamber. Leukocoria (white pupil) is the most common presenting finding. Other presentations include strabismus, decreased vision, ocular inflammation, and family history. Diagnosis is made during indirect ophthalmoscopic examination with a characteristic finding of a chalky white-gray retinal mass that is soft and friable. If the diagnosis is in doubt, aqueous paracentesis may be helpful. Once the diagnosis is made, therapeutic options include enucleation, external beam radiation therapy, radioactive plaques, cryotherapy, laser photoablation and chemotherapy.

G. Corneal disorders may also result in hypopyon. Bacterial keratitis occurs in contact lens wearers and may rapidly progress to corneal ulceration with hypopyon. Dry ocular surfaces, topical corticosteroid use, and immunosuppression may also predispose to bacterial keratitis. Patients present with a corneal opacity or infiltrate along with red eye, photophobia, foreign body sensation and mucopurulent discharge. The infiltrate or ulcer will stain with fluorescein and may be seen with a penlight and does not require a slit-lamp for identification. After obtaining cultures, promptly treat with topical broad spectrum antibiotics.

H. Contact lens-related infectious keratitis may also result in a hypopyon that is a sterile inflammatory reaction in response to the overlying corneal inflammation. Upon slit-lamp examination, white infiltrates are seen in the anterior stroma, usually in the peripheral cornea near the limbus. Diagnosis is usually made during routine eye examination in contact lens wearers. These sterile infiltrates respond well to topical antibiotic coverage and a short course of topical steroids along with temporary elimination of contact lens wear. Tight-fitting contact lenses may also cause sterile hypopyon and corneal stromal edema with small peripheral infiltrates. Treatment is removal of the contact lens along with a short course of artificial tears, topical steroids, and topical antibiotic coverage.

BIBLIOGRAPHY

1. Abramson DH, Frank CM, Susman M, et al. Presenting signs of retinoblastoma. J Pediatr. 1998;132:505-8.
2. Bates AK, Morris RJ, Stapleton F, et al. 'Sterile' corneal infiltrates in contact lens wearers. Eye. 1989;3:803-10.
3. Clark WL, Kaiser PK, Flynn HW Jr, et al. Treatment strategies and visual acuity outcomes in chronic postoperative Propionibacterium acnes endophthalmitis. Ophthalmology. 1999;106:1665-70.
4. Endophthalmitis Vitrectomy Study Group. Results of the endophthalmitis vitrectomy study: A randomized trial of immediate vitrectomy and of intravenous antibiotics for the treatment of postoperative bacterial endophthalmitis. Arch Ophthalmol. 1995;113:1479-96.
5. Evereklioglu C. Ocular Behcet disease: Current therapeutic approaches. Curr Opin Ophthalmol. 2011;22:508-16.
6. Lingappan A, Wykoff CC, Albini TA, et al. Endogenous fungal endophthalmitis: Causative organisms, management strategies, and visual acuity outcomes. Am J Ophthalmol. 2012;153:162-6.
7. Ramsay A, Lightman S. Hypopyon uveitis. Surv Ophthalmol. 2001;46:1-18.
8. Taban M, Behrens A, Newcomb RL, et al. Acute endophthalmitis following cataract surgery: A systematic review of the literature. Arch Ophthalmol. 2005;123:613-20.
9. Tugal-Tutkun I, Onal S, Altan-Yaycioglu R, et al. Uveitis in Behçet disease: An analysis of 880 patients. Am J Ophthalmol. 2004;138:373-80.
10. Wykoff CC, Flynn HW Jr, Miller D, et al. Exogenous fungal endophthalmitis: Microbiology and clinical outcomes. Ophthalmology. 2008;115:1501-7.
11. Zaidi AA, Ying GS, Daneil E, et al. Hypopyon in patients with uveitis. Ophthalmology. 2010;117:366-72.

Microphthalmos

Johan Zwaan

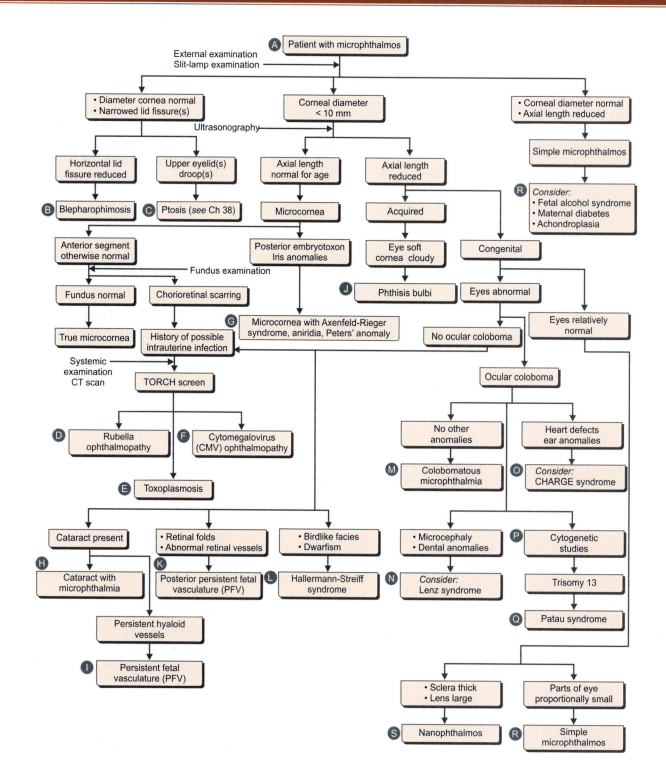

30

Microphthalmos is defined as an eye that is congenitally smaller than the norm. This means an axial length of less than 21 mm in an adult or less than 16 mm in a newborn. The anomaly consists of a group of diverse disorders, which is classified as simple (no other ocular anomalies) or complex (combination with other eye anomalies, cataract or vitreoretinal disease). The complex category is further divided in colobomatous and noncolobomatous.

A. When a patient or parent reports that an eye appears smaller than normal, true microphthalmos may be present or the eye may have microcornea. A microcornea has a horizontal diameter of less than 10 mm in the adult or less than 9 mm in an infant. Although usually occurring in combination, microphthalmos can be present with a normal-sized cornea and vice versa. Narrowing of the lid fissure may cause the eye to look smaller than it is.

B. The blepharophimosis syndrome is characterized by shortening of the horizontal lid fissure, ptosis, telecanthus and epicanthus inversus. There are two types with autosomal inheritance, in one of which the affected women are infertile. It may also occur sporadically and is often secondary to anophthalmos or extreme microphthalmos, in which orbital and eyelid growths are reduced.

C. Ptosis may give the impression that the eye on the involved side is small, particularly when the ptosis is one-sided or asymmetric (chapter 38).

D. Several intrauterine infections can affect eye size. Infections with the rubella virus in the first trimester cause infection of the embryo in 50% of cases. In the rubella syndrome, microphthalmos may be combined with cataracts and pigmentary "salt-and-pepper" retinopathy. The retinopathy usually does not reduce vision significantly. Glaucoma and keratitis are less common. Systemic problems include congenital heart defects, sensorineural deafness, and growth and mental retardation.

E. The offspring of women who become infected with toxoplasmosis in the first trimester have the most severe manifestations of the disease. Although infections later in pregnancy may give minimal or no abnormalities, some neonates who have initially negative examinations may later develop the syndrome. Microphthalmos is always accompanied in this syndrome by chorioretinitis, which is the most common expression of the syndrome. Other findings include intracranial calcifications, hydrocephalus, microcephalus, seizures and jaundice. The intracranial abnormalities may cause blindness more often than the chorioretinitis, which will reduce vision, particularly when the macular area is involved, but not abolish it.

F. Cytomegalovirus (CMV) infects up to 2–3% of newborns, making it the most common intrauterine infection. However, less than one-fifth of the infected babies develop congenital anomalies. Microphthalmos is relatively mild. Chorioretinitis, which causes less pigmented scars than toxoplasmosis, and optic atrophy develop in 6% of the fetuses of women having a primary CMV infection during pregnancy. Microcephalus, hydrocephalus, cerebral calcifications that are typically located periventricularly, and cerebral atrophy may be present. Less common eye manifestations are cataract, glaucoma and keratitis.

G. All of the anterior segment dysgenesis syndromes, as well as aniridia, may be associated with microcornea.

H. Nuclear cataracts often are found together with microcornea. This combination may be autosomal dominant. The microcornea and small anterior chamber make lensectomy or lens aspiration more difficult.

I. Anterior persistent hyperplastic primary vitreous (PHPV) or persistent fetal vasculature (PFV) is characterized by persistence of the hyaloid vasculature. A fibrovascular membrane covers the posterior surface of the lens and sometimes invades the lens. It is connected to the optic disc or less commonly to retinal vessels by a stalk containing the hyaloid artery. Contraction of the membrane pulls the ciliary processes under the lens, resulting in a highly characteristic pigmented fringe behind the lens periphery. This same contraction moves the lens-iris diaphragm forward, narrowing the anterior chamber angle and eventually leading to angle-closure glaucoma, which is difficult to treat. Most cases are sporadic and involve only one eye, although bilateral and familial PFV have been reported. Visual outcome after surgery is

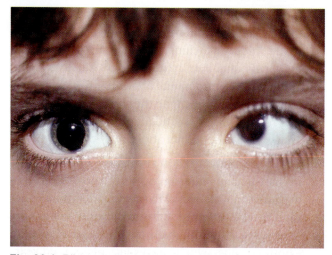

Fig. 30.1: Bilateral microphthalmia, left more than right, due to large chorioretinal colobomas.

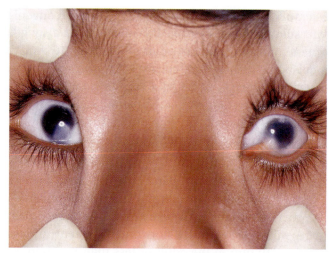

Fig. 30.2: Colobomatous microphthalmia, with X-linked inheritance.

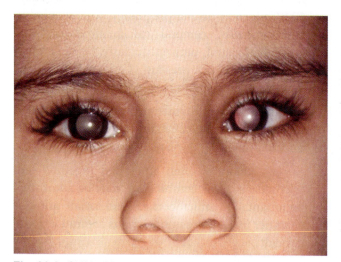

Fig. 30.3: Child with nanophthalmic eyes.

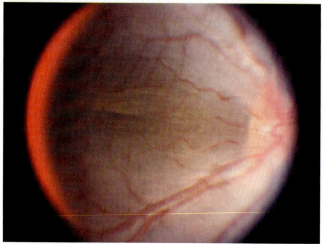

Fig. 30.4: Retinal folding in nanophthalmic eye.

often surprisingly good and depends partially on the extent of retinal involvement and on the patient's age at surgery. In less severe cases, the fibrovascular membrane is limited to a peripheral sector of the lens and the vascular stalk inserts into the peripheral retina.

J. Chronic uveitis or hypotony may lead to atrophy of the eye. The eye shrinks and the contents become disorganized. This is called phthisis bulbi. Tumors may be present in such an eye and need to be excluded. In young children retinoblastoma can occur, whereas in adults uveal melanomas may be present.

K. Posterior PFV is also called congenital retinal fold. There is a fold of retina and condensed vitreous running from the disc to the periphery, sometimes up to the ora serrata. Abnormal blood vessels are seen within the fold, presumably remnants of anastomoses between hyaloid and retinal vasculature. The eye is microphthalmic, and there is no cataract, unlike in anterior PFV. Because of macular involvement, the vision is usually poor and esotropia and nystagmus may result.

L. Patients with Hallermann-Streiff syndrome have a birdlike face with hypotrichosis, dental abnormalities and short stature. The eyes are severely microphthalmic, with small corneae and cataracts, which often reabsorb spontaneously. The inheritance pattern is unclear.

M. Colobomas are the most common cause of microphthalmos. They may be isolated or part of a syndrome with systemic abnormalities. The inheritance is autosomal dominant with variable expression, although recessive and rarely X-linked inheritance has been reported. Many cases are sporadic. Vision is always reduced because the chorioretinal colobomas have to be large for the eye to become microphthalmic.

N. In Lenz syndrome, microphthalmia is combined with vertebral, dental and urogenital anomalies and with heart defects. Inheritance is X-linked.

O. CHARGE syndrome stands for coloboma, heart defects, choanal atresia, retarded growth, genital anomalies, and ear anomalies. It usually is sporadic, although rare familial occurrences have been reported.

P. A variety of chromosomal anomalies may be associated with colobomatous microphthalmia. Common syndromes are Patau syndrome (trisomy 13), cat eye syndrome (trisomy or tetrasomy 22pter), Wolf-Hirschhorn syndrome (4p-) and triploidy. There are numerous other rare associations.

Q. The main characteristics of Patau syndrome are colobomas, cleft lip and palate and polydactyly. The colobomas are extensive and involve the iris, ciliary body, retina/choroid and optic disc. The eye is usually microphthalmic, although not always. The retina is dysplastic, and cartilage develops in the eye. Almost all organ systems can be involved. Severe cardiac and central nervous system (CNS) anomalies limit life expectancy. Only 5% of the infants survive beyond age 3 years.

R. Various reports indicate that 50–80% of patients with simple microphthalmos have a systemic disease such as fetal alcohol syndrome, fetal exposure to other toxins (vitamin A, thalidomide, warfarin) or to maternal diabetes mellitus, fetal infections (rubella and others), or a large variety of inherited syndromes.

S. Nanophthalmos is a rare form of microphthalmos in which the eye is proportionally smaller in all directions. The axial length is 16.0–18.5 mm and the eye is very hyperopic (10 or more diopters). The lens is large relative to eye size, and the cornea is small. This causes the iris to bow forward, resulting in a very shallow anterior chamber and a narrow chamber angle. Angle closure glaucoma often follows. The sclera is thicker than usual, impeding venous outflow through the vortex veins. This causes uveal effusions and choroidal detachments spontaneously, but in particular during and after intraocular surgery. The detachments also contribute to angle-closure glaucoma.

BIBLIOGRAPHY

1. Fowler KB, Stagno S, Pass RE, et al. The outcome of congenital cytomegalovirus infection in relation to maternal antibody status. N Engl J Med. 1992;326:663-7.
2. Koppe JG, Loewer-Sieger DH, Roever-Bonnet H. Results of 20-year follow-up of congenital toxoplasmosis. Lancet. 1986;1:254-6.
3. Mullaney PB, Karcioglu ZA, AI Mesfer SA, et al. Presentation of retinoblastoma as phthisis bulbi. Eye. 1997;11:403-8.
4. Pollard Z. Treatment of persistent hyperplastic primary vitreous. J Pediatr Ophthalmol Strabismus. 1985;22:180-3.
5. Warburg M. Classification of microphthalmos and coloboma. J Med Genet. 1993;30:664-9.
6. Weiss AH, Kousseff BG, Ross EA, Longbottom J. Complex microphthalmos. Arch Ophthalmol. 1989;107:1619-24.
7. Weiss AH, Kousseff BG, Ross EA, Longbottom J. Simple microphthalmos. Arch Ophthalmol. 1989;107:1625-30.

Macrophthalmos

31

Johan Zwaan

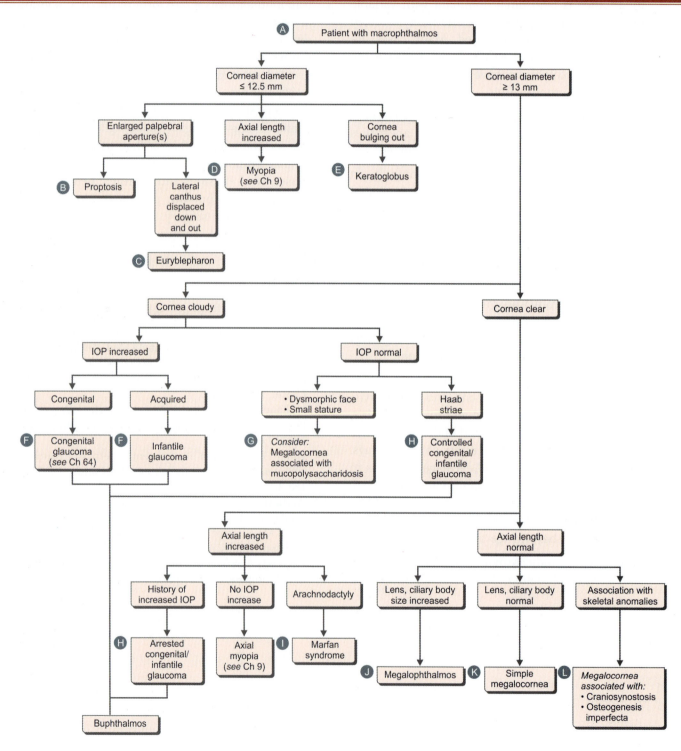

An eye that is larger than the norm expected for a patient's age is called *macrophthalmos*. The size of the normal eye changes dramatically during the first few years of life. Axial length averages 16–17 mm at term. Because of the very rapid postnatal growth phase it gains 3.5–4 mm in the next 18 months. Growth slows down to 1.1 mm from age 2 to 5 years and even more from age 5 to 13 years (1.3 mm). After the age of 13, growth is negligible. The average axial length from this time on is 23 mm.

A. Certain conditions give the appearance of macrophthalmos even when the ocular size is normal. The corneal diameter may be increased or the eye may be more prominent than usual because of exophthalmos or retraction of the eyelids. Measurement of the diameter of the cornea by slit lamp examination or with calipers and of the ocular axial length by ultrasonography may be necessary to differentiate megalocornea and anterior megalophthalmos from true macrophthalmos. The normal cornea has a horizontal diameter of 9.5–10 mm at birth. At 1 year of age it has grown to 11.5–12 mm and at age 3 years and beyond the diameter is 12 mm. If the cornea is adult size at birth (12.5 mm or 13 mm at age 2 years and beyond), it is considered enlarged and called *megalocornea*.

B. When the eye is proptotic because of thyroid orbitopathy (Chapter 46), or another orbital pathologic condition, when the orbits are shallow as seen in craniofacial anomalies, such as Apert or Crouzon syndrome, or in eyelid retraction, patients or parents often believe that the globe is enlarged. Standard clinical examination is usually adequate to lay this idea to rest.

C. Euryblepharon is a congenital abnormality of the eyelids. The lateral canthus is displaced downward and outward, and the lower eyelid downward. The palpebral fissure is enlarged. This may give the erroneous impression that the eye is larger than normal. The abnormality may be autosomal dominant. It is sometimes seen in Down syndrome and in craniofacial anomalies.

D. In myopia, the cornea usually is normal in diameter. Refraction or cycloplegic retinoscopy will give the diagnosis.

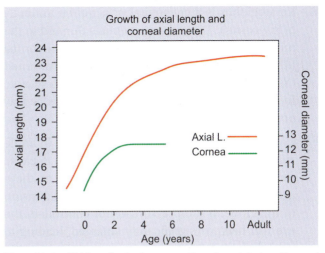

Fig. 31.1: Table displaying growth of axial length and corneal diameter.

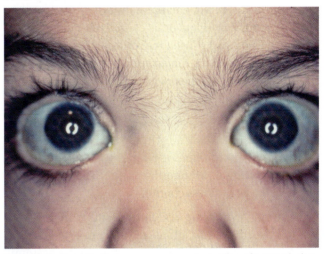

Fig. 31.2: Seemingly large eyes are in reality of normal size, due to euryblepharon.

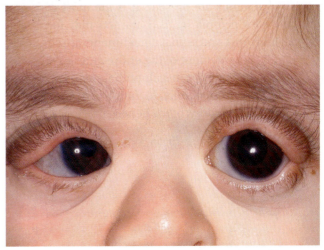

Fig. 31.3: Gigantism of the left eye in a patient with neurofibromatosis type 1.

E. Keratoglobus is a congenital or acquired anomaly of the cornea. The corneal stroma is thinned in the mid-periphery, leading to a bulging out of the cornea in a globular configuration. It may be inherited (X-linked) or occur in association with blue sclerae. In Down and Rubinstein-Taybi syndromes, it may occur acutely as a form of hydrops.

F. Congenital glaucoma is present at birth; infantile glaucoma occurs in the first year of life. Because the sclera and cornea are more elastic at these ages, increased ocular pressure causes expansion of the globe. If the pressure is not controlled, the eye will become significantly enlarged, leading to buphthalmos.

G. Mucopolysaccharidoses cause clouding of the cornea and rarely enlargement of the cornea. Rule out secondary glaucoma caused by thickening of the cornea and consequent anterior chamber angle narrowing and/or the accumulation of metabolites in the trabecular meshwork.

H. If congenital or infantile glaucoma is controlled early enough by surgical or medical means, the corneal diameter may still be within normal limits. If the control is borderline or poor, elongation of the eye may continue. Monitoring of the axial length is a useful way to assess control.

I. Marfan syndrome is autosomal dominant. It is caused by mutations of the fibrillin gene on chromosome 15q 21.1. In addition to the systemic findings of cardiac and skeletal anomalies, ocular abnormalities are present. It is the most common cause for ectopia lentis. Cataracts may form, and high myopia and retinal detachments are common. Rarely, enlargement of the entire anterior segment is present (anterior megalophthalmos). Expression may vary from family to family because of the different mutations of the gene.

J. In (anterior) megalophthalmos, the ciliary ring and the lens-iris diaphragm are enlarged as well as the cornea. Iridodonesis, iris transillumination, lens dislocation and high myopia/astigmatism can result. This may be an isolated condition, but it has been found in association with Apert syndrome, Marfan syndrome and mucolipidosis type 2.

K. Simple megalocornea is an X-linked disorder, although other inheritance patterns have been reported. The cornea is clear, and thickness and endothelial cell density are normal. The diameter may be as large as 18 mm. It is differentiated from congenital glaucoma because the cornea is clear and intraocular pressure (IOP) is normal, as is the optic nerve.

L. Megalocornea may be associated with a variety of systemic disorders, such as Alport syndrome, craniofacial anomalies, Marfan syndrome, facial hemihypertrophy, mucolipidosis type 2 and Down syndrome.

BIBLIOGRAPHY

1. Curtin BJ. The Myopias: Basic Science and Clinical Management. Philadelphia: Harper & Row; 1985.
2. Egbert JE, Kushner BJ. Excessive loss of hyperopia. A presenting sign of juvenile aphakic glaucoma. Arch Ophthalmol. 1990;108:1257-9.
3. Hoskins HD, Shaffer RN, Hetherington J. Anatomical classification of developmental glaucomas. Arch Ophthalmol. 1984;102:1331-6.
4. Hoyt CS, Billson FA. Buphthalmos in neurofibromatosis: is it an expression of regional gigantism? J Pediatr Ophthalmol. 1977;14:228-34.
5. Mackey DA, Buttery RG, Wise GM, et al. Description of X-linked megalocornea with identification of the gene locus. Arch Ophthalmol. 1991;109:829-33.
6. Maumenee IH. The Marfan syndrome is caused by a point mutation in the fibrillin gene. Arch Ophthalmol. 1992;110:472-3.

32

Painful Orbital Swelling

Constance L Fry

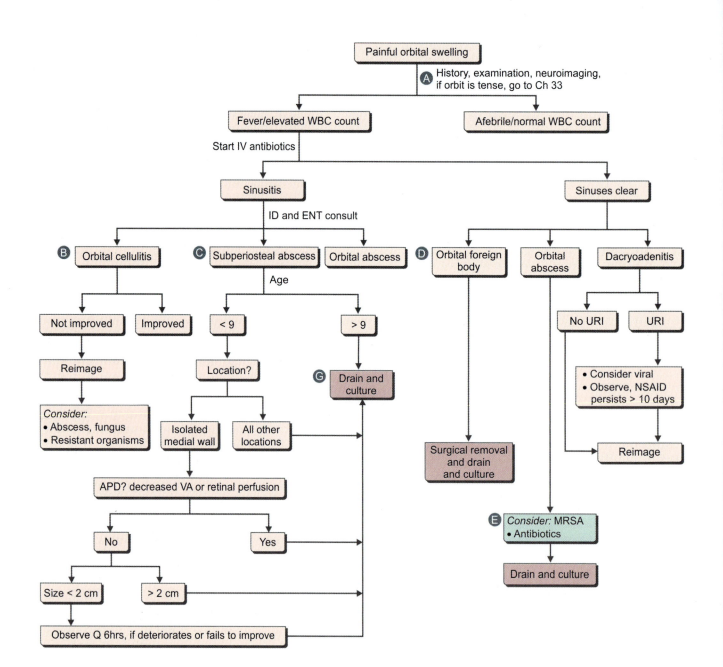

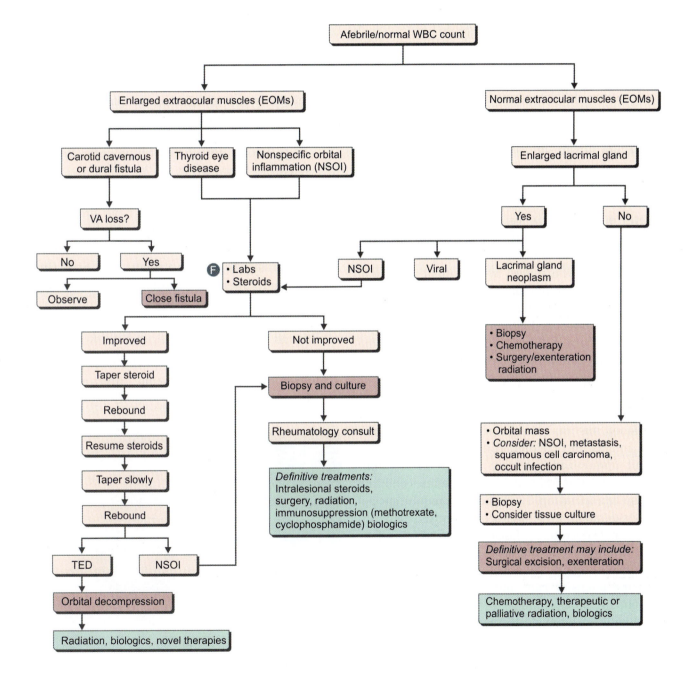

A. The evaluation of a patient with painful orbital swelling requires a comprehensive history, and a complete eye examination paying particular attention to the vision, pupils, palpation of the orbit, adenopathy and extraocular motility. If the patient appears toxic, the temperature and white blood cell count should be evaluated. The presence of adenopathy points toward a malignancy, viral etiology or rarely a gonococcal infection. A contrasted computed tomography (CT) scan of the orbits and sinuses is performed acutely. CT scans image the bone well and are ideal in the setting of trauma. In the absence of retained metallic foreign body or other contraindications, magnetic resonance imaging (MRI) is superior to CT in imaging fungal infections, the orbital apex and retained wooden foreign bodies. Painful swelling of the lids without orbital involvement is most commonly a preseptal cellulitis.

B. Over 90% of orbital cellulitis is associated with sinusitis. Typically, these patients are admitted for intravenous antibiotics until improvement is seen and then managed by outpatient therapy in the absence of immunosuppression or atypical presentations. Orbital cellulitis in adults and teenagers associated with sinusitis is usually caused by mixed flora, thus broad-spectrum antibiotics are indicated. Certain instances require special antibiotic coverage including: exposure to freshwater after a bite, associated dental abscesses, diabetics and otherwise immunocompromised patients. In infants, maternal mastitis should be considered. In infants and children consult the pediatrician, and immunization history against *Haemophilus influenzae* should be queried. Sometimes children require a spinal tap. Two conditions require special consideration in immunocompromised patients. The first, necrotizing fasciitis is characterized by rapid progression and facial numbness. This may require surgical debridement and stabilization in the intensive care unit as mortality rates are high. The other is fungal infection. Fungal orbital cellulitis can be an elusive diagnosis. Neuroimaging abnormalities may be subtle and the clinical examination should dictate treatment.

C. The vast majority of subperiosteal abscesses (SPA) and all orbital abscesses require urgent drainage.

The only SPA that can be managed expectantly in the hospital is in a child less than 9 years old with an isolated medial wall abscess that is less than 2 cm and is without an afferent pupillary defect (APD). If the fever lasts more than 36 hours on intravenous antibiotics, if the patient deteriorates after 48 hours or fails to improve after 72 hours, drainage is required (Figs. 32.1 to 32.3).

D. Nonmetallic orbital foreign bodies may be difficult to diagnose and the history should guide therapy. MRI is superior to CT to image wood. Green wood and plastic are often not directly seen. Signs of orbital foreign bodies include a draining fistula and linear tracks of air in the orbit. Symptomatic foreign bodies typically need to be removed. Metallic foreign bodies are often asymptomatic and can usually be observed (Fig. 32.4).

E. When draining orbital infections obtain tissue for tissue culture. If antibiotics have already been started, the laboratory should hold the specimen a minimum of 5 days to improve the chance of determining the causative organism(s). Send Gram stain and cultures for aerobic, anaerobic, fungus and acid-fast bacilli and possibly fungal stains. Fungal and anaerobic organisms can be particularly difficult to isolate.

F. Methicillin-resistant *Staphylococcus aureus* infections present differently and are rarely associated with sinusitis. A third presents with

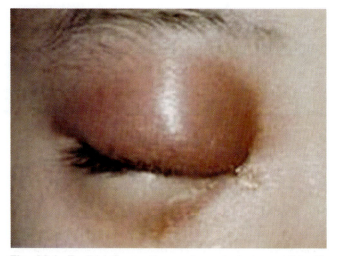

Fig. 32.1: Eyelid inflammation and proptosis in a child with medial wall subperiosteal abscess.

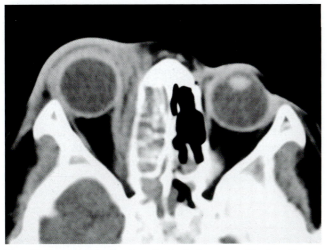

Fig. 32.2: Medial wall subperiosteal abscess with sinusitis.

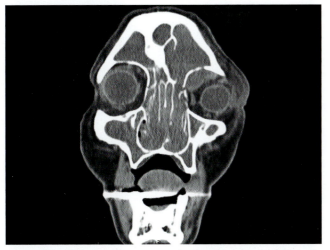

Fig. 32.3: Superior subperiosteal abscess with pansinusitis and *Streptococcus* and *Klebsiella* bacteremia.

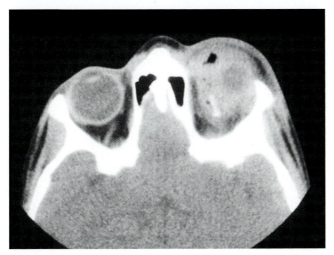

Fig. 32.4: Orbital foreign body with orbital cellulitis, linear tracks of air.

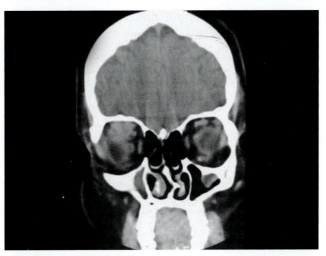

Fig. 32.5: Superior myositis, nonspecific orbital inflammation.

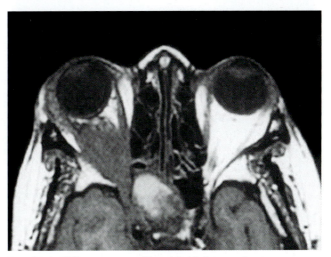

Fig. 32.6: Diffuse nonspecific orbital inflammation.

lacrimal gland infections and a third with multiple abscesses. The overwhelming majority requires surgery.

G. Prior to starting steroids, obtain laboratory studies including complete blood count, angiotensin converting enzyme, sedimentation rate, lysozyme, cytoplasmic antineutrophil cytoplasmic antibodies, perinuclear antineutrophil cytoplasmic antibodies, serum protein electrophoresis and quantiferon gold. Tuberculosis should be excluded. Care should be taken to attempt to avoid use of steroids in atypical fungal infections, obtaining tissue in unclear cases. Other conditions prompting caution are peptic ulcer disease, diabetes, hypertension, psychiatric disorders, osteoporosis, hypothyroidism and hepatic dysfunction. Internal medicine consultation is advisable (Figs. 32.5 and 32.6).

BIBLIOGRAPHY

1. Cockerham KP, Cockerham GC, Zwick OM. Orbital inflammation. Focal Points. 2007;25(3)1-16.
2. Dewan MA, Meyer DR, Wladis EJ. Orbital cellulitis with subperiosteal abscess: demographics and management outcomes. Ophthal Plast Reconstr Surg. 2011;27(5):330-2.
3. Garcia GH, Harris GJ. Criteria for nonsurgical management of subperiosteal abscess of the orbit: analysis of outcomes 1988-1998. Ophthalmology. 2000;107(8):1454-6.
4. Glatt HJ, Custer PL, Barrett L, et al. Magnetic resonance imaging and computed tomography in a model of wooden foreign bodies in the orbit. Ophthal Plast Reconstr Surg. 1990;6(2):108-14.
5. Mathias MT, Horsley MB, Mawn LA, et al. Atypical presentations of orbital cellulitis caused by methicillin-resistant *Staphylococcus aureus*. Ophthalmology. 2012;119(6):1238-43.

Orbital Compartment Syndrome

33

Constance L Fry, Barrett G Haik

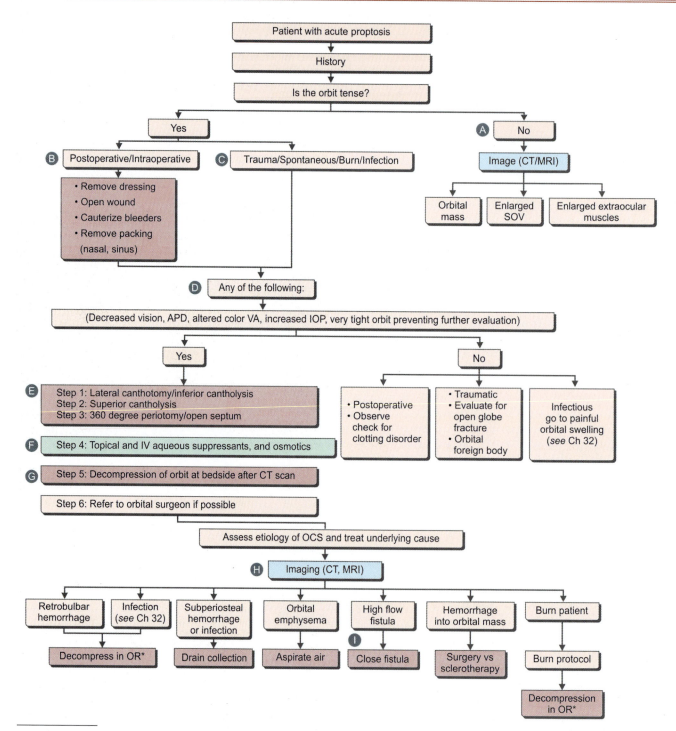

Patient with acute proptosis

History

Is the orbit tense?

Yes — No **A**

B Postoperative/Intraoperative — **C** Trauma/Spontaneous/Burn/Infection — Image (CT/MRI)

• Remove dressing
• Open wound
• Cauterize bleeders
• Remove packing (nasal, sinus)

Orbital mass | Enlarged SOV | Enlarged extraocular muscles

D Any of the following:

(Decreased vision, APD, altered color VA, increased IOP, very tight orbit preventing further evaluation)

Yes — No

E Step 1: Lateral canthotomy/inferior cantholysis
Step 2: Superior cantholysis
Step 3: 360 degree periotomy/open septum

F Step 4: Topical and IV aqueous suppressants, and osmotics

G Step 5: Decompression of orbit at bedside after CT scan

Step 6: Refer to orbital surgeon if possible

• Postoperative
• Observe check for clotting disorder

• Traumatic
• Evaluate for open globe fracture
• Orbital foreign body

Infectious go to painful orbital swelling (*see* Ch 32)

Assess etiology of OCS and treat underlying cause

H Imaging (CT, MRI)

Retrobulbar hemorrhage | Infection (*see* Ch 32) | Subperiosteal hemorrhage or infection | Orbital emphysema | High flow fistula | Hemorrhage into orbital mass | Burn patient

Decompress in OR* | Drain collection | Aspirate air | **I** Close fistula | Surgery vs sclerotherapy | Burn protocol

Decompression in OR*

*Rarely necessary

A. Acute proptosis in the absence of orbital compartment syndrome (OCS) rarely occurs in patients with orbital tumors (most commonly acute episodes of intralesional hemorrhage), carotid-cavernous fistulas, dural cavernous fistulas and other orbital disorders such as thyroid eye disease or inflammatory disorders. These conditions more commonly present with subacute or chronic proptosis.

B. In the postoperative patient with OCS, first the wound should be opened and the location of the bleeding vessels identified and coagulated (Fig. 33.1).

C. For infectious causes of OCS, relieve the tense orbit and begin treatment of the infection [(See Chapter 32) (Fig. 33.2)].

D. A tense orbit with signs of visual compromise is a clinical diagnosis that necessitates emergent treatment often in advance of neuroimaging. Most commonly, this will be in the emergency room, recovery room or operating room. The patient may be intubated, intoxicated or otherwise unable to give subjective information. If the patient has been given narcotics for pain, the pupils may be miotic and relatively nonreactive. Thus, the examiner may not be able to assess parameters other than intraocular pressure or resistance to retropulsion. Rarely, OCS will be so severe that the lids cannot be opened adequately to even assess intraocular pressure.

E. Once the diagnosis of OCS is made, prompt action is indicated. This begins with a lateral canthotomy and inferior cantholysis. After each intervention, the parameter(s) prompting intervention should be re-evaluated to assess whether the therapy was effective or whether the next step should be undertaken. It may take a few minutes for the elevated orbital pressure to be alleviated. The next step, if indicated, is a superior cantholysis. In the majority of cases, a canthotomy and cantholysis will adequately decompress the orbit. If not, the orbital septum can be opened via the lateral canthal incision or a lid crease incision and a 360° periotomy can also be performed (Figs. 33.3 and 33.4).

F. Osmotics (such as mannitol, isosorbide or glycerin) and aqueous suppressants (such as topical β-blockers and α-adrenergic agonists, and topical or oral carbonic anhydrase inhibitors) may be tried,

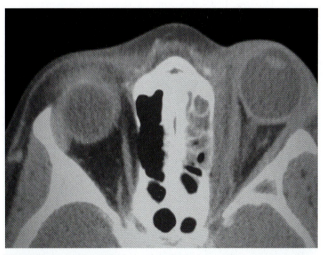

Fig. 33.2: Left orbital compartment syndrome due to a subperiosteal infection showing a subtle V-sign at the insertion of the optic nerve into the globe from the proptosis stretching the nerve (*Source*: Byron Wilkes, MD).

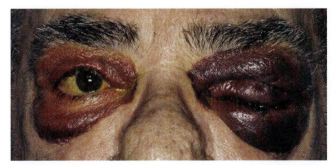

Fig. 33.1: Left-sided orbital compartment syndrome due to retrobulbar hemorrhage after four lid blepharoplasty. The vision was decreased to 20/200 with a left afferent pupillary defect (APD). Treatment consisted of opening incisions on left, identifying and coagulating bleeding vessels in the orbicularis and evacuating the orbital hemorrhage with blunt dissection.

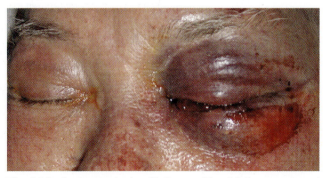

Fig. 33.3: Acute proptosis of left eye with orbital compartment syndrome necessitating canthotomy and inferior cantholysis (*Source*: Olga Shif, MD).

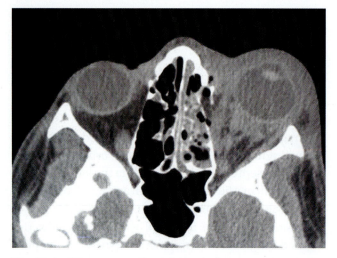

Fig. 33.4: CT scan revealing left retrobulbar hemorrhage after blunt trauma.

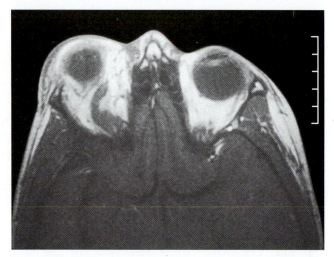

Fig. 33.5: CT demonstrating enlarged superior ophthalmic vein with acute proptosis on the right. The vision was decreased to 20/200 with an afferent pupillary defect due to a traumatic carotid cavernous fistula. An acute canthotomy and inferior cantholysis were performed to stabilize patient until coil embolization.

but the evidence of their efficacy is incomplete. The underlying disease process should be treated, such as intravenous antibiotics for infection and possibly intravenous steroids for inflammation.

G. At the bedside, two types of orbital decompression may be attempted. The floor may be out fractured inferomedially into the maxillary sinus, taking care to avoid the neurovascular bundle. Blunt spreading in the inferolateral quadrant may be cautiously attempted to remove trapped blood or air if present in this region. With either of these maneuvers, care should be taken to avoid globe perforation.

H. The choice of imaging modality will be determined by history (computed tomography is preferable for trauma patients), risk of metallic foreign body [magnetic resonance imaging (MRI) is contraindicated] and whether a vascular malformation is likely (MRI allows for better visualization).

I. Orbital compartment syndrome in the setting of enlarged extraocular muscles and an enlarged superior ophthalmic vein is most commonly seen with a carotid-cavernous fistula. If there is visual compromise, an arteriogram with an interventional neuroradiologist, may determine the connections requiring surgery or coil embolization (Fig. 33.5).

BIBLIOGRAPHY

1. Burkat CN, Lemke BN. Retrobulbar hemorrhage: inferolateral anterior orbitotomy for emergent management. Arch Ophthalmol. 2005;123:1260-2.
2. Lima V, Burt B, Leibovitch I, et al. Orbital compartment syndrome: the ophthalmic surgical emergency. Surv Ophthalmol. 2009;54:441-9.
3. Liu D. A simplified technique of orbital decompression for severe retrobulbar hemorrhage. Am J Ophthalmol. 1993;116:34-7.

Eye Trauma

Johan Zwaan

34

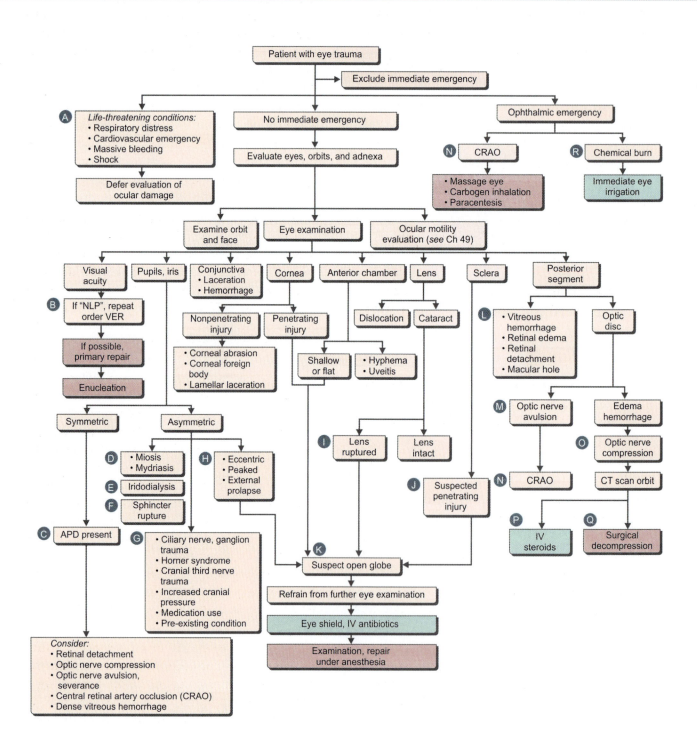

The initial evaluation of a patient with eye trauma should be as complete as possible because decisions about diagnostic and treatment options hinge on it. At the same time, the evaluation should not worsen the ocular condition. A careful history is extremely important in directing the required therapeutic interventions. Emergency situations should be recognized and treated immediately with the remainder of the examination being postponed if necessary. If the patient is cognizant, a visual acuity should be obtained for prognostic and legal reasons.

A. If the initial evaluation reveals any life-threatening conditions, then the treatment of those takes precedence over the treatment of any eye injury.

B. If no light perception is present in a severely traumatized eye and enucleation is contemplated, it may be preferable to do a primary repair, repeat the visual acuity measures, obtain a visually evoked response, and possibly get a second opinion. As long as the enucleation is done within 2 weeks after the initial injury, the rare complication of sympathetic ophthalmia can be avoided. Consider primary enucleation if a second general anesthesia puts the patient at risk.

C. An afferent pupillary defect (APD) implies dysfunction of the optic nerve or the retina. Whether dense media opacities, such as a vitreous hemorrhage, can cause an APD in the absence of optic nerve or retina damage is still being debated.

D. After a blunt injury, the pupil first reacts with spastic miosis. Then, the spasm relaxes and traumatic mydriasis sets in.

E. Stretching at the iris root, usually by blunt trauma, may damage the circular iris blood vessels and cause a hyphema. The iris root can be torn off, leading to iris dialysis. Other sequelae are angle recession and rarely a cyclodialysis cleft. Initial treatment of any of these abnormalities is generally conservative, with definitive surgical repair postponed until the swelling has subsided.

F. Minimal sphincter rupture merely causes mild anisocoria with the sphincter function remaining intact. Severe trauma may lead to a dilated, nonreactive pupil. If the rupture is localized, a teardrop or sector deformity can result. A teardrop-shaped pupil may also result from prolapse, and if one is found, the presence of an open globe should be excluded.

G. Asymmetry of the pupil does not necessarily indicate trauma to the eye *per se*. A variety of neurologic insults may be the cause, some of which may indicate intracranial injury. If photographs dating to before the accident are available, they are useful in excluding pre-existing conditions. Pharmacologic causes for pupillary asymmetry may be obtained from the history.

H. If there is overt prolapse of the iris or the pupil is eccentric or peaked, corneal or scleral integrity may have been compromised and an open globe may be present. Defer further examination of the eye until an examination under anesthesia can be performed.

I. A ruptured lens leads to liberation of lens material into the anterior chamber, where it may induce phacoanaphylactic uveitis or phacolytic glaucoma. Lens removal (usually by aspiration) at the time of primary repair is indicated. A fibrinoid anterior chamber reaction can be prominent, particularly in children, and can mimic the release of lens proteins. It should be differentiated from lens rupture. Hydration of the lens through the capsular rupture can cause lens swelling and lead to pupillary block. The decision to remove a traumatic cataract or dislocated lens at the time of initial repair depends on visual acuity, the presence of other eye problems (e.g. hyphema, lens swelling), and other potential complications of the cataract (e.g. pupillary block). In many cases primary removal is not necessary, and a secondary procedure can be contemplated under more controlled conditions. Implantation of a posterior chamber intraocular lens in the capsular bag, if possible, or in the sulcus as part of the primary repair is becoming more common. Vitreous loss is common during removal of a traumatic cataract or dislocated lens and must be prepared for.

J. A conjunctival laceration or foreign body, a subconjunctival hemorrhage, conjunctival chemosis, a shallow anterior chamber in the absence of a corneal laceration, and a soft eye should lead to the suspicion of a scleral laceration. Shotgun pellet and other injuries to the eyelids may appear small and inconsequential externally, but they may have penetrated the globe through the eyelid. A high index of suspicion is necessary to avoid overlooking scleral lacerations. Ultrasonography (through the eyelids) and computed tomography (CT) scanning are useful auxiliary tools. If any doubt exists about a possible scleral laceration, careful surgical exploration is mandatory.

K. Even the smallest pressure on an open globe can lead to extrusion of ocular contents. If an open globe is diagnosed or even suspected, manipulation may lead to increased damage and should therefore be avoided. Cover the eye with a shield for protection. If deemed necessary, give antibiotics intravenously rather than topically to avoid introduction of high and potentially toxic concentrations into the eye. When the patient is taken to the operating room, use general anesthesia rather than local anesthesia so that anesthetic solution is not injected into the eye. Once the patient has been anesthetized, muscle contractions are relaxed and the risk for squeezing ocular contents out of the eye lessens.

L. If possible, perform indirect ophthalmoscopy early so that continued hemorrhage does not blur the image. Avoid scleral depression until an open globe has been excluded. The pupil needs to be dilated for the examination, and this should be recorded clearly on the chart to avoid confusion with neurologic reasons for a dilated pupil.

M. If the vasculature is compromised with the optic nerve avulsion, which is usually the case, the disk and retina will be edematous. Blood may be present on the disc. A hole or crater may be seen at the level of the disc where the nerve was torn.

N. In central retinal artery occlusion (CRAO), vision is lost within seconds, usually because of embolization of the artery. Thrombosis, vasculitis, spasm and dissecting aneurysm can also cause CRAO. There is an APD, and the retina is pale and edematous with a cherry-red macula. Treatment within 60 minutes after onset may restore vision. The treatment aims at dislodging the embolus to a more peripheral arteriole by increasing arterial diameter (by carbogen inhalation) or reducing intraocular pressure [paracentesis, massage and intravenous (IV) acetazolamide].

O. Optic nerve injuries of any type are relatively uncommon. Compression of the nerve may result from displaced bone fragments of the sphenoid or, more commonly, from edema or hemorrhage. Imaging studies, in particular CT scanning, are essential in reaching the proper diagnosis.

P. Treatment of optic nerve injuries is controversial. IV steroids are helpful, if given early.

Q. Consider decompression of the compressed optic nerve if IV steroids do not improve the clinical condition.

R. A chemical burn, especially an alkali burn, is an ophthalmic emergency. Start treatment by lavage immediately, even before the exact nature of the burn is known.

▌BIBLIOGRAPHY

1. Alfaro DV, Liggett PE (Eds). Vitreoretinal Surgery of the Injured Eye. Philadelphia: Lippincott, Williams & Wilkins; 1998.
2. Kuhn F, Morris R, Witherspoon CD, et al. A standardized classification of ocular trauma. Ophthalmology. 1996;103: 240-3.
3. Kylstra JA, Lamkin JC, Runyan DK. Clinical predictors of scleral rupture after blunt ocular trauma. Am J Ophthalmol. 1993;115:530-5.
4. MacCumber MW. Management of Ocular Injuries and Emergencies. Philadelphia: Lippincott-Raven; 1998. pp. 55-77.
5. Shingleton BJ, Hersh PS, Kenyon KR (Eds). Eye Trauma. St Louis: Mosby; 1991.

35

Intraocular Calcium Density

Marilyn C Kincaid, Frank W Scribbick

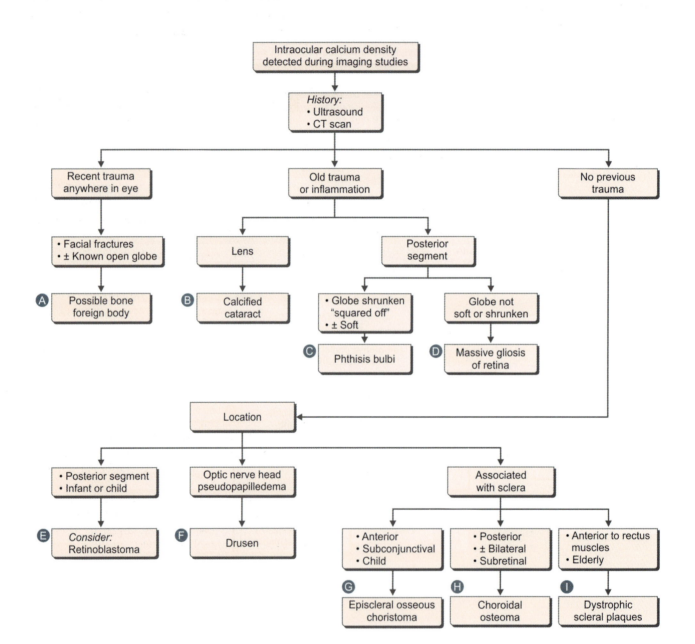

A. Penetrating injuries of the globe, particularly when hidden by intact conjunctiva, often result in relatively minor patient complaints despite the presence of a retained intraocular foreign body. When a CT scan indicates fracture of the orbital bones, check the image of the globe for the possibility of an intraocular bone fragment. Ultrasound is also useful to identify intraocular foreign bodies in the setting of periocular trauma and opaque media.

B. Traumatic cataracts often develop calcification over time, especially when the original injury occurred in childhood. Mature cataracts without a history of trauma can also undergo dystrophic calcification. The location of the calcification on CT or ultrasound scan along with a clinically evident opaque lens helps make the diagnosis.

C. Phthisis bulbi is shrinkage and total internal disorganization of the globe. Often, it is hypotonous as well, although later this may be less evident because of fibrosis and intraocular ossification. The shrunken globe also takes on a 'squared off' appearance because of the remodeling action of the rectus muscles. Intraocular bone forms from osseous metaplasia of the retinal pigment epithelium. Eyes with opaque media can harbor occult intraocular neoplasms and should be evaluated with ultrasound or CT scan.

D. Massive gliosis of the retina describes a posterior segment mass composed of proliferating glial cells disorganizing and replacing the retina. This damaged retina can also undergo dystrophic calcification, and may appear as calcium or bone on diagnostic imaging.

E. Most retinoblastomas demonstrate small, diffuse foci of calcification on CT or ultrasound. Histologically, these calcific foci are found in areas of focal necrosis. Although calcification is characteristic of retinoblastoma, its absence does not rule it out. Less common causes of congenital/childhood intraocular calcium are Trisomy 13 and teratoid medulloepithelioma.

F. Optic nerve head drusen can simulate papilledema, but CT or ultrasound readily discloses the drusen. Drusen are also highly autofluorescent, and can be visualized on the red-free photos during fluorescein angiography.

G. Episcleral osseous choristomas are extremely rare and typically found in the interpalpebral region and are completely benign. The confirmation of dense calcification can allay the family's fears.

H. Choroidal osteomas are classically found in the choroid posteriorly in women. The cause is obscure. They are elevated and yellowish and can simulate a melanoma or metastatic tumor. However, the presence of dense calcification on CT or high reflectivity on ultrasound confirms the diagnosis of osteoma.

I. Scleral plaques anterior to the rectus muscles, especially the horizontal recti, are common in older persons. No therapy is indicated.

▌BIBLIOGRAPHY

1. Atta HR. Imaging of the optic nerve with standardized echography. Eye (Lond). 1988;2:358-66.
2. Henke V, Philip W, Naumann GO. Intraocular ossification in clinically unsuspected malignant melanoma of the uvea in phthisis bulbi. Klin Monatsbl Augenheilkd. 1986;189:243-6.
3. Mansour AM, Barber JC, Reinecke RD, Wang FM. Ocular choristomas. Surv Ophthalmol. 1989;33:339-58.
4. Shields CL, Shields JA, Augsburger JJ. Choroidal osteoma. Surv Ophthalmol. 1988;33:17-27.

SECTION 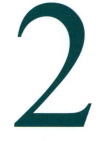 2

Oculoplastics

Eyelid Swelling

David EE Holck, Dimitrios Sismanis

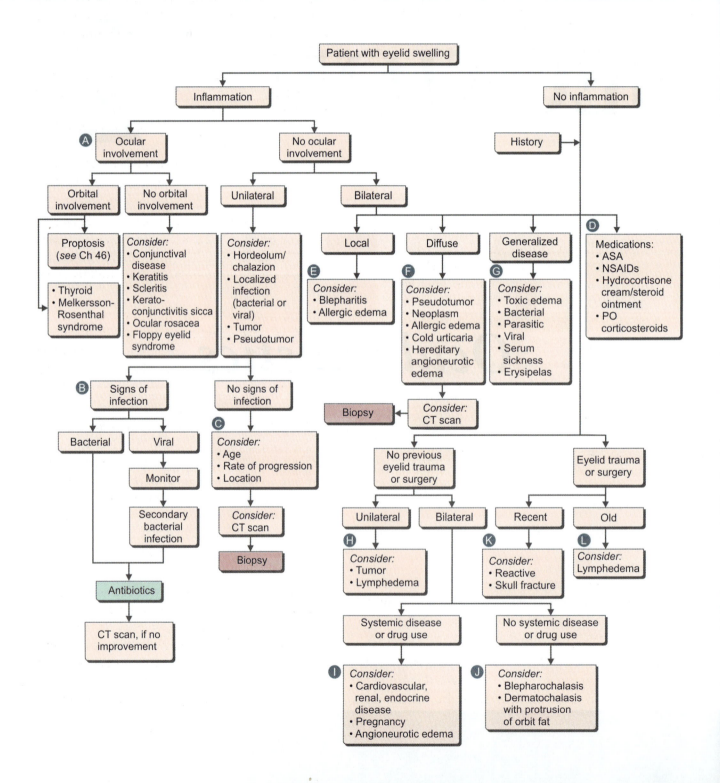

With the unique anatomy and aging changes of eyelid soft tissue, this area easily accumulates fluid and masses. Eyelid skin is the thinnest in the body and the orbital septum stretches with age allowing herniation of orbital fat into the eyelid. Lesions affecting the eyelid or orbital compartments allow expansion of the eyelid soft tissues. Eyelid swelling may result from lesions, inflammation, fluid accumulation or a combination. Eyelid edema is a sign of a local or systemic pathologic process resulting in accumulation of fluid. With eyelid swelling, the skin is often smooth and tense. With resolution, fine wrinkling of the skin is often seen with decreased elasticity.

A. A complete ophthalmic evaluation is necessary to determine, if ocular involvement is present. Inflammatory conditions may secondarily involve the eyelids. Abaxial globe displacement suggests an orbital process. Orbital processes including thyroid disease and Melkersson-Rosenthal syndrome (consisting of the triad of facial nerve palsy, facial edema and lingua plicata) may cause eyelid swelling. Ocular involvement of conjunctival disease, keratitis, floppy lid syndrome, keratoconjunctivitis sicca and ocular rosacea may results in eyelid edema.

B. Localized infectious processes may clinically appear as unilateral eyelid swelling. Dacryocystitis may involve the lower eyelid, and present as a mass below the medial canthal tendon (cautions for lacrimal sac tumor, if a mass is palpable above the medial canthal tendon). Periorbital sinus disease may present as upper or lower eyelid swelling. Viral etiologies, while often self-limited, may progress (especially herpetic infections) and require therapy.

C. Patient age, location of eyelid swelling and progression are important historical elements in creating a differential diagnoses for swelling. Pediatric rhabdomyosarcoma may mimic eyelid swelling. Sebaceous cell carcinoma may mimic inflammatory processes, including chalazia and blepharoconjunctivitis.

D. Medications may also induce eyelid edema and swelling. Aspirin, nonsteroidal anti-inflammatory medications and corticosteroids are commonly used to treat swelling, but may result in worsening of eyelid edema.

E. The eyelids are commonly involved in ocular allergy. Contact dermatitis (atopic type IV hypersensitivity reactions) from local or topical agents, to insect bites may involve the upper or lower eyelids. More generalized reactions from IgE urticarial or drug reactions may also involve the surrounding face as well.

F. The spectrum of lymphoid processes from pseudotumor to malignant lymphoma may present uni- or bilaterally. Imaging may define the lesion, if biopsy is planned. Immunological markers and flow cytometry are helpful to evaluate lymphomatous lesions. Cold urticaria and hereditary angioneurotic edema are diffuse disorders that may also result in eyelid edema.

G. Generalized infectious processes of bacterial, viral, or parasitic etiologies may produce toxins or an allergic edematous process. Erysipelas and serum sickness may similarly cause swelling of the eyelid.

H. Tumors may present as unilateral or bilateral eyelid swelling (lymphangiomas, hemangiomas, neurofibromas). History and clinical examination may narrow a differential diagnoses. Imaging and consideration of biopsy may be necessary for definitive diagnoses.

I. Fluid and edematous processes are often seen in cardiovascular, renal, or endocrine abnormalities. Edema may also be seen in pregnancy. Angioneurotic edema is an idiopathic chronic vasomotor condition affecting the subcutaneous eyelid tissue. This may result in cyclic or irregular episodes lasting days to weeks. A history of atopic disease, allergies, or endocrine abnormalities may be discovered in these patients.

J. Blepharochalasis is an idiopathic condition associated with recurrent bouts of transient painless eyelid edema. It may appear at any time from infancy to adulthood but is most commonly seen in the second decade of life. It has a female predilection. After recurrent episodes, fine wrinkling and permanent eyelid changes including pigmentation may result. Usually, this is a bilateral condition but unilateral cases have been reported.

K. Trauma frequently produces edema, swelling or hemorrhage. Skull fractures commonly produce swelling of the eyelids from blood extending along the floor of the orbit into the eyelids.

L. Any local cause that impedes lymphatic drainage from the eyelid can produce chronic edema. Scarring from surgery or trauma may impair drainage, especially in the temporal legion. Malignant processes, chronic skin disease and irradiation to the periocular region can also impede lymphatic outflow causing edema.

BIBLIOGRAPHY

1. Duke-Elder S, MacFaul PA. System of Ophthalmology, Vol 13, pt 1: The Ocular Adnexa: Diseases of the Eyelids. St Louis: Mosby; 1974. pp. 11-23.
2. Orentreich DS, Orentreich N. Dermatology of the eyelids. In: Smith BC, Nesi FA, Lisman RD, Levine MR (Eds). Ophthalmic, Plastic, and Reconstructive Surgery. St Louis: Mosby; 1998. pp. 485-530.
3. Sami MS, Soparkar CNS, Patrinely JR, et al. Eyelid edema. Semin Plast Surg. 2007;21:24-31.
4. Starr MB. Infectious and hypersensitivity of the eyelids. In: Smith BC, Nesi FA, Lisman RD, Levine MR (Eds). Ophthalmic Plastic and Reconstructive Surgery. St Louis: Mosby; 1998. pp. 531-56.

Retraction of the Upper Eyelid

37

Christopher M DeBacker, David EE Holck

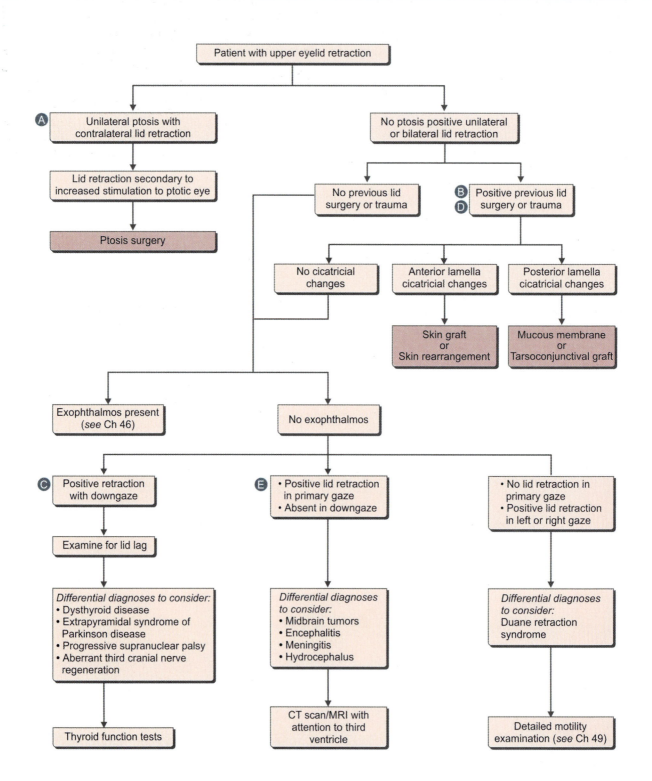

Eyelid retraction occurs when the upper eyelid margin rests at or above the superior corneoscleral limbus, often leading to superior scleral show. The normal upper eyelid rests 1–2 mm below the superior corneoscleral limbus.

A. Hering law may manifest as eyelid retraction in a patient with contralateral blepharoptosis. Alternate cover test or observing the retracted eyelid as the contralateral ptotic eyelid is lifted will aid in diagnosis.

B. Surgical overcorrection of blepharoptosis repair may cause upper eyelid retraction. Overly aggressive skin excision in upper blepharoplasty may manifest as upper eyelid retraction, particularly, if scar tissue occurs at the level of the orbital septum. Most of these patients will also manifest lagophthalmos.

C. The most common cause of unilateral and bilateral upper eyelid retraction is thyroid eye disease (Fig. 37.1). Lid lag is a very sensitive marker for thyroid eye disease and will often accompany upper eyelid retraction in this population. A delay in upper eyelid downward excursion in downgaze defines lid lag.

D. Recession of the superior rectus muscle can lead to upper eyelid retraction.

E. Central nervous system pathology may cause eyelid. Parinaud (dorsal midbrain) syndrome manifests bilateral and symmetric upper eyelid retraction (Collier sign), upgaze palsy, and pupillary light-near dissociation. The upper eyelid retraction is

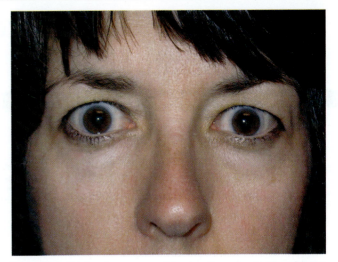

Fig. 37.1: Bilateral upper eyelid retraction due to thyroid eye disease.

absent in downgaze, in contrast to thyroid eyelid retraction.

▌BIBLIOGRAPHY

1. Bartley GB. The differential diagnosis and classification of eyelid retraction. Ophthalmology. 1996;103: 168-76.
2. Meyer DR, Wobig JL. Detection of contralateral eyelid retraction associated with blepharoptosis. Ophthalmology. 1992;99:366-75.
3. Putterman AM. Surgical treatment of thyroid-related upper eyelid retraction. Graded Müller's muscle excision and levator recession. Ophthalmology. 1981;88: 507-12.

Drooping of Upper Eyelid (Blepharoptosis)

38

Constance L Fry, Mary Kelly Green, Kenneth L Piest*

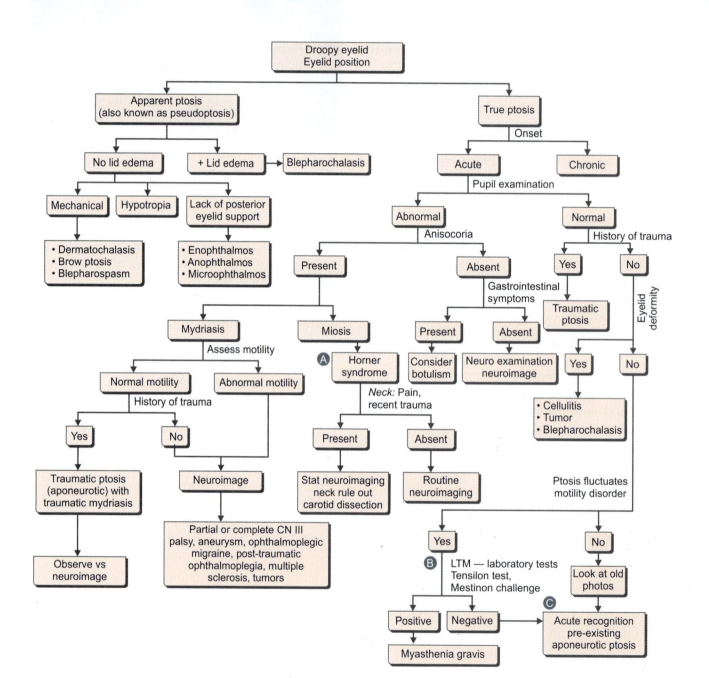

*Deceased

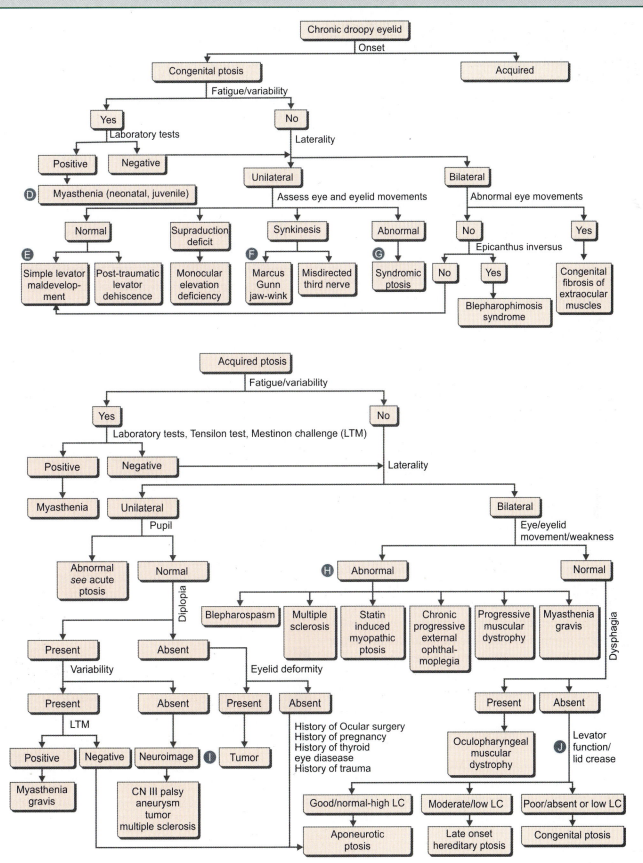

Blepharoptosis refers to drooping of the upper eyelid. Ptosis is classically categorized as levator maldevelopment (congenital), other myogenic causes, aponeurotic ptosis, neurogenic causes, and mechanical and apparent ptosis (also known as pseudoptosis). The onset, associated medical conditions, and the physical examination are utilized in a decision tree fashion in order to determine the cause of the ptosis. While the vast majority of cases will either be levator maldevelopment or aponeurotic ptosis, it is important to identify those rare cases that are acutely precipitated by serious systemic conditions that require prompt intervention as well as other causes of secondary ptosis of gradual onset.

A. Acute onset of Horner syndrome with headache in the setting of trauma requires emergent neuroimaging. The presence of neck pain or recent neck trauma necessitates emergent evaluation for a dissecting aneurysm of the carotid artery. While Horner syndrome may be caused due to a lesion anywhere along the sympathetic pathway, the majority does not involve the central nervous system (CNS) and thus neuroimaging should initially focus on the chest and neck. Exceptions are in the setting of headache and/or brainstem or spinal cord symptoms, then evaluation of the CNS pathway should occur first.

B. Myasthenia gravis is characterized by variability and fatigability. The ptosis may be unilateral or bilateral. The disease may be localized ocular myasthenia or systemic myasthenia gravis. If the patient reports difficulty in breathing or has muscle weakness (particularly the neck muscles), emergent referral may be necessary. A variety of tests may be performed to attempt to diagnose the disorder including: the ice glove test (80% sensitive), laboratory studies for acetylcholine antibody receptors, genetic testing [for congenital myasthenic syndromes (*see* D)], injections of intravenous edrophonium (Tensilon®), intramuscular neostigmine (uncommon), oral therapeutic trials with pyridostigmine (Mestinon®), and electromyography (EMG). Single fiber EMG is particularly useful in ocular and congenital myasthenia. Acetylcholine antibody receptors may be negative in up to 60% of patients and, similarly, a negative Tensilon® test does not categorically exclude the disease. It is important to follow appropriate precautions when performing a Tensilon® test and be aware that cardiac disease and bronchial asthma are relative contraindications to the procedure (Fig. 38.1).

C. Aponeurotic ptosis is the second most common cause of ptosis and is characterized by normal levator function, a high lid crease and a thin eyelid (Fig. 38.2).

D. Myasthenia gravis is uncommon in childhood, but should be considered in cases of variable ptosis. Three forms of ptosis are seen in children: transient neonatal myasthenia, persistent neonatal myasthenia and juvenile myasthenia (*see* section B).

E. Simple levator maldevelopment (congenital) ptosis is due to a developmental dystrophy of the levator muscle and comprises over 50% of all ptosis cases (Fig. 38.3).

F. The Marcus Gunn jaw-winking syndrome occurs in 5% of patients with congenital ptosis. It is the most common cause of congenital synkinetic ptosis. In some patients, the ptosis is more symptomatic, while in others, the jaw-wink is more severe and this affects management choices.

G. Ptosis may occur in a variety of developmental syndromes such as: Crouzon, fetal alcohol and Goldenhar syndromes.

H. Acquired myogenic ptosis is the result of local or diffuse muscular disease. The history, family history and examination direct the evaluation

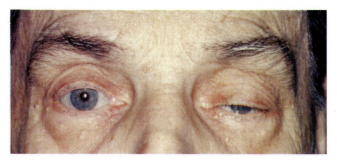

Fig. 38.1: Unilateral severe ptosis in a patient with myasthenia gravis.

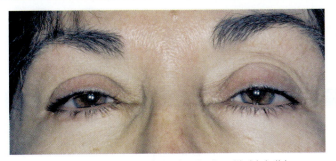

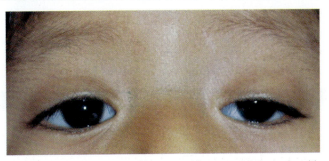

Fig. 38.2: Asymmetric aponeurotic ptosis with high lid crease more noticeable on the left upper eyelid.

Fig. 38.3: Marked bilateral asymmetric congenital ptosis with frontalis overaction and absent eyelid creases.

which may include laboratory studies, occasionally genetic testing and EMG as well as evaluation by a neurologist familiar with the disorders. Certain disorders, such as Kearns-Sayre syndrome associated with chronic progressive external ophthalmoplegia, have cardiac conduction defects.

I. A thickened or misshaped eyelid suggests a ptosis associated with an eyelid or orbital tumor. Neurofibromatosis type 1 may affect the lid creating an S-shaped deformity from a neurofibroma. Additionally, mucoceles and tumors involving the superior orbit or lacrimal gland may induce a secondary ptosis.

J. The optimal management of ptosis is determined by the amount of ptosis, levator function, the protective mechanisms of the eye (Bell phenomenon, cranial nerve seven function, lagophthalmos, and tear film status), as well as the etiology of the ptosis and co-existing eye diseases such as glaucoma and ocular motility disorders. In patients presenting with unilateral ptosis, the presence of Hering phenomenon masking a bilateral asymmetric ptosis should be sought. In the healthy eye, surgical correction of simple levator maldevelopment and aponeurotic ptosis is dictated by the amount of ptosis, the onset (congenital versus acquired) and the levator function. Patients with a poor levator function (less than 5 mm) will require a frontalis suspension; those with moderate levator function require a levator resection. Patients with good levator function may benefit from a levator advancement, mullerectomy or Fasanella-Servat tarsomyectomy procedure. The preferred method of surgery for other causes of ptosis is beyond the scope of this review.

BIBLIOGRAPHY

1. Callahan MA, Beard C. Beard's Ptosis, 4th Edition. Birmingham, AL: Aesculapius Publishing Co; 1990.
2. Putnam JR, Nunery WR, Tanenbaum M, et al. Blepharoptosis. In: McCord Jr CD, Tanenbaum M, Nunery WR (Eds). Oculoplastic Surgery, 3rd Edition. New York: Raven Press; 1995. pp. 175-220.

Acquired Ectropion

Christopher M DeBacker, David EE Holck

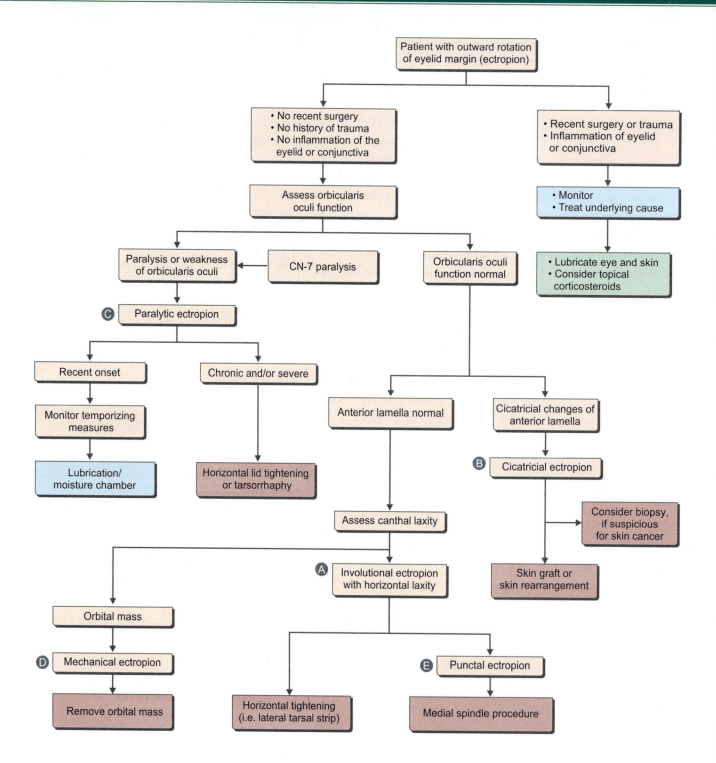

39

Patient with outward rotation of eyelid margin (ectropion)

- No recent surgery
- No history of trauma
- No inflammation of the eyelid or conjunctiva

- Recent surgery or trauma
- Inflammation of eyelid or conjunctiva

Assess orbicularis oculi function

- Monitor
- Treat underlying cause

Paralysis or weakness of orbicularis oculi

CN-7 paralysis

Orbicularis oculi function normal

- Lubricate eye and skin
- Consider topical corticosteroids

C Paralytic ectropion

Recent onset

Chronic and/or severe

Anterior lamella normal

Cicatricial changes of anterior lamella

Monitor temporizing measures

B Cicatricial ectropion

Lubrication/moisture chamber

Horizontal lid tightening or tarsorrhaphy

Assess canthal laxity

Consider biopsy, if suspicious for skin cancer

A Involutional ectropion with horizontal laxity

Skin graft or skin rearrangement

Orbital mass

D Mechanical ectropion

E Punctal ectropion

Remove orbital mass

Horizontal tightening (i.e. lateral tarsal strip)

Medial spindle procedure

A. Involutional lower eyelid ectropion occurs as a result of horizontal laxity. This may be a result of lateral canthal tendon attenuation, medial canthal tendon attenuation, tarsal laxity (i.e. floppy eyelid syndrome), or a combination thereof (Figs. 39.1A and B). The 'snap test' and the 'lid distraction test' are useful maneuvers to assess etiology.

B. Cicatricial ectropion is caused by a vertical deficiency of anterior lamellar eyelid tissue (predominantly skin). This may be a result of trauma, overzealous lower blepharoplasty or other eyelid surgery, burns, irradiation, inflammatory skin conditions, and cicatrizing malignancies. Mild versions may be helped with aggressive skin conditioning (petrolatum and corticosteroids) and horizontal tightening; however, most will require replacement of the deficient skin via skin grafts together with horizontal eyelid tightening (Figs. 39.2A and B).

C. Paralytic ectropion may be due to acute or chronic Bell palsy or trauma to the upper facial branches of the facial nerve. Aggressive lubrication is necessary

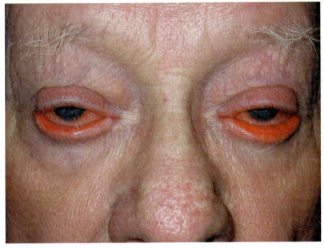

Fig. 39.1A: Acquired ectropion of the lower eyelids with conjunctival injection and exposure keratoconjuctivopathy.

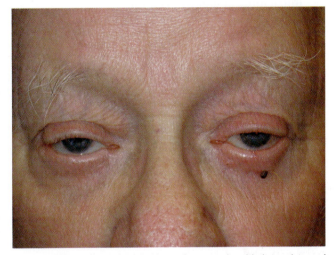

Fig. 39.1B: Acquired ectropion after repair with lateral tarsal strip and full-thickness eyelid sutures.

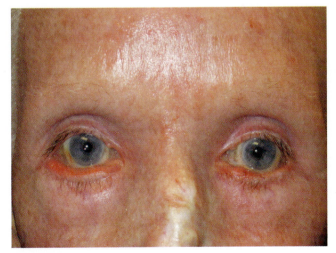

Fig. 39.2A: Cicatricial lower eyelid ectropion.

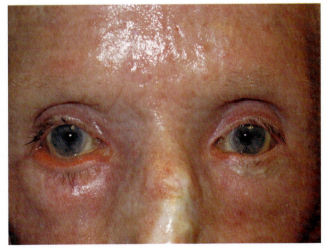

Fig. 39.2B: Cicatricial ectropion repair with full-thickness left lower eyelid skin graft.

as most of these will be accompanied by some degree of paralytic lagophthalmos with attendant exposure keratoconjunctivopathy. Surgical intervention may be required via lower lid tightening.

D. Mechanical ectropion is caused by bulky tumors weighing down the lower eyelid. Treatment in these cases is aimed at removal of the causative mass.

E. Punctal ectropion may accompany any type of ectropion. If the lower punctum is not reapposed to the globe despite having addressed all of the horizontal and vertical factors present, a medial spindle procedure will aid in rotating the punctum into a more anatomic position.

BIBLIOGRAPHY

1. DeBacker CM (2011). Entropion and ectropion repair. Medscape Reference: Drugs, Diseases & Procedures. [online] Available from http://emedicine.medscape.com/article/1844045-overview. [Accessed September 2011].
2. Jordan DR, Anderson RL. The lateral tarsal strip revisited. The enhanced tarsal strip. Arch Ophthalmol. 1989;107:604-6.
3. McCord CD, Ellis DS. The correction of lower lid malposition following lower lid blepharoplasty. Plast Reconstr Surg. 1993;92:1068-72.
4. Nowinski TS, Anderson RL. The medial spindle procedure for involutional medial ectropion. Arch Ophthalmol. 1985;103:1750-3.

Acquired Entropion

Christopher M DeBacker, David EE Holck

40

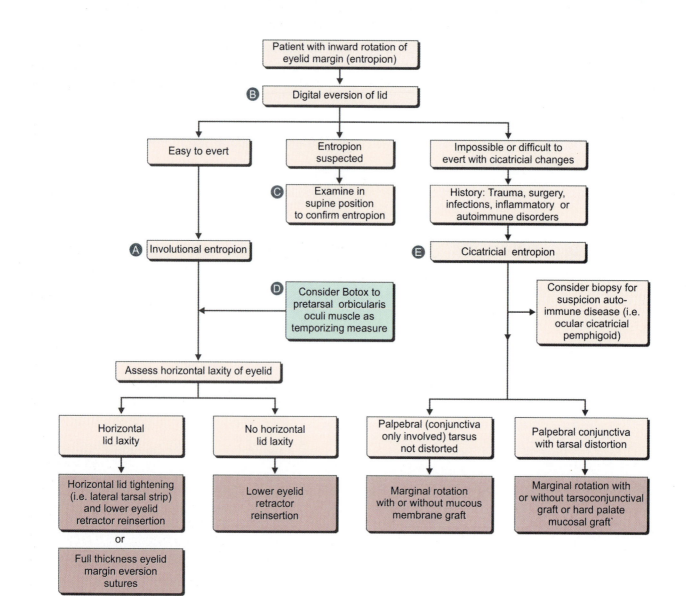

A. Involutional entropion presents as inturning of the lower eyelid margin with lashes and skin abrading the ocular surface. Relative enophthalmos is a common association and is manifest by an accompanying deep superior sulcus. Horizontal eyelid laxity is usually present, and dehisced/attenuated lower eyelid retractors lead to unopposed orbicularis oculi action with a visibly 'over-riding' muscle (Figs. 40.1A and B).

B. The 'digital eversion' test is helpful to distinguish involutional entropion from cicatricial entropion.

The lid margin will evert with pressure on the tarsus and globe inferiorly with involutional entropion but not with cicatricial entropion. Eversion of the lower lid will also reveal visible dehiscence of the whitish lower eyelid retractors in many cases of involutional entropion, whereas cicatricial entropion will show scar tissue of the palpebral conjunctiva, tarsus, or both.

C. For the patient in whom there is a high suspicion of entropion, but it is not manifest in primary gaze in the upright sitting position, it is helpful to lay the patient

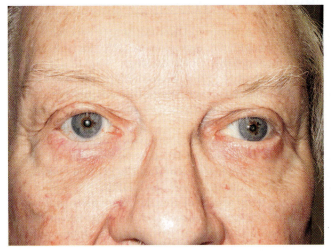

Fig. 40.1A: Involutional entropion right lower eyelid.

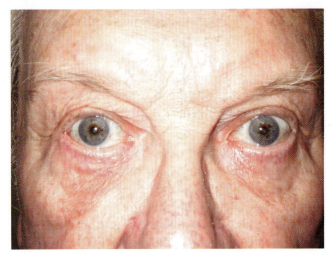

Fig. 40.1B: Repair of involutional entropion right lower eyelid with horizontal tightening (lateral tarsal strip) and lower eyelid retractor reinsertion.

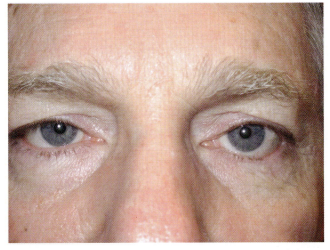

Fig. 40.2A: Left lower eyelid cicatricial entropion with lower eyelid retraction.

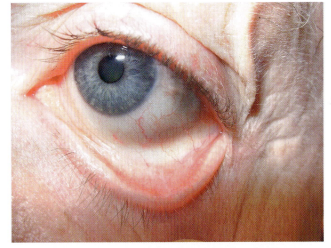

Fig. 40.2B: Left lower eyelid posterior lamellar cicatrix.

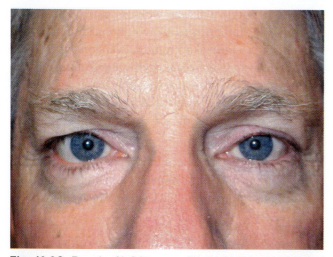

Fig. 40.2C: Repair of left lower eyelid cicatricial entropion and retraction with cicatrix release and hard-palate mucosal graft.

supine before examining. The lid will often invert with this maneuver as the globe settles back into the socket (enhancing the relative enophthalmos).

D. A vicious cycle of spastic entropion and ocular irritation may be caused by ocular inflammation. Treatment of the underling ocular condition along with taping of the lower eyelid inferiorly may break the cycle. Botox (off-label use) is effective when injected at low dose into the central and lateral pretarsal orbicularis oculi muscle.

E. Cicatricial entropion may be caused by trauma or postsurgical scarring. All causes lead to vertical shortening of the posterior lamella of the eyelid. Concomitant scarring of the middle lamellar of the lower eyelid may also result in lower eyelid retraction (Figs. 40.2A to C). Inflammatory, infectious, and autoimmune causes, such as Stevens-Johnson syndrome, herpes zoster, and ocular cicatricial pemphigoid, should be considered in the differential diagnosis. Ocular cicatricial pemphigoid is a progressive disease that requires ongoing chemotherapy to quell the inflammation and halt progression of the scarring.

BIBLIOGRAPHY

1. Barnes JA, Bunce C, Olver JM. Simple effective surgery for involutional entropion suitable for the general ophthalmologist. Ophthalmology. 2006;113:92-6.
2. DeBacker CM (2011). Entropion and ectropion repair. Medscape Reference: Drugs, Diseases and Procedures. Available on http://emedicine.medscape.com/article/ 1844045-overview.
3. DeBacker CM (2011). Entropion. Medscape Reference: Drugs, Diseases and Procedures. Available on http:// emedicine.medscape.com/article/1212456-overview.
4. Heiligenhaus A, Shore JW, Rubin PA, Foster CS. Long-term results of mucous membrane grafting in ocular cicatricial pemphigoid. Implications for patient selection and surgical considerations. Ophthalmology. 1993;100:1283-8.
5. Quickert MH, Rathbun E. Suture repair of entropion. Arch Ophthalmol. 1971;85:304-5.

Upper Eyelid Reconstruction

41

David EE Holck, Dimitrios Sismanis

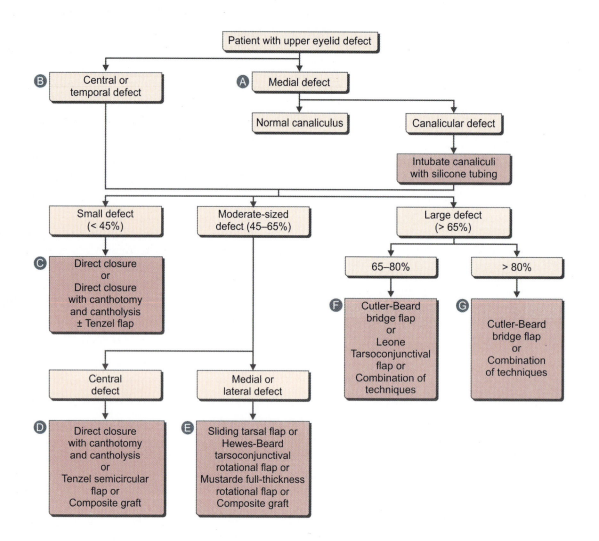

In reconstruction of eyelid defects, structural integrity of the segment is critical in order to adequately protect the globe. When analyzing an upper eyelid defect, it is critical to define the missing segment in terms of anterior and posterior lamella. The posterior lamella consists of the conjunctiva, upper eyelid retractors, and upper eyelid structural support with a tarsal substitute. The anterior lamella consists of the skin and orbicularis oculi muscle. Adequate reconstruction avoids vertical retraction to minimize the risk of lagophthalmos and ocular exposure. In this way, form follows function, and an adequate functional closure often provides acceptable cosmesis.

A. If a medial upper eyelid deficit is present, the surgeon must rule out canalicular involvement. If present, reconstruction should be accomplished using mono-canalicular or bicanalicular silicone stent intubation and canalicular repair. Plastic repair of the canalicular segment to an adjoining segment is optimal. If a large segment of the canalicular system is absent, it is still useful to intubate the remaining system. Epithelialization around the tube is still possible. Loupe magnification or a surgical microscope may be helpful in repairing these defects. Reconstruction of the medial canthal attachments requires posterior fixation to maintain lid-globe contact.

B. To maintain lateral canthal tendon integrity, reattachment to the residual canthal tendon and distal tarsal plate is optimal. Otherwise, posterior fixation must be accomplished to the periosteum near the lateral orbital tubercle. If inadequate tissue remains, a periosteal flap originating from the external orbital rim and based in its medial aspect may offer additional structural support with a posterior vector of pull. Anterior placement results in the lid margin displaced away from the globe.

C. For small or medium sized full thickness defects, the wounds may be freshened and closed directly in layers depending upon the amount of eyelid laxity present. If tension is present, canthotomy and cantholysis may be useful in reconstructing the area without excess tension.

D. If adequate tarsus is present on either side of the defect, additional anterior lamellar tissue may be obtained using a Tenzel semicircular rotational flap. The curve of the flap is directed inferiorly to repair upper eyelid defects.

E. Isolated medial or lateral defects may be closed using adjacent tissue from the upper eyelid. The remaining tarsus and conjunctiva is slid or rotated to close the posterior lamellar defect. The anterior lamella may be repaired with a full thickness skin graft or an adjacent skin-muscle flap. A lateral defect may also be closed using a lid-sharing Hewes-Beard tarsoconjunctival flap. In this technique, a tarsoconjunctival strip is taken from the lower eyelid and swung into the upper eyelid posterior lamellar defect. The blood supply comes from the lateral hinge. The anterior lamellar defect is again closed with a free skin graft or an adjacent myocutaneous flap. Another technique involves using a full thickness pedicle flap from the lower eyelid that is rotated into the upper eyelid defect. This technique provides function as well as eyelashes in the reconstructed segment. The lower eyelid is then reconstructed with side-to-side closure and an adjacent rotational flap. Still another alternative involves taking a composite graft, which is a free graft harvested from the contralateral upper eyelid. The musculocutaneous layer is removed, but the lid margin and lashes are preserved. The anterior lamella is reconstructed with a skin-muscle flap, which provides a blood supply to the free graft.

F. The Cutler-Beard flap is useful for large full thickness defects of the upper eyelid. This lid sharing procedure is a staged procedure, and the flap will need to be severed after several weeks. This technique does not bring tarsal support, and a structural tarsal substitute is necessary (cartilage or other donor materials). The Leone tarsoconjunctival flap is a modification of using residual upper eyelid tissue in a recessed fashion with a donor lower eyelid flap. This technique requires opening of the flap at a later date and may be suboptimal in monocular patients.

G. Defects involving more than 80% of the upper eyelid pose a difficult challenge in reconstruction, and may require a combination of techniques.

▌BIBLIOGRAPHY

1. Frueh BR. Upper eyelid reconstruction. In: Stewart WB (Ed). Ophthalmic, Plastic and Reconstructive Surgery. San Francisco: American Academy of Ophthalmology; 1984. pp. 258-64.
2. Kohn R. Textbook of Ophthalmic, Plastic and Reconstructive Surgery. Philadelphia: Lea & Febiger; 1988.
3. Kwitko EM, Nesi FA. Eyelid and ocular adnexal reconstruction. In: Smith BC, Nesi FA, Lisman RD, Levine MD (Eds). Ophthalmic, Plastic, and Reconstructive Surgery. St Louis: Mosby; 1998. pp. 576-608.
4. McCord CD, Wesley R. Reconstruction of the upper eyelid and medial canthus. In: McCord CD, Tanenbaum M (Eds). Oculoplastic Surgery. New York: Raven; 1987. pp. 73-93.

Lower Eyelid Reconstruction

Christopher M DeBacker, David EE Holck

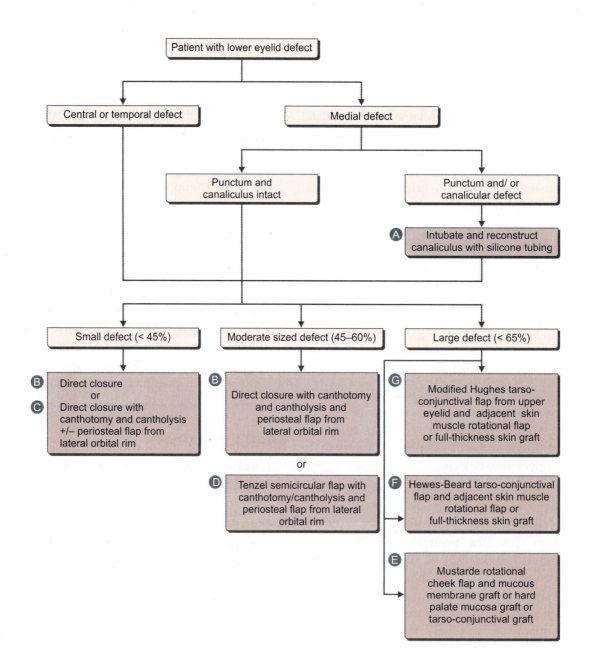

Patient with lower eyelid defect

Central or temporal defect

Medial defect

Punctum and canaliculus intact

Punctum and/ or canalicular defect

Ⓐ Intubate and reconstruct canaliculus with silicone tubing

Small defect (< 45%)

Moderate sized defect (45–60%)

Large defect (< 65%)

Ⓑ Direct closure
or
Ⓒ Direct closure with canthotomy and cantholysis +/– periosteal flap from lateral orbital rim

Ⓑ Direct closure with canthotomy and cantholysis and periosteal flap from lateral orbital rim

or

Ⓓ Tenzel semicircular flap with canthotomy/cantholysis and periosteal flap from lateral orbital rim

Ⓖ Modified Hughes tarso-conjunctival flap from upper eyelid and adjacent skin muscle rotational flap or full-thickness skin graft

Ⓕ Hewes-Beard tarso-conjunctival flap and adjacent skin muscle rotational flap or full-thickness skin graft

Ⓔ Mustarde rotational cheek flap and mucous membrane graft or hard palate mucosa graft or tarso-conjunctival graft

For purposes of reconstruction, the lower eyelid needs to be viewed as a bilamellar structure; the anterior lamella consists of skin and orbicularis oculis muscle while the posterior lamella consists of palpebral conjunctiva, tarsus, capsulopalpebral fascia and the sympathetic muscle. The orbital septum and orbital fat separate the two lamellae. Reconstructive procedures are aimed at repairing these two structures to allow for adequate protection of the globe as well as to optimize cosmesis.

A. The puncto-canalicular system needs to be assessed in all reconstructive procedures. Available options include mono- and bi-canalicular intubation via intubation of the nasolacrimal duct, as well as pigtail placement of silicon tubes for purely canalicular intubation. Large medial canthal defects involving the entire upper nasolacrimal drainage system are best addressed at a future date with conjunctival-dacryocystorhinostomy and Jones tube placement.

B. The canthi need to be assessed for involvement. Deep canthal suture fixation may suffice for defects under minimal horizontal tension, while periosteal flaps may be required for closure under excessive horizontal tension.

C. Defects of up to 40% of the horizontal lower eyelid may be closed primarily, depending upon the degree of tension. Additional laxity can be gained by release of the inferior crus of the lateral canthal tendon.

D. Larger defects (up to 60%) can be repaired with a semicircular rotational flap of anterior lamellar tissue combined with complete release of the inferior crus of the lateral canthal tendon. Adjunctive periosteal flap creation from the lateral orbital rim should be utilized for lateral lid support or significant chemosis will result.

E. Defects, which involve a significant amount of vertical and horizontal eyelid tissue, may be closed with Mustarde-type rotational cheek flaps for anterior lamellar reconstruction, and free tarso-conjunctival grafts for posterior lamellar reconstruction.

F. When greater than 60% of the horizontal lower eyelid is missing, a lid sharing procedure will generally be required. An exception to this is perhaps a broad shallow defect with substantial vertical skin laxity. In these cases, free tarso-conjunctival grafts may be utilized with a sliding myocutaneous flap for anterior lamellar reconstruction.

G. Lid sharing procedures, i.e. the modified Hughes tarso-conjunctival flap, combined with a skin graft or myocutaneous advancement flap are particularly useful for large lower eyelid full-thickness defect (Figs. 42.1A and B). This is a two-stage procedure, which will require transection of the flap 4–6 weeks

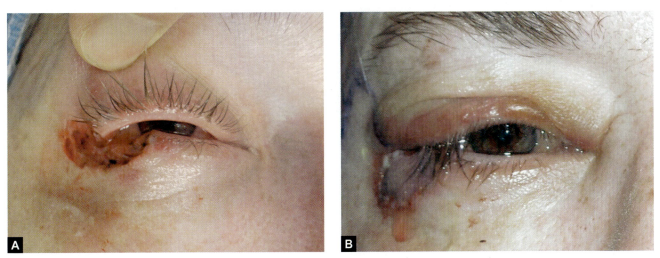

Figs. 42.1A and B: (A) Right lower eyelid full-thickness defect following excision of basal cell carcinoma; (B) Immediate appearance of reconstructed eyelid following tarso-conjunctival flap from right upper eyelid and full-thickness skin graft from retro-auricular area.

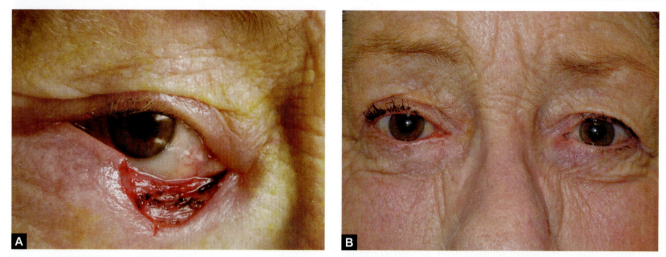

Figs. 42.2A and B: (A) Full-thickness right lower eyelid defect following skin cancer removal. The punctum is intact; (B) Two month postoperative appearance of right lower eyelid following tarso-conjunctival flap and full-thickness skin graft.

after the initial reconstruction (Figs. 42.2A and B). This is not a procedure that should be used in children in the amblyopic age range. Monocular adults should be given other options to consider in addition to lid sharing procedures .

BIBLIOGRAPHY

1. Hewes EH, Sullivan JH, Beard C. Lower eyelid reconstruction by tarsal transposition. Am J Ophthalmol. 1976;81:512-4.
2. Hughes WL. Total lower lid reconstruction: technical details. Trans Am Ophthalmol Soc. 1976;74:321-9.
3. Leone CR Jr, Hand SI Jr. Reconstruction of the medial eyelid. Am J Ophthalmol. 1979;87:797-801.
4. Mustardé JC. Repair and Reconstruction in the Orbital Region: A Practical Guide. Edinburgh: Churchill-Livingstone; 1971.
5. Tenzel RR. Reconstruction of the central one half of an eyelid. Arch Ophthalmol. 1975;93:125-6.
6. Weinstein GS, Anderson RL, Tse DT, et al. The use of a periosteal strip for eyelid reconstruction. Arch Ophthalmol. 1985;103:357-9.

Blepharospasm

43

Christopher M DeBacker, David EE Holck

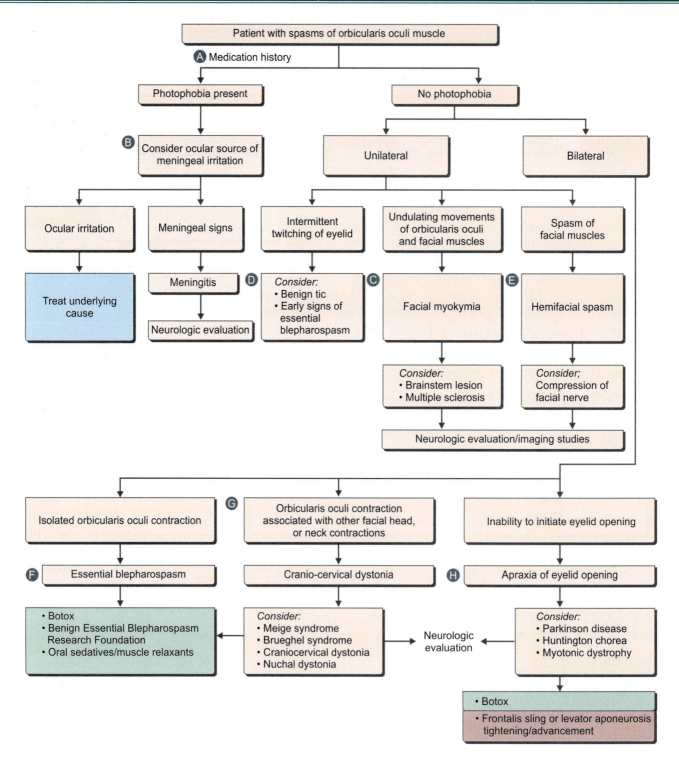

A. A medication history should be obtained to rule out drug reactions as a cause of blepharospasm. Dopaminergic, antidopaminergic and antipsychotic medications can cause blepharospasm although they will usually be accompanied by characteristic movements of tardive dyskinesia.

B. Reflex blepharospasm may be caused by keratopathy, iritis, dry eyes or posterior subcapsular cataracts.

C. Ocular facial myokymia causes rapid, fine, undulating movement of orbicularis oculi muscle and facial muscle fibers. No tonic spasms are present. Transient, intermittent forms of myokymia are usually benign and linked to stressors, such as lack of sleep and excess caffeine intake. If these movements become persistent, brainstem lesions, multiple sclerosis and Guillain–Barré syndrome should be considered.

D. Benign tics are habitual twitches of the facial muscles and eyelids. These may be related to stress or fatigue but are of no neurologic significance.

E. Hemifacial spasm is a unilateral process characterized by intermittent synchronous contractures of the entire side of the face (Fig. 43.1). It may be progressive in nature. It is usually caused by compression of the facial nerve at the cerebellopontine angle by an enlarged blood vessel. Neurosurgical decompression of the nerve root may be curative. Contrast-enhanced magnetic resonance imaging (MRI) will image the aberrant blood vessel as well as less common causes of hemifacial spasm, such as a pontine glioma. Aberrant regeneration of the facial nerve following Bell palsy causes a similar clinical picture of hemifacial spasm. This may be associated with ipsilateral facial weakness. As opposed to essential blepharospasm, the contracture of hemifacial spasm is present during sleep.

F. Benign essential blepharospasm is a bilateral focal dystonia affecting the orbicularis oculi muscles, procerus muscles and corrugator muscles. The disease generally progresses from mild twitching to forceful contractures often rendering the patient functionally blind. Women are affected

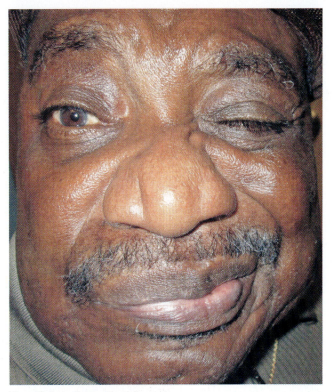

Fig. 43.1: Left hemifacial spasm.

more than men. The etiology is unclear but appears to be of central origin in the basal ganglia. Botulinum toxin is effective in lessening spasms in most individuals, although morbidity from the disease can be psychologically and socially significant. Adjunctive oral medications, such as Klonopin, baclofen and Artane, may be helpful in those patients not deriving adequate relief with Botox. Surgical myectomy may be indicated in severe cases. The Benign Essential Blepharospasm Research Foundation (BEBRF) has been an invaluable support system for individuals suffering from the disease, as well as their families.

G. Blepharospasm may occur as part of a spectrum of cervico-cranial dystonias. Meige syndrome manifests lower facial dystonia along with blepharospasm. Torticollis is a manifestation of neck muscle involvement, while oromandibular dystonia may involve the tongue, pharynx, neck and respiratory muscles. All of these diseases probably represent different manifestations of the same underlying pathophysiology.

H. Apraxia of eyelid opening is characterized by an inability to open the eyelids in the absence of detectable spasms of the orbicularis oculi muscle.

BIBLIOGRAPHY

1. Anderson RL, Patel BC, Holds JB, Jordan DR. Blepharospasm: past, present, and future. Ophthal Plast Reconstr Surg. 1998;14:305-17.
2. Dutton JJ, Buckley EG. Long-term results and complications of botulinum: A toxin in the treatment of blepharospasm. Ophthalmology. 1988;95:1529-34.

Orbital Floor Fracture (Blowout Fracture)

44

David EE Holck, Dimitrios Sismanis

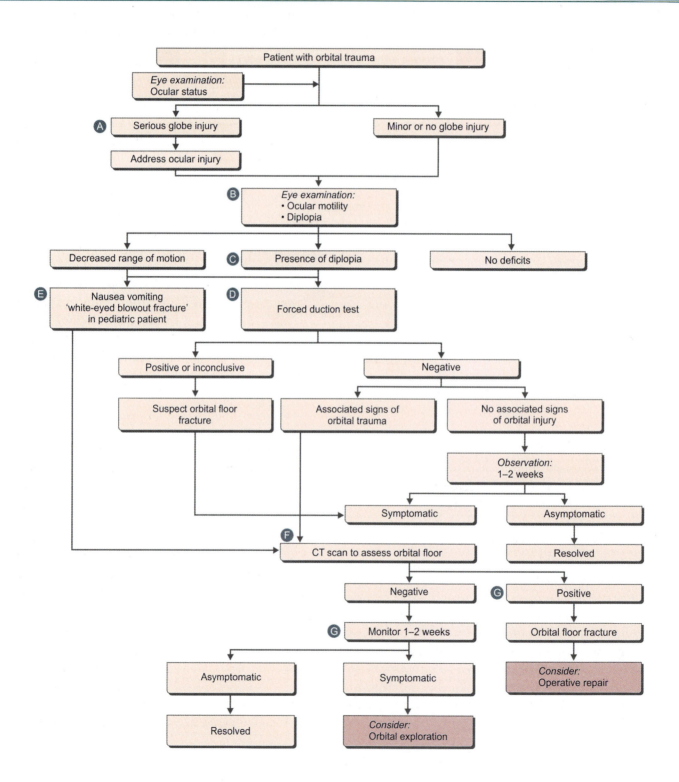

Trauma to the eye or orbit is responsible for a significant volume of all acute care visits in the United States each year. The orbital floor is the most common wall of the orbit to fracture. Mechanisms of injury of the orbital floor include a hydraulic theory and a buckling theory. The former involves increased orbital soft tissue pressure causing the orbital floor to break at the weakest point (usually the posteromedial orbital floor). The latter involves direct trauma to the inferior orbital rim causing the floor to buckle and fracture into the maxillary sinus.

The orbital floor is not flat. The floor slopes up-ward toward the optic canal from its lowest point, approximately one centimeter posterior to the inferior orbital rim. The floor consists of the maxillary bone, with a small contribution posteriorly from the palatine bone, and bordered anterolaterally from the zygomatic bone. The thinnest portion in the floor overlies the infraorbital canal, housing the infraorbital neurovascular bundle (maxillary division of the trigeminal nerve). This makes this location a common area for fractures to occur.

A. Ocular and central nervous system injuries take precedence over repair of an orbital floor fracture. Prior to consideration of orbital fracture repair, a complete ophthalmic evaluation should be un-dertaken to evaluate the integrity of the globe. Ruptured globe repair, retinal detachment repair or other globe injury takes precedence over orbital fracture repair. Additionally, central nervous system involvement necessitates clearance by the neuro-surgeon prior to fracture repair.

B. Clinical signs of orbital floor fracture include perior-bital ecchymosis, edema, subcutaneous emphyse-ma, enophthalmos or exophthalmos, subconjunc-tival hemorrhage, globe dystopia and infraorbital nerve anesthesia or dysesthesia.

C. Complaints of binocular vertical diplopia are commonly noted in orbital floor fractures. This may be noted in up gaze, down gaze, or in primary position. It may be accompanied with or without pain during sursumduction. This vertical diplopia may be due to mechanical restriction of the orbital septa (or less commonly entrapment of the inferior rectus muscle). Occasionally, and even less commonly, the diplopia may be a result of cranial nerve palsy.

D. In addition to a complete ophthalmic examination, specific attention to ocular motility is useful to not only document initial disability, but to evaluate resolution over time. Clinically, motility can be measured in prism diopters, and by using diplopia visual fields. Photographic documentation in all cardinal fields of gaze is also useful. In cases where differentiating between paretic and restrictive motility disturbances is critical, forced ductions and generations are useful, both preoperatively and intraoperatively.

E. The pediatric population represents a subpopula-tion that may demonstrate unique features in orbital floor fractures. Jordan and colleagues described the 'white- eyed blowout fracture', in which a history of blunt trauma to the orbit may have little clinical evidence of trauma, but have dramatic limitation in vertical gaze. This may also be associated with a marked vagal response of nausea and vomiting. CT scanning often demonstrates minimal bony displacement or soft tissue herniation. The increased flexibility of bones of the orbital floor in the pediatric population creates a trapdoor incarceration of orbital soft tissue. This may result in a compartment syndrome that results in aggressive fibrosis and ischemia of the entrapped tissue. This population requires urgent surgical reduction of the herniated tissue to prevent long-term complications.

F. Computed tomography (CT) scanning is the most valuable imaging technique, as it visualizes bone and soft tissue, including the extraocular muscles. Optimal results are obtained with direct coronal and thin axial sections. Spiral CT scanning can now obtain accurate, high-resolution images. Tradi-tional Waters radiographs are rarely used today. Magnetic resonance imaging is useful to view orbital soft tissue, but less so orbital bony structures. Other fractures including medial wall fractures that are seen with floor fractures should be evaluated on the CT scan.

G. In a literature review on isolated orbital floor fractures, Burnstine made recommendations based upon the importance to clinical outcome as well as supportive evidence. Immediate surgical intervention is indicated in early enophthalmos, hypophthalmos and 'white-eyed blowout fractures'.

Surgical intervention within two weeks of injury includes symptomatic diplopia with evidence of entrapped extraocular muscle or soft tissue, large floor fractures, hypophthalmos and progressive infraorbital nerve hypoesthesia. Observation may be indicated in patients with good motility and without significant diplopia, enophthalmos or vertical globe dystopia. Authors have debated the importance of operating within two weeks of orbital injury and have found similar beneficial results waiting additional periods. However, these reviews are useful for determining early repair, delayed repair or observation of fracture patients.

BIBLIOGRAPHY

1. Burnstine MA. Clinical recommendations for repair of isolated orbital floor fractures: An evidence-based analysis. Ophthalmology. 2002;109:1207-10.
2. Chang A, Carter KD, Nerad JA. Orbital floor fractures. In: Holck DEE, Ng JD, (Eds). Evaluation and Treatment of Orbital Fractures: A Multidisciplinary Approach. Philadelphia: Elsevier; 2006.
3. Jordan DR, Allen LH, White J, et al. Intervention within days for some orbital floor fractures: The white-eyed blowout. Ophthalmol Plast Reconstr Surg. 1998;14:37.
4. Simon GJ, Syed HM, McCann JD, et al. Early versus late repair of orbital blowout fractures. Ophthalmic Surg Lasers Imaging. 2009;40:141-8.

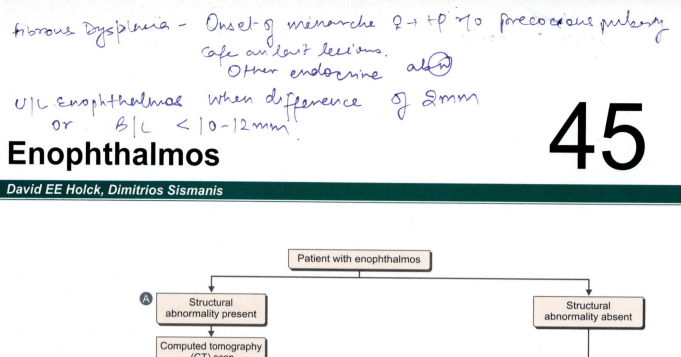

Fibrous Dysplasia – Onset of menarche ♀ → +P 70 precocious puberty
cafe aulait lesions.
Other endocrine ab(n)

U/L enophthalmos when difference of 2mm
or B/L < 10-12mm

Enophthalmos

45

David EE Holck, Dimitrios Sismanis

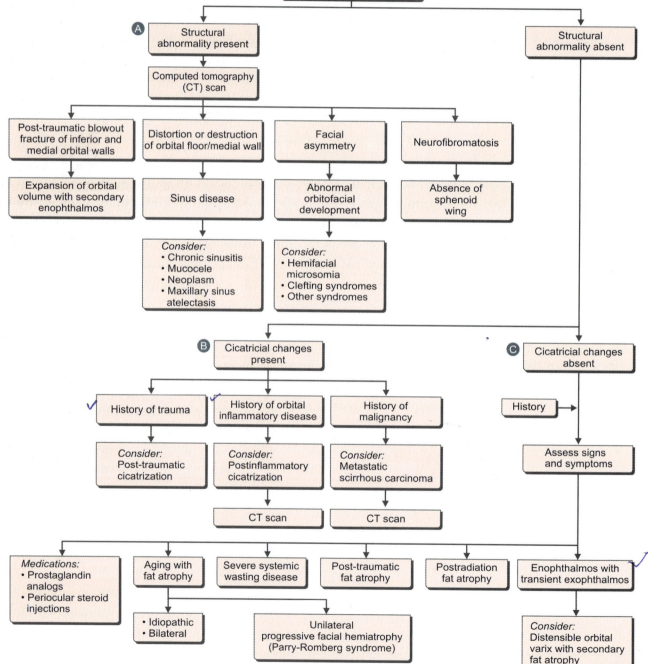

Hertel's . not accurate if asymmetry b/w lateral orbital rims
Naugle's Orbitometer — rest on superior & inferior rims

Enophthalmos is a posterior axial displacement of the globe relative to the contralateral globe or the orbital rims. It may be a critical sign that is often overlooked or underdiagnosed. Multiple mechanisms may result in enophthalmos, and these are anatomically based. Expansion of the bony orbit allows the orbital soft tissue volume to settle into the larger volume. Atrophy of orbital fat within the orbital walls may also cause progressive sinking in of the orbital contents. Finally, cicatrizing (scarring) processes of the orbital soft tissue may cause a tractional pull and posterior displacement. These mechanisms may be separate or in combination:

A. If an orbital structural abnormality is evident or suspected, then computed tomography scanning is indicated to evaluate the bony architecture and compare the symmetry between the orbits. Trauma with bony orbital fractures, especially the orbital floor and medial walls produce an increase in orbital volume (blowout of the orbital walls). This increased orbital volume allows the orbital fat and soft tissue to settle into the expanded boundaries, producing the enophthalmos. Other bony orbital destructive processes that expand the orbital volume may include chronic sinusitis, maxillary sinus atelectasis (silent sinus syndrome), sinus mucocele, as well as invasive malignancies. The absence of the greater wing of the sphenoid bone in neurofibromatosis may result in enophthalmos or exophthalmos. Additionally, several congenital syndromic conditions may be associated with symmetric or asymmetric enophthalmos.

B. Cicatrizing (scarring) processes may cause progressive enophthalmos. Classically, breast carcinoma may be associated with enophthalmos, as well as metastatic adenocarcinoma. Primary sites include lung, prostate and gastric carcinomas. Orbital inflammatory syndromes (sclerosing pseudotumor) as well as post-traumatic conditions may result in cicatrization of the orbital soft tissue and enophthalmos. Dysmotility may be seen in these situations, and imaging with computed tomography or magnetic resonance imaging is helpful to elucidate the abnormalities.

C. Fat atrophy from many causes may also result in clinical enophthalmos. Aging changes may result in atrophy and secondary enophthalmos, as well as idiopathic conditions resulting in asymmetric atrophy (unilateral progressive facial hemiatrophy, Parry-Romberg syndrome). Wasting diseases may result in total body fat atrophy, including the orbits. Medications including steroid injections as well as prostaglandin analog eyedrops used in glaucoma therapy may result in fat atrophy (the latter may be reversible upon discontinuation of the prostaglandin drop). Orbital or facial radiation for neoplastic or inflammatory conditions may also result in fat atrophy and enophthalmos. Orbital varices may also cause enophthalmos secondary to compression fat atrophy or hemorrhage resulting in resorption.

BIBLIOGRAPHY

1. Filippopoulos T, Paula JS, Torun N, et al. Periorbital changes associated with topical bimatoprost. Ophthal Plast Reconstr Surg. 2008;24:302-7.
2. Jackson IT. Enophthalmos. In: Hornblass A, (Ed). Oculoplastic Orbital and Reconstructive Surgery. Baltimore: Williams & Wilkins; 1990. pp. 1299-312.
3. Rootman J. Diseases of the Orbit. Philadelphia: JB Lippincott; 1988.
4. Soparkar CN, Patrinely JR, Cuaycong MJ, et al. The silent sinus syndrome: a cause of spontaneous enophthalmos. Ophthalmology. 1994;101:772-8.

46

Exophthalmos

Christopher M DeBacker, David EE Holck

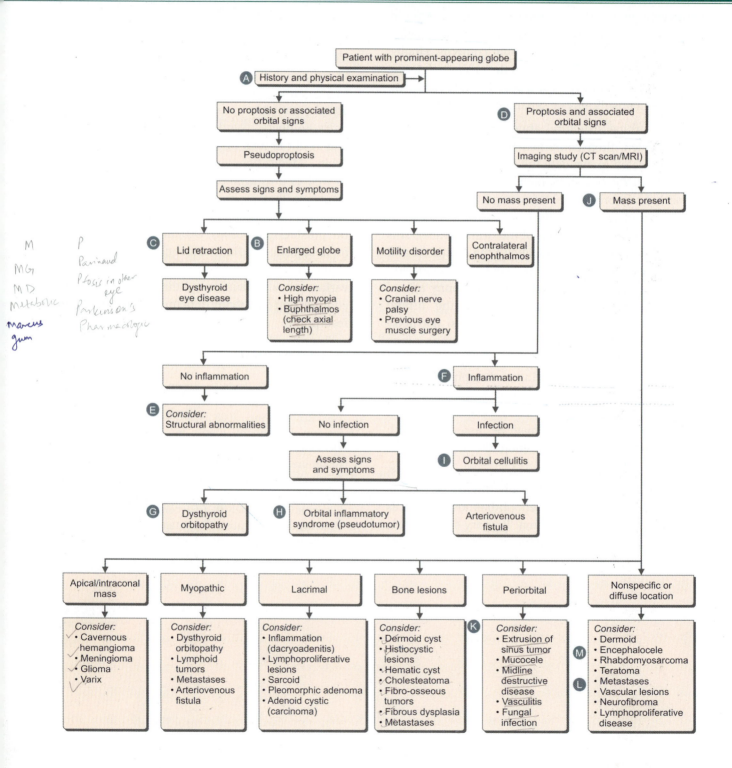

M
MG
MD
Metabolic

marcus
gunn

P
Parinaud
Ptosis in other eye
Parkinson's
Pharmacologic

The presence of a prominent globe may be indicative of a space-occupying lesion in the orbit. Infections and neoplasms must always be considered given their potential for morbidity and mortality. The most common cause of proptosis is orbital cellulitis in children, and thyroid eye disease in adults. The most common benign orbital tumors in children are capillary hemangiomas and dermoid cysts, and cavernous hemangiomas in adults. The most common cause of bilateral proptosis in children is metastatic neuroblastoma and leukemia (chloroma), and thyroid eye disease in adults. The most common orbital malignancy is rhabdomyosarcoma in children, and secondary tumors from adjacent sinuses in adults.

A. A thorough medical history is imperative in the workup of the patient with exophthalmos, as is evident from the high association with systemic processes. An eye examination and head and neck examination is important. Visual acuity needs to be assessed, as well as color vision. The presence or absence of an afferent pupillary defect should be noted, and cranial nerve and motility testing need to be performed. The presence of pain, erythema, edema and pulsations should also be noted.

B. High myopes with eyes having long axial lengths can simulate exophthalmos as can eyelid retraction (pseudoproptosis), and should be included in the differential diagnosis.

C. A common finding with thyroid eye disease is eyelid retraction, which can give the impression of proptosis. The most sensitive finding in thyroid eye disease is 'lid lag' (the upper eyelid lags behind the globe in down gaze).

D. Protrusion of the globe greater than 21 mm or asymmetry greater than 2 mm between the two eyes is indicative of proptosis. Various exophthalmometers exists and most are based on measurements taken from the lateral orbital rim to the corneal apex. The Naugle exophthalmometer is useful for individuals with asymmetric positioning of the lateral orbital rims. An imaging study is critical to assess the orbit when proptosis is evident.

E. Structural abnormalities can decrease orbital volume, producing secondary exophthalmos. This is common in craniofacial syndromes such as Crouzon disease. Post-traumatic conditions may produce a similar situation. Both of these conditions require orbital and midface advancement to increase orbital volume.

F. Orbital inflammatory conditions comprise about 60% of all orbital disease, and are broken down further into infectious and noninfectious etiologies. Presentation is usually acute or subacute, with variable eyelid erythema, edema, conjunctival injection and chemosis along with orbital signs and symptoms.

G. Thyroid eye disease may precede, proceed, or present concurrently with systemic thyroid disease (Fig. 46.2). Unilateral or bilateral exophthalmos, eyelid retraction, chemosis, ocular injection, strabismus and optic neuropathy may be present. A thyroid stimulating immunoglobulin (TSI) level is helpful to assess and follow the presence or absence of the active inflammatory stage of thyroid eye disease.

H. Orbital inflammatory syndrome (OIS) or 'orbital pseudotumor' typically presents with pain, in addition to other orbital signs and symptoms. It may present as a myositis (involving the tendinous insertion of the extraocular muscles, in contrast to thyroid eye disease), dacryoadenitis, scleritis or diffuse orbital inflammation. Approximately, half of children have bilateral involvement, whereas in adults bilaterality is suspicious for a systemic lymphoproliferative disease or systemic vasculitis. OIS is usually quite sensitive to systemic corticosteroids.

I. Orbital cellulitis is usually secondary to an adjacent sinusitis. Endogenous sources and exogenous spread from a preseptal cellulitis may also occur. Imaging with a computed tomography (CT) scan is necessary to assess the periorbital sinuses and the possibility of a subperiosteal or intraorbital abscess. Hospital admission with intravenous antibiotics is necessary, and abscess drainage may be required if clinical or radiologic response is not evident or if vision is threatened.

J. Orbital neoplasms account for about 20% of orbital disease. Medical history, patient age, presenting signs and symptoms, and imaging characteristics

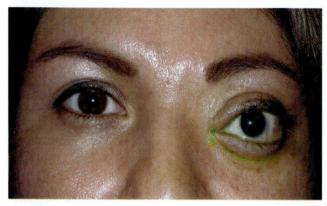

Fig. 46.1: Low-flow venous malformation of the left orbit with proptosis.

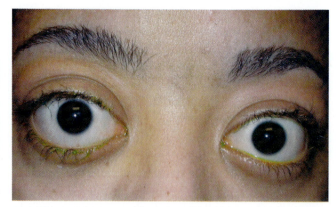

Fig. 46.2: Bilateral proptosis due to thyroid eye disease.

will be helpful in narrowing the differential diagnosis. An orbitotomy may be required for diagnosis and treatment.

K. Contiguous spread of disease from the eyelids and adnexal structures, periorbital sinuses and intracranial compartment is the most common cause of orbital malignancy in adults. The patients' medical history is important for making a diagnosis, and orbital imaging studies [CT scan and magnetic resonance imaging (MRI)] is necessary.

L. Vascular lesions of the orbit may present in children and adults. Capillary hemangiomas of the orbit will often have associate cutaneous lesions. Lymphangiomas may present with rapid growth during upper respiratory infections causing sudden increase in proptosis due to intralesional hemorrhage. Post-traumatic carotid-cavernous sinus fistulas and varices are examples of high and low-flow lesions of adults (Fig. 46.1), which may cause proptosis. Appropriate imaging with contrast-enhanced MRI, magnetic resonance angiogram, and CT-angiogram in consultation with a neuro-radiologist is helpful for diagnosis.

M. Rhabdomyosarcoma must always be considered in children presenting with orbital disease, even though the clinical history may be muddled by a recent traumatic event. Rapid diagnosis and treatment are imperative to limit mortality and ocular morbidity.

BIBLIOGRAPHY

1. Dutton JJ, Haik BG. Thyroid Eye Disease: Diagnosis and Treatment. New York, USA: Informa Healthcare; 2002
2. Garrity JA, Henderson JW, Cameron JD. Henderson's Orbital Tumors. Philadelphia: Lippincott Williams & Wilkins; 2006.
3. Leone CR Jr, Lloyd WC 3rd. Treatment protocol for orbital inflammatory disease. Ophthalmology. 1985;92:1325-31.
4. Rootman J, (Ed). Diseases of the Orbit: A Multidisciplinary Approach. Philadelphia: Lippincott Williams & Wilkins; 2003.

Symblepharon

Dimitrios Sismanis, David EE Holck

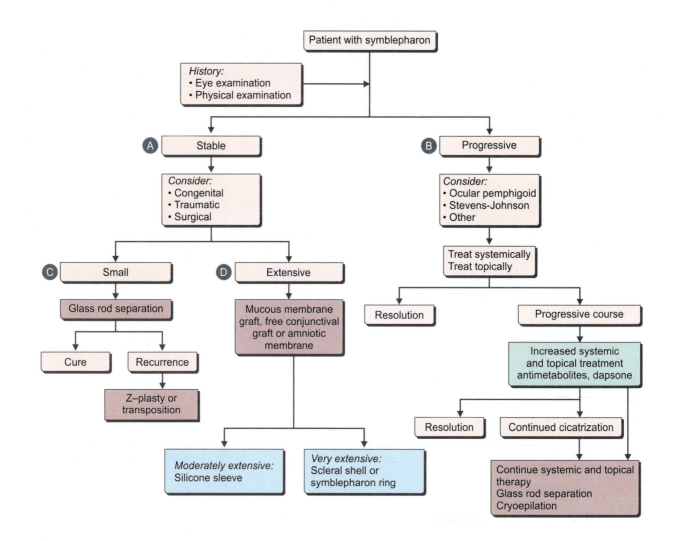

47

A symblepharon is an adhesion between conjunctival surfaces or between the conjunctiva and the cornea. When mucosal surfaces are abraded and come in contact with each other, they can become adherent. Etiologies include congenital, traumatic, postsurgical or inflammatory causes. While the first three etiologies present as a stable adhesion, inflammatory symblepharon may show a progressive course.

ETIOLOGY OF SYMBLEPHARON

A. Stable Symblepharon

Congenital Symblepharon

A congenital symblepharon is rare and may be associated with Goldenhar syndrome or a forme fruste of that disease. Dermolipomas and limbal dermoids, which occur commonly in this syndrome, can rarely be associated with abnormal adhesions. These patients may also experience postsurgical symblepharon (*see* below) when these tumors are removed. Treatment of congenital symblepharon is surgical. Treatment of congenital symblepharon should be implemented early, particularly if extraocular muscle movement is restricted or a strabismus results. Otherwise, amblyopia could ensue.

Traumatic Symblepharon

Symblepharon may occur after trauma, when a malpositioning of tissues or a loss of conjunctiva associated with denuded epithelial surfaces adjacent to each other can promote adhesions. It is thus important to avoid being too aggressive in debridement and save as much traumatized tissue as possible. Chemical exposures, though traumatic in nature, should be considered inflammatory in the acute period; however, symblepharon occurring after the acute inflammatory episode has occurred may be managed as traumatic symblepharon. The treatment for traumatic symblepharon is surgical. Adequate time should be given from the initial trauma to allow for healing to occur.

Postsurgical Symblepharon

Postsurgical symblepharon occurs most often after pterygium excision. In this situation, raw surfaces are created on the cornea, limbus and sclera, which together with conjunctival shortening and shrinkage, produce adhesions, which may also involve the inner aspects of both the upper and lower eyelids. This may also occur after any conjunctival excision, particularly aggressive removal of dermolipomas. After removal of large eyelid tumors, there can be a paucity of conjunctiva to cover the reconstructed area, and bare epithelial surfaces may adhere. Symblepharon was also common after scleral buckling procedures, when the 360° conjunctival incisions were made several millimeters from the limbus. However, most retina surgeons now use limbal incisions. The mainstay of treatment of postsurgical symblepharon is prevention. Appropriate surgical technique should be implemented including meticulous wound closure and avoidance of exposed de-epithelialized tissue. However, if postsurgical symblepharon occurs treatment is surgical as for traumatic symblepharon. Realignment of malpositioned tissue may be rectified in the immediate postoperative period if it is recognized. If it is not recognized in the immediate postoperative period, it is likely best to wait 6 months before addressing the postoperative symblepharon surgically.

B. Progressive Symblepharon

Ocular Cicatricial Pemphigoid

Ocular pemphigoid is a bilateral autoimmune inflammatory conjunctival disease with progressive, relentless shrinkage of the mucosal surfaces. It affects women twice as often as men and usually occurs after the age of 60 years. Diagnosis is made histopathologically with immunostaining. Cicatrizing conjunctivitis can cause a decrease in tear and goblet cell secretion, symblepharon and may even result in restricted ocular motility. Additional sequelae include cicatricial entropion and trichiasis. As with postsurgical symblepharon, the treatment of inflammatory symblepharon is prevention. Progressive inflammatory symblepharon is treated medically to reduce the amount of inflammation and cicatrization. Systemic and topical corticosteroids (in suspension or ointment form) are used. Topical cyclosporine may be administered as well in the acute inflammatory process to reduce inflammation, in addition to treating the associated chronic dry eye. Aggressive lubrication in the form of preservative free tears and ointment should be used. Particularly in Stevens-Johnson syndrome routine sweeping of the fornices should be performed to prevent adhesion formation. Placement of scleral shells in the fornices also separates the palpebral from the bulbar conjunctiva but is sometimes traumatic and irritating to an eye that is already inflamed. Further, it may not retard the process in the long run.

In ocular pemphigoid, antimetabolites (e.g. cyclophosphamide) are used together with corticosteroids. Another adjunctive treatment for ocular cicatricial pemphigoid is dapsone, an antibacterial used to treat leprosy. Care should be taken to avoid dapsone use in patients with glucose 6-phosphate dehydrogenase deficiency as this may precipitate hemolysis and resultant anemia.

Otherwise, treatment for extensive symblepharon is surgical, as is the treatment for cicatricial entropion and trichiasis that may accompany the symblepharon.

Stevens-Johnson Syndrome

Stevens-Johnson syndrome (erythema multiforme) is an acute inflammatory vesicular reaction of the skin and mucous membranes. Although potentially fatal, this disease is self-limited, as opposed to ocular pemphigoid. However, during the acute stage there can be conjunctival shrinkage, surface membrane destruction and permanent keratitis sicca. This condition is thought to occur most often as a result of drug sensitivity to sulfonamides, salicylates or penicillin. Treatment is similar as above.

Other Causes of Inflammatory Symblepharon

Inflammatory etiologies of symblepharon include chemical exposure, membranous conjunctivitis, chronic topical medication use, atopic keratoconjunctivitis, radiation treatment and rarely malignancy. Inflammatory symblepharon is the most frustrating and difficult to treat because its activity may persist and any surgical intervention, although successful at first, may fail later. Treatment is similar as above.

C. Surgical Correction of Mild Symblepharon

The goal of surgical correction of symblepharon is to lyse adhesions between the bulbar and palpebral conjunctiva, to reconstruct the fornices, to replace as much conjunctiva as necessary to cover the ocular surface and to allow for proper mobility of the globe. If the symblepharon is small, glass rod separation may be first attempted. If this is inadequate, a Z-plasty can be done to increase the fornix depth. Another technique is to separate the symblepharon from the globe, and then mobilize the bulbar conjunctiva on either side of the symblepharon excision site. Next, slide the two sides toward each other and suture them together, and then transpose the remaining symblepharon, which is still attached to the palpebral conjunctiva, into the fornix and secure it with a full thickness lid suture which is tied on the outside of the lid (transposition).

D. Surgical Correction of Severe Symblepharon

For the more severe symblepharon associated with shrinkage, a split-thickness buccal mucosal graft (0.5 mm thickness) or a free conjunctival graft should be used to cover the raw surfaces after the symblepharon has been completely released, and the globe and eyelids are fully mobile. Amniotic membrane may be used as an alternative to autologous mucous membrane. The entire ocular surface as well as the lid margin should be covered. The mucosal graft may be secured with suture, or with fibrin glue. A scleral shell or a symblepharon ring may then be used to keep the fornices intact and should be left in for 1–2 weeks. If the area is not too extensive, a thin silicone sleeve (0.5 mm thickness) can be draped over the lid margin, one surface on the fornix side and other on the cutaneous side, with a through-and-through suture to stabilize it. Surgical treatment of cicatricial entropion and the resultant trichiasis is beyond the scope of this chapter. Briefly, cicatricial entropion is corrected by lengthening the posterior lamella as described above. Trichiasis is usually addressed with cryoepilation.

▌BIBLIOGRAPHY

1. Belin MW, Hannush SB. Mucous membrane abnormalities. In: Abhott RL, (Ed). Surgical Intervention in Corneal and External Disease. Orlando: Grune and Stratton; 1987. pp. 159-76.
2. Gregory, Darren. Acute Stevens-Johnson syndrome: ophthalmologic evaluation and management. In: Mannis MJ (Ed). Vision Pan-America. Sacrament. Arlington: Pan-American Association of Ophthalmology; 2010.
3. Leone CR. Treatment of conjunctival diseases and chalazia. In: Stewart W, (Ed). Ophthalmic Plastic Surgery and Reconstructive Surgery. San Francisco: American Academy of Ophthalmology; 1984.

SECTION 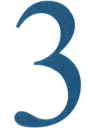 3

Pediatric Ophthalmology and Strabismus

Treatment of Amblyopia Secondary to a Refractive Error

48

James L Mims III

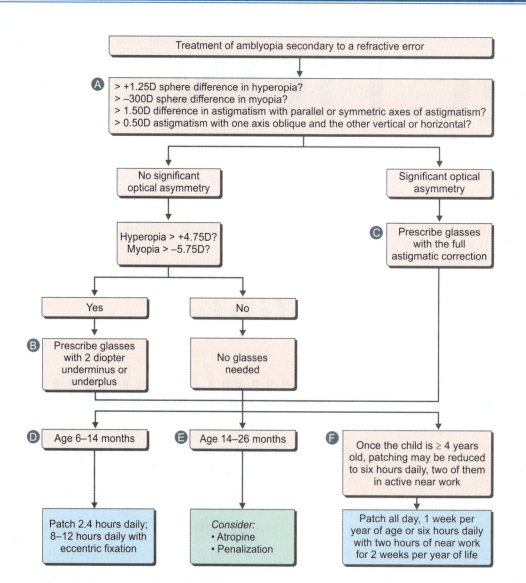

A. The degree of anisometropia that is likely to cause amblyopia is only moderately well known. The following is based on American Academy of Ophthalmology and American Association for Pediatric Ophthalmology and Strabismus recommendations and the author's experience— you should provide optical correction for these degrees of anisometropia: (1) greater than +1.25 D difference in hyperopia, (2) greater than −3.00 D sphere difference in myopia, (3) greater than 1.50 D difference in parallel or symmetric axes of astigmatism,* and greater than 0.50 D

---

*Parallel axes can be judged simply by looking at the refractor, phoropter, or trial frame and judging whether the axis of astigmatism of one eye is within 20° of parallel with the axis of astigmatism of the other eye. Symmetric axes of astigmatism refer to mirror image astigmatism (e.g. 45° in one eye and 135° in the other eye). If the axes are 30° or more away from parallel or mirror image symmetry, a very minor amount of astigmatism will cause amblyopia, even if the amount of astigmatism is the same in each eye

astigmatism with one axis oblique and the other axis vertical or horizontal.

B. Children with bilateral hyperopia of greater than +4.75 D sphere will have bilateral refractive amblyopia if they do not start wearing glasses by age 7 years, even if there is no anisometropia. If they are given the full correction, divergence fusional amplitudes will be reduced and iatrogenic accommodative esotropia can result. (My child was not cross-eyed without glasses until he started wearing the glasses you prescribed, Doctor). Giving 2 D less than the full spherical equivalence is safe in anticipation of patching, unless the child has a tiny esotropia ('flick ET', or a monofixation syndrome), in which case the full hyperopic correction should be given. An obsolete rule was to give 50% of a highly hyperopic correction. I have seen more than one child with +8.00 D hyperopia whose accommodative esotropia began when 50% of the full plus was prescribed by another practitioner. This left the child with +4.00 D residual, enough to produce accommodative esotropia. Children with bilateral myopia of –5.75 D sphere also need glasses to prevent bilateral refractive amblyopia but if they are given in the full myopic correction, they may reject it because of the new demands being made on their accommodative abilities. Also, a few may become esotropic as a result of new stimulation of accommodative convergence provided by the full myopic correction. Finally, there is evidence that in highly myopic children, a widely dilated pupil after cycloplegia may give an excessively high myopic reading on retinoscopy because of aberrations in the peripheral lens (children usually have larger pupils after cycloplegia than adults). These are three good reasons to underminus a highly myopic child's first pair of glasses, generally by about 2 D. In moderate myopia, overcorrection by 0.50 D is preferred by some practitioners, anticipating that the myopia will worsen.

C. Because adults may develop headaches or other symptoms of asthenopia when they are first given an optical correction for their astigmatism, many practitioners do not realize the importance of giving the full astigmatic correction to a child. Not only can the child readily adapt to the full correction but it is required if amblyopia is to be treated effectively.

D. Once the determination has been made whether glasses should be prescribed, the next question is how to occlude the better eye. Babies 6–14 months old are extremely sensitive to patching, and severe iatrogenic amblyopia can result from overpatching in infancy. Alternate patching is no longer recommended. Babies 6–14 months of age should be patched 2–4 hours daily, unless the nondominant eye has eccentric fixation. If the nondominant eye has eccentric fixation, then 8–10 waking hours may be appropriate if the infant can be monitored no less frequently than every 2 weeks.

E. When a child reaches 14 months of age, he or she enters the developmental period known as the 'terrible two's (a poll of 18 pediatricians and 2 pediatric specialists led to the unanimous response that the terrible two's starts at age 14 months and ends at age 27–36 months). During this period, seriously consider atropine penalization.

F. After the third birthday, patching all but 2 hours daily, 1 week per year of age, is standard. Many eye care practitioners do not routinely prescribe enough hours of patching each day. When the amblyopia is severe in a child aged 6–9 years, the dominant eye should be patched all waking moments for a full 10 weeks. If no improvement occurs after the 10 weeks, it is reasonable to stop patching. When patching is discontinued, it should be withdrawn gradually, reducing the hours of patching each week by 1 hour daily. Calendar sheets given to the parents are helpful. It has been demonstrated that if the original visual acuity at the start of patching was very poor (20/100 or worse) or if the best visual acuity obtained after prolonged patching was 20/50 or worse, maintenance patching 2 hours daily after school until the tenth birthday is important to prevent a return of severe amblyopia. When the amblyopia is severe, it may be unreasonable to ask one adult to initiate patching. Having one parent set-up a schedule of several concerned adults (e.g. grandparents) so that each one can spend an hour with the child on a Saturday (simply keeping him or her from touching the patch) is more effective than elaborate restraints, punishments, and so on, when the patching is started. Filling up a large desk pad calendar with the patches as they are removed and giving a reward for each week of good patching behavior is another effective technique. Once the child is 4 years old or older, patching may be reduced to 6 hours daily if the child can be persuaded to enthusiastically pursue 'near work activities' such as video games or arts and crafts for 2 of the 6 hours daily.

BIBLIOGRAPHY

1. Attebo K, Mitchell P, Cumming R, et al. Prevalence and causes of amblyopia in an adult population. Ophthalmology. 1998;105:154-9.
2. The Pediatric Eye Disease Investigator Group. A randomized pilot study of near activities vs. non-near activities during patching therapy for amblyopia. J AAPOS 2005;129-36.
3. The Pediatric Eye Disease Investigator Group. A randomized trial of atropine regimens for treatment of moderate amblyopia in children. Ophthalmology 2004;111:2076-85.

49

The Diagnosis of Strabismus

Johan Zwaan

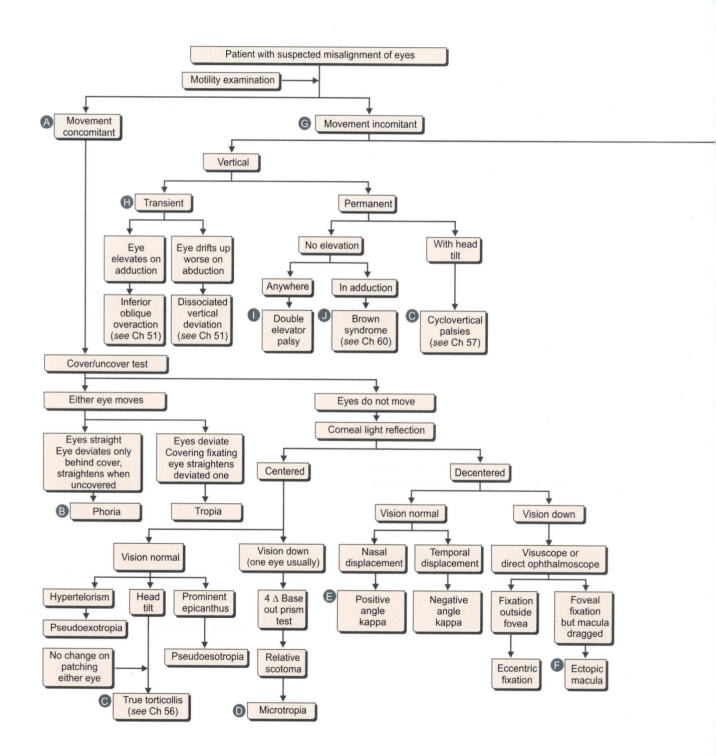

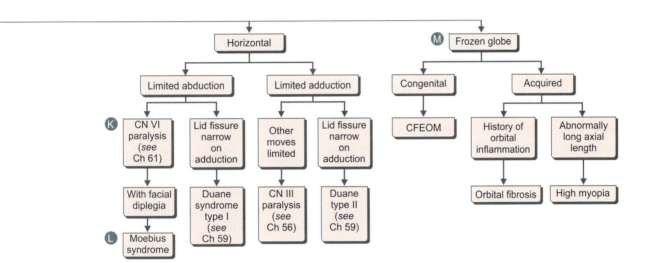

When a parent brings a child with a suspected misalignment of the eyes to the ophthalmologist, a complete eye examination, including a dilated fundus examination and cycloplegic retinoscopy or refraction, is imperative. Attention needs to be paid to significant refractive errors, to abnormalities in the media (Chapter 67), and to possible lesions of the fundus. As noted elsewhere (Chapter 71), one in five children with retinoblastoma presents with strabismus. Once the causes of secondary strabismus have been eliminated, the examiner can concentrate on the ocular motility problem.

The diagnostic scheme proposed here is somewhat dogmatic. It does not take into account that conditions may coexist. For instance, a positive angle kappa, giving an appearance of exotropia, may be combined with a true esotropia, which then is more difficult to detect. Alternatively, esotropia is commonly associated with overaction of the inferior oblique muscles, which turns a primarily comitant strabismus transiently into an incomitant one, mostly in adduction.

A. Misalignment of the visual axes with full motility and basically the same deviation in all directions of gaze occurs by far in the largest group of children with strabismus. The epidemiology of strabismus is rather deficient, but up to 5% of the entire population may have a form of strabismus. In addition, children with pseudostrabismus also have comitant and full motility.

B. Sometimes, a phoria is difficult to bring out with the cover and uncover test. Repeated alternate cover testing may be needed to break up fusion.

C. A head tilt indicates a cyclovertical muscle palsy or a disorder of the sternocleidomastoid muscle or cervical spine. Their differentiation is important (Chapters 56 and 57) for the institution of proper treatment. If a child with a fourth cranial nerve palsy is unnecessarily treated by surgery or physical therapy, as if the torticollis were caused by a sternocleidomastoid abnormality, amblyopia can be induced.

D. Microstrabismus·covers a range of abnormalities in which the deviation is so small that it is difficult to demonstrate a shift of the eye with the usual cover test. One type is characterized by a minimal misalignment with a complete sensory adaptation. Unilateral amblyopia is often caused by anisometropia and parafoveal fixation. Peripheral fusion and modest stereoacuity are demonstrable.

E. The angle kappa is the angle between the visual axis (from point of fixation to fovea) and the pupillary axis (through the center of the pupil perpendicular to the cornea). Its interest lies mainly in the confusion it may cause in the recognition of strabismus. It can simulate an exodeviation or esodeviation or obscure a true strabismus in the opposite direction.

F. Ectopia of the macula by dragging is mostly caused by severe retinal scarring seen with retinopathy of prematurity. It may be bilateral. It can also be associated with the retinitis caused by *Toxocara canis* infection and with familial exudative vitreoretinopathy.

G. The limited data available indicate that perhaps only 1 in 1,000 strabismus patients has an incomitant type (excluding the rather common overaction of the inferior obliques and dissociated vertical deviation).

H. The transient vertical deviations seen in association with congenital (infantile) esotropia and sometimes exotropia (i.e. overaction of the inferior obliques and dissociated vertical deviations) are perhaps the most common reason for a vertical deviation. They are discussed in detail elsewhere (Chapter 51).

I. Double elevator palsy is demonstrated by an inability to elevate the eye in any direction of gaze. Although this disability may result from a paralysis of both superior rectus and inferior oblique muscle, more likely the paralysis of the superior rectus causes contraction of the inferior rectus, which then mechanically limits upgaze in all directions.

J. Brown syndrome is congenital or acquired. Its hallmark is an inability to elevate the eye in adduction, which becomes progressively better, the more the eye is abducted. It is accompanied by overaction of the contralateral superior rectus muscle, which is the more obvious sign. The congenital variety may be caused by an anomaly of the superior oblique tendon (too short) or by an abnormality of the trochlea or tendon sheath. All types mechanically restrict elevation. The acquired variety can be caused by inflammation, trauma, or rarely other causes such as a metastasis. Sometimes it occurs periodically with a flare-up of juvenile idiopathic arthritis.

K. The differential diagnosis of cranial nerve sixth palsies can be confusing. The most common type is Duane syndrome type I, in which the palsy is combined with retraction of the eye and narrowing of the lid fissure on adduction. Congenital isolated palsy of the sixth cranial nerve is often benign and transient, resolving before age 2 months. In the absence of other neurologic abnormalities, the prognosis is excellent. An acquired sixth cranial nerve palsy can also be benign and transient. It may occur a few weeks after a febrile illness, after immunization, or without a recognized precipitating factor, and it may recur. The paralysis generally recovers within 2–3 months, but recovery may take several months. Persistence of the palsy for several months without any improvement is a reason for concern and neurologic and otolaryngologic evaluations, CT and/or MRI scanning should be done. Hydrocephalus and pseudo tumors may be associated with sixth cranial nerve palsy, but a tumor, usually a pontine glioma, must be excluded.

L. In Moebius syndrome congenital palsies of the sixth cranial nerve are combined with facial diplegia (due to facial nerve palsy), resulting in a flat expressionless face. Other cranial nerve palsies may be present. Other neurologic and other anomalies may be present.

M. Frozen globes with little or no motility can be the result of congenital fibrosis of the extraocular muscles, of which several varieties exist. Recent research has shown that the most common type, with the eyes fixed in downgaze and associated with ptosis, is caused by an autosomal dominant locus on chromosome 12. A second type with the eyes frozen in exotropia, mild hypotropia, and with ptosis is caused by an autosomal recessive gene on chromosome 11q13. In both types the third cranial nerve and its nucleus is (partially) absent. Other causes for frozen globes include orbital fibrosis, following severe orbital pseudotumor, and very high myopia.

BIBLIOGRAPHY

1. Afifi AK, Bell WE, Bale JF, et al. Recurrent lateral rectus palsy in childhood. Pediatr Neurol. 1990;6:315-8.
2. Brodsky MC, Pollock SC, Buckley EG. Neural misdirection in congenital ocular fibrosis syndrome: implications and pathogenesis. J Pediatr Ophthalmol Strabismus. 1989;26: 159-61.
3. Clarke WN, Noel LP. Stereoacuity testing in the monofixation syndrome. J Pediatr Ophthalmol Strabismus. 1990;27:161-3.
4. Helveston EM. Classification of superior oblique muscle palsy. Ophthalmology. 1992;99:1609-15.
5. Hotchkiss MG, Miller NR, Clark AW, et al. Bilateral Duane's retraction syndrome. A clinical-pathological case report. Arch Ophthalmol. 1980;98:870-4.
6. Metz HS. Double elevator palsy. J Pediatr Ophthalmol Strabismus. 1981;18:31-5.
7. Raab EL. Clinical features of Duane's syndrome. J Pediatr Ophthalmol Strabismus. 1986;23:64-8.
8. Wang SM, Zwaan J, Mullaney PB, et al. Congenital fibrosis of the extraocular muscles type 2, an inherited exotropic strabismus fixus, maps to distal 11q13. Am J Hum Genet. 1998;63:517-25.
9. Wilson ME, Parks MM. Primary inferior oblique overaction in congenital esotropia, accommodative esotropia, and intermittent exotropia. Ophthalmology. 1989;96:950-5.

Infantile Esotropia

James L Mims III

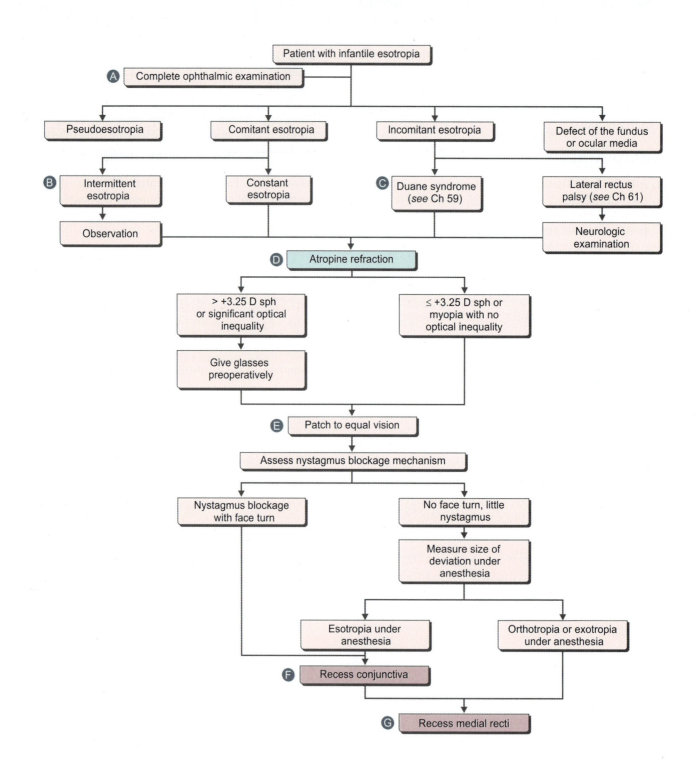

50

A. Infants believed by referring physicians, nurses or family to have esotropia should be examined by age 5 months to rule out defects of the fundi or ocular media, including retinoblastoma. Primary care physicians should be taught to use the red reflex test with the direct ophthalmoscope, as well as the corneal reflection test (Hirschberg) when esotropia is suspected. Many infants with esotropia have only a small or intermittent deviation by age 6 months, which grows into a large, constant deviation by age 10 months.

B. A deviation in infants that is intermittent or spasmodic and less than 25 prism diopters (PD) in size may simply resolve with no treatment and deserves several months of simple observation.

C. Incomitant esotropia with limited abduction of one eye may be a sign of Duane syndrome if the palpebral fissure narrows on adduction and the degree of esotropia is relatively small compared with the severity of the limitation of abduction. True lateral rectus palsies, with a 25–35 PD esotropia combined with severe limitation of abduction and little or no narrowing of the palpebral fissure on adduction, are less common than Duane syndrome, require neurologic examination and may clear spontaneously in 6 weeks.

D. Atropine refraction is mandatory unless office drops in a blue-eyed child indicate significant myopia. Glasses are prescribed if the spherical equivalent is +3.25 D hyperopic or if there is a significant optical difference between the two eyes (Ch 48). Preoperative glasses generally do not straighten the eyes in infantile esotropia, but if glasses prove to be needed postoperatively, the parents will never say, "Doctor, my child did not need glasses until you did your surgery".

E. Patching to equal vision means free alternation of fixation, or at least maintenance of fixation of the cross-fixating eye until at least the midline as it follows a horizontally moving target.

Table 50.1: Amounts of medial rectus recession	
Diopters of preoperative esotropia	Millimeters of bilateral medial rectus recession (each eye)
15	3.5
20	4.2
25	4.7
30	5.1
35	5.5
40	5.7
45	6.1
50	6.3
55	6.5
60	6.7
65	6.9
70	7.1
75	7.2

F. Avoid cul-de-sac technique and recess conjunctiva if preoperatively the fixing eye is in adduction to null nystagmus with a face turn or if the esotropia persists under anesthesia.

G. Recess the medial recti according to a dose-response curve. Amounts of medial rectus recession in classic textbooks have previously been too small (Table 50.1).

BIBLIOGRAPHY

1. Ing MR. Early surgical alignment for congenital esotropia. J Pediatr Ophthalmol Strabismus. 1983;20:11-8.
2. Kushner BJ, Lucchese NJ, Morton GV. Should recessions of the medial recti be graded from the limbus or the insertion? Arch Ophthalmol. 1989;107:1755-8.
3. Mims JL III, Treff G, Kincaid M, et al. Quantitative surgical guidelines for bimedial recession for infantile esotropia. Binocular Vision. 1985;1:7-22.
4. Tran HM, Mims JL 3rd, Wood RC. A new dose-response curve for bilateral medial rectus recessions for infantile esotropia. J AAPOS. 2002;6:112-9.

Overaction of the Inferior Oblique Muscles and Dissociated Vertical Deviation

51

James L Mims III

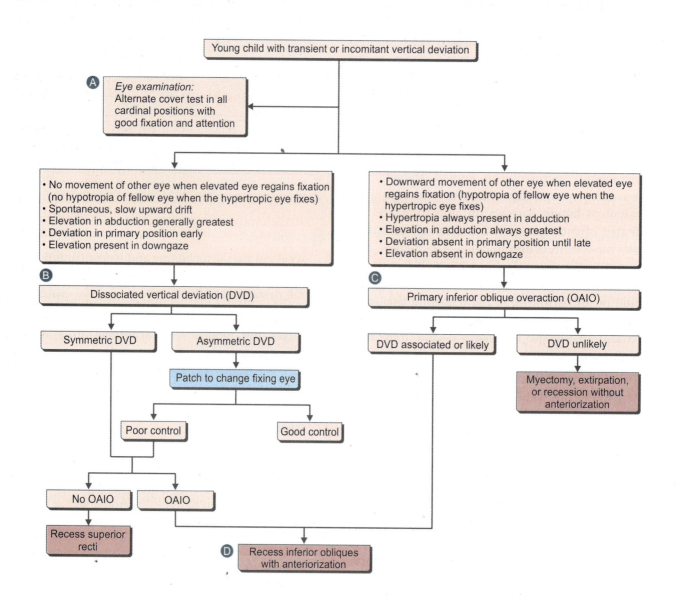

A. The most common disorders producing transient or incomitant vertical deviation in a young child are dissociated vertical deviation (DVD) and primary overaction of the inferior obliques (OAIO). Both are common in children who have (had) infantile esotropia. Numerous remote-controlled toys at the end of a 20-foot eye lane and several toys for near fixation are essential to obtain good alternate cover test measurements in all cardinal positions with good fixation and attention. In DVD, the other eye does not move when the elevated eye regains fixation (no hypotropia of the fellow eye when the hypertropic eye fixes). In primary OAIO, however, the other eye moves downward when the elevated eye regains fixation (hypotropia of the fellow eye when the hypertropic eye fixes). DVD occurs as a slow, upward drift of the affected eye, often with some extorsion as the eye drifts upward. It may be spontaneous or may occur only behind cover. In OAIO, a hypertropia of the fixing eye always occurs in adduction. In DVD, the elevation in abduction is generally (not always) greatest; in OAIO the elevation in adduction is always greatest. DVD is intermittently manifest in the primary (straight-ahead) position early, whereas in OAIO the deviation is not present in the primary position until late in the course of the disorder. The vertical deviation of DVD is present (and may be greatest) in downgaze; the vertical deviation of OAIO is usually absent in downgaze. If there is no elevation of the adducting eye on direct sidegaze in the patient who has significant upshoot of the adducting eye when the fixing abducted eye looks up and into abduction, suspect a variant of the co-contraction syndromes (e.g. Duane syndrome; Ch 59). In this case bilateral lateral rectus recessions with supraplacement are the appropriate surgical therapy.

B. Once the diagnosis of DVD has been made, give careful attention to the spectacle correction. In many cases, optical correction of astigmatism controls the DVD. If the deviation is uncontrolled with glasses and the DVD is much worse in one eye than in the other, the eyes of some children less than 5 years of age may be patched so thoroughly that the eye with the greater tendency to DVD can be made to become the fixing (dominant) eye. If this can be accomplished, the DVD remains latent. If the DVD is symmetric or objectionably large in both eyes even after glasses and patching, carefully look for an association of OAIO. If even a little OAIO is present, recession of the inferior obliques with anteriorization to a point 1 mm anterior to the lateral end of the inferior rectus insertion eliminates both the DVD and the OAIO. If simply no OAIO is present, the most popular procedure is bilateral 10-mm recession of the superior recti. This may be done by the "hang loose" technique, which is technically easy and leaves the superior rectus on the nasal side of the vertical axis of Fick, a detail important in the prevention of the secondary exotropia that could otherwise be produced by a large superior rectus recession. One complication of the hang loose technique has been lack of adherence of the superior rectus to the globe, especially if it falls over the superior oblique tendon. A more reliable procedure is to attach the end of the superior rectus directly to the globe with a 10-mm recession and 3–4 mm of nasal transposition. Whatever technique of superior rectus recession is used, it is essential to dissect the dorsal surface of the superior rectus 16–18 mm posterior to its insertion to sever the frenulum that connects the superior rectus to the levator. If this connection is not severed, severe lid retraction can result postoperatively.

C. If the incomitant vertical deviation has been determined primarily to be OAIO, some DVD is often also present. If the child has had infantile esotropia, DVD may develop in the future, occasionally as late as age 11 years. If any DVD is present, or if there is a history of infantile esotropia, it is wise to recess the inferior obliques with anteriorization to 1 mm anterior to the lateral ends of the inferior recti. If there is no history of infantile esotropia, and the OAIO is not associated with any DVD, the author favors recession of the IO 14 mm along its natural pathway with triangular myectomy of the posterior insertional fibers, and reattachment of the anterior insertional fibers 5 mm posterior to the lateral end of the IO insertion. This is effective for the OAIO, and the IO remains available in the unlikely event that it will have to be anteriorly transposed in the future as part of treatment for DVD.

D. Recession of the inferior obliques with anteriorization to a point 1 mm anterior to the lateral end of the inferior rectus insertion eliminates not only the OAIO but also the DVD. It should never be done unilaterally; unilateral anteriorization produces a significant restrictive hypotropia.

BIBLIOGRAPHY

1. Kushner BJ. Pseudoinferior oblique overaction associated with Y and V patterns. Ophthalmology. 1991;98:1500-5.
2. Magoon E, Cruciger M, Jampolsky A. Dissociated vertical deviation: an asymmetric condition treated with large bilateral superior rectus recession. J Pediatr Ophthalmol Strabismus. 1982;19:152-6.
3. Mims JL, Wood RC. Bilateral anterior transposition of the inferior obliques. Arch Ophthalmol. 1989;107:41-4.
4. Mims JL, Wood RC. Antielevation syndrome after bilateral anterior transposition of the inferior oblique muscles: incidence and prevention. J AAPOS. 1999; 3:333-6.

Recurrent Esotropia After Bimedial Recession for Infantile Esotropia

52

James L Mims III

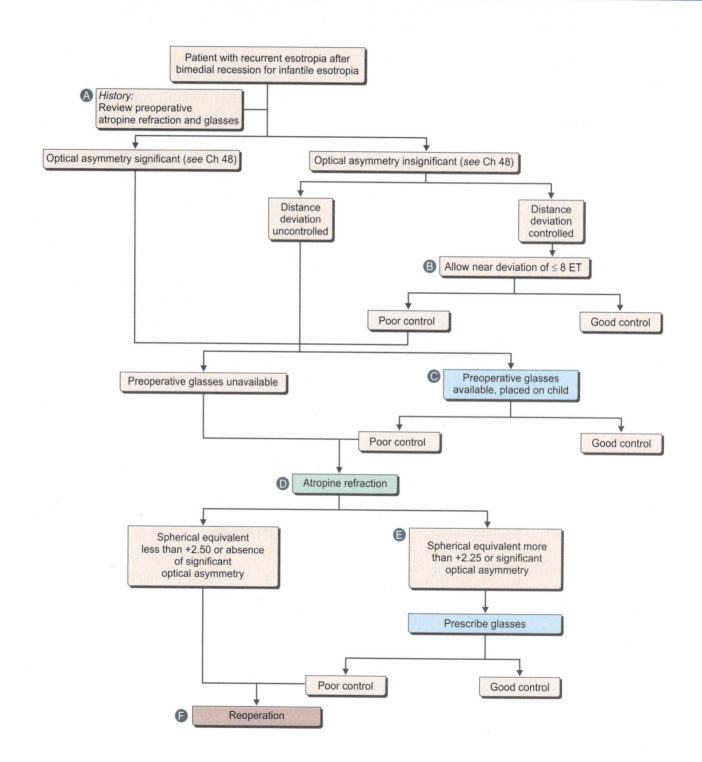

- Patient with recurrent esotropia after bimedial recession for infantile esotropia

A *History:* Review preoperative atropine refraction and glasses

- Optical asymmetry significant (*see* Ch 48)
- Optical asymmetry insignificant (*see* Ch 48)
  - Distance deviation uncontrolled
  - Distance deviation controlled
    - **B** Allow near deviation of ≤ 8 ET
      - Poor control
      - Good control

- Preoperative glasses unavailable
- **C** Preoperative glasses available, placed on child
  - Poor control
  - Good control

- **D** Atropine refraction
  - Spherical equivalent less than +2.50 or absence of significant optical asymmetry
  - **E** Spherical equivalent more than +2.25 or significant optical asymmetry
    - Prescribe glasses
      - Poor control
      - Good control

- **F** Reoperation

A. In the first 2 months after strabismus surgery, the preoperative atropine refraction (retinoscopy) generally is closer to the refraction the child is likely to have after healing is complete then a repeat cycloplegic retinoscopy performed early after surgery, because there may be temporary changes in astigmatism the first few weeks after strabismus surgery. Significant optical asymmetry is more than +1.25 sphere difference in hyperopia, more than −3.00 sphere difference in myopia, more than 1.50 difference in astigmatism is symmetric or parallel axes of astigmatism, and more than 0.50 difference in astigmatism with one axis oblique and the other axis vertical or horizontal.

B. Floropryl, recommended in the previous edition for recurrent high accommodative convergence/accommodation (AC/A) ratio esotropia (ET) in infants, is no longer available, and other miotics are not safe for infants. Fortunately, it has recently been realized that the currently popular large bilateral medial rectus (MR) recessions require 3 months to reach their full effect. Also, a child with less than 10 prism diopters (PD) of ET at near will preserve stereopsis.

C. Lack of availability of preoperative glasses or poor control of the distance or near deviation after placement of the preoperative glasses onto the child should lead to a repeat atropine refraction.

D. If the atropine refraction is to be repeated, once-daily administration of a tiny drop of 1% atropine ophthalmic ointment given each of 2 days before the office visit is adequate. This is usually most convenient at bed time each of the 2 days prior to the visit. Atropine overdose leading to late-night phone calls from anxious parents can be eliminated by teaching the parents to put a tiny dab of the ointment directly into the cul-de-sac. Because the previous bilateral MR recession has led to some contracture of the antagonist lateral recti, glasses with a spherical equivalent of only +2.50 may eliminate residual esodeviation, *even* if the AC/A ratio is clinically high (10 PD greater esodeviation at near than at distance). Bifocals do not preserve stereopsis and are no longer recommended.

E. If glasses for significant optical asymmetry or +2.50 or more are not sufficient to reduce the recurrent ET to 8 PD or less, then a second surgery should be performed.

F. The most common second surgery for recurrent esotropia has become resection of one lateral rectus (LR), with the size of the unilateral LR resection determined by the size of the *near* deviation. This is generally 5 mm for 10 ET, 6 mm for 12 ET, 7 mm for 14 ET, 8 mm for 16 ET and 9 mm for 18 ET. For recurrent 25–35 ET, re-recession of one MR should be considered, but avoid putting the new insertion of the re-recessed MR more than 7.2 mm posterior to its original insertion to avoid a high incidence of consecutive exotropia. Bilateral lateral rectus resections may be done, with reduction according to the original amount of bilateral MR recession performed, and according to the size of the residual or recurrent ET.

▌BIBLIOGRAPHY

1. Freeley DA, Nelson LB, Calhoun JH. Recurrent esotropia following early successful surgical correction of congenital esotropia. J Pediatr Ophthalmol Strabismus. 1983;20:68-71.
2. Mims JL, Wood RC. A method for graduated re-recession of the medial recti for late recurrent esotropia: results in 25 cases. Binocular Vision. 1988;3:77-84.
3. Mims JL, Wood RC. A three dimensional surgical dose-response schedule for lateral rectus resections for residual congenital/infantile esotropia after large bilateral medial rectus recessions. Binocul Vis Strabismus Q. 2000;15:20-8.
4. Olitsky SE, Kelly C, Lee H, et al. Unilateral rectus resection in the treatment of undercorrected or recurrent strabismus. J Pediatr Ophthalmol Strabismus. 2001;38:349-53.

Surgical Treatment of Consecutive Exotropia

53

James L Mims III

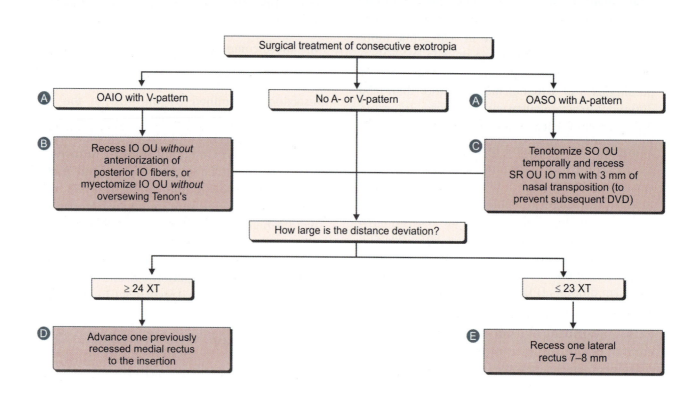

Consecutive exotropia (XT) after bilateral medial rectus recession is common, occurring in up to 1 in 5 infantile esotropes and 1 in 10 acquired esotropes. Half of the cases occur in the first 2 years after the first surgery; the remainder can occur up to 20 years later. This chapter is based on a personal series of 136 patients treated surgically for consecutive XT, as well as on the listed references. Success rate is greater than 90% at 6-months follow-up with this protocol.

A. About one-third of children with consecutive XT will have a significant V- or Y-pattern with overaction of the inferior oblique (OAIO) or a significant A-pattern with overaction of the superior oblique (OASO). Alternating hypertropias as the child looks back and forth across the primary plane are the hallmark of both OAIO and OASO.

B. Weakening of the inferior oblique (IO) is indicated if hypertropia is seen as the child looks to the side greater than 20°. Most surgeons prefer recessions. In the context of consecutive XT with a V- or Y-pattern, it is important to remember that anteriorization of the posterior fibers of the IO will not collapse the V- or Y-pattern in one-third of cases. Thus, the posterior fibers must be reattached to the globe along the lateral edge of the inferior rectus, generally directly posterior to the point where the anterior fibers of the IO are reattached to the globe, to ensure collapse of the pattern. If the surgeon prefers myectomy, the collapse of the pattern is ensured but oversewing Tenon's capsule may produce a powerful weakening effect on the IO, causing the superior oblique (SO) to overact years later.

C. If no hypertropias are seen in extreme sidegazes, the 'OASO' appearance seen on the testing of versions may be simply the result of the vertical dimension of the orbital outlet being wider in the middle than at the sides, as pointed out by Guyton, and no SO tenotomies may be needed. This phenomenon has been called pseudo-OASO. If they are truly needed (as indicated by left hypotropia on extreme right gaze and right hypotropia on extreme left gaze), the tenotomies should be effective and on the temporal side. Silicone spacers will collapse the pattern but will not normalize the versions and may be associated with restrictive hypertropias on downgaze. (Wright silicone spacers are recommended for Brown syndrome.) In a child with a history of infantile esotropia or in any child with enough instability of ocular alignment that consecutive XT with OASO has developed, dissociated vertical deviation will be made significantly worse after SO tenotomy. Thus, simultaneous with the SO tenotomies, the surgeon should almost always perform a bilateral superior rectus (SR) recession of 10 mm with 3 mm of nasal transposition. The nasal transposition prevents worsening of the consecutive XT because the secondary action of the SR is adduction. The SR should be directly sewn to the surface of the globe using a Parks crossed swords or similar technique. Using a hang-back can result in lack of adherence of the SR to the globe (lost muscle) because of the SO tendon in this area. This complex surgery has had an 80% success with 1-year follow-up in 14 cases.

D. About one-fourth of the cases, those with a distance deviation of ≥ 24 XT, are well treated with advancement of one medial rectus to the insertion in addition to whatever surgery is needed on the cyclovertical muscles for A- or V-pattern. This remarkably successful surgical plan was discovered only in the last 10 years. Many years ago, it was discovered that advancement of both medial recti to the insertion led to a return of the original esotropia, even for consecutive XT angles as large as 45 XT. This distressing result led Cooper (1961) to recess lateral recti (LR) for consecutive XT and to 'Cooper's Dictum', in which he advocated treating the consecutive XT as a new case, emphasizing recessions of one or two LR. This dictum is now obsolete in regard to bilateral LR recessions for consecutive XT; bilateral LR recessions have a low success rate with long-term follow-up. In an occasional case with a significant A-pattern without good evidence of OASO, advancement of one medial rectus will be successful, if the near deviation is at least 15 XT.

E. About half of the cases will return (or present) when the distance deviation is ≤ 23 XT because an XT of ≥8 XT is noticeable by most lay observers. These are well treated with recession of one lateral rectus in addition to whatever surgery is needed on the cyclovertical muscles for the A- or V-pattern. Recess one LR 7 mm for 10–12 XT, recess one LR 7.5 mm for 13–16 XT and recess one LR 8 mm for 17–20 XT.

BIBLIOGRAPHY

1. Bradbury JA, Doran RM. Secondary exotropia: a retrospective analysis of matched cases. J Pediatr Ophthalmol Strabismus. 1993;30:163-6.
2. Cooper EL. The surgical management of secondary exotropia. Trans Am Acad Ophthalmol Otolaryngol. 1961;65:595-608.
3. Mims JL, Wood RC. Outcome of a surgical treatment protocol for late consecutive exotropia following bilateral medial rectus recession for esotropia. Binocul Vis Strabismus Q. 2004;19:201-6.
4. Ohtsuki H, Hasebe S, Tadokoro Y, et al. Advancement of medial rectus muscle to the original insertion for consecutive exotropia. J Pediatr Ophthalmol Strabismus. 1993;30:301-5.

Intermittent Exotropia

James L Mims III

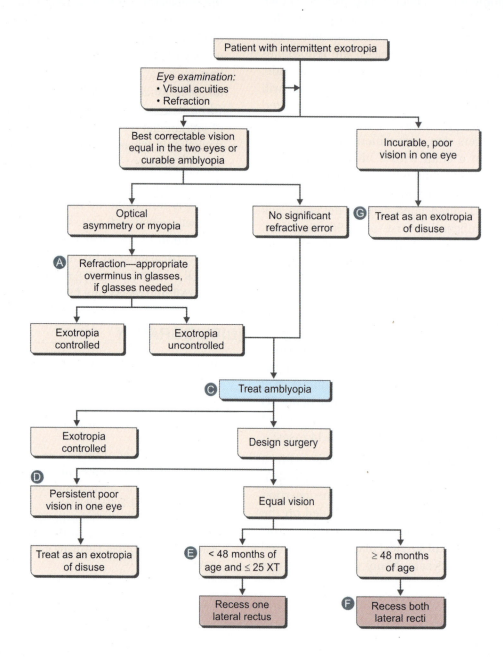

A. Intermittent exotropia (XT) of childhood may be first observed by the parent or other caregiver as early as 10 months of age or as late as 9 years of age. Alert referring pediatricians will refer the children as young as 1 year of age based on the reported observations of the parent, even though the primary care physician has not observed the deviation. Frequently, remote-controlled toys in a 20-foot eye lane will allow measurement of an intermittently manifest deviation not observed by the pediatrician, because the deviation is almost always manifest initially only with distance fixation.

B. A few children with intermittent XT may respond to stimulation of their accommodative convergence with small amounts of overminus in the glasses prescription. At age 2–6 years, a child with –1.00 D myopia may be given –2.00 D, a child with –2.00 D myopia may be given –2.75 D, and a child with –3.00 D myopia may be given –3.50 D. Children in this age group with myopia of ≥ 4.00 or ≤–0.75 and those with hyperopia generally do not tolerate overminus in glasses more than briefly.

C. If amblyopia is present and an intermittent deviation is less than 11 prism diopters, patching with appropriate compensation of optical asymmetry in glasses can, in a few cases, be curative (Ch 48).

D. Persistent poor vision in one eye (20/80 or worse) is an indication for limiting strabismus surgery to the poorer eye.

E. Recession of one lateral rectus 8.5–10 mm has now become almost universally recognized as the most effective treatment for children under 48 months of age with deviations of 10–22 XT. Lysis of an extensive frenulum connecting the dorsal surface of the inferior oblique to the inner surface of the lateral rectus may be helpful. For the 20% who have a recurrent XT in the years after the first surgery, recession of the other lateral rectus (even if the same eye is going out again) 8–9 mm has a much higher success rate than resection of the (ipsilateral) medial rectus.

F. For the child greater than 48 months of age, unilateral lateral rectus recessions are favored by some surgeons if the deviation is less than 22 XT, but many specialists favor bilateral lateral rectus recessions in these slightly older children. For 16–19 XT, 5 mm; for 20 XT, 5.5 mm; for 25 XT, 6 mm; for 30 XT, 7 mm; for 40 XT, 8 mm. Add 1 mm to these guidelines ("augmented lateral rectus recessions") if the near deviation is more than 10 XT or more than 50% of the distance deviation. (This author takes the position that augmented lateral rectus recessions are more successful and better tolerated than recess-resect for "Basic" exotropic deviations with larger near deviations). The observation that the near deviation is corrected as much or more than the distance deviation with large lateral rectus recessions (or, previously, with tenotomies) is over 170 years old. For recurrent XT developing in the years after bilateral lateral rectus recessions, a 5 mm resection of one medial rectus is curative permanently in 80%. Note: This entire chapter assumes that overacting superior or inferior obliques are either not present, or are simultaneously surgically ameliorated.

G. If anatomic abnormality, disease or amblyopia unresponsive to standard treatment is present and the poorer eye has 20/80 or worse acuity, consider limiting surgery to the poorer eye. Very large unilateral lateral rectus recessions of 10 mm may be all that is needed to correct up to 30 XT if the XT is of "disuse".

BIBLIOGRAPHY

1. MacKenzie W. The Cure of Strabismus by Surgical Operation. Appendix to a Practical Treatise on the Diseases of the Eye, 3rd Edition. (with 1st Edition. appendix). London: Longman, Orne, Brown, Green, and Longmans; 1840. p. 20 (appendix).
2. Mims JL III. Outcome of 5 mm resection of one medial rectus extraocular muscle for recurrent exotropia. Binocul Vis Strabismus Q. 2003;18:143-50.
3. Nelson LB, Bacal DA, Burke MJ. An alternative approach to the surgical management of exotropia—the unilateral lateral rectus recession. J Pediatr Ophthalmol Strabismus. 1992;29:357-60.
4. Weakley DR, Stager DR. Unilateral lateral rectus recessions in exotropia. Ophthalmic Surg. 1993;24: 458-60.

Acquired Esotropia of Childhood

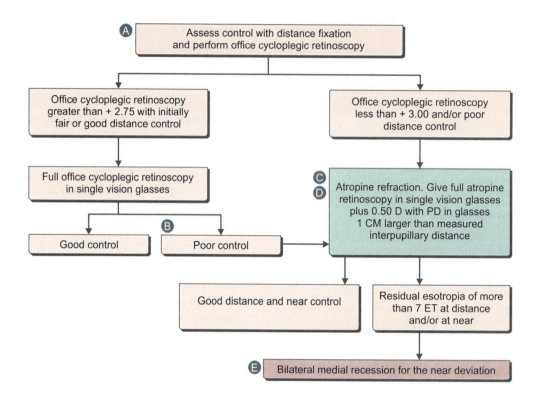

James L Mims III

Success in management of acquired esotropia (ET) of childhood depends as much on care and vigilance in nonsurgical therapy as on performing the 'right amount' of surgery.

A. Office cycloplegic retinoscopy follows instillation of a mixture that includes 0.5% cyclopentolate, 2.5% phenylephrine and 0.5% tropicamide. This mixture is created by mixing higher percentage drops with each other (15 cc of 2% cyclopentolate, 15 cc of 10% phenylephrine and 30 cc of 1% tropicamide). If the distance deviation was controlled (8 ET or less) or infrequently intermittent at the first visit prior to the application of glasses, then the full office

cycloplegic should be prescribed without resorting to an atropine refraction.

B. If the distance and near deviations are not adequately controlled (< 8 ET) after 6 weeks of full-time wear of the glasses, then the atropine refraction visit is essential.

C. Once-daily administration of a tiny dab of 1% ophthalmic ointment for 2 or 3 days before the office visit is adequate. Atropine overdose leading to late-night phone calls from anxious parents can be prevented by teaching parents to place a tiny dab of the ointment onto the fingertip and to place the dab directly into the cul-de-sac of the lower lid as it is retracted by pulling downward on the cheek.

D. If the spherical equivalent is above +2.75 or if there is significant optical asymmetry (+1.25 difference on the hyperopic side, –3.00 difference on the myopic side, astigmatism difference of +1.50 with axes that are symmetric or astigmatism difference of +1.00 if the axis of one eye is vertical and the axis of the other eye is oblique), single vision glasses are prescribed according to the full hyperopic correction found after instillation of atropine.

E. If the distance or/and the near deviation is/are not controlled with the full hyperopic correction, then surgery should be considered. In a few patients with hyperopia over +5.00 whose only residual deviation as they wear the glasses is a small angle near deviation of 12 ET or less, increasing the full hyperopic correction by an arbitrary +0.50 and prescribing an interpupillary distance (the distance between the optical centers of the lenses) of a full cm (10 mm) larger than the measured distance may reduce the effective near deviation to a tolerable level (the artificially large PD is an inexpensive way to provide 5 diopters of base-out prism to the +5.00 diopter hyperope). The amount of bilateral medial rectus recession may be taken from the following table, which was generated as the least-squares exponential curve fitted to a large sample of patients (N = 68) with acquired ET (Table 55.1).

Table 55.1: Acquired esotropia

Diopters of preoperative esotropia	Millimeters of bilateral medial rectus recession (each eye)
15 D	3.7 mm
20 D	4.3 mm
25 D	4.7 mm
30 D	5.0 mm
35 D	5.3 mm
40 D	5.5 mm
45 D	5.8 mm
50 D	6.1 mm
55 D	6.3 mm
60 D	6.4 mm
65 D	6.5 mm

BIBLIOGRAPHY

1. Kushner BJ, Preslan MW, Morton GV. Treatment of partly accommodative esotropia with a high accommodative convergence-accommodation ratio. Arch Ophthalmol. 1987;105:815-8.
2. James L Mims III, Treff G, Wood RC. Variability of strabismus surgery for acquired esotropia. Arch Ophthalmol. 1986;104:1780-2.
3. James L Mims III, Wood RC. The maximum motor fusion test: a parameter for surgery for acquired esotropia. J AAPOS. 2000;4:211-6.
4. Olitsky SE, Kelly C, Lee H, et al. Unilateral rectus resection in the treatment of undercorrected or recurrent strabismus. J Pediatr Ophthalmol Strabismus. 2001;38:349-53.

Diagnosis of Head Tilts and Face Turns in Children

James L Mims III

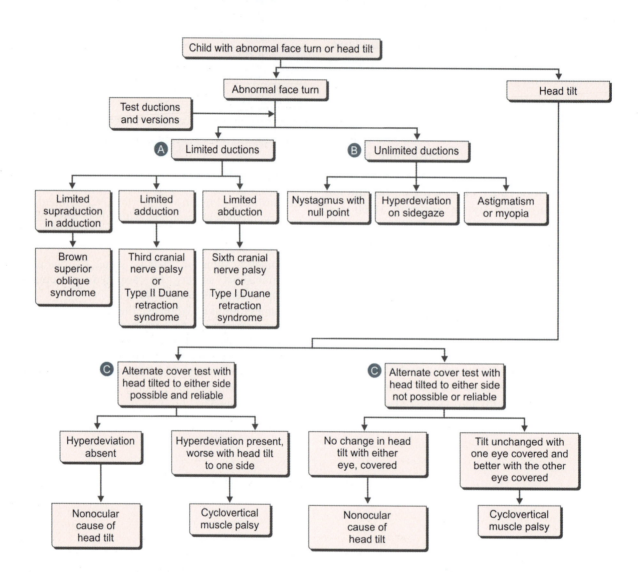

A. The ophthalmic examination of any child greater than 6 months of age should begin with a study of the ductions and versions. This can be done with a series of interesting toys held in various cardinal positions. The versions (both eyes together and binocular) are checked first; if there is an abnormality in the versions, the examiner can then study the ductions (one eye and monocular) by holding his or her hand just in front of one eye without touching the child. At times, the mother's hand may be needed to cover one eye. If the (monocular) ductions are limited in supraduction and in adduction, the child probably has Brown superior oblique syndrome from either poor slippage of the superior oblique tendon through the trochlea or an abnormality of length or insertion of the superior oblique tendon. Children with progressive Brown syndrome may also have a progressive face turn and an increasing exodeviation with time. Only if the face turn or chin elevation is handicapping or progressive should children with Brown syndrome receive superior oblique surgery. Limited adduction may be caused by a third cranial nerve palsy or by type II Duane retraction syndrome. Exotropia is associated with both third cranial nerve palsies and with type II Duane syndrome, but only the third cranial nerve palsy may occur with hypotropia. The palpebral fissure narrows on attempted adduction in Duane syndrome; the palpebral fissure stays the same or widens on attempted adduction in third cranial nerve palsies. Third cranial nerve palsies in children mandate examination by a neurologist. If abduction is limited, the child may have a sixth cranial nerve palsy or type I Duane retraction syndrome. The esotropia of a sixth cranial nerve palsy is typically much larger than that associated with most cases of type I Duane syndrome. Narrowing of the palpebral fissure (caused by co-contraction of the horizontal recti in the eye with Duane syndrome) occurs on attempted adduction in Duane syndrome but not in sixth cranial nerve palsies. Sixth cranial nerve palsies in children may resolve without treatment in 6 weeks if caused by postinfectious neuritis, but the innocuous nature of computed tomography (CT) scanning has led to widespread use of CT soon after the acute onset of sixth cranial nerve palsies. This allows early detection of the uncommon case with significant abnormality of the central nervous system (CNS).

B. If the versions (both eyes) are normal, the ductions (one eye) are also normal. The three most common causes of an abnormal face turn in a child with unlimited ductions are nystagmus with a null point in extreme sidegaze, hyperdeviation on gaze to one side absent or less on gaze to the other side, and refractive errors (astigmatism or myopia). The nystagmus may be grossly worse when the child's attention is forced toward the nonpreferred direction of gaze, or only micronystagmus may be present, necessitating direct ophthalmoscopy (and a cooperative patient) to confirm nystagmus as the cause of the face turn. More than 90% of children with congenital nystagmus have a disorder of the visual sensory system; children with acquired nystagmus may have CNS tumors. Hyperdeviation on gaze to one side absent or less on gaze to the other side commonly is caused by superior oblique palsy, less commonly by dissociated vertical deviation, and rarely by asymmetric primary inferior oblique overaction. Refractive errors such as astigmatism or myopia should not be overlooked as causes of face turns in children. The child may be using the edge of his or her nose to produce a pinhole camera effect to improve vision. If a child with some nystagmus is given glasses to correct the astigmatism and/or the myopia and the face turn persists to the extent that the child has difficulty using the glasses, a Kestenbaum or augmented Anderson procedure (10-mm recession of the medial rectus of the eye that is adducted during the preferred face turn, combined with 12-mm recession of the lateral rectus of the eye that is abducted during the preferred face turn) is indicated for the nystagmus.

C. A head tilt in a child may be the result of ocular or nonocular causes, such as spastic torticollis. If the child cooperates for alternate cover testing with the head tilted to either side, cyclovertical muscle palsy is diagnosed. A less cooperative child may allow patching of one eye for a time. If there is no change in the head tilt with either eye covered, the cause of the tilt is nonocular. If the tilt is little changed with one eye covered and improves significantly with the other eye covered, a cyclovertical muscle palsy is probably present.

BIBLIOGRAPHY

1. Harley RD. Paralytic strabismus in children. Etiologic incidence and management of the third, fourth, and sixth nerve palsies. Ophthalmology. 1980;87:24-43.
2. Kushner BJ. Ocular causes of abnormal head postures. Trans Am Acad Ophthalmol Otolaryngol. 1979;86:2115-25.
3. Mitchell PR, Wheeler MB, Parks MM. Kestenbaum surgical procedure for torticollis secondary to congenital nystagmus. J Pediatr Ophthalmol Strabismus. 1987;24:87-93.
4. Weiss AH, Biersdorf WR. Visual sensory disorders in congenital nystagmus. Ophthalmology. 1989;96:517-23.

Diagnosis of Cyclovertical Muscle Palsies

57

James L Mims III

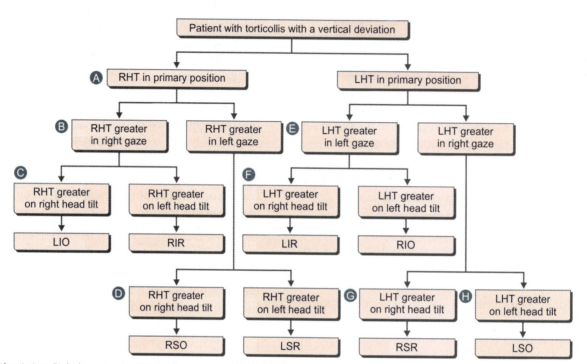

Abbreviations: Right hypertropia, RHT; Left hypertropia, LHT; Left inferior oblique, LIO; Right inferior rectus, RIR; Left inferior rectus, LIR; Right inferior oblique, RIO; Right superior oblique, RSO; Left superior rectus, LSR; Right superior rectus, RSR; Left superior oblique, LSO

Bielschowsky and Parks have popularized a three-step test for the diagnosis of cyclovertical muscle palsies. This test works only when the cause of the hyperdeviation is a paresis of a single cyclovertical muscle in a patient who has had no surgery. The first step is to determine whether the hypertropia is a right hypertropia (RHT) or a left hypertropia (LHT). The second step is to identify whether the hypertropia increases in right gaze (dextroversion) or in left gaze (levoversion). Finally, the third step is to determine whether the vertical deviation increases on tilting the head to the right or to the left.

A. If there is an RHT in the primary position, either the depressors of the right eye [the right inferior rectus (RIR) and the right superior oblique (RSO)] or the elevators of the left eye [the left superior rectus (LSR) and the left inferior oblique (LIO)] are paretic.

B. Among these four muscles, right gaze is the field in which the LIO and the RIR are acting more powerfully in the vertical direction and in which the other two muscles are acting more as tortors.

C. When the head is tilted to the right, there is a tendency toward extorsion of the left eye. The extortors of the left eye are the LIO and the left inferior rectus (LIR). A paretic LIO would be opposed by a normal LIR as these extortors were acting, thus increasing the RHT. When the head is tilted to the left, there is a tendency toward extorsion of the right eye. The extortors of the right eye are the RIR and the right inferior oblique (RIO). A paretic RIR would be opposed by a normal RIO, thus increasing the RHT.

D. Again, when there is an RHT in the primary position, either the depressors of the right eye (the RIR and the RSO) or the elevators of the left eye (the LSR and the LIO) are paretic. Among these four muscles, left gaze is the field in which the RSO and the LSR are acting more powerfully in the vertical direction and in which the other two muscles are acting more as tortors. When the head is tilted to the right, there is a tendency toward intorsion of the right eye. The intortors of the right eye are the RSO and the right superior rectus (RSR). A paretic RSO would be opposed by a normal RSR as these intortors were acting, thus increasing the RHT. When the head is tilted to the left, there is a tendency toward intorsion of the left eye. The intortors of the left eye are the LSR and the left superior oblique (LSO). A paretic LSR would be opposed by a normal LSO, thus increasing the RHT.

E. An LHT could be caused by the left eye depressors, LIR or LSO or by the right eye elevators RSR or RIO.

F. Among these four muscles, the LIR and the RIO act more powerfully in the vertical direction in left gaze.

G. On right head tilt, the left eye extortors LIR and LIO are stimulated, thus increasing the LHT if the LIR is paretic. On left head tilt, the right eye extortors RIO and RIR are stimulated, thus increasing the LHT if the RIO is paretic.

H. With an LHT greater in right gaze, the two suspect muscles are the RSR and the LSO. On right head tilt, the right eye intortors RSR and RSO are stimulated, thus increasing the LHT if the RSR is paretic. On left head tilt, the left eye intortors LSO and LSR are stimulated, thus increasing the LHT if the LSO is paretic.

BIBLIOGRAPHY

1. Kushner BJ, Kraft S. Ocular torsional movements in normal humans. Am J Ophthalmol. 1983;95:752-62.
2. Parks MM. Isolated cyclovertical muscle palsy. AMA Arch Ophthalmol. 1958;60:1027-35.
3. Scott AB. Extraocular muscles and head tilting. Arch Ophthalmol. 1967;78:397-9.
4. von Noorden GK. Atlas of Strabismus, 4th Edition. St Louis: Mosby; 1983. pp. 148-55.

Choice of Surgery for Unilateral Superior Oblique Palsy

58

James L Mims III

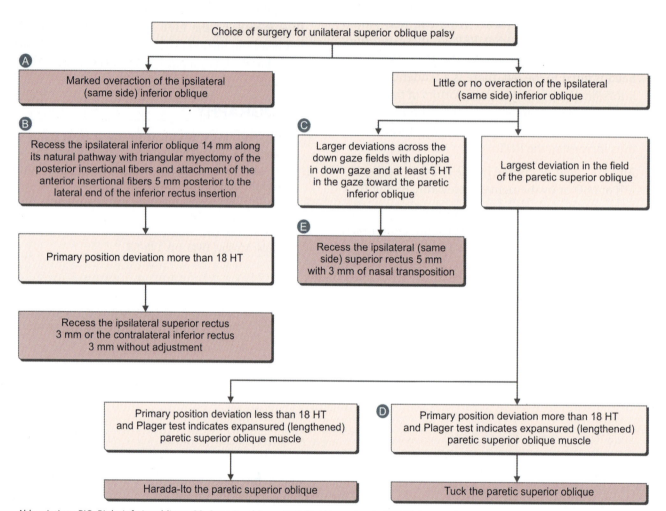

Choice of surgery for unilateral superior oblique palsy

A Marked overaction of the ipsilateral (same side) inferior oblique

Little or no overaction of the ipsilateral (same side) inferior oblique

B Recess the ipsilateral inferior oblique 14 mm along its natural pathway with triangular myectomy of the posterior insertional fibers and attachment of the anterior insertional fibers 5 mm posterior to the lateral end of the inferior rectus insertion

C Larger deviations across the down gaze fields with diplopia in down gaze and at least 5 HT in the gaze toward the paretic inferior oblique

Largest deviation in the field of the paretic superior oblique

Primary position deviation more than 18 HT

E Recess the ipsilateral (same side) superior rectus 5 mm with 3 mm of nasal transposition

Recess the ipsilateral superior rectus 3 mm or the contralateral inferior rectus 3 mm without adjustment

Primary position deviation less than 18 HT and Plager test indicates expansured (lengthened) paretic superior oblique muscle

D Primary position deviation more than 18 HT and Plager test indicates expansured (lengthened) paretic superior oblique muscle

Harada-Ito the paretic superior oblique

Tuck the paretic superior oblique

Abbreviations: RIO: Right inferior oblique; SO: Superior oblique; RHT: Right hypertropia; RSR: Right superior rectus

A, B. By far the most common pattern in congenital or acquired superior oblique (SO) palsy is overaction of the ipsilateral (same side) inferior oblique (IO) seen on the testing of versions. The most effective, yet controlled, IO weakening procedure is a 14 mm recession along the natural pathway of the IO, with a 4 mm triangular myectomy of the posterior insertional fibers and attachment of the anterior insertional fibers

5 mm posterior to the lateral end of the inferior rectus (IR). Myectomies are effective, but not reversible. In some very young children, this will eliminate up to 30 PD hypertropia (HT) in the primary position. For patients older than 5 years with deviations larger than 18 HT in the primary position, recession of the IO may be augmented by a small (3 mm) fixed (not adjustable) recession of the ipsilateral (same side) superior

rectus (SR) or the contralateral (opposite side) IR. This author has tabulated a series of more than 18 adjustable IR recessions in publications and/or presentations by other surgeons which have resulted in progressive overcorrections with consequent troublesome diplopia. In contrast, a small 3 mm recession of the contralateral (opposite side) IR can successfully augment an ipsilateral (same side) IO recession in the less common patient with a primary position deviation of more than 18 HT.

C. For patients with a primary position deviation less than 18 HT, but who have little or no overaction of the ipsilateral (same side) IO and who have 5 HT or more in straight contralateral gaze, recession of the ipsilateral (same side) SR 5 mm with 3 mm of nasal transposition [nasal transposition to avoid exotropia (XT) in upgaze] will be greatly appreciated and eliminate pre-operative diplopia in downgaze.

D. Patients with maximal deviation in contralateral downgaze should have a SO "strengthening" procedure of the ipsilateral (same side) SO, either a Harada-Ito as described by Ken Wright or a SO tuck as described by Richard Saunders. If the primary position is above 18 HT, consider a simultaneous recession of the ipsilateral (same side) IO, but keep in mind that Alan Scott has stated that most of the patients with enough postoperative problems to be presented at a strabismus Grand Rounds had both a SO tuck and an IO weakening procedure simultaneously (to that I would add or an adjustable contralateral (opposite side) IR recession). In general, SO tucks or Harada-Ito procedures should be avoided unless intraoperatively it can be demonstrated that the SO tendon is "floppy" as described by David Plager. This can be demonstrated by drawing the eye up and in with a pair of five-toothed Lester forceps placed at the 1:30 o'clock and 7:30 o'clock positions on the scleral side of the limbus for the left eye, and the 4:30 and 10:30 o'clock positions on the scleral side of the limbus for the right eye.

E. Normally, when under general anesthesia the eye is drawn up and in, the inferolateral limbus cannot be drawn upward and inward more than the upper lid speculum level, unless the tendon is "floppy" (the tendon may be congenitally loose, or, in longstanding SO palsies, the floppy tendon is actually an expansured—the opposite of contractured—SO muscle body which has become relatively flaccid). Do not perform a tuck or a Harada-Ito unless this test as described by David Plager indicates that it will not produce a substantial Brown's syndrome. In longstanding SO palsies, a Family Album Tomogram (FAT) scan, as described by neuro-ophthalmologist J Lawton Smith, can be extremely helpful. If the head tilt has been present since childhood as confirmed by the FAT scan, then you can expect the SO tendon to be loose enough that a SO strengthening procedure will not produce a Brown's syndrome. Also, as originally described by Ed Wilson, if an imaginary dotted line connecting the lateral canthi extended laterally converges with another imaginary dotted line connecting the corners of the mouth to the side of the habitual head tilt, then the SO tendon will probably be loose enough to allow a SO strengthening procedure without producing a Brown with an overcorrection (this test as described by Ed Wilson is a subtle indicator of unilateral facial hypoplasia due to the head tilt having been present from early childhood).

BIBLIOGRAPHY

1. Helveston EM. Surgical Management of Strabismus: An Atlas of Strabismus Surgery, 4th Edition. Mosby: St Louis; 1993. pp. 465-88.
2. Mims JL 3rd. The Triple Forced Duction Test(s) for diagnosis and treatment of superior oblique palsy—with an updated flow chart for unilateral superior oblique palsy. Binocul Vis Strabismus Q. 2003;18:15-24.
3. Saunders RA. Treatment of superior oblique palsy with superior oblique tendon tuck and inferior oblique muscle myectomy. Ophthalmology. 1986;93:1023-7.
4. Sprunger DT, Helveston EM. Progressive overcorrection after inferior rectus recession. J Pediatr Ophthalmol Strabismus. 1993;30:145-8.

Choice of Surgery for Duane Retraction Syndrome

James L Mims III

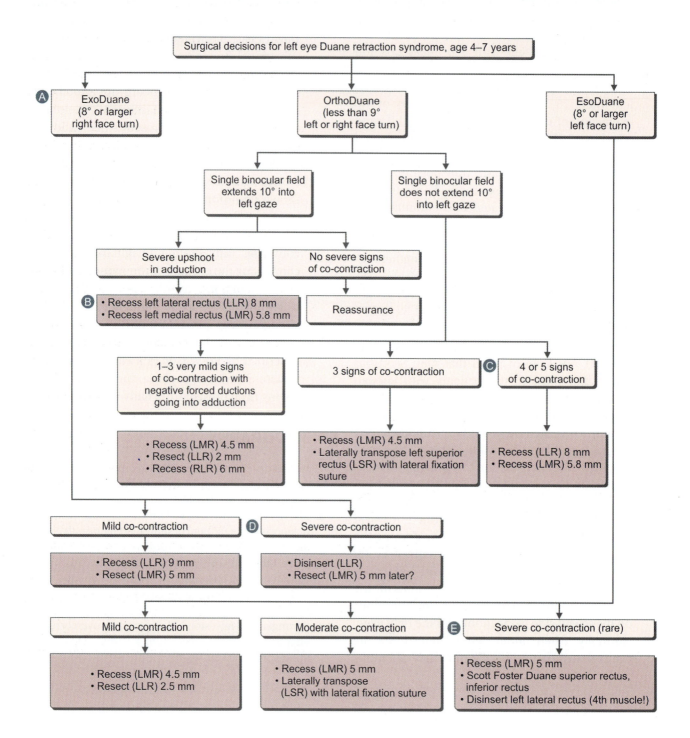

Surgical decisions for left eye Duane retraction syndrome, age 4–7 years

A ExoDuane (8° or larger right face turn)

OrthoDuane (less than 9° left or right face turn)

EsoDuane (8° or larger left face turn)

Single binocular field extends 10° into left gaze

Single binocular field does not extend 10° into left gaze

Severe upshoot in adduction

No severe signs of co-contraction

B
- Recess left lateral rectus (LLR) 8 mm
- Recess left medial rectus (LMR) 5.8 mm

Reassurance

1–3 very mild signs of co-contraction with negative forced ductions going into adduction

3 signs of co-contraction

C 4 or 5 signs of co-contraction

- Recess (LMR) 4.5 mm
- Resect (LLR) 2 mm
- Recess (RLR) 6 mm

- Recess (LMR) 4.5 mm
- Laterally transpose left superior rectus (LSR) with lateral fixation suture

- Recess (LLR) 8 mm
- Recess (LMR) 5.8 mm

Mild co-contraction

D Severe co-contraction

- Recess (LLR) 9 mm
- Resect (LMR) 5 mm

- Disinsert (LLR)
- Resect (LMR) 5 mm later?

Mild co-contraction

Moderate co-contraction

E Severe co-contraction (rare)

- Recess (LMR) 4.5 mm
- Resect (LLR) 2.5 mm

- Recess (LMR) 5 mm
- Laterally transpose (LSR) with lateral fixation suture

- Recess (LMR) 5 mm
- Scott Foster Duane superior rectus, inferior rectus
- Disinsert left lateral rectus (4th muscle!)

A. Patients with all types of Duane retraction syndrome (DRS) have co-contraction of the medial and lateral recti on adduction and narrowing of the palpebral fissure on adduction. The narrowing of the palpebral fissure is caused by innervation of the inferior compartment of the lateral rectus (LR) with fibers of the medial rectus (MR) subnucleus of the third cranial nerve. Most patients with Duane syndrome have it in the left eye and most are "Type I", with limited abduction of the Duane eye. A few patients with Duane syndrome have "Type II" with full abduction owing to the Duane LR receiving normal innervation from the sixth cranial nerve, and also the abnormal innervation from the MR subnucleus of the third cranial nerve. This Flow chart is designed around the primary position deviation: ExoDuane, OrthoDuane, and EsoDuane; because two-thirds of patients with DRS have it in the left eye, the Flow chart is for a left eye Duane syndrome. Rarely, patients with Duane syndrome will have a chin depression due to exotropia in down gaze. These are well treated with infraplacement of the lateral recti. Similarly, patients with exotropias only in up gaze (Kushner syndrome) are well treated with supraplacement of the lateral recti.

B. If the single binocular field extends 10° or more into the side of the Duane eye and there is no severe upshoot in adduction, the patient should simply be reassured regarding the diagnosis and no surgery is indicated. If there is disfiguring upshoot in adduction, recession of the Duane MR 5.8 mm and the Duane LR 8 mm will reduce this to a tolerable level in almost all cases.

C. If the single binocular field does not extend at least 10° into the side of the Duane eye, then the patient is frequently functionally handicapped, even if there is no large face turn. The five signs of co-contraction are conveniently listed as follows: (1) narrowing of the palpebral fissure 1 mm or more on adduction, (2) defective adduction by observing a corneal light reflex more than 1 mm inside lateral corneal limbus on full attempted adduction of the Duane eye (Urist test of adduction), (3) exotropia of more than 3 PD exotropia in contralateral gaze, (4) near point of convergence beyond 10 cm, (5) upshoot or downshoot of the Duane eye on adduction. The severity of co-contraction dictates, which procedure the surgeon, has the privilege of performing to enhance abduction of the Duane eye. If the co-contraction is truly mild, the philosophy of "creating an exotropia and curing it at the same surgery" may be employed by recessing the Duane MR 4.5 mm, resecting the Duane LR 2 mm and recessing the LR of the other eye 6 mm. A recession of more than 6 mm will increase the co-contraction of the Duane eye, and about one in six patients receiving this surgery in this context will have to have a subsequent takedown of the resected Duane LR. Caveat: Do not resect the Duane LR if the forced ductions going into adduction of the Duane eye under anesthesia are positive. An intriguing future possibility would be to replace the resection of the Duane LR with a lateral transposition of the superior rectus (SR) with lateral fixation suture (1/2 of a Scott Foster procedure), as is recommended in this Flow chart under three signs of co-contraction. Incidentally, the reason that the inferior rectus does not have to be laterally transposed is that the inferior innervation compartment of the Duane LR receives the fibers from the Duane MR third nerve subnucleus, but the superior innervation compartment of the Duane LR does not and is differentially atrophic on MRI. This is also the reason that many esoDuane syndrome patients have a face turn on distance viewing but no face turn in reading down gaze, where their field of single binocular vision is more nearly normal and centralized. If the co-contraction is the main issue, then this may be relieved by a recess-resect of the horizontal recti of the Duane eye, but this will not enhance abduction of the Duane eye.

D. In the patient with exoDuane, the co-contraction may be mild enough that both the exodeviation and the co-contraction will be relieved by a 9 mm recession of the Duane LR. This may be augmented by a 5 mm resection of the Duane MR without fear of making the co-contraction worse. If the co-contraction is severe, OB Jackson and Susan Berry have independently presented cases for whom they disinserted the offending Duane LR and made the patient much happier. In one case, Berry subsequently resected the Duane MR.

E. The most common Duane syndrome patient who can benefit from strabismus surgery is the esoDuane with a face turn. A recess-resect of the Duane eye may be done if the preoperative signs of co-contraction are truly mild. The Duane LR is stiff, the resection should be limited to 2.5 mm at most, and the resection of the Duane LR should be avoided if there is any positivity on forced ductions going into adduction for the Duane eye at the start of surgery. If this positivity is present, change to the formulation presented under "moderate co-contraction", a recession of the Duane MR 5 mm with lateral transposition of the Duane SR with lateral fixation suture. In two of 94 cases of Duane operated by this author, four-muscle surgery was justified on the Duane eye, including disinsertion of the offending Duane LR, replacement of its function with a lateral transposition of both vertical recti with lateral fixation sutures (Scott Foster procedure), and subsequent modest recession of the Duane MR if necessary at a second procedure.

BIBLIOGRAPHY

1. Duane A. Congenital deficiency of abduction associated with impairment of adduction, retraction movements, contraction of the palpebral fissure and oblique movements of the eye. Arch Ophthalmol. 1905;34: 133-59.
2. Mahendale RA, Dagi LR, Wu C, et al. Superior rectus transposition and medial rectus recession for Duane syndrome and sixth nerve palsy. Arch Ophthalmol. 2012;130:195-201.
3. Miller NR, Kiel SM, Green WR, et al. Unilateral Duane's retraction syndrome (type 1). Arch Ophthalmol. 1982; 100:1468-72.
4. Morad Y, Kraft SP, Mims III JL. Unilateral recession and resection in Duane syndrome. J AAPOS. 2001;5:158-63.

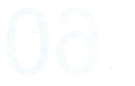

Choice of Surgery for Limited Supraduction in a Child

James L Mims III

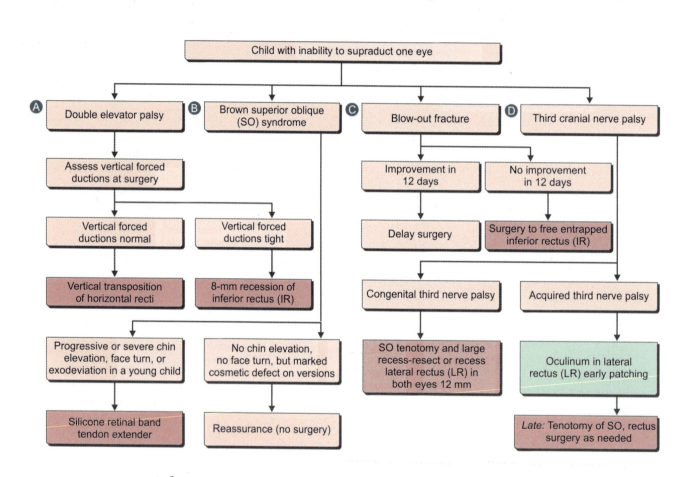

A. The cause of double elevator palsy (DEP) is clearly supranuclear; the DEP eye can be seen to supraduct during stage II general anesthesia, and this has been reported with photographic documentation. A patient with a paralyzed superior rectus (SR) with a normal inferior oblique cannot elevate the eye convincingly even in adduction; it is useful to think of a DEP as an SR palsy. Indeed, vertical saccades are often subnormal in this disorder. Children with DEP have limitation of elevation in up, up-and-left, and up-and-right ductions and a consequent hypotropia in the involved eye that increases in up gaze. They may have a chin-up position with fusion in down gaze (more common) or amblyopia in the hypotropic-affected eye. Ptosis or pseudoptosis may be present in the primary position. As with other vertical deviations; it is important to level the eyes before considering ptosis surgery. In some patients with DEP, the primary defect is restriction of the inferior rectus (IR); in others, the primary defect is the SR palsy. If the vertical forced ductions are tight (positive going into supraduction) at surgery, the best procedure is an 8-mm recession of the IR with adequate separation of the IR from the underlying tissues and suspension of the palpebral head of the IR to prevent lid retraction. If the vertical forced ductions are normal, the accepted procedure is a vertical transposition of the horizontal recti as popularized by Knapp. This generally corrects 25 prism diopters (PD) of vertical deviation.

B. Brown superior oblique (SO) syndrome includes inability of the patient to look up-and-in with positive forced ductions in this direction. In more severe cases, the patient demonstrates depression on adduction of the involved eye and normal or near-normal elevation when the eye is in abduction. Positive forced ductions bringing the Brown SO syndrome eye up-and-in are a defining characteristic of Brown SO syndrome. When the patient demonstrates chin elevation and a face turn away from the Brown eye habitually to fuse, a 6 mm Wright silicone spacer (#240 retinal silicone band) is indicated. When placing this spacer, it is critical that a fascial shelf be preserved between the inferior surface of the spacer and the superior surface of the globe (sclera). Otherwise, severe scarring can occur and make the Brown worse. The more experienced the strabismus surgeon, the more that surgeon is hesitant to operate on Brown, because a progressive SO palsy can ensue. Complete SO tenotomy is almost never indicated in Brown SO syndrome. The progressive SO palsy after SO tenotomy can require two subsequent surgeries, including posterior fixation suture on the contralateral IR, or even a rotational procedure involving supraplacement of the medial rectus and infraplacement of the lateral rectus. If there is no chin elevation and no face turn, reassurance concerning the modest limitation of duction in Brown SO syndrome is the best medicine.

C. The treatment of traumatic blowout fracture of the orbital floor remains controversial, but most surgeon/authors agree that some delay is appropriate to see whether the patient improves spontaneously. Although the mechanism probably does not involve deformation of the globe, up to 30% of patients with blowout fractures also have serious intraocular abnormality. The IR muscle may have become paretic, and a hypertropia may result after freeing the muscle from the fracture. This can be predicted by preoperative saccadic velocities. In many cases, this paresis of the IR improves temporarily.

D. The key to success for surgery for third cranial nerve palsies is tenotomy of the SO on the involved side. In an acquired third nerve palsy, injection of botulinum A toxin (Oculinum) into the LR and patching early may speed recovery. Beware of the MR in congenital third nerve palsies; it may have a very stiff length-tension curve, even stiffer than the Duane LR. Avoid resections when possible. If the MR is not fibrotic and stiff with positive forced ductions in abduction, a large recess-resect can work well. If the MR is stiff and fibrotic, 12-mm bilateral LR recessions are appropriate.

BIBLIOGRAPHY

1. Metz HS. Double elevator palsy. Arch Ophthalmol. 1979;97:901-3.
2. Mims III JL. Double elevator palsy eye supraducts during stage II general anesthesia supporting hypothesis of (supra) nuclear etiology. Binocular Vision & Strabismus Quarterly. 2005;20:199-204.
3. Wilkins RB, Havens WE. Current treatment of blowout fractures. Ophthalmology. 1982;89:464-7.
4. Wright DW. Superior oblique silicone expander for Brown syndrome. J Pediatr Ophthalmol Strabismus. 1991;28:101-7.

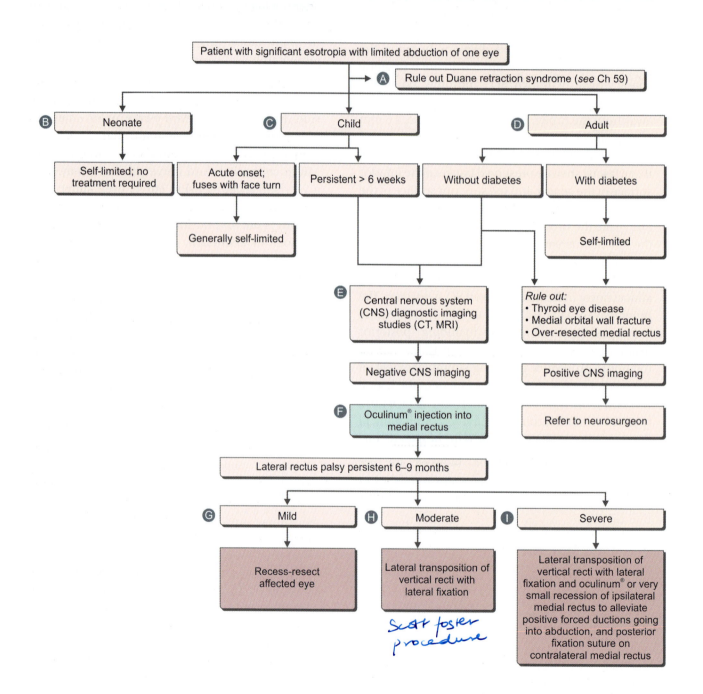

A. Limited abduction of one eye is most commonly Duane retraction syndrome; surgical options for this condition are covered in another chapter (*See* Chapter 59). The experienced ophthalmologist usually makes a diagnosis of type I Duane syndrome in the first 10 seconds of the examination. Usually, the examiner is impressed by the severe lack of abduction of one eye in the presence of a relatively small angle of esotropia. The diagnosis is confirmed by the narrowing of the palpebral fissure on adduction of the affected eye. Upshoots or downshoots in adduction, V-patterns, limitation of adduction of the affected eye, and reduced saccadic velocity on adduction as well as on abduction of the affected eye are commonly seen in Duane syndrome.

B. Congenital sixth nerve palsies in the neonate are almost always self-limited and resolve without treatment. Infantile esotropia usually develops at age 4–7 months, not earlier. Large-angle infantile esotropia may have limited abduction of both eyes, and conjunctival recessions may be indicated to improve results of bimedial recessions in such infants. After successful recession of both medial recti, abduction is full and a diagnosis of bilateral lateral rectus palsy is no longer entertained.

C. Children with acute-onset lateral rectus palsies who fuse with a face turn generally have a benign postinfectious neuritis of the nerve that spontaneously resolves by 6 weeks after onset. If such a child begins to lose his or her face turns and fusion, part-time patching of the nonaffected eye may be indicated (2–5 hours daily). If the palsy is persistent for 6 weeks, diagnostic imaging studies of the central nervous system [computed tomography (CT) or magnetic resonance imaging (MRI)] and consultation with a neurologist are mandatory. Some neurologists advocate obtaining imaging studies earlier.

D. Sixth nerve palsies in adults require consultation with a neurologist. Diabetic sixth nerve palsies are self-limited, but diabetes is so common that diabetic sixth nerve palsy is a diagnosis of exclusion. In adults, be careful to rule out thyroid eye disease, medial orbital wall fracture, and an over-resected medial rectus (or a lost lateral rectus) from previous strabismus surgery. Hypertrophy of the medial rectus may be seen on CT in thyroid eye disease. A lost lateral rectus is associated with widening of the palpebral fissure on attempted abduction.

E. Central nervous system diagnostic imaging studies are mandatory in all adults with sixth nerve palsies (even diabetic adults) and among all children whose acute-onset sixth nerve palsy has persisted beyond 6 weeks. Obviously, a positive finding leads to consideration of neurosurgical intervention.

F. If the diagnostic imaging studies are negative and the lateral rectus palsy is less than 3-months-old, the antagonist medial rectus may be injected with botulinum A toxin (Oculinum®), which causes a temporary weakening of muscles. Oculinum in this context can be a great convenience to the adult, who may return to work with some binocularity, and it may help maintain binocular function in selected pediatric patients. In some patients, the Oculinum causes an over effect for several months; the best results are generally seen 4–8 months after injection.

G. A patient with mild sixth nerve palsy retains some abduction, but the amount of sclera still showing at the lateral limbus on attempted abduction is distinctly more on the affected side. Saccadic velocities shows 20% reduction in adduction-abduction comparisons. A large recess-resect of the affected eye is indicated.

H. A moderate sixth nerve palsy shows little abduction beyond the midline with a moderately large esotropia. Lateral transposition of the vertical recti with lateral fixation sutures 8 mm posterior to the new insertions of the vertical recti (the Scott Foster procedure) gives the best results. Include only the inferior 25% of the transposed superior rectus and only the superior 25% of the transposed inferior rectus. Avoid induced hypertropias by placing the new insertion of the superior rectus 2 mm posterior and 2 mm superior to the superior end of the paretic lateral rectus, while placing the superior end of the new insertion of the transposed inferior rectus just at the inferior end of the insertion of the paretic lateral rectus. Do not simultaneously recess the ipsilateral medial rectus or weaken it with

Oculinum®; doing so will result in overcorrections of moderate sixth nerve palsies.

I. A severe sixth nerve palsy, with inability to abduct even to the midline and a large angle esotropia, should similarly be treated with a Scott Foster lateral transposition of the vertical recti with lateral fixation sutures, and simultaneously with either a very small (3.5 mm) ipsilateral medial rectus recession (if the forced ductions going into abduction are really positive) or Oculinum® injection to the ipsilateral medial rectus. This may be augmented with a posterior fixation suture on the contralateral medial rectus.

BIBLIOGRAPHY

1. Foster RS. Vertical muscle transposition augmented with lateral fixation. J AAPOS. 1997;1:20-30.
2. Metz HS, Scott AB, Scott WE. Horizontal saccadic velocities in Duane's syndrome. Am J Ophthalmol. 1975;80:901-6.
3. Rosenbaum AL, Foster RS, Ballard E, et al. Complete superior and inferior rectus transposition with adjustable medial rectus recession for abducens palsy. In: Reinecke RD (Ed). Strabismus II, Proceedings of the Fourth Meeting of the International Strabismological Association. California: Grune & Stratton; 1982. pp. 599-605.
4. Scott AB. Botulinum toxin injection into extraocular muscles as an alternative to strabismus surgery. Ophthalmology. 1980;87:1044-9.

Choice of Surgery for A- and V-Pattern Strabismus

James L Mims III

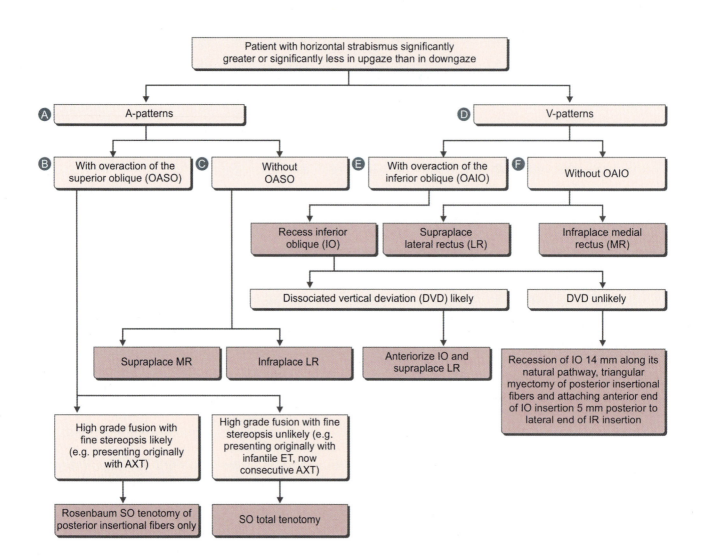

Up to 25% of patients with a horizontal strabismus have an A- or a V-pattern, a horizontal deviation that changes in size with upgaze and downgaze. Fairly extreme positions of upgaze and downgaze (25 degrees) are best for measuring the patterns; usually, the patient's chin is elevated for downgaze and depressed for upgaze. A clinically significant A-pattern has a difference between upgaze and downgaze of 10 prism diopters (PD). A clinically significant V-pattern has a difference between upgaze and downgaze of 15 PD.

A. Patients with A-patterns have increasing convergence (decreasing divergence) in upgaze. For all patients with A-pattern horizontal strabismus, it is important to look for overaction of the superior oblique (OASO) muscles. In downgaze, the superior oblique (SO) muscles have a powerful abducting capacity because the SO tendon unwraps from the globe as the eye looks down, and the effective point of contact of the SO tendon is more and more posterior to the vertical axis of Fick as the tendon unwraps from the globe.

B. A-patterns with OASO require surgery on the SO for correction. If there is only low-grade fusion (generally a late consecutive exotropia years after a bilateral medial rectus recession in a patient who originally presented with infantile esotropia), then a bilateral SO tenotomy is the most effective, although this will sometimes result in an innocuous small angle esotropia in downgaze. Bilateral total SO tenotomies will correct 30–45 PD of up-down difference, and may increase the variability of the effect of simultaneous horizontal surgery, but on average do not have a predictable undercorrecting or overcorrecting effect on simultaneous horizontal surgery. If the patient originally presented with A-pattern intermittent exotropia with OASO and a capacity for high-grade fusion with fine stereopsis is probable, then total tenotomy of the SO should be avoided; it can produce a head tilt due to asymmetric iatrogenic SO palsies. Where a capacity for high-grade fusion is likely, then the best procedure is a bilateral Rosenbaum tenectomy of the posterior fibers of the SO insertion, leaving only the anterior 1 mm of insertion intact. This also avoids an overcorrection (esotropia) in downgaze, which in the patient presenting with exotropia could result in annoying diplopia in downgaze.

C. A-patterns without OASO may be treated with supraplacement of the medial recti (MR) or infraplacement of the lateral recti (LR) with the expectation of correcting approximately 15 PD of the upgaze-downgaze difference. Patients undergoing bilateral MR recessions for esotropia with A-pattern should not have greater than 2 mm of supraplacement of the MR. Supraplacement more than this usually, in time, produces a secondary exotropia. LR may be infraplaced 4 mm with good result. Why does supraplacement or infraplacement work? Recession of a rectus muscle decreases the pull of a muscle by shortening it, and placing it lower on its length-tension curve. After recession and infraplacement of an LR muscle, the

LR becomes even shorter as the eye moves into downgaze; thus increasing the effect of the recession in downgaze. In nondominant eyes, the MR may be supraplaced, and the LR may be infraplaced as part of a recess-resect procedure.

D. Patients with V-patterns have increasing divergence (decreasing convergence) in upgaze. For all patients with V-pattern horizontal strabismus, look for overaction of the inferior oblique (OAIO) muscles. In upgaze the inferior oblique (IO) muscle and tendon unwrap from the globe as the eye looks up, and the effective point of contact of the IO is more and more posterior to the vertical axis of Fick as it unwraps from the globe.

E. V-pattern strabismus with OAIO should have a weakening procedure of the IO. If dissociated vertical deviation (DVD) is present or likely to develop in the future (as in infantile esotropia), anteriorize the IO, placing them at the lateral ends of the inferior recti. If future development of DVD is unlikely, simply perform a triangular myectomy of the posterior insertional fibers, and attach the remaining anterior end of the IO insertion 5 mm posterior to the lateral end of the inferior recti (resulting in a 14 mm recession along the natural pathway of the IO, with added myectomy of the posterior insertional fibers; upublished technique of Monte Stavis). It is a truism that 'you get what you need' from IO recessions; both severe and mild OAIO are eliminated by recessions.

F. For V-patterns without OAIO, supraplacement of the LR 4 mm or infraplacement of the MR 4 mm will correct 15–20 PD of upgaze-downgaze difference.

▌BIBLIOGRAPHY

1. Knapp P. A- and V-patterns. In: Symposium on Strabismus. Transactions of the New Orleans Academy of Ophthalmology. St Louis: Mosby; 1971. pp. 242-54.
2. Mims JL Ill, Wood RC. Bilateral anterior transposition of the inferior obliques. Arch Ophthalmol. 1989;107:41-4.
3. Shin GS, Elliott RL, Rosenbaum AL. Posterior superior oblique tenectomy at the scleral insertion for collapse of A-pattern strabismus. J Pediatri Ophthalmol Strabismus. 1996;33:211-8.
4. von Noorden GK. A- and V-patterns. In: Binocular Vision and Ocular Motility. 4th edition. St Louis: Mosby; 1990:351-65.

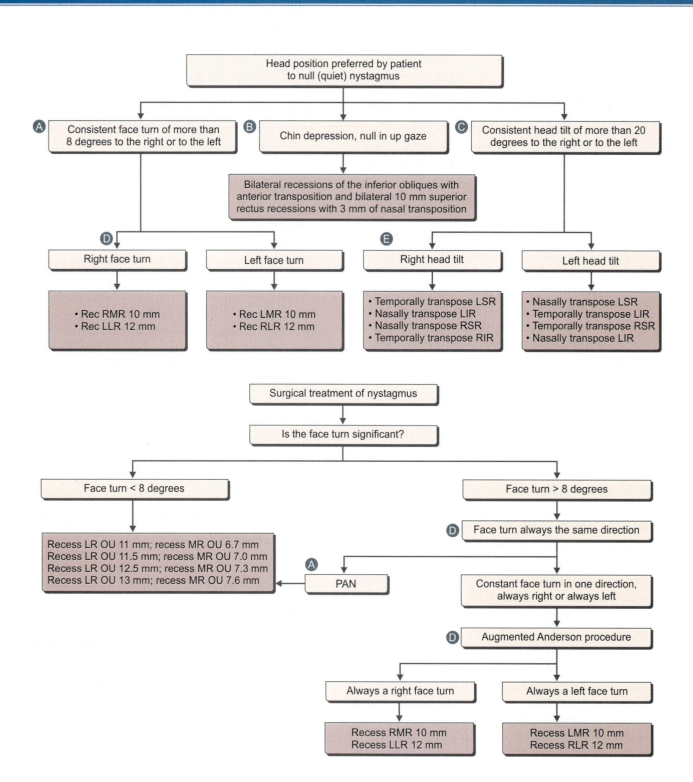

The surgical treatment of nystagmus remains controversial in regard to large recessions of all four horizontal recti to reduce the intensity of the nystagmus. Surgical treatment to improve face turns, head tilts, and chin depressions used by the patient to null (quiet) nystagmus is universally accepted as usually substantially beneficial to the patient and with acceptable risk/benefit ratios. Generally, such surgery is postponed until the child is at least 4 to 6 years old, to allow firm binocularity to develop prior to surgery to reduce a face turn, head tilt, or chin depression used to null nystagmus. A family history may reveal that other family members improved their nystagmus as late as 6 years of age, another reason to postpone the surgery.

A. If the patient tends to turn his or her face to null nystagmus, the clinician must be certain that the patient always has a face turn in the same direction, always right, or always left. Periodic alternating nystagmus (PAN) is not rare, and may require up to 20 minutes of patient observation to be certain that PAN is present or not. The usual periodicity of extreme right gaze changing to extreme left gaze in PAN is 4 minutes, but this author has observed one case that required 7 minutes to change face turn. If the face turn to null nystagmus is less than 10 degrees, the patient may not be troubled enough by the face turn to warrant surgery. The best method to measure the face turn is to use a good distance fixation target, such as a small cartoon movie or video appealing to the child. Older children may be asked to read letters or to name the Allen figures. Standing behind and above the child as the child sits in the exam chair, a laser, or other pointer may be used to project a spot on the wall 20 feet (6 meters) distant as the pointer is aligned with the occipital vertex and the center of the forehead of the child. Classical trigonometry reveals that with the small movie screen or other fixation target 20 feet away, 21 inches to one side of the fixation target corresponds to a face turn of 5 degrees (to the right or to the left, depending on the direction of the face turn), 42 inches to one side corresponds to a face turn of 10 degrees, and 64 inches to one side corresponds to a face turn of 15 degrees. Also, an orthopedic goniometer may be held above the child's head.

B. If the child nulls in down gaze, no surgery is usually indicated, because all school works and studying are done in down gaze. A chin elevation to see well in the distance will not be needed frequently, and such patients are best served by no surgery at all. In marked contrast, if the child nulls in sharp up gaze, the child may erroneously be consigned to special education or even inappropriate psychiatric therapy. In addition to surgery, such children will need extensive communication by the physician with the schoolteachers, and book stands will still be needed for all near work. The surgery should include bilateral recessions of the inferior obliques with anterior transposition and bilateral 10 mm superior rectus recessions with 10 mm of nasal transposition. The nasal transposition is necessary to prevent exotropia in up gaze. In about 50% of such cases, the patient will subsequently null with a large face turn and require an Augmented Anderson (*see* paragraph D).

C. Head tilts to null nystagmus are uncommon, and the risk of inducing a new strabismus requiring additional strabismus surgery is significant. Therefore, the patient should be allowed to have their tilt unless it is more than 20 degrees to either side, and surgery should be postponed until the age of 6 years to take advantage of the chance that the nystagmus will improve spontaneously. The more established surgical procedure (multiple respected surgeons) uses the vertical recti to rotate the eyes in the direction of the preferred head tilt, a maneuver in principle similar to other nystagmus surgery where the goal is to move the eyes to the primary (straight ahead) position from wherever the eyes tend to be when the patient is using a head position to null nystagmus. A newly published (and not yet verified) approach is to use the oblique muscles. For a right head tilt, the anterior 50% of the RSO is tenectomized at the insertion, and the yoke LIO is maximally recessed. For a left head tilt, the anterior 50% of the LSO is tenectomized at the insertion, and the yoke RIO is maximally recessed.

D. Once it has been confirmed that the patient always turns the face in the same direction, an Augmented Anderson is reliably helpful. For a right face turn, the right medial rectus is recessed 10 mm and the yoke left lateral rectus is recessed 12 mm. For a left face turn, the left medial rectus is recessed 10 mm and the yoke right lateral rectus is recessed 12 mm. This routinely reduces the face turn by an average of only 11 degrees when tested several months after surgery, but the parents almost always report that they almost never see the face turn now postoperatively. In about 10% of cases, the patient will eventually turn the face the other way, and the Augmented Anderson will be needed for the new face turn. In about 5% of cases, the Augmented Anderson will prove to be insufficient, and resections of the antagonists may be performed further to improve the face turn. The parents should be informed, however, that large recessions are associated with small improvements in visual function, but that resections are merely useful to change the face turn.

E. The most highly verified method (multiple respected surgeons) to reduce a large head tilt used to null nystagmus uses the vertical recti to rotate the eyes so that they will be vertically aligned with the vertical axis of the face. This is in principle similar to other nystagmus surgery where the goal is to move the eyes to the primary (straight ahead) position from wherever the eyes tend to be when the patient is using a head position to null nystagmus. The transpositions should be along the spiral of Tilleaux and should be no more than 7 mm to prevent iatrogenic vertical deviations. Whenever this author performs this surgery, he prepares a paper with large print than can be shown to him by the circulating nurse during the surgery. For a right head tilt, temporally transpose the LSR, nasally transpose the LIR, nasally transpose the RSR, and temporally transpose the RIR. For a left head tilt, nasally transpose the LSR, temporally transpose the LIR, temporally transpose the RSR, and nasally transpose the LIR.

BIBLIOGRAPHY

1. Lueder GT, Galli M. Oblique muscle surgery for treatment of nystagmus with head tilt. J AAPOS. 2012;16:322-6.
2. Reinecke RD. Costenbader lecture. Idiopathic infantile nystagmus: Diagnosis and treatment. J AAPOS. 1997;2:67-82.
3. Roberts RA, Saunders RA, Wilson ME. Surgery for vertical head position in null point nystagmus. J Pediatr Ophthalmol Strabismus. 1996; 33:219-4.
4. von Noorden GK, Jenkins RH, Rosenbaum AL. Horizontal transposition of the vertical rectus muscles for treatment of ocular torticollis. J Pediatr Ophthalmol Strabismus. 1993;30:8-14.
5. von Noorden GK. Binocular Vision and Ocular Motility: Theory and Management of Strabismus, 5th Edition. St. Louis, MO: Mosby-Year-Book; 1996. p 493.

Developmental Glaucoma

64

Ankur Gupta, Johan Zwaan, Peter A Netland

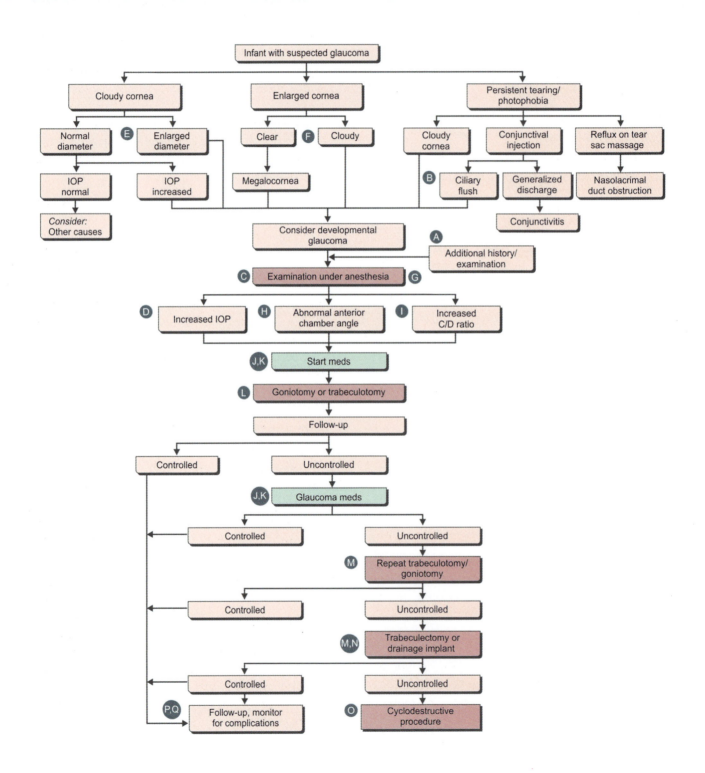

The developmental glaucomas are a heterogenous group of disorders in which the aqueous outflow system is anatomically abnormal, leading to an increase in intraocular pressure (IOP) and subsequent damage to the optic nerve. The most common type is primary developmental glaucoma, which results from maldevelopment of the trabecular meshwork. Secondary developmental glaucoma results from defects of the anterior chamber angle due to ocular or systemic abnormalities, usually genetic in nature. The symptoms, signs, and initial treatment are very similar regardless of the etiology (*see* Flow chart). However, ophthalmic and systemic comorbidities are considered in the long-term management of secondary disease.

A. When an infant presents with significant photophobia, persistent tearing, blepharospasm, and a hazy or enlarged cornea, developmental glaucoma should always be considered. A history of increasing haziness and of the eye 'getting bigger' is helpful. Many types of developmental glaucomas are inherited, making the family history important. The clinician should also note the presence of other congenital defects, and obtain a thorough birth history including information about any maternal perinatal infections. Examination of the child with classic symptoms in the clinic is usually adequate to make a preliminary diagnosis, even if an accurate IOP measurement cannot be obtained. Pacifying the infant with a bottle, or administration of chloral hydrate sedation, may facilitate IOP determination in the clinic.

B. Although the conjunctiva may be diffusely injected in the developmental glaucoma, more commonly the deep perilimbal vessels are involved around the cornea, a pattern known as the ciliary flush. There may also be a blue appearance to the sclera from scleral expansion and thinning due to increased IOP.

C. Examination under anesthesia should be the next step in evaluation. Intravenous and mask anesthesia are sufficient for brief examination, whereas endotracheal intubation is required for longer examinations, or concomitant surgery. The examination should include measurement of horizontal and vertical corneal diameter, a recording of the clarity of the cornea, the status of the anterior chamber with gonioscopy, ophthalmoscopy to determine the cup/disk ratio (C/D), and refraction.

D. During an examination under anesthesia, anesthetic agents may influence the IOP measurements. While succinylcholine and cyclopropane increase the IOP, both halothane and sevoflurane reduce it. Pressure readings should be taken early and under light anesthesia, before intubation. IOP < 21 mm Hg may be used as a reference point but IOP must be interpreted in the context of other examination findings. Because the infant eye is distensible, the IOP does not rise as high as it does in acute glaucoma in adults. Thus, a normal IOP by itself is not enough to exclude a diagnosis of glaucoma if other signs are present.

E. The normal horizontal diameter of a newborn cornea is 10.0–10.5 mm, increasing by 0.5–1 mm in the first year of life. Because the cornea and sclera of the infant eye are thinner and less rigid than in the adult, increased IOP will lead to expansion of the size of the eye and thus to enlarged corneal diameter and axial length. A corneal diameter greater than 12 mm is highly suspicious for glaucoma. If the IOP remains uncontrolled, the diameter of the cornea may reach 15–16 mm. Increasing corneal size is a useful indicator that the glaucoma is not controlled, regardless of normal or close to normal IOP readings. Enlarged corneal diameter by itself does not prove that glaucoma is present. The cornea is also larger, although clear, in megalocornea.

F. Corneal edema in early disease indicates simple epithelial edema resulting from increased IOP. If left untreated, this progresses to permanent stromal edema with scarring. The increased IOP also causes breaks in Descemet membrane visible on slit lamp examination known as Haab striae.

G. Ultrasonography is a useful tool in measuring the axial length, both for diagnosis and follow-up of the enlarged glaucomatous globe. Normal axial length in the infant ranges from 17.5–20 mm, with growth up to 22 mm at 1 year. In congenital glaucoma, the myopia associated with increased axial length can also be assessed with streak retinoscopy. These measurements are most easily done a part of the evaluation.

H. The anterior chamber angle is always abnormal in developmental glaucoma. The iris has a flat appearance and inserts more anterior than usual, in front of the scleral spur, or it may sweep up to cover the trabecular meshwork. The ciliary body is obscured by this anterior insertion. Other anomalies often visible are thinning of the peripheral iris from stretching, exaggerated Schwalbe line or posterior embryotoxon, iris processes inserting into Schwalbe line, and abnormalities of the iris stroma.

I. A normal cup to disc (C/D) ratio of the infant optic nerve is less than 0.3. A difference in value between the two eyes is also highly suspicious for glaucoma. Cupping develops early and rapidly in infants. Control of IOP with surgery will often lead to marked reversal of cupping, as opposed to the irreversible optic nerve damage seen in adult glaucoma. Increase in cup size between examinations indicates poor control.

J. While developmental glaucoma is a surgical disease, medical therapy can be started as soon as the diagnosis is reached. Topical and systemic medications can be useful for reducing or preventing further damage while prompt surgical arrangements are made. These medications may also be necessary for long-term management of complex cases that have not responded adequately to surgery. Clinicians must take into account the increased risk of systemic side effects with topical medications in pediatric patients due to their decreased body mass, and decreased blood volume.

K. Primary drug therapy for infantile glaucoma includes carbonic anhydrase inhibitors (CAIs), beta blockers, and prostaglandin analogs. CAIs are available in topical and systemic formulations with both being commonly prescribed and well tolerated. Timolol is an effective drug for developmental glaucoma but can cause respiratory, cardiovascular, and other side effects. Studies have shown a moderate hypotensive effect with the use of latanoprost, and patients should be additionally advised about the potential for local side effects. Sympathomimetic (brimonidine) and parasympathomimetic agents (pilocarpine, choline esterase inhibitors) are generally not considered first-line for the treatment of congenital glaucoma but they can be used as adjunct agents with other medications. Alpha-2 agonists (brimonidine) should be used with caution in young children due to the risk of respiratory suppression.

L. The mainstay of treatment for congenital glaucoma is surgery. Goniotomy and trabeculotomy have been found to be equally effective initial surgical options for developmental glaucoma. Advantages of goniotomy include less conjunctival scarring and a shorter operating time. Goniotomy, however, requires a clear cornea, and is technically more challenging. Trabeculotomy can be performed with a cloudy cornea, and can potentially treat the entire angle through a single incision with a 360 degree suture technique. Endoscopic goniotomy does not require a clear cornea but requires specialized equipment and has not yet been extensively studied.

M. Follow-up consists of repeated office examinations and examinations under anesthesia as needed, with the above-mentioned techniques to assess IOP control. Repeat trabeculotomy or goniotomy is the common approach if the primary surgery did not succeed. Combined trabeculotomy/trabeculectomy has been advocated for those patients with poor prognoses, or those who have failed previous surgery.

N. Glaucoma drainage tube implants are generally reserved for patients, who are refractory to primary surgery in which other approaches have failed. Popular devices include the Molteno and Baerveldt (nonvalved) implants and the Ahmed glaucoma valve (valved). Success with these devices has been shown to be as high as 90% at 6–12 months but decreases with long-term follow-up. There is also a higher rate of implant-related complications in these patients, particularly a risk of hypotony with nonvalved devices. Two-stage implantation of drainage implants can reduce the risk of hypotony-related complications. The decision to proceed with tube implant versus trabeculectomy is left to the discretion of the surgeon, as there are few comparative studies in the pediatric population, and a lack of definitive consensus on which approach is superior.

O. Cyclodestructive procedures are indicated when other methods to control the IOP have failed, or when the potential for useful vision is very low. There is a risk for vision loss or phthisis bulbi.

P. There are many reasons why children with glaucoma need to be followed closely. Because glaucomatous infant eyes are often highly myopic, refractions and amblyopia treatment, if indicated, are an essential yet often overlooked aspect of care. Corneal decompensation can be caused by edema, scarring or amyloid deposition, necessitating corneal surgery. Genetic counseling for the family regarding recurrence risks should not be forgotten.

Q. Long-term visual prognosis varies depending on the subtype of glaucoma. Primary congenital glaucoma offers the best chance of normal vision, with one study showing that just under 70% of eyes achieved visual acuity of at least 20/70. Factors such as poor vision at diagnosis, unilateral disease, multiple surgeries, and ocular comorbidities worsen prognosis. Amblyopia is the most common cause for long-term visual impairment. Children with poor visual outcomes may benefit from rehabilitation and vision aids, as well as parental counseling.

BIBLIOGRAPHY

1. Aponte EP, Diehl N, Mohney BG. Medical and surgical outcomes in childhood glaucoma: A population-based study. J AAPOS. 2011;15:263-7.
2. Khitri MR, Mills MD, Ying GS, et al. Visual acuity outcomes in pediatric glaucomas. J AAPOS. 2012;16:376-81.
3. Lawrence SD, Netland PA. Trabeculectomy versus combined trabeculotomy-trabeculectomy in pediatric patients. J Pediatr Ophthalmol Strabismus. 2012;49:359-65.
4. Lawrence SD, Netland PA. Primary surgical treatment for developmental glaucomas. In: Spaeth GL, Danesh-Meyer HV, Goldberg I, Kampik A (Eds). Ophthalmic Surgery Principles and Practice, 4th Edition. New York: Elsevier; 2012. pp. 294-301.
5. Lawrence SD, Mandal AK, Netland PA. Pediatric glaucoma. In: Wright KW, Strube YNJ (Eds). Pediatric Ophthalmology and Strabismus. 3rd Edition. New York, NY: Oxford University Press; 2012. pp. 801-26.
6. Mandal AK, Netland PA. The Pediatric Glaucomas. Edinburgh, UK: Elsevier; 2006.
7. Mullaney PB, Selleck C, Al-Awad A, et al. Combined trabeculotomy and trabeculectomy as an initial procedure in uncomplicated congenital glaucoma. Arch Opthalmol. 1999;117:457-60.

Conjunctivitis of the Newborn (Ophthalmia Neonatorum)

65

Johan Zwaan

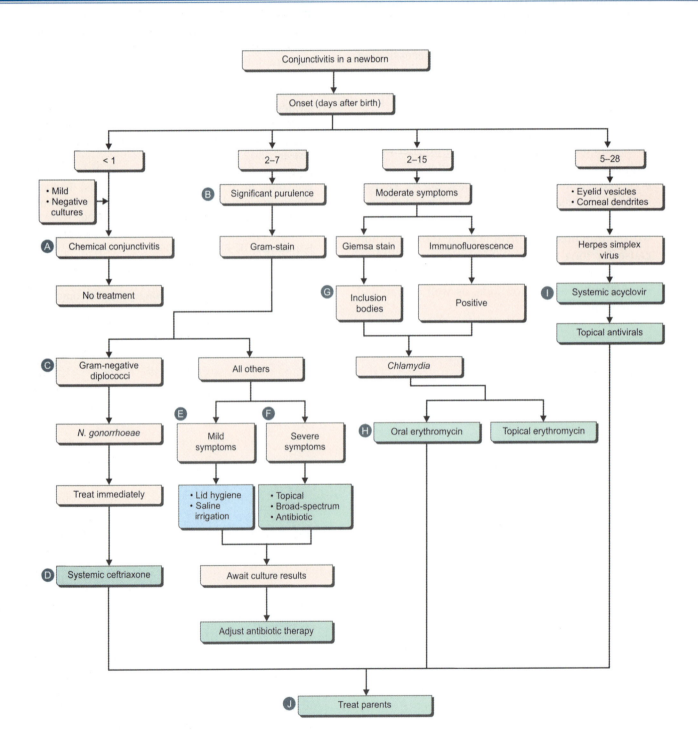

Conjunctivitis in the first few weeks of life, with purulent discharge, lid edema, conjunctival hyperemia and occasionally preauricular adenopathy, is common. In the United States, 1–2% of newborns may be affected. In less developed countries, the incidence is much higher and the pathogens are different. The time of onset after birth and the clinical characteristics of the conjunctivitis are helpful adjuncts in reaching a tentative diagnosis. However, there is a large overlap in time periods and clinical manifestations, and laboratory studies are essential in establishing the exact diagnosis, particularly when the infection does not improve with the initial empirically chosen antibiotics. Polymerase chain reaction and immunofluorescence techniques offer a much faster diagnosis than cultures, with high specificity and sensitivity (See Flow Chart).

A. The administration of 1% silver nitrate in the eye to prevent gonococcal conjunctivitis is mildly irritating and often causes some hyperemia and chemosis of the conjunctiva. Rarely, the cornea is affected, leading to a chemical keratitis. The conjunctivitis always occurs within 24 hours of birth and is mild and self-limiting (3–5 days). No treatment is required. Irrigation of the eyes may cause more irritation and should be avoided. The incidence of this problem is decreasing with the increasing use of erythromycin ointment or povidoneiodine for prophylaxis.

B. Bacterial conjunctivitis occurs mostly in the 1st week of life. It is fairly severe and characterized by purulent discharge. Gram and Giemsa stains of conjunctival scrapings should be done, and cultures and sensitivities initiated.

C. If Gram-negative diplococci are found in a conjunctival scraping, the most likely diagnosis is gonococcal conjunctivitis, although *Neisseria meningitidis* infection presents the same way. In either case urgent treatment is indicated, and one should not await the results of cultures. The clinical findings are dramatic, and corneal ulceration and even perforation develop rapidly if appropriate treatment is not instituted. The *Meningococcus* can also penetrate intact tissues and rapidly cause disseminated disease, including meningitis.

D. Penicillin-resistant *Neisseria gonorrhoeae* is now endemic, and the use of systemic penicillin for gonococcal ophthalmia neonatorum is no longer a choice. Instead, third generation cephalosporin can be used for 7 days. Infants at risk, because they are born from a mother known to have gonorrhea, should be given a single 25–50 mg/kg dose of ceftriaxone shortly after birth. Adjunctive topical treatment with erythromycin or bacitracin may be helpful. Hourly irrigation with saline may reduce the bacterial load.

E. Mild bacterial conjunctivitis is usually self-limited, and postponement of treatment is acceptable until a specific diagnosis is available. Indeed, in many patients lid hygiene and saline washes are adequate therapy. However, antibiotics may shorten the course of the infection and prevent recurrence and spread.

F. More severe conjunctivitis should be treated with a topical broad spectrum antibiotic until a targeted choice of therapy can be made. Chloramphenicol gives broad coverage and is still popular in other countries, but in the United States, it is no longer used as a primary medication because of the very small risk of aplastic anemia. Neosporin (polymyxin-bacitracin-neomycin) is a good choice, but it tends to cause allergic reactions. Bacitracin and erythromycin are usually effective. Gentamicin can be used for Gram-negative infections, although resistant strains of *Haemophilus influenzae* and *Pseudomonas aeruginosa* are common. Topical medications with broad coverage and few adverse reactions are polytrim (trimethoprim-polymyxin) and fluoroquinolones such as ciloxan (ciprofloxacin).

G. Mild to moderate conjunctivitis in the first few weeks of life, often starting in one eye and then spreading to the second eye, points to *Chlamydia trachomatis* as a cause. In babies treated with prophylactic erythromycin ointment, the onset may be delayed more. Chlamydia is now the most important cause of ophthalmia neonatorum in the United States. In contrast to the situation in adults, in whom a work-up is often negative, the positive yield of laboratory tests in infants is high. Intracytoplasmic basophilic inclusion bodies on Giemsa preparations are typical. Immunofluorescent techniques are available and allow a rapid and accurate diagnosis.

H. Oral erythromycin is the drug of choice for chlamydial ophthalmia because it also treats the nasopharyngeal colonization, which can lead to reinfection. A 2-week course of 50 mg/kg per day in four divided doses is now the standard. It may prevent the chlamydial pneumonia syndrome. Tetracycline should not be used because of its deleterious effects on growing bones and teeth. Adjuvant treatment with topical erythromycin is beneficial.

I. Recognition of conjunctivitis caused by herpes simplex virus is important because of the possibility of disseminated infection with central nervous system involvement. Systemic treatment with acyclovir may reduce the risk for a generalized infection. In addition, topical idoxuridine or vidarabine is helpful. Up to 50% of babies with herpes simplex conjunctivitis develop keratitis with typical dendrites or punctate staining. If the keratitis is severe, cycloplegics are indicated.

J. Many, if not most, of the cases of ophthalmia neonatorum are caused by infection during passage through the birth canal. Thus, the clinician must think of these diseases as a family problem rather than just an infection of an individual baby. Asymptomatic parental colonization with Chlamydia can be a source for reinfection of the infant. The parents should be treated with oral erythromycin or tetracyclin. The latter should not be given to nursing mothers; however, maternal (and paternal as well) gonococcal infections must be treated with a single dose of 1 g of ceftriaxone intramuscularly. Maternal venereal herpes simplex is of particular concern because of the risk for neonatal disseminated infection. Central nervous system involvement can lead to severe psychomotor retardation of the baby. While prophylaxis is too late for the newborn with herpes simplex ophthalmia, subsequent deliveries should be done by cesarean section to avoid infection of additional children.

BIBLIOGRAPHY

1. Grosskreutz C, Smith LB. Neonatal conjunctivitis. Int Ophthalmol Clin. 1992;32:71-9.
2. Haase DA, Nash RA, Nsanze H, et al. Single-dose ceftriaxone therapy of gonococcal ophthalmia neonatorum. Sex Transm Dis. 1986;13:53-5.
3. Haimovici R, Roussel TJ. Treatment of gonococcal conjunctivitis with single-dose intramuscular ceftriaxone. Am J Ophthalmol. 1989;107:511-4.
4. Isenberg SJ, Apt L, Wood M. A controlled trial of povidoneiodine as prophylaxis against ophthalmia neonatorum. N Engl J Med. 1995;332:562-6.
5. Sandström I. Treatment of neonatal conjunctivitis. Arch Ophthalmol. 1987;105:925-8.
6. Sandström KI, Bell TA, Chandler JW, et al. Microbial causes of neonatal conjunctivitis. J Pediatr. 1984;105: 706-11.
7. Winceslaus J, Goh BT, Dunlop EM, et al. Diagnosis of ophthalmia neonatorum. Br Med J (Clin Res Ed). 1987;295:1377-9.
8. Zwaan J. Ophthalmia neonatorum. In: Dershewitz RA (Ed). Ambulatory Pediatric Care, 3rd Edition. Philadelphia: Lippincott-Raven; 1999. pp. 535-8.

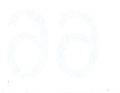

Does This Baby See?

Johan Zwaan

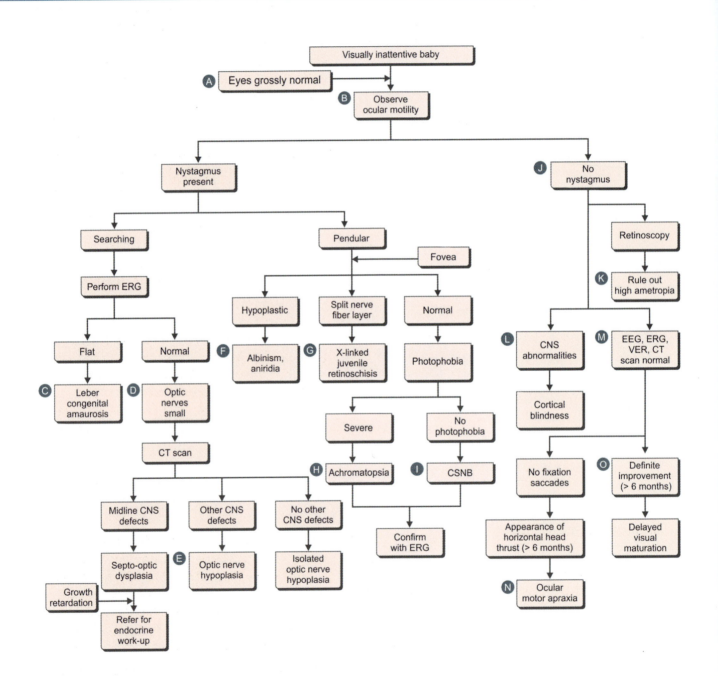

A. Although the acuity in Snellen equivalents in a newborn baby is low, around 20/1000, normal development progresses rapidly, and at 1 month, vision increases to 20/600. By 4 months, acuity is 20/200, and at 1 year, at least 20/50. At 6–8 weeks and often even earlier, clear fixation and following reflexes should be present. Before this age, it may be unclear whether the baby sees or not. However, parents are quite aware if the visual development deviates from the norm, and this is obviously a reason for major concern. Relatively few ocular conditions cause apparent blindness in babies with normal appearing eyes: achromatopsia, all types of albinism, retinal degeneration, and bilateral optic nerve hypoplasia (ONH). The poor vision may have a central mechanism. Babies may also be 'pseudo-blind.'

B. The scheme proposed here, based on eye movements, is useful as a starting point, but in all patients with suspected blindness, perform a complete examination, often including electro-physiology (EEG), electroretinogram (ERG), visually evoked response (VER). CT scan and/or MRI can be helpful. Close cooperation with the pediatric neurologist, pediatrician, and geneticist may be indicated. Because it may be difficult to reach a diagnosis immediately, it is better to postpone a definitive answer to the parents until the clinical picture is unequivocal. Nothing is worse than to inform parents that their baby is blind (or normal) and to be forced later to reach the opposite conclusion.

C. In Leber congenital amaurosis (LCA), the fundus first appears entirely normal, although a pigmentary retinopathy may eventually develop. High hyperopia is typical in uncomplicated LCA, in which the abnormalities are restricted to the eye. Pupillary reactions are sluggish or even para-doxical. The ERG is extinguished in both light- and dark-adapted conditions. Other retinal degenera-tions may have similar effects, but they are usually not evident in the neonate.

D. Although diagnosing hypoplasia of the optic nerves seems simple, the changes can be subtle and are sometimes overlooked. The small disc is often surrounded by a yellow halo, the "double-ring" sign. The nerve fiber layer is thinner than usual, and the foveal reflex may be decreased. Sometimes, the hypoplasia is segmental. The latter is particu-larly true for the children of diabetic mothers.

E. Severe ONH causes random eye movements, if bilateral. It may be isolated or combined with CNS abnormalities. The classical combination is

with sagittal midline defects, such as agenesis of the anterior commissure and septum pellucidum. Septo-optic dysplasia is often associated with hypopituitarism; therefore, endocrine evaluation is essential. Early recognition and appropriate hormonal replacement therapy allow reversal of the growth retardation commonly seen in these patients. Other often-associated anomalies are hydranencephaly, anencephaly, and encepha-loceles. There is evidence that some cases of ONH may be caused by environmental factors. Drugs, such as anticonvulsants and quinidine, and maternal diabetes mellitus have been implicated.

F. At least 10 syndromes are characterized by oculo-cutaneous or ocular albinism. All have reduced pigmentation of the ocular pigment epithelia, hypoplasia of the *fovea*, reduced vision, and nystagmus. Their differentiation is beyond the scope of this chapter. However, a precise diagnosis is important because some types are associated with systemic disorders of significant morbidity. It is also required for genetic counseling. Foveal hypoplasia is also seen in aniridia.

G. Juvenile retinoschisis is almost always X-linked and thus manifested only in males. It has rarely been found in females, compatible with autosomal-recessive inheritance. There is a splitting of the nerve fiber layer at the posterior pole and in the peripheral retina. The macular changes can be subtle and difficult to detect. The expression is variable, and vision may be as good as 20/50. Vitreous abnormalities may be present. The ERG is helpful: A *waves* are normal, but the amplitudes of both scotopic and photopic B *wave* are usually reduced.

H. Vision is severely reduced in achromatopsia. Color vision is lost. Almost pathognomonic is severe photophobia. The disease is rare and is autosomal-recessive. The ERG flicker response is absent; photopic flash response is reduced, but the scoto-pic response is normal. The nystagmus has a very low amplitude and at times is difficult to detect.

I. Congenital stationary night blindness (CSNB) is hereditary, although all three major inheritance patterns have been described, indicating genetic heterogeneity. In the X-linked variety, vision is reduced and nystagmus, as well as (moderately) high myopia, is present. Color vision is normal. The ERG shows a reduced scotopic B *wave*. Autosomal-dominant CSNB does not show reduced vision and nystagmus; the autosomal-recessive type is variable.

J. If no nystagmus is present, babies fall into two major groups once large refractive errors have been excluded and corrected. The first group has evidence of CNS abnormalities; the second has a negative history and essentially normal examination.

K. Very high degrees of myopia or hyperopia can lead to behavior that makes one suspect blindness. Therefore, always perform retinoscopy. In addition, some other causes of reduced vision are typically associated with refractive errors, such as myopia in CSNB or hyperopia in LCA.

L. Premature birth and/or low birth weight, a history of perinatal asphyxia, developmental anomalies, or a seizure disorder may all indicate possible damage to the occipital cerebral cortex. CT scan, MRI, and referral to the pediatric neurologist are necessary.

M. If all test results are normal in a seemingly blind baby, the natural history may help. Waiting until the baby is 6-month-old or so may yield a diagnosis.

N. Ocular motor apraxia is usually congenital, but can be acquired. Because of the lack of oculomotor response, the apraxia is often mistaken for visual unresponsiveness, particularly in the first several months, when the typical horizontal head jerks (to change fixation) have not yet appeared. The syndrome is characterized by a failure to elicit saccades on command, although saccades may be initiated by some visual reflexes (i.e., optokinetic stimulation). In the congenital variety, only the horizontal saccades are involved. The congenital condition improves with time.

O. Delayed visual maturation (DVM) may occur in babies whose ocular and systemic examinations are otherwise normal. EEG and ERG are normal, but pattern onset/offset visual-evoked responses may be mildly delayed. Most of these children will have 'caught up' by the age of 6 months, and their subsequent development (visual, neurologic, and otherwise) should be entirely normal. Premature babies or babies with psychomotor retardation may also show DVM. Finally, children with an ocular abnormality, explaining a reduction in sight, may have much poorer vision than expected on the basis of the eye findings. Although the prognosis for the last two groups is not as favorable as for the patients with isolated DVM, vision often improves with time.

BIBLIOGRAPHY

1. Catalano RA. Nystagmus. In: Nelson LB, Calhoun JH, Harley RD (Eds). Pediatric Ophthalmology, 3rd Edition. Philadelphia: WB Saunders, 1991.
2. Hoyt C, Nickel B, Billson F. Ophthalmological examination of the infant. Surv Ophthalmol. 1982;26:177-89.
3. Lambert SR, Kriss A, Taylor D. Delayed visual maturation, a longitudinal clinical and electrophysiological assessment. Ophthalmology. 1989;96:524-9.
4. Lambert SR, Taylor D, Kriss A. The infant with nystagmus, normal appearing fundi, but an abnormal ERG. Surv Ophthalmol. 1989;34:173-86.
5. O'Donnell FE, Green WR. The eye in albinism. In: Duane TD, Jaeger EA (Eds). Clinical Ophthalmology. Philadelphia: Harper & Row, 1988.
6. Rosenberg ML, Wilson E. Congenital ocular motor apraxia without head thrusts. J Clin Neurol Ophthalmol. 1987;7:26-8.
7. Teller D, McDonald M, Preston K, et al. Assessment of visual acuity in infants and children: The acuity card procedure. Dev Med Child Neurol. 1986;28:779-90.

Leukocoria

Johan Zwaan

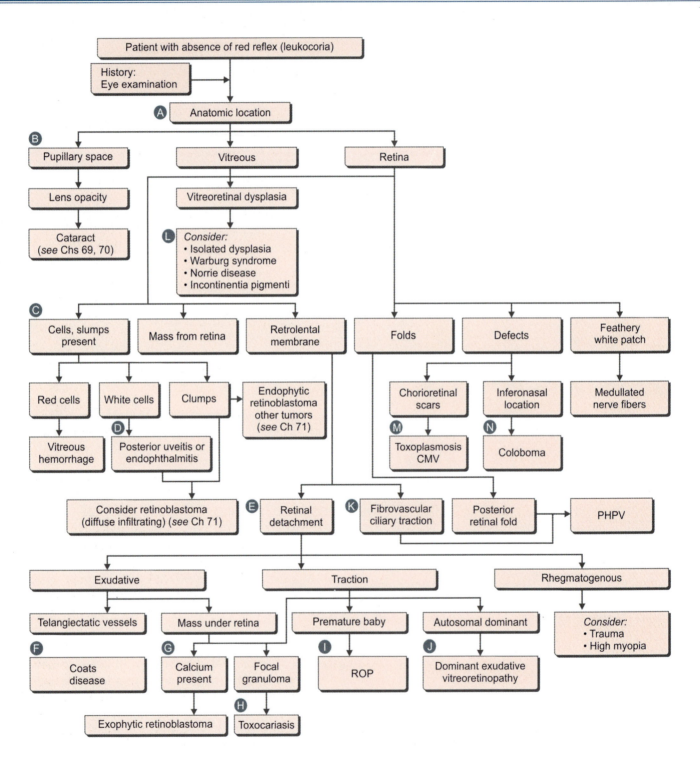

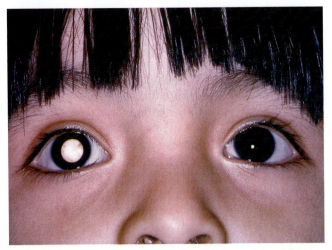

Fig. 67.1: A 3-year-old girl with retinoblastoma of the right eye.

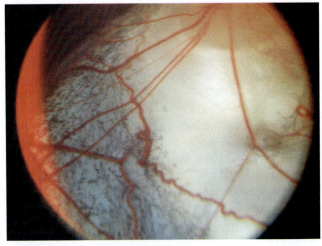

Fig. 67.2: A large chorioretinal coloboma.

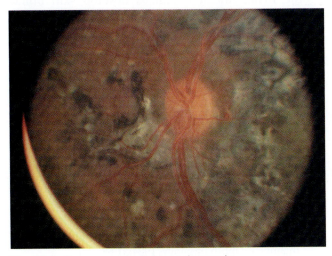

Fig. 67.3: Severe congenital toxoplasmosis.

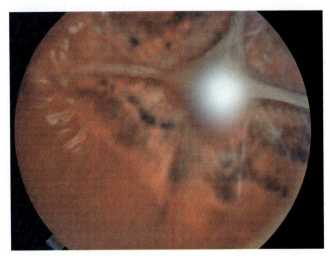

Fig. 67.4: Intra-ocular Toxocara, with a large granuloma and gliotic bands stretching out from it.

Leukocoria in a child requires urgent attention, primarily because in most patients with retinoblastoma, it is the first sign noticed. A white pupil indicates a severely amblyopiogenic condition, which may be treatable. The history, including that of the family, can be extremely helpful in the differential diagnosis. In addition to eye examinations, special tests, such as ultrasonography, computed tomography (CT) scanning, and magnetic resonance imaging (MRI), may be required.

The scheme presented here is oversimplified because there is significant overlap in the pathologic expression of the multiple causes of leukocoria. Moreover, the findings depend on the stage of the clinical problem. Each patient should be evaluated individually, taking into account all information provided by history, eye and systemic examinations, and special tests.

A. Anatomic location is important in the differential diagnosis of leukocoria. The "vitreous" category includes structures displaced into the normal location of the vitreous gel (i.e. detached retinas).

B. Normally, only the lens is found immediately behind the pupil, so an opacity here indicates a cataract. Advanced cases of persistent hyperplastic primary vitreous (PHPV) can also present with a posterior or total cataract (*see* paragraph K). A cataract does not exclude other causes of leukocoria, therefore thoroughly examine the remainder of the eye.

C. Cells or clumps in the vitreous indicate hemorrhage, infection, or tumor, in particular retinoblastoma. Although seedlings from an endophytic retinoblastoma are not easily missed, the diffuse infiltrating type is insidious and often misdiagnosed as uveitis or endophthalmitis.

D. There are many causes for posterior uveitis in children such as cytomegaly virus (CMV), *Toxocara canis* or *Toxocara catis,* and rarely *Candida albicans* (in immunosuppressed children) and congenital syphilis, sympathetic ophthalmia, and sarcoidosis. The most common expression of the congenital toxoplasmosis syndrome is chorioretinitis.

E. Retinal detachments commonly present as leukocoria in children. There often is an overlap between the types of detachment. For instance, dominant exudative vitreoretinopathy has exudates, yet the associated detachment is usually caused by traction.

F. Coats disease is almost always unilateral and occurs primarily in older boys, although it sometimes occurs at an early age and in females. At late stages, subretinal lipid and cholesterol crystals may be seen.

G. Calcium in a retinal mass is highly typical for retinoblastoma, although not entirely pathognomonic.

H. *T. canis,* or rarely *T. catis,* can cause a chorioretinal granuloma in the peripheral retina or the macula, or it can masquerade as endophthalmitis. Systemic manifestations are rare. The Enzyme/linked immunosorbent assay (ELISA) test for *Toxocara* has its limitations: 10% of patients with the disease have a negative test, and the test can be positive when *Toxocara* is not present. It does not differentiate between live or dead organisms. A definite diagnosis requires a pathological examination of a specimen.

I. The serious forms (stage 3–5) of retinopathy of prematurity (ROP) affect mostly premature babies, whose birth weight is <1500 g ("micropremies"). In stage 3, extraretinal neovascularization is seen, and in stage 4, a subtotal retinal detachment, tractional or exudative.

J. The appearance of dominant exudative vitreoretinopathy is similar to that of ROP, but there is an autosomal-dominant inheritance pattern and the children are not premature.

K. The hallmarks of PHPV are persistent hyaloid vessels and a retrolental fibrovascular membrane with traction, which pulls the ciliary processes behind the lens, making them visible. Persistent fetal vessels have been proposed as a more general term, but most authors still use the term PHPV. The lens may be cataractous, the posterior capsule may be ruptured, and blood vessels may invade the lens. The eye is usually microphthalmic. In posterior PHPV, the retina is folded from the disc to the periphery, at times all the way to the ora serrata. Abnormal vessels are seen in the fold, and the adjacent vitreous is condensed.

L. The ocular manifestations of the different vitreoretinal dysplasias are similar, and a definitive diagnosis cannot be made on the basis of the eye examination alone. Systemic examination and history provide the major clues. Warburg syndrome is autosomal recessive and combines brain and eye malformations. Brain abnormalities include agyria, hydrocephalus, and, variably, encephalocele; there is severe mental retardation. Ocular findings include retinal dysplasia. Because Norrie disease is X-linked recessive, it is found in males only. The vitreoretinal dysplasia usually is progressive and leads to total retinal detachment and blindness. Many affected patients are retarded; others have hearing loss. Incontinentia pigmenti is X-linked dominant and presumed lethal in the male. Affected females develop skin bullae postnatally, which leave a pattern of pigmented lines upon resolution.

M. Both *Toxoplasma gondii* and CMV cause indistinguishable atrophic chorioretinal scars, surrounded by pigmentation.

N. Chorioretinal colobomas vary from very small to encompassing most of the fundus and optic nerve. They are always located inferonasally, reflecting the embryonic position of the choroidal fissure. If the coloboma is large, the eye is usually microphthalmic.

BIBLIOGRAPHY

1. Char DH, Hedges TR, Norman D. Retinoblastoma CT diagnosis. Ophthalmology. 1984;91:686-95.
2. Ellis GS, Pakalnis VA, Worley G, et al. Toxocara canis infection: Clinical and epidemiological associations with seropositivity in kindergarten children. Ophthalmology. 1986;93:1032-7.
3. Flynn JT, Bancalari E, Bachynski BN, et al. Retinopathy of prematurity: Diagnosis, severity, and natural history. Ophthalmology. 1987;94:620-9.
4. Goldberg MF. Clinical manifestations of ectopia lentis et pupillae in 16 patients. Ophthalmology. 1988;95:1080-7.
5. Katz NK, Margo CE, Dorwart RH. Computerized tomography with histopathological correlation in children with leukocoria. J Pediatr Ophthalmol Strabismus. 1984; 21:50-7.
6. Lieberfarb RM, Eavey RD, Delong GR, et al. Norrie's disease: A study of two families. Ophthalmology. 1985; 92:1445-51.
7. Noble K, Carr R. Disorders of the fundus: Toxoplasma retinochoroiditis. Ophthalmology. 1982;89:1289-91.
8. Zwaan J. Leukocoria. In: Dershewitz RA (Ed). Ambulatory Pediatric Care, 3rd Edition. Philadelphia, PA: Lippincott-Raven; 1999. pp. 562-5.

Cloudy Cornea in a Neonate

Johan Zwaan

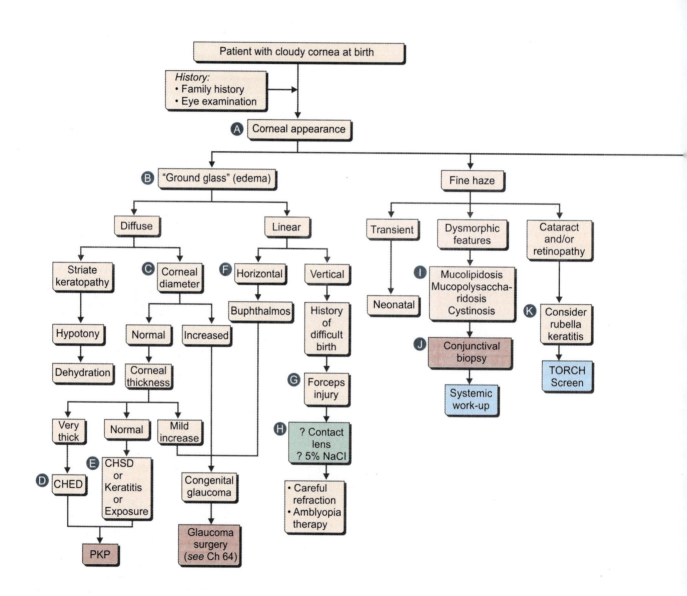

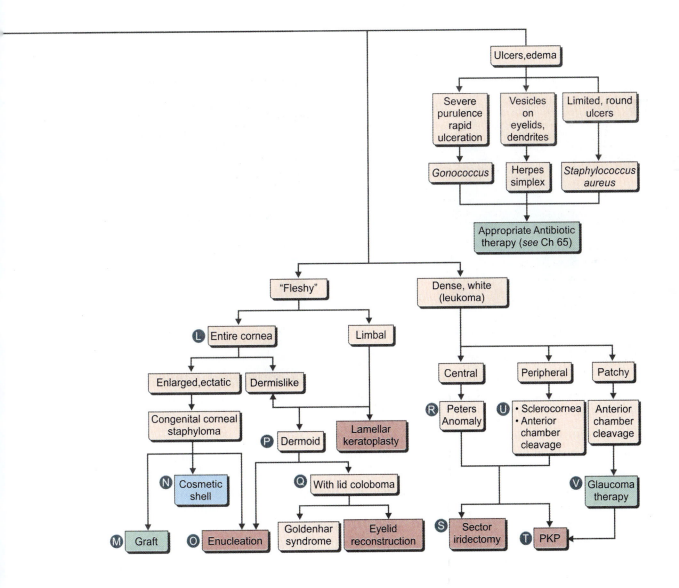

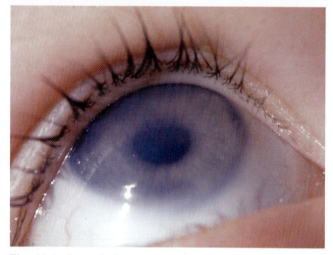

Fig. 68.1: Ground glass appearance of the cornea of a child with congenital hereditary endothelial dystrophy.

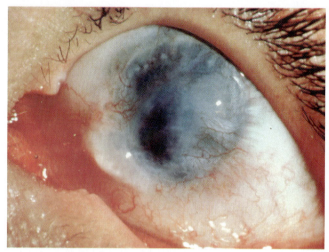

Fig. 68.2: Sclerocornea.

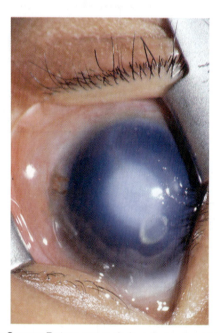

Fig. 68.3: Severe Peters anomaly in a 3-month-old infant.

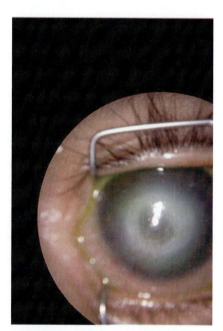

Fig. 68.4: Infantile glaucoma with corneal edema and corneal ectasia.

A cornea cloudy at birth, if not *very* transient, always indicates a significant ocular problem. Although some of the underlying causes do not require immediate intervention, a detailed history and eye examination should be given immediately to identify babies who need treatment, such as congenital glaucoma patients. The prognosis for visual development depends greatly on the pathogenesis of the corneal opacity.

The corneal abnormality can be a tip-off for the existence of systemic or genetic disease.

A. The appearance of the corneal opacity is one of the most important indications of the underlying pathogenesis.

B. A ground glass appearance almost always indicates edema. It is important to differentiate the three major causes—congenital glaucoma, congenital hereditary endothelial dystrophy (CHED), and forceps injury–because the first requires immediate treatment.

C. The corneal diameter is enlarged in congenital glaucoma, unless the disease is in an early stage. Additional tests are required for a definitive diagnosis: measurement of the intraocular pressure (IOP), inspection of the anterior segment (gonioscopy), and examination of the optic nerves (optic cup size). The enlarged cornea in glaucoma should not be confused with megalocornea (Chapter 31).

D. Tremendously increased corneal thickness is the hallmark of CHED. This is an autosomal-recessive condition characterized by absence or insufficiency of the corneal endothelium, resulting in massive corneal edema. It is rare in the United States but much more common in the Middle East. The abnormally thick cornea often results in what appears to be a moderately elevated IOP. This makes the differentiation from congenital glaucoma even more difficult. It is helpful that the corneal diameter does not increase, even in the presence of greatly increased thickness. If goniotomy or trabeculotomy is erroneously performed, the corneal edema will not improve in patients with CHED, whereas it usually will, when congenital glaucoma is surgically controlled.

E. Congenital hereditary stromal dystrophy (CHSD) is autosomal dominant and not progressive. The stroma has a ground glass appearance at birth or may be flaky white. Congenital syphilis can cause an interstitial keratitis, but this is almost never present at birth; the child usually is several years old before the problem manifests. Rubella can cause a congenital corneal haze, which may be more or less severe (*see* section "K"). Exposure, usually from eyelid abnormalities, is not apparent immediately at birth but shows up quickly, particularly if a portion of the lid is missing (*see* section "Q"). Immediate protection of the cornea with lubricants and patching is mandatory. Follow this as soon as practical by surgical eyelid reconstruction.

F. Horizontal breaks in the endothelium and Descemet membrane (Haab striae) are typical for congenital glaucoma. Even if the disease is arrested, the enlarged corneae of these patients,

with or without Haab striae, are always at risk for endothelial decompensation and often, later in life, become edematous.

G. Endothelial cracks from forceps deliveries are generally vertically or obliquely oriented because they are caused by compression of the eye against the superior orbital rim. The diagnosis is facilitated by the birth history and the presence of other signs of facial injury.

H. The use of contact lenses or hypertonic saline ointment may reduce the edema that follows the injury to the corneal endothelium. Because this edema resolves spontaneously in a few weeks to months when the endothelium heals, the actual benefit of these treatments is difficult to prove. In these babies, significant astigmatism and myopia development in the affected eye and careful refraction and amblyopia therapy are most important.

I. With the exception of tyrosinemia, metabolic genetic diseases, such as mucopolysaccharidoses, mucolipidoses, and cystinosis, uncommonly cause a congenitally cloudy cornea. If such a diagnosis is suspected, other findings such as dysmorphic features or psychomotor retardation are usually more important.

J. Conjunctival biopsy, combined with electron microscopy of the specimen, can often accurately pinpoint the diagnosis of these metabolic diseases. It is a simple procedure with low morbidity and is not used enough.

K. The congenital rubella syndrome can be associated with a keratopathy, which presents as a more or less dense haze. The cloudiness generally clears spontaneously in a few months. It should be differentiated from congenital glaucoma, which can occur in up to 10% of babies with rubella.

L. If the entire cornea is replaced with an ectatic and opaque structure or with a dermoid-like choristoma, the prognosis for restoration of useful vision is guarded.

M. Grafting should be considered, particularly when both eyes are affected, even though the outcome of penetrating keratoplasty (PKP) in children is not as favorable as in adults. In addition, performing the surgery *very* early helps in minimizing amblyopia. There is also an indication that the rejection rate is less if the keratoplasty is performed when the child is no more than a few months old. In some cases, a lamellar keratoplasty gives a good cosmetic result.

N. A cosmetic shell or a painted contact lens may be used if the corneal lesion is not too elevated.

O. Enucleation should rarely be necessary. If the eye does not see and is unsightly, replacement with a hydroxyapatite implant or a dermis-fat graft can be considered. Effects of enucleation on orbital growth should be taken into account.

P. Limbal dermoids can be treated by simple excision (lamellar keratectomy). Occasionally, they take up the entire thickness of the cornea or sclera, and the surgeon must be prepared to do a corneal patch graft. Careful examination, including gonioscopy, warns the clinician of this possibility in most cases, if not all.

Q. If the dermoid is associated with an eyelid coloboma, the latter needs to be repaired to prevent exposure keratitis.

R. Peters anomaly is characterized by a central corneal leukoma with a relatively clear periphery. It often occurs bilaterally, in which case surgical treatment is indicated in at least one eye. Before the attempted repair, do a full evaluation, including ultrasound and perhaps CT scanning, to find the extent of iris and lens involvement and the possible presence of persistent hyperplastic primary vitreous, which may cloud the prognosis.

S. Surgical treatment of these patients is controversial because the results have been limited. With or without treatment, vision is usually severely reduced. If both eyes are involved, an attempt at surgical improvement of the vision is warranted, as long as the parents understand that the prognosis is guarded. If congenital glaucoma is also present, it should be controlled first. In many patients, an optical sector iridectomy will allow them to look around the corneal opacity. This much less invasive procedure does not require the intensive follow-up necessary after PKP.

T. Penetrating keratoplasty (PKP) in patients with Peters anomaly is often complicated by adhesions between the cornea and the iris or lens. This may necessitate lensectomy and anterior vitrectomy, which further diminishes an already poor prognosis.

U. In sclerocornea, the peripheral cornea is opaque; the center is clear or at least less opaque.

V. In anterior chamber cleavage syndromes, other than Peters anomaly, corneal opacities are usually mild and do not require therapeutic intervention. Glaucoma is often present and must be treated.

BIBLIOGRAPHY

1. Ahmad M, Barber JC, Reinecke RD, et al. Ocular choristomas. Surv Ophthalmol. 1989;33:339-58.
2. Angell LK, Robb RM, Berson FG. Visual prognosis in patients with ruptures in Descemet's membrane due to forceps injuries. Arch Ophthalmol. 1981;99:2137-44.
3. Cotran PR, Bajart AM. Congenital corneal opacities. Int Ophthalmol Clin. 1992;32:93-105.
4. Kenyon KR. Lysosomal disorders affecting the ocular anterior segment. In: Nicholson DH, (Ed). Ocular Pathology Update. New York, NY: Masson, 1980.
5. Kirkness CM, McCartney A, Rice NS, et al. Congenital hereditary corneal oedema of Maumenee: Its clinical features, management and pathology. Br J Ophthalmol. 1987;71:130-45.
6. Mulet M, Caldwell DR. Corneal abnormalities. In: Wright KW, (Ed). Pediatric Ophthalmology and Strabismus. St Louis, MO: Mosby; 1995. pp. 321-48.
7. Parmley VC, Stonecipher KG, Rowsey JJ. Peters' anomaly: A review of 26 penetrating keratoplasties in infants. Ophthalmic Surg. 1993;24:31-5.
8. Stein RM, Cohen EJ, Calhoun JH, et al. Corneal birth trauma managed with a contact lens. Am J Ophthalmol. 1987;103:596-7.

Johan Zwaan

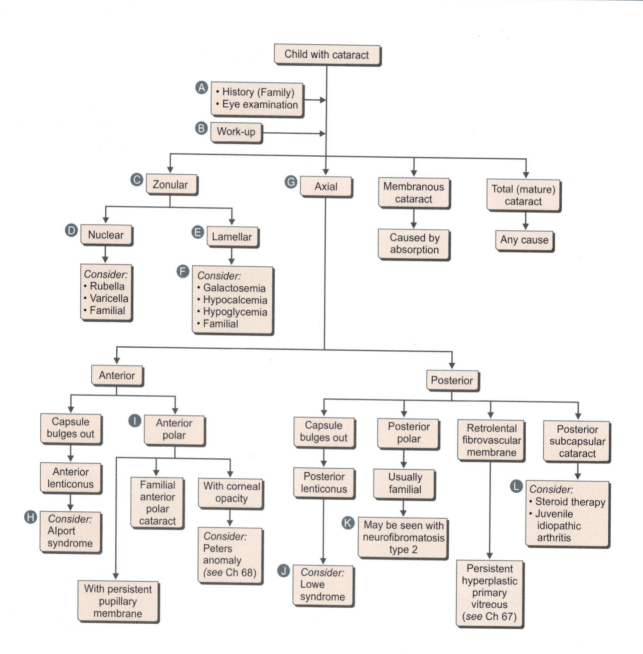

A congenital cataract is found in about one in 250 live-births. Roughly, one-third is associated with a syndrome or metabolic disease, one-third is clearly hereditary, and the cause of the remainder is unknown. Congenital cataract is still one of the leading causes of blindness in children (20%).

A. A family history and particularly a careful eye examination of parents and other family members can be very helpful in establishing a diagnosis.

B. A work-up normally needs not be extensive. If a baby has a cataract secondary to a metabolic deficiency, the child also fails to thrive, is sickly, and has come to the attention of the pediatrician well before the diagnosis of cataract is made. There is one exception to this: galactokinase deficiency can result in lens opacification in an otherwise perfectly healthy child. It is usually more than adequate to obtain a fasting blood sugar (hypoglycemia), urine for reducing sugars (galactosemia), serum calcium, and phosphate (hypoparathyroidism, severe vitamin D deficiency), and urinary amino acids (Lowe syndrome). If an infectious process is suspected, order a TORCH screen and a VDRL.

C. Zonular cataracts are restricted to certain zones within the lens, although they may be accompanied by "riders." Most are either nuclear or lamellar, although sutural, stellate, floriform, and other morphologic types also fall under this category. The position of the cataract gives to an extent an indication of the timing of cataractogenesis,

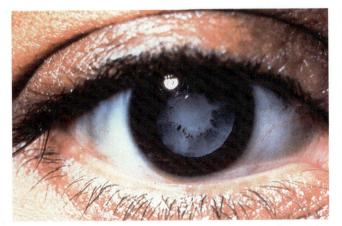

Fig. 69.1: Pediatric nuclear cataract with "spoke-like" opacities and lamellar capacity.

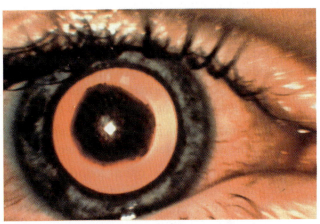

Fig. 69.2: Nuclear cataract in retro-illumination.

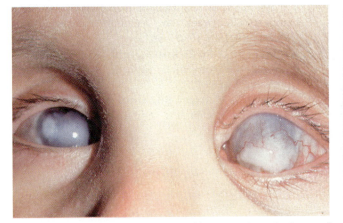

Fig. 69.3: Lowe syndrome patient with cataracts and advanced glaucoma.

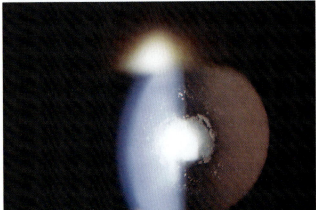

Fig. 69.4: Posterior lenticonus within associated cataract.

reflecting the way in which the lens fibers are laid down during development. A nuclear cataract dates back to early embryogenesis, and lamellar cataracts (typically with a clear nucleus inside and a clear cortical shell outside) originate later in prenatal or postnatal Iife.

D. A nuclear cataract is often familial. In a sick infant, it should lead to the suspicion of rubella, although other viruses, notably varicella, can cause a similar lens opacity.

E. Lamellar lens opacities are often autosomal dominant. The cataracts associated with metabolic diseases are usually lamellar.

F. Galactosemia comes in two distinct types. In galactokinase deficiency, children have no systemic illness, whereas children with a deficiency of galactose-1-phosphate uridyltransferase are quite ill. The cataract appears the same in both; an oil drop configuration in the center of the lens is caused by a refractive change in the nucleus. It is secondary to osmotic changes and is reversible in an early stage. More permanent lamellar opacities appear, if galactose is not removed from the diet.

G. Axial cataracts, as the name indicates, are located around the anteroposterior axis of the lens.

H. Anterior lenticonus is often found in Alport syndrome (chronic renal failure and sensorineural deafness). Other eye findings include a flecked retina and corneal arcus.

I. Anterior polar cataracts are often small and until recently were thought to be nonprogressive. However, some progress to a point at which they interfere greatly with vision, making removal necessary.

J. Lowe syndrome shows severe lens anomalies. In addition to having posterior lenticonus, the lens is often shaped-like a flat disc and is always cataractous. The syndrome is X-linked recessive; carriers have fine punctate lens opacities.

The children are severely retarded and have a dysmorphic face with chubby cheeks.

K. Patients with neurofibromatosis type 2 (bilateral central acoustic neuromas) have a high incidence (at least 80% in our series) of posterior subcapsular cataracts, often somewhat off-center, or sectorial cataracts. This finding may be a useful marker for genetic counseling.

L. Steroid therapy can cause posterior subcapsular cataracts. In an early stage, these cataracts have little effect on vision. Given the choice of developing a cataract or omitting an often lifesaving therapy, the answer is clear. If the cataract interferes significantly with visual performance, it can always be removed. Juvenile idiopathic arthritis, which can occur at an early age, may result in posterior subcapsular cataracts.

BIBLIOGRAPHY

1. Amaya L, Taylor D, Russell-Eggitt I, et al. The morphology and natural history of childhood cataracts. Surv Ophthalmol. 2003;48:125-44.
2. Brocklebank JT, Harcourt RB, Meadows SR. Corticosteroidsinduced cataracts in idiopathic nephrotic syndrome. Arch Dis Child. 1982;57:30-5.
3. Cibis GW, Waeltermann JM, Whitcraft CT, et al. Lenticular opacities in carriers of Lowe's syndrome. Ophthalmology. 1986;93:1041-6.
4. Crouch ER, Parks MM. Management of posterior lenticonus complicated by unilateral cataracts. Am J Ophthalmol. 1978;85:503-7.
5. Govan JAA. Ocular manifestations of Alport's syndrome. Br J Ophthalmol. 1983;67:493-503.
6. Jaafar MS, Robb RM. Congenital anterior polar cataract: a review of 63 cases. Ophthalmology. 1984;91:249-51.
7. Lambert SR, Drack AV. Infantile cataracts. Surv Ophthalmol. 1996;40:427-58.
8. Lambert SR, Taylor D, Kriss A, et al. Ocular manifestations of the congenital varicella syndrome. Arch Ophthalmol. 1989;107:52-6.
9. Wheeler DT, Mullaney PB, Awad A, et al. Pyramidal anterior polar cataracts. Ophthalmology. 1999;106:2362-7.

70

Cataract in a Child: Treatment

Mary A O'Hara, Johan Zwaan

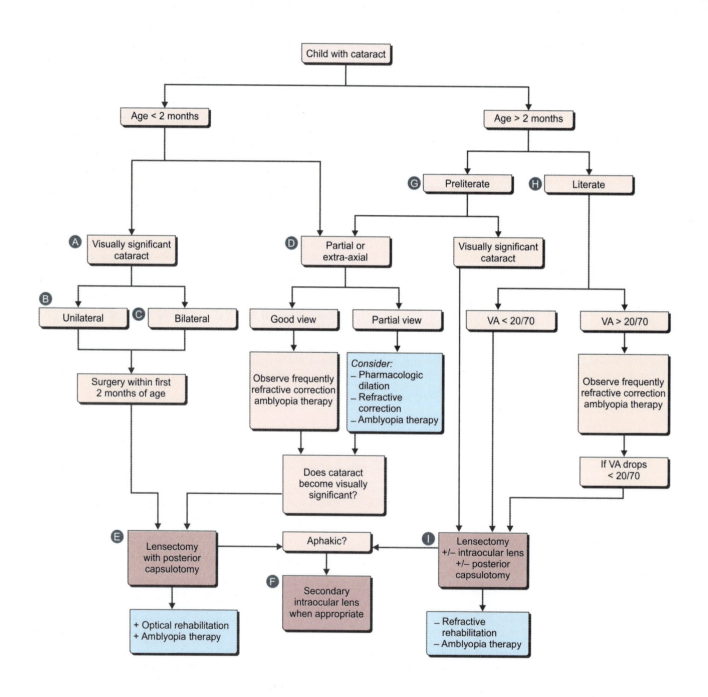

The treatment of pediatric cataracts continues to evolve. Many techniques used in adult cataract surgery have translated to the surgical removal of pediatric cataracts. Recent research has revealed the benefits and limitations of certain treatments when applied to the pediatric eye. However, visual outcome in pediatric cataract surgery still depends on the age of the patient when the cataract became visually significant, the timeliness of intervention and, most importantly, the commitment of the family in caring for the patient in the postoperative period.

A. Fixation behavior is inconsistent in the first 2 months of life. Therefore, the visual significance of a cataract is determined by whether or not the undilated pupil affords a view of the retinal details. It is estimated that when retinal details are obscured by a cataract, the visual potential of that eye is less than 20/60. By the same token, a dense central cataract of 3 mm or more will obscure the retinal view through the average infant pupil of 2 mm.

B. Preoperative care of the unilateral cataract may include bilateral light occlusion. Short periods of bilateral patching prior to cataract surgery may prolong the critical period of visual development and decrease the amount of postoperative amblyopia in the cataractous eye. This technique is controversial and should be used for less than 2 weeks before cataract surgery. The risk of bilateral amblyopia and nystagmus during this critical period precludes long-term use of this technique.

C. In general, bilateral cataracts have a better postoperative visual outcome than unilateral cataracts. If the child has a significant anesthetic risk, simultaneous surgery may be preferred. Most surgeons will treat simultaneous surgery as two separate cases under one anesthetic, using separate surgical prep, hand washing and gowning, and instruments, for each eye. Sequential cases are usually done within 1 or 2 weeks if the cataracts are symmetrical.

D. A partial or extra-axial cataract may be amenable to treatment with noncycloplegic dilating agents such as phenylephrine or tropicamide. These agents dilate the pupil, thus allowing the infant to 'look around' the cataract. Stronger agents such as cyclogyl or atropine may be used for longer periods of dilation. Frail infants may be susceptible to systemic side effects such as paralytic ileus from the use of these drops. In addition to a longer period of dilation, these agents also cycloplege the eye. Bifocal or progressive-add spectacles are needed for the older child when these agents are used. If asymmetry between the cataracts in each eye exists, it may be helpful to prophylactically patch the less-involved eye a few hours per day. Frequent and careful follow-up is imperative.

E. Lensectomy results in aphakia, which is as amblyopiogenic as the previous cataract. Prompt refractive rehabilitation is important in the treatment of amblyopia. Contact lens remains the most common method of refractive correction of infant aphakia. Young infants are usually overcorrected 2–3 diopters because the majority of their visual experience is at near. As the child matures to a toddler, the contact lenses are corrected for distance and the child wears bifocals or progressive-add spectacles for near and intermediate focus. Aphakic spectacles have been used when contact lens use is not practical. Intraocular lenses have been placed in special cases, but are usually not implanted before 6 months of age because of increased risk of complications.

F. Secondary intraocular lenses are widely accepted for use after 2 years of age. The decision to implant a secondary intraocular lens is based on contact lens intolerance, compliance issues, and parental concerns.

G. The assessment of visual significance of a cataract in the older infant and preliterate child is aided by observation of fixation behavior and the presence of strabismus that indicates loss of binocularity. Nystagmus denotes a poor prognosis for vision.

H. In the literate child, a corrected visual acuity of 20/70 or worse is a generally accepted indication for surgical intervention. The higher visual threshold for surgery in a child versus an elderly adult is due to the attendant loss of accommodation that occurs in pediatric cataract surgery. Surgery is deferred until the vision is 20/70 or worse so that the child's ability to focus at near and intermediate distances is preserved as long as possible.

I. Lensectomy in an older infant or child is more likely to include primary implantation of an intraocular lens. Bag placement is preferred. The management of the posterior capsule is age dependent. Since most posterior capsules will opacify with time, a posterior capsulotomy becomes necessary. In the young child, this is done at the time of the original surgery. The older, more cooperative child may undergo YAG laser posterior capsulotomy at a later date.

BIBLIOGRAPHY

1. Dave H, Phoenix V, Becker ER, et al. Simultaneous vs sequential bilateral cataract surgery for infants with congenital cataracts. Arch Ophthalmol. 2010;128:1050-4.

2. Plager DA, Lynn MJ, Buckley EG, et al. Complications, adverse events, and additional intraocular surgery 1 year after cataract surgery in the Infant Aphakia Treatment Study. Ophthalmology. 2011;118:2330-4.

3. Russell BC, Ward MA, Lynn M, et al. The Infant Aphakia Treatment Study contact lens experience: One-year outcomes. Eye Contact Lens. 2012;38:234-9.

4. Wilson ME Jr, Trivedi RH, Pandey SK. Pediatric Cataract Surgery: Techniques, Complications and Management. Philadelphia, PA: Lippincott, Williams and Wilkins, 2005.

5. Wright KW. Lens abnormalities. In: Wright KW, Strube YNJ, (Eds). Pediatric Ophthalmology and Strabismus, Third edition. New York, NY: Springer-Verlag; 2012.

6. Wright KW, Wehrle MJ, Urrea PT. Bilateral total occlusion during the critical period of visual development. Arch Ophthalmol. 1987;103:321.

Retinoblastoma

71

Timothy P Cleland, Johan Zwaan, Lina Marouf

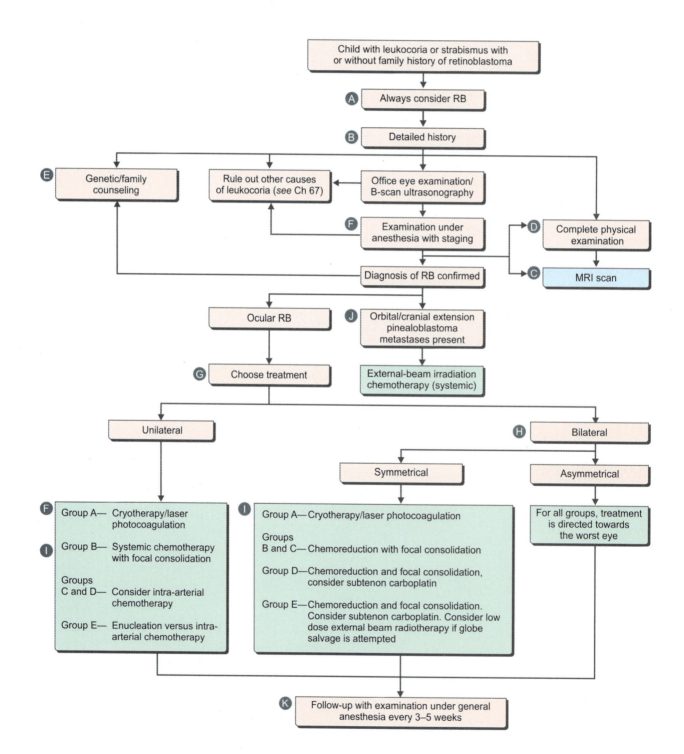

Retinoblastoma (RB) is relatively rare, with a worldwide incidence of about 11 cases per one million children less than 5 years of age. Among various worldwide populations, the incidence of the heritable form remains constant, indicating environmental factors play little role in its etiology. In the United States, there are an estimated 250–350 new cases per year. RB is the most common intraocular malignancy in childhood. The alert pediatrician or family physician plays the most important role in early detection. Although, the diagnosis is occasionally made later than desirable, the combination of aware primary care providers, improved diagnostic methods, and newer, more aggressive treatment has yielded a cure rate of >90%. The care of these patients is best concentrated in centers where experienced pediatric oncologists, interventional radiologists, genetic counselors, and ocular oncologists are readily available.

The International Classification System was introduced to better describe the likelihood of globe salvage when systemic chemotherapy (as opposed to external beam radiotherapy) is used as the primary treatment (Table 71.1). The risk of loss of the eye due to RB is 'very low' for Group A eyes and increases to 'very high' to Group E eyes. Prognostically, it is important to note that with this classification system absolute tumor size is less important than other factors such as the presence of vitreous or subretinal seeds.

A. About 60% of children with RB present with leukocoria and another 20% with strabismus, equally divided between esotropia and exotropia. In infants with these signs, always consider RB, especially if the child has a positive family history. Atypical clinical presentations include hypopyon, hyphema, glaucoma, and preseptal cellulitis. A timely diagnosis is critical.

B. A detailed history can reveal important diagnostic information. Although a positive family history is helpful, some parents are unsure of their own ocular history. Some parents may not associate a history of 'white pupil' with RB.

C. During the office examination, contact B-scan ultrasonography can usually be performed. Routine CT scanning is not recommended, especially in children less than 1 year of age. MRI (with gadolinium enhancement) of the brain and

Table 71.1: International classification for intraocular retinoblastoma

Group A—Very low risk
Small discrete intraretinal tumors away from the foveola and disc
- All tumors are 3 mm or smaller in greatest dimension, confined to the retina
- All tumors are located farther than 3 mm from the foveola and 1.5 mm from the optic disc

Group B—Low risk
All remaining discrete retinal tumors without seeding
- All tumors confined to the retina not in group A
- Any tumor size and location with no vitreous or subretinal seeding

Group C—Moderate risk
Discrete local disease with minimal focal subretinal or vitreous seeding
- Tumor(s) must be discrete
- Subretinal fluid, present or past, without gross seeding, involving up to one quadrant of retina
- Local subretinal seeding, present or past, less than 5 mm from the tumor
- Focal fine vitreous seeding close to discrete tumor

Group D—High risk
Diffuse disease with significant vitreous and/or subretinal seeding
- Tumor(s) may be massive or diffuse
- Subretinal fluid, present or past, up to total retinal detachment
- Diffuse subretinal seeding may include subretinal plaques or tumor nodules
- Diffuse or massive vitreous disease may include 'greasy' seeds or avascular tumor mass

Group E—Very high risk
Presence of any one or more of these poor prognosis features
- Tumor touching the lens
- Neovascular glaucoma
- Tumor anterior to anterior vitreous face involving ciliary body or anterior segment
- Diffuse infiltrating retinoblastoma
- Opaque media from hemorrhage
- Tumor necrosis with aseptic orbital cellulitis
- Phthisis bulbi

Modified from: Shields CL, Mashayekhi A, Au Ak, et al. The International Classification of Retinoblastoma Predicts Chemoreduction Success. Ophthalmology. 2006;113(12):2276-80.

orbits is typically performed to evaluate whether extraocular extension and/or optic nerve invasion is present. MRI cuts through the pineal gland will reveal a 'trilateral' RB, if present.

D. A general physical examination helps in the differential diagnosis and, in advanced cases, may aid in the diagnosis of metastatic disease. Children suspected of having RB with a deletion of chromosomal region 13q14 show developmental delay and facial dysmorphism.

Table 71.2: Risk for recurrence of RB in family members of affected patients

	Bilateral tumors or positive family history (%)	Unilateral tumors and no family history (%)
Patient's child	50	8
Patient's brother or sister	5	0.8
Child of unaffected sibling	0.5	0.08
First cousin	0.05	0.008
Identical twin	100	15
Nonidentical twin	5	0.8

Modified from: Musarella MA, Gallie BL. A simplified scheme for genetic counseling in retinoblastoma. J Pediatr Ophthalmol Strabismus. 1987; 24:124-5.

E. Although detailed counseling need not and probably should not be done immediately after the diagnosis is made, parents should be told that RB may be a genetic disease. RB behaves as an autosomal-dominant disease with a very high penetration rate. About 25% of patients have a positive family history; they are assumed to have the genetic disease. For the remaining 75% of patients, it is important to determine whether they had a germinal mutation and risk passing the RB gene to their children. Patients with multiple tumors and with bilateral disease have had a germinal mutation. Most patients with a single, unilateral tumor probably had a somatic mutation, but 10–15% may still have the genetic disease. Genetic testing for the RB1 germline mutation is available.

Table 71.2 assumes 100% penetrance and is useful for determining the approximate recurrence risk in family members of RB patients.

F. An examination under anesthesia is performed to properly stage the disease. For Group E eyes, enucleation is usually not performed at this point, as most parents require time to understand and accept the need. A complete inspection of both the anterior and posterior segments is critical. Detailed retinal drawings are made. B-scan ultrasonography can be performed (or repeated) if unsuccessful during the office exam. Photodocumentation has become very useful in documenting response to treatment. Fine-needle aspiration is rarely indicated. Spinal taps, bone marrow biopsy or aspiration, and bone scans are no longer routinely obtained by most practitioners, unless metastases are suspected.

G. The treatment plan is individualized and dictated by bilaterality and the extent of ocular involvement. Advanced, unilateral disease can now be successfully treated with intra-arterial chemotherapy (IAC). One hundred percent tumor control for Group C and Group D eyes has been reported. Rare side effects of IAC include choroidal atrophy, retinal artery occlusion, and ophthalmic artery occlusion.

H. Advanced bilateral disease is typically treated with three-agent chemotherapy (vincristine, etoposide, and carboplatin), followed by focal consolidation.

Systemic chemotherapy is thought to play a role in reducing the risk of 'trilateral' RB as well as minimizing the incidence of second cancers in patients with the germline mutation.

I. 'Focal consolidation' refers to the use of either cryotherapy or laser photocoagulation to the residual tumor mass following initial systemic chemotherapy. Cryotherpy involves a triple freeze-thaw technique and is useful for Group A tumors anterior to the equator. Cryotherapy is not the treatment of choice if vitreous seeds are seen overlying the tumor. Laser photocoagulation (either the 532 nm green or the 810 nm infrared) is performed by first surrounding then completely covering the tumor mass.

J. Enucleation should be delayed until the response to systemic chemotherapy is fully evaluated in both eyes. If upon pathologic examination, retrolaminar and/or choroidal involvement is seen, six cycles of adjuvant chemotherapy is recommended.

K. Effects of treatment should be evaluated in 3–5 weeks. This requires examination under anesthesia. Additional treatment may be applied at this time if viable tumor is still present. The frequency of examinations depends on the success of the treatment.

Up to ages 3-4 years, perform examination under anesthesia every 4 months, and from age 5-6 every 6 months. Yearly examinations after the age of 6 years may still require general anesthesia. After the age of 8 years, clinical examinations with scleral depression are usually tolerated and should be done yearly. Patients with heritable RB are at significant risk for other malignancies. Although some authors have recommended periodic CT scans or bone scans to rule out these tumors, this practice may not be necessary because clinical symptoms are usually present well before these tests yield results. Moreover, the received radiation may be tumorigenic itself. Annual MRI scanning might be considered, but its value for periodic screening has not been established.

BIBLIOGRAPHY

1. Abramson DH, Frank CM, Susman M, et al. Presenting signs of retinoblastoma. J Pediatr. 1998;132:505.
2. Finger PT, Harbour JW, Karcioglu ZA. Risk factors for metastasis in retinoblastoma. Surv Ophthalmol. 2002;47:1.
3. Harbour JW. Molecular basis of low-penetrance retinoblastoma. Arch Ophthalmol. 2001;119:1699.
4. Levy C, Doz F, Quintana E, et al. Role of chemotherapy alone or in combination with hyperthermia in the primary treatment of intraocular retinoblastoma: Preliminary results. Br J Ophthalmol. 1998;82:1154.
5. Murphree AL, Gomer CJ, Sato J. Carboplatin and hyperthermia in the management of posterior pole retinoblastoma. The Franceschetti Lecture, Seventh International Symposium on Retinoblastoma. Sienna, Italy, 1992.
6. Murphree AL, Villablanca JG, Deegan WF 3rd, et al. Chemotherapy plus local treatment in the management of intraocular retinoblastoma. Arch Ophtahlmol. 1996; 114:1348.
7. Pendergrass TW, Davis S. Incidence of retinoblastoma in the United States. Arch Ophthalmol. 1980;98:1204.
8. Rodriguez-Galindo C, Wilson MW, Haik BG, et al. Treatment of metastatic retinoblastoma. Ophthalmology. 2003;110:1237.
9. Shields CL, Bianciotto CG, Ramasubramanian A, et al. Intra-arterial chemotherapy for retinoblastoma: I. Control of tumor, subretinal seeds, and vitreous seeds. Arch Ophthalmol. 2011;129:1399-406.
10. Shields CL, Honavar SG, Meadows AT, et al. Chemoreduction in unilateral retinoblastoma. Arch Ophthalmol. 2002;120:1653.
11. Shields CL, Shields JA. Retinoblastoma management: Advances in enucleation, intravenous chemoreduction, and intra-arterial chemotherapy. Curr Opin Ophthalmol. 2010;21:203-12.
12. Shields JA, Parsons H, Shields CL, et al. The role of cryotherapy in the management of retinoblastoma. Am J Ophthalmol. 1989;108:260.
13. Strong LC, Knudson AG Jr. Letter: Second cancers in retinoblastoma. Lancet. 1973;2:1086.

Uncorrectable Poor Vision in a Child

Johan Zwaan

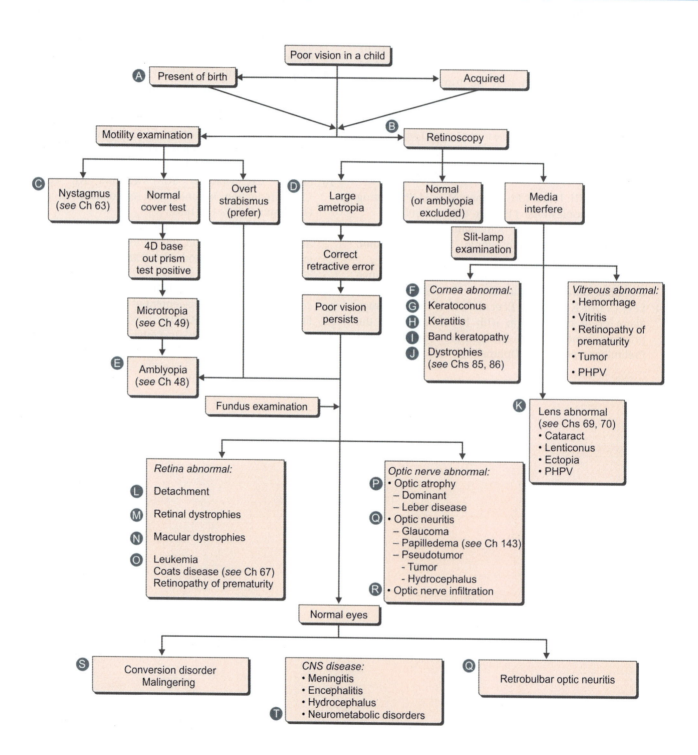

72

When one is confronted with a child with apparently uncorrectable poor vision, it is important to determine the duration of the condition. Congenital anomalies of the visual system often go unrecognized until later in life, particularly when only one eye is involved. A young child does not complain of decreased vision unless the loss is acute and bilateral. The earlier the loss, the more effective the compensatory mechanisms are. About half of pediatric vision loss is caused by genetic disease.

A. The time of onset of vision loss is important in the differential diagnosis. A careful history should be taken to determine if the presumed acquired problem actually may have been present since birth. In addition to structural abnormalities, such as a large chorioretinal coloboma, there are other not so obvious causes of decreased vision from birth (*see* Chapter 66).

B. Retinoscopy is extremely useful, not only for refraction but also for quick detection of abnormalities in the media. For instance, very early keratoconus is often first detected by a distortion of the retinoscopic reflection. Opacities in the media are easily seen as well.

C. Nystagmus is associated with reduced visual acuity, moderately so in congenital motor nystagmus and more severely in secondary nystagmus associated with such disorders as albinism (*see* Chapter 66) or unoperated or late operated congenital cataract (*see* Chapter 69). The existence of nystagmus gives some indication of the age at which the visual problem arose. Before age 2 years nystagmus will result, after age 6 definitely not; in between it can go either way. Nystagmus does not appear until about 2–3 months after birth.

D. A refractive error may be found in combination with strabismus. Microtropia is often associated with anisometropia. Similarly, a difference in refractive error between the two eyes may trigger a preference for one eye and amblyopia in the other.

E. For simplicity's sake, refractive errors and amblyopia and other causes of reduced vision are separated here, yet they often are combined. For instance, patients with retinal dystrophies commonly also have significant refractive errors, and the reduction in vision caused by optic nerve hypoplasia or cataract may be compounded by amblyopia or refractive errors.

F. Corneal problems are discussed in more detail in Chapters 74–87.

G. Keratoconus frequently has its onset in the early teens, with increasing amounts of myopia and astigmatism.

H. Acute forms of keratitis are easily detected; syphilitic interstitial keratitis with characteristic stromal blood vessels and 'ghost' vessels must be separated from Cogan syndrome, in which interstitial keratitis is combined with vestibular hearing loss.

I. Band keratopathy indicates ocular inflammation or systemic disease such as sarcoidosis. Juvenile idiopathic arthritis (JIA), previously labeled juvenile rheumatoid arthritis (JRA), is insidious in its course, and band keratopathy may be the first sign of the disease. By then the low grade uveitis of JIA may have done severe damage to the eye.

J. Epithelial and stromal corneal dystrophies rarely show decreased vision in childhood. This contrasts with endothelial dystrophies [congenital hereditary endothelial dystrophy (CHED) and posterior polymorphous endothelial dystrophy (PPMD)], which can significantly interfere with normal vision (*see* Chapter 68).

K. For lens abnormalities, *see* Chapters 69 and 70.

L. Retinal detachments may occur in high myopia, retinopathy of prematurity, and some vitreoretinal dystrophies and dysplasias, among others. Also consider trauma, including child abuse.

M. Retinal dystrophies rarely present with reduced vision as a primary complaint. More commonly, night vision, peripheral vision and color perception may be disturbed. Relatively few neurometabolic disorders affecting both brain and eyes first present with reduced vision as a primary complaint.

N. Macular dystrophies (e.g. Best vitelliform dystrophy, Stargardt disease) often present with vision loss. Particularly in Stargardt disease, the early retinal changes may be so subtle that they are overlooked and the patient may be considered 'functionally' blind.

O,R. Leukemia may cause retinal hemorrhages, white patches and even infarctions. It can also infiltrate the optic nerve, resulting in a picture difficult to separate from papilledema from other causes.

P. Dominant optic atrophy has its onset usually around 10 years of age. Leber disease is more commonly found in young adulthood. The latter is preponderantly seen in young men and is the result of mitochondrial inheritance, possibly combined with an external factor. Several autosomal-recessive syndromes are characterized by optic atrophy. An example is DIDMOAD or Wolfram syndrome, combining optic atrophy with diabetes mellitus and diabetes insipidus. Deafness may also occur.

Q. Optic neuritis presents with profound and acute vision loss. The picture can be dramatic. There is an afferent pupillary defect, and the optic disk is swollen. If it is not, retrobulbar optic neuritis may be present. Computed tomography or magnetic resonance imaging scans and cerebrospinal fluid studies should clarify the diagnosis. The visually evoked response is most helpful. Both the visual and systemic prognoses are good; most children with this disorder have good visual recovery and no neurological sequelae.

S. Reduced vision resulting from a conversion disorder (this term is considered preferable to hysterical blindness) is a diagnosis of exclusion. If all testing is negative, this possibility can be entertained. Children with this problem may have some social difficulties (at home or at school) but are generally normal without evidence for psychiatric disease. The prognosis is excellent: Münchausen syndrome and clear malingering are rare in children. An exception is seen in kids, who want glasses because they consider them 'cool' or a friend was given glasses. Several tests are available for the diagnosis of conversion disorder. Most are based on making the child believe that he or she is using the 'good' eye, whereas in reality the 'bad' one is being used.

T. Neurometabolic disorders often show eye abnormalities, but the systemic findings overshadow the visual ones. Exceptions are juvenile Batten disease, juvenile metachromatic leukodystrophy, adrenoleukodystrophy, and sialidosis type 1, in which at least initially reduced vision is the major symptom.

BIBLIOGRAPHY

1. Droste PJ, Archer SM, Helveston EM. Measurement of low vision in children and infants. Ophthalmology. 1991;98:1513-8.
2. Good VD. Non-organic visual disorders. In: Taylor D, Hoyt CS (Eds). Pediatric Ophthalmology, 3rd Edition. Elsevier, Saunders; 2005. pp. 687-93.
3. Kerrison JB, Howell N, Miller NR, et al. Leber hereditary optic neuropathy. Electron microscopy and molecular genetic analysis of a case. Ophthalmology. 1995;102:1509-16.
4. McDonald MA. Assessment of visual acuity in toddlers. Surv Ophthalmol. 1986;31:189-210.
5. Repka MX, Miller NR. Optic atrophy in children. Am J Ophthalmol. 1988;106:191-3.

Nasolacrimal Duct Obstruction in Children

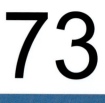

Johan Zwaan

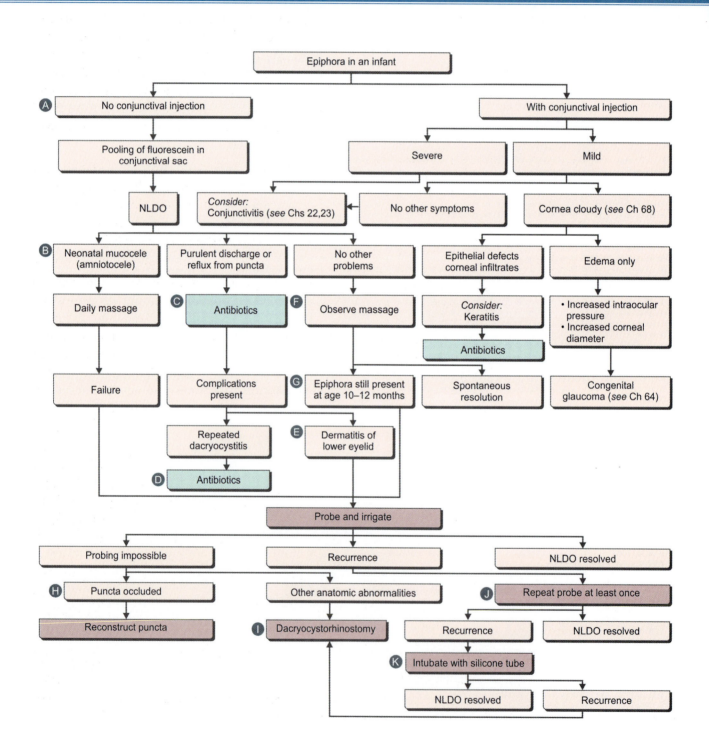

Nasolacrimal duct obstruction (NLDO) is present in about 5% of newborn infants. Tear production is not fully developed at birth, and epiphora may not be obvious until the child is a few weeks old. NLDO results from a blockage anywhere in the nasolacrimal drainage system, which may be caused by an incomplete opening of the duct between the inner canthus and the inferior turbinate of the nasal cavity or, rarely, by the absence of parts of the system. In most patients, it results from an obstruction at the lower end of the nasolacrimal duct, where the duct joins the nasal mucosa at the valve of Hasner. The infant presents with an overflow of tears, and the eye looks wet. A variable amount of mucopurulent discharge may be present. Although the diagnosis should be self-evident, it is commonly mistaken for conjunctivitis, particularly by non-ophthalmologists, even though the conjunctiva is usually quiet. Rare causes of epiphora, such as congenital glaucoma, must be excluded.

A. Clinical signs are usually enough to make the diagnosis of NLDO, but it may be helpful to test the lacrimal drainage by instilling fluorescein in the conjunctival sac. If the yellow solution does not clear from the eye in a few minutes or if the clearance lags considerably behind that of the fellow eye, a complete or partial NLDO is present. A formal Jones test (*see* Chapter 17) is not practical in children. There is usually no need to perform sophisticated diagnostic work-up such as dacryoscintigraphy.

B. Occasionally, a newborn has a bluish swelling in the area of the nasolacrimal sac. Kinking of the canaliculi prevents backflow from the sac, and a clear mucoid fluid accumulates. This mucocele, also called *congenital dacryocystocele* or *amniotocele* should not be mistaken for a hemangioma or a midline encephalocele. Sometimes, the mucocele drains spontaneously or after massage, but if drainage does not occur within a few days, do a probing to prevent secondary infection. If such an infection occurs, hospitalization for treatment with systemic antibiotics is usually necessary to control the dacryocystitis and the commonly associated preseptal cellulitis.

C. If evidence for infection is present, initiate proper antibiotic treatment. Currently, the author prefers to use polytrim drops, three times daily for 5 days. This can be repeated as needed. Some ophthalmologists prefer to use an antibiotic chronically.

D. If the tear sac becomes infected, the resulting abscess may drain through the skin or the infection may spread, causing a cellulitis of the periorbita. Systemic and topical antibiotics are required. Probing can be performed after the infectious process has quieted down. To prevent fistula formation, avoid surgical drainage by a stab incision through the skin or through the inferonasal conjunctival cul-de-sac deep to the canaliculi.

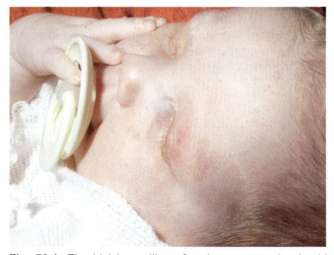

Fig. 73.1: The bluish swelling of a dacryocystocele should not be confused with an anterior encephalocele or a capillary hemangioma.

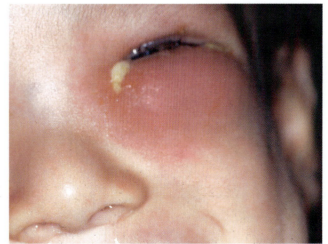

Fig. 73.2: Dacryocystitis with purulent discharge and lower eyelid cellulitis.

E. Chronic wetness of the lower eyelid and toxic effects of mucopurulent discharge can cause dermatitis of the lid, which is very irritating (a 'diaper rash' of the eyelid). A barrier cream or even simple vaseline on the lid to protect the skin may be helpful. If the rash is severe, early probing is indicated.

F. Although some physicians probe all infants with NLDO early, the author prefers to wait because ≥ 90% of the obstructions resolve spontaneously by the age of 1 year. Massage of the nasolacrimal sac helps decompress it and reduce the amount of discharge. Massage can be curative when the distal obstruction 'pops' as the contents of the sac are driven through the duct.

G. If NLDO is still present at age 10–12 months, it will probably not clear on its own. The disadvantage of waiting is that probing requires general anesthesia in the older child. An infant < 6 months can be mummified, and probing can be done safely in the office under topical anesthesia. Nevertheless, the high spontaneous resolution rate justifies being patient and thereby saving most infants from an unnecessary procedure. Of course, this reasoning applies only, if the NLDO is uncomplicated.

H. Rarely, other anatomic abnormalities cause epiphora. Occluding puncta can be opened by rupturing the occluded membrane or by snipping the tissues between the distal end of the canaliculus and the cul-de-sac. It may be possible to intubate the canaliculi retrograde from a dacryocystotomy incision. Usually, a conjunctivo-dacryocystorhinostomy (DCR) becomes necessary if parts of the nasolacrimal drainage system are missing.

I. Well-done probings are almost always successful in infants with NLDO. Patients requiring a DCR should be the exception rather than the rule.

J. If the first probing does not work, one or two repetitions are called for. The repeat procedure is sometimes combined with fracturing of the inferior turbinate, as it may block the lower opening of the nasolacrimal duct. I have not found this to be useful. There is little evidence that the use of balloon catheter dilation is more successful than standard probing and it adds significant cost to the procedure.

K. Silicone tubes of different design are available for mono- or bicanalicular use.

BIBLIOGRAPHY

1. Becker BB, Berry FD, Koller H. Balloon catheter dilatation for treatment of congenital nasolacrimal duct obstruction. Am J Ophthalmol. 1996;124:304-9.
2. Faget B, Katowitz WR, Racy E, et al. Pushed monocular intubation: an alternative stenting system for the management of congenital nasolacrimal duct obstructions. JAAPOS. 2012;16:468-72.
3. Mansour AM, Cheng KP, Mumma JV, et al. Congenital dacryocele: a collaborative review. Ophthalmology. 1991;98:1744-51.
4. Robb RM. Probing and irrigation for congenital nasolacrimal duct obstruction. Arch Ophthalmol. 1986;104:378-9.
5. Zwaan J. The anatomy of probing and irrigation for congenital nasolacrimal duct obstruction. Ophthalmic Surg Lasers. 1997;28:71-3.
6. Zwaan J. Treatment of congenital nasolacrimal duct obstruction before and after the age one year. Ophthalmic Surg Lasers. 1997;28:932-6.

SECTION 4

Corneal Disorders

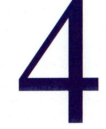

Punctate Corneal Staining

74

Lisa Vogel, Daniel A Johnson

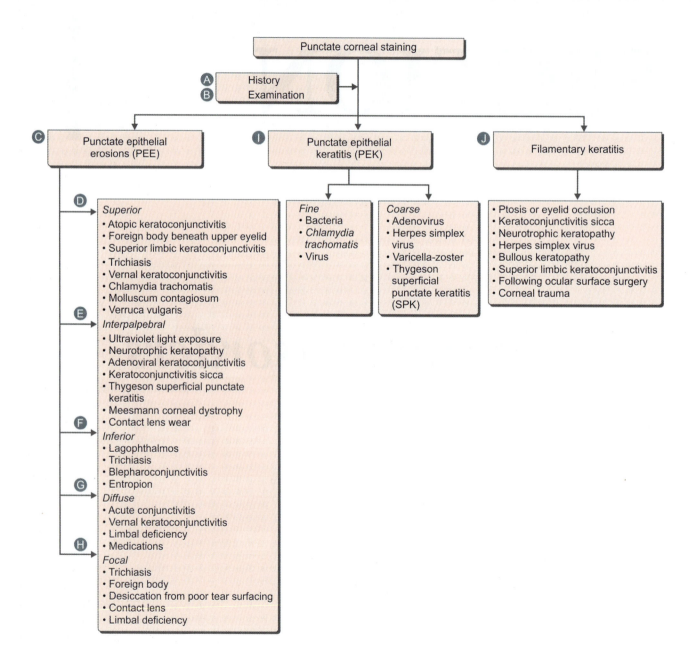

A. Vital dye staining of the cornea with fluorescein, rose bengal, or lissamine green is useful to identify the presence of ocular surface epithelial damage. To identify the cause of the staining, it is necessary to elicit a detailed history including severity, onset, and modifying factors. Past history, including past medical history, use of medications (particularly ophthalmic), use of contact lenses, ocular surgeries, and ocular trauma should be obtained. Ophthalmic medications and over-the-counter eyedrops may contain preservatives that are harmful to the corneal epithelium, whereas other medications may have side effects such as reduced tear production that can damage the cornea.

B. An examination of the eyelids and periocular area should be performed to determine the presence of rosacea or other forms of dermatitis, molluscum lesions, trichiasis, distichiasis, ptosis, ectropion, entropion, or lid retraction, all of which predispose to corneal staining. Raised lesions on the bulbar conjunctiva such as pterygia, pingueculae, or conjunctival tumors may cause focal desiccation of the cornea. Conjunctival follicles, or lymphoid aggregates, suggest a chemical or microbial cause of the corneal staining. Papillae, which are focal dilated conjunctival vessels associated with edema and inflammatory cells, are a nonspecific sign of inflammation most often from a bacterial, allergic, toxic, or mechanical cause.

Vital staining abnormalities can range from miniscule punctate lesions to large areas encompassing multiple regions of the cornea. Slit lamp examination is necessary to differentiate between the entities that display punctate staining: punctate epithelial erosions (PEE) and punctate epithelial keratitis (PEK). The location and characteristics of the lesions often suggest a specific disease process and can facilitate making a diagnosis.

C. Punctate epithelial erosions (Fig. 74.1) are focal areas of disruption of the junctions between epithelial cells. They are visualized as small green dots on slit lamp examination when stained with fluorescein and viewed with cobalt blue illumination. These lesions are restricted to the epithelial surface, and may be indiscernible without vital dye staining. The patient may have signs and symptoms including lacrimation, photophobia, reactive blepharospasm, and foreign body sensation; however, the patient may be asymptomatic. The pattern of punctate staining aids in the differential diagnosis.

D. Punctate erosions of the superior cornea suggest conditions affecting the upper eyelid or conjunctiva. These conditions include superior limbic keratoconjunctivitis (SLK), atopic and vernal

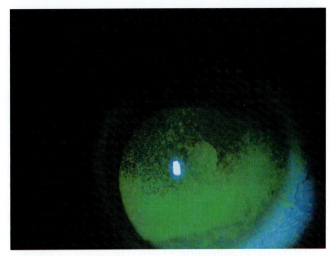

Fig. 74.1: Confluent punctate epithelial erosions on the interpalpebral cornea from keratoconjunctivitis sicca.

keratoconjunctivitis, and ocular infection with *Chlamydia trachomatis*, *Molluscum contagiosum*, or *Verruca vulgaris*. Trichiasis from an upper eyelid lash and a foreign body retained beneath the upper eyelid can produce punctate erosions superiorly, especially if focal.

E. Central or interpalpebral erosions are common manifestations of contact lens overwear, ultraviolet (UV) light damage, keratoconjunctivitis sicca/dry eye, neurotrophic keratopathy, and early adenoviral conjunctivitis. Thygeson superficial punctate keratitis (SPK) may have either fine central PEE or coarse PEK. Meesmann corneal dystrophy, with surface irregularities and epithelial cysts, should also be considered. Boaters and skiers who do not wear adequate eye protection may present with interpalpebral erosions due to epithelial cell damage from UV light reflected from water or snow, respectively. A similar process affects welders that do not wear adequate eye protection.

F. Punctate erosions on the inferior cornea suggest disorders that prevent normal eyelid closure and hinder surfacing of the tears. Lagophthalmos is seen not only in anatomical lid abnormalities but also in neurogenic processes such as Parkinson disease or Bell palsy. Additional causes of inferior corneal staining include blepharoconjunctivitis, trichiasis, and entropion.

G. Diffuse punctate erosions are most often caused by toxicity or prolonged use of topical medications, such as antibiotics, antiviral agents, cycloplegics, glaucoma medications, ophthalmic solutions with preservatives, and systemic chemotherapeutic agents. Even lubricant eyedrops used for dry eyes can produce diffuse staining if they contain preservatives and are used in excess. Vernal keratoconjunctivitis and early bacterial or viral conjunctivitis also produce a generalized pattern of erosions. Limbal stem cell deficiency, which leads to conjunctivalization of the cornea, chronic inflammation, vascularization, and destruction of epithelial integrity may show signs of corneal irregularity and diffuse PEE.

H. Focal erosions are suspicious for mechanical trauma from a foreign body or from trichiasis. Linear, vertically oriented erosions suggest a foreign body retained beneath the upper eyelid with the linear defects caused by the blinking action of the eyelid. Focal erosions at the limbus may be associated with corneal intraepithelial neoplasia (CIN) or corneal desiccation adjacent to areas of elevated conjunctiva as can be seen with pinguecula, pterygia, conjunctival tumors, and following conjunctival surgery. Such areas of conjunctival elevation hinder the normal surfacing of the tears that produces the associated corneal staining. Staining at 3:00 and 9:00 may be seen with contact lens wear.

I. Punctate epithelial keratitis (PEK) is characterized by raised abnormal epithelial cells surrounded by an inflammatory infiltrate. These abnormal cells appear as gray-white lesions that stain with both fluorescein and rose bengal. The appearance of the lesions, whether fine or course, has diagnostic significance. The differential diagnosis of fine PEK includes conjunctivitis with bacteria, including *Chlamydia trachomatis,* and some viruses. The differential diagnosis of coarse PEK includes adenovirus, herpes simplex, varicella-zoster, and Thygeson SPK.

J. Filamentary keratitis (Fig. 74.2) is a nonspecific finding that results from small, filamentary deposits of epithelial cells and mucous attached to the corneal epithelium by one end. Symptoms include foreign body sensation, photophobia, and increased blinking. Filaments may be characterized by number, location, and chronicity and stain with

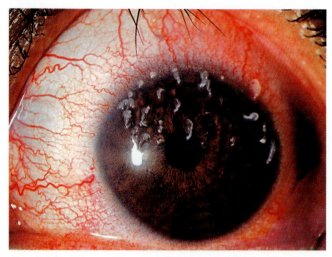

Fig. 74.2: Filamentary keratitis in a patient with kerato-conjunctivitis sicca and floppy eyelid syndrome.

both rose bengal and fluorescein. They may be temporary after patching or surgery, or chronic and recurrent after conditions such as dry eye, neurotrophic keratopathy, bullous keratopathy, and superior limbic keratoconjunctivitis (SLK). SLK causes PEE and occasional corneal filaments on the superior cornea. It is associated with hyperemia of the superior bulbar conjunctiva, papillary hypertrophy of the superior tarsal conjunctiva, keratinization of the superior limbal conjunctiva, and micropannus. The association between SLK and thyroid dysfunction requires thyroid evaluation in patients diagnosed with SLK.

BIBLIOGRAPHY

1. Arffa R (Ed). Grayson's Diseases of the Cornea, 4th Edition. St Louis, MO: Mosby; 1997. pp. 44-8, 196-7.
2. Burman S, Sangwan V. Cultivated limbal stem cell transplantation for ocular surface reconstruction. Clin Ophthalmol. 2008; 2:489-502.
3. Coster D. Superficial Keratopathy. Duane's Ophthalmology. CD-ROM. Lippincott Williams and Wilkins; 2006.
4. Gumus K, Lee S, Yen MT, et al. Botulinum toxin injection for the management of refractory filamentary keratitis. Arch Ophthalmol. 2012; 130:446-50.
5. Krachmer JH, Mannis MJ, Holland EJ (Eds). Cornea, 2nd Edition. Philadelphia, PA: Mosby; 2005. pp. 229-32, 526.
6. Pettit TH, Meyer KT. The differential diagnosis of superficial punctate keratitis. Int Ophthalmol Clin. 1984;24:79-92.
7. Roy FH, Fraunfelder FW, Fraunfelder FT. Roy and Fraunfelder's Current Ocular Therapy, 6th Edition. China: Saunders Elsevier; 2008. p. 434.
8. Yanoff M, Duker JS. Ophthalmology, 3rd Edition. China: Mosby; 2009. p. 291.

75

Corneal Dendritic Lesions

Brian P Schallenberg, Daniel A Johnson

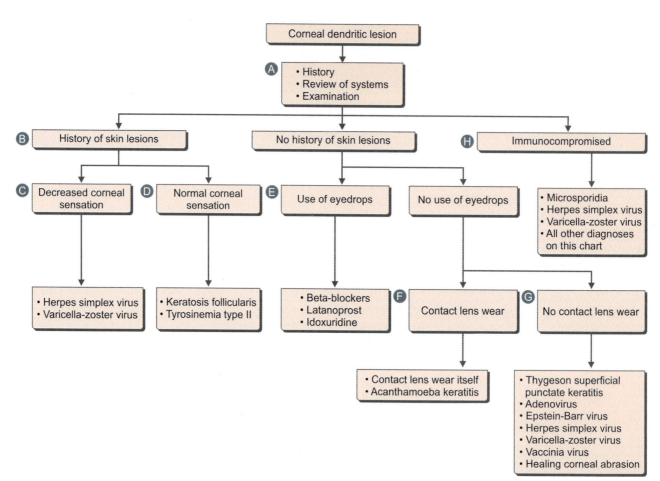

Adapted from: Shields CK, Yee RW. Corneal dendritic lesions. In: van Heuven WAJ, Zwaan J (Eds). Decision Making in Ophthalmology, 1st edition.

A. Corneal dendritic lesions are areas of abnormal corneal epithelium in a branching pattern. While epithelial keratitis from herpetic disease is the classic cause of these lesions, the differential diagnosis is extensive. This differential diagnosis can be narrowed by the history and physical exam. Any history of dermatologic disease, ocular trauma, ocular surgery, medications, and contact lens use should be elicited.

B. Concurrent or prior dermatologic disease suggests either the classic cause of herpetic disease or the uncommon disorders of keratosis follicularis (Darier disease) or tyrosinemia type II.

C. Both herpes simplex virus (HSV) and varicella-zoster virus (VZV) are capable of forming corneal dendritic lesions; however, they are usually distinguishable by their clinical appearance and the associated cutaneous involvement. Dendrites of HSV stain (Fig. 75.1) with both fluorescein (along the ulcerations that run the length of the branches) and rose bengal (along the outer walls of the branches) and contain terminal bulbs. The

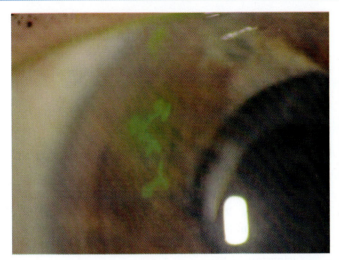

Fig. 75.1: Herpes simplex virus. Note the presence of terminal bulbs.

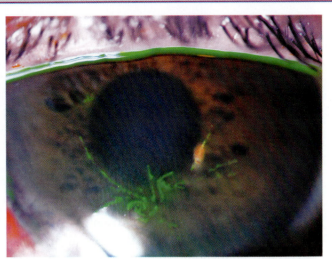

Fig. 75.2: Varicella-zoster virus. Note absence of the terminal bulbs.

term *dendrite* is used classically in reference to the lesions caused by HSV, whereas *pseudodendrite* is used for corneal dendritic lesions from other causes. Pseudodendrites in herpes-zoster ophthalmicus (HZO) (Fig. 75.2), caused by the reactivation of VZV, stain poorly with fluorescein (since there is no central ulceration), stain intensely with rose bengal, and do not have terminal bulbs. In addition, those of HZV are more stellate in appearance. Both disorders can produce corneal anesthesia and a vesicular rash; however, not all patients will have a history or evidence of cutaneous involvement. In HSV, the distribution of the rash is not dermatomal, the vesicles generally heal without scarring, and postherpetic neuralgia and postherpetic itch do not occur. In HZO, the rash involves the V1 dermatome of the trigeminal nerve, the vesicles may produce scarring, and postherpetic neuralgia and postherpetic itch are common. Generally, ocular involvement with VZV is more common when cutaneous involvement affects the side of the tip of the nose, also known as "Hutchinson sign."

D. Keratosis follicularis, also known as Darier or Darier—White disease is a rare autosomal-dominant disorder of keratinization with high penetrance and variable expressivity. It is caused by abnormalities of the *ATP2A2* gene on chromosome $12q^{23}$-$q^{24.1}$ encoding a calcium pump, abnormalities of which can lead to faulty intercellular desomosomes. The cutaneous lesions appear as yellow-brown or skin-colored greasy, scaly papules on the forehead, scalp line, sides of the nose, behind the ears, chest, neck, and back. Mucous membrane and nail changes may occur. Corneal involvement with keratosis follicularis includes peripheral corneal opacities, Salzmann-like nodules, and central irregular epithelium.

Tyrosinemia type II, also known as Richner-Hanhart syndrome, is an autosomal-recessive defect in tyrosine aminotransferase, encoded by a gene on chromosome 16q22.1-q22.3, which leads to elevated levels of tyrosine in the urine and blood. The cutaneous involvement is notable for hyperkeratotic lesions. The corneal dendritic lesions do not stain well with fluorescein or rose bengal and can be associated with recurrent erosions, corneal scarring, and neovascularization.

E. Medications reported to cause dendritic lesions include topical beta-blockers, latanoprost, and idoxuridine. The lesions resolve upon discontinuing the offending medication.

F. Dendritic lesions associated with contact lens include contact lens wear itself, and infection with *Acanthamoeba*. Soft contact lens wear has been reported to cause mid-peripheral dendritic lesions with patchy fluorescein staining and no terminal bulbs. These resolve upon discontinuation of contact lens wear and have been suggested to be immunologically mediated. Similarly, corneal infection with *Acanthamoeba* can produce corneal dendritic lesions that have been misdiagnosed as HSV keratitis. Dendritic lesions from *Acanthamoeba* may have associated stromal inflammation but do not have terminal bulbs.

G. Additional disorders that can produce corneal dendritic lesions include Thygeson superficial punctate keratitis (TSPK), adenovirus, Epstein-Barr virus, and healing corneal epithelial defects. TSPK is an epithelial process of unknown etiology characterized by recurrent episodes of ocular surface irritation. The process is usually bilateral but can be asymmetric. Examination reveals irregular corneal epithelium and associated superficial stromal inflammatory cells but no significant conjunctival reaction. The epithelial lesions are raised and may have a stellate appearance. Viral processes reported to cause corneal dendritic processes include Epstein-Barr virus, adenovirus, and Vaccinia virus. The epithelial ridge of a healing epithelial defect may have a dentritiform appearance with patchy staining but no terminal bulbs.

H. Microsporidia is an intracellular protozoan known to cause stromal keratitis in immunocompetent individuals and an epithelial keratitis that can appear dendritic in patients who are immunocompromised. Risk factors include travel to the tropics and contact with birds and cats. Light microscopy may identify the gram-positive intraepithelial spores; however, transmission electron microscopy and polymerase chain reaction studies are potentially more sensitive and specific. Electron microscopy should reveal polar tubules that are coiled, a characteristic that distinguishes them from other protozoa. Polymerase chain reaction will likely identify the microsporidia species as *Vittaforma corneae* in patients with keratitis.

▌BIBLIOGRAPHY

1. Arffa RC, Grayson M. Grayson's Diseases of the Cornea, 4th Edition. St Louis, MA: Mosby; 1997.
2. Berger CA, White CR. Exudative papulosquamous diseases. In: Sams WM Jr, Lynch PJ (Eds). Principles and Practice of Dermatology. New York: Churchill Livingstone; 1996.
3. Hamrah P, Cruzat A, Dastjerdi MH, et al. Unilateral herpes zoster ophthalmicus results in bilateral corneal nerve alteration. Ophthalmology. 2013;120:40-7.
4. Kaufman HE, Rayfield MA, Gebhardt BM. Herpes simplex viral infections. In: Kaufman HE, Barron BA, McDonald MB (Eds). The Cornea, 2nd Edition. Boston, MA: Butterworth-Heinemann; 1998. pp. 247-78.
5. Krachmer JH, Mannis MJ, Holland EJ. Cornea, 3rd Edition (Vol. 2). Philadelphia, PA: Elsevier; 2011.
6. Margulies LJ, Mannis MJ. Dendritic lesions associated with soft contact lens wear. Arch Ophthalmol. 1983;101:1551-3.
7. Pavan-Langston D. Viral disease of the cornea and external eye. In: Albert DM, Miller J, Azar D, Blodi B (Eds). Albert and Jakobiec's Principles and Practice of Ophthalmology, 3rd Edition. Philadelphia, PA: Elsevier/Saunders; 2008. pp. 681-2.
8. Reddy AK, Balne PK, Gaje K, et al. PCR for the diagnosis and species identification of microsporidia in patients with keratitis. Clin Microbiol Infect. 2011;17:476-8.

Marginal Corneal Ulcer

76

Anhtuan H Nguyen, Kent L Anderson

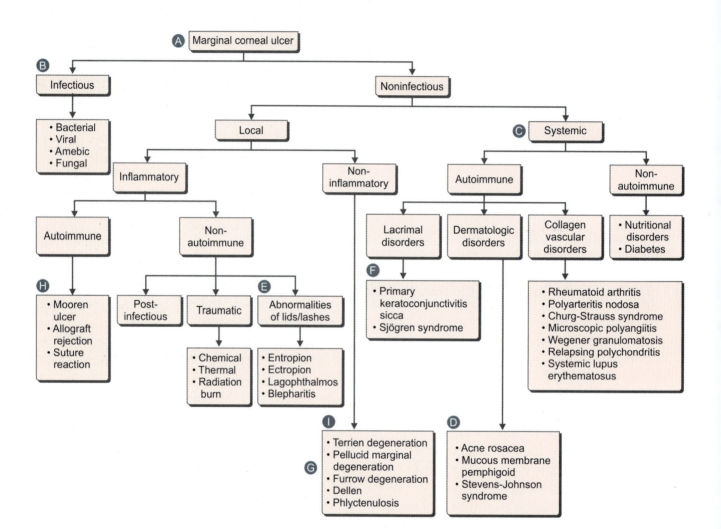

INTRODUCTION

Marginal corneal ulcers may form as a result of infection, peripheral ulcerative keratitis (PUK), which may be associated with systemic disease, local insults, and other idiopathic etiologies. Patients present with ocular redness, pain, tearing, photophobia, and in advanced cases, decreased vision. Examination shows corneal opacity and variable depth of peripheral corneal thinning. Severe cases may present with corneal perforation. Adjacent conjunctiva, episclera, and sclera may be inflamed.

Initial Management

A. Evaluation consists of history, physical examination, and systemic assessment. If infection is suspected, obtain special staining, perform culture with confocal microscopy if suspicious for fungal or parasitic infection, and initiate fortified antibiotics for gram-positive coverage and the fourth-generation fluoroquinolone for gram-negative coverage. If associated systemic disease is suspected, test for rapid plasma reagin, antinuclear antibodies, rheumatoid factor, anti-citrullinated protein antibodies, erythrocyte sedimentation rate, anti-SSA and anti-SSB autoantibodies, and complete blood count. A bandage soft contact lens should not be used for infectious etiology. Preservative-free lubricating agents should be initiated to promote removal of inflammatory proteins and mediators on the ocular surface. If there is significant thinning or perforation, corneal gluing with cyanoacrylate glue should be attempted. Surgical therapy includes amniotic membrane transplantation, conjunctival flap, and keratoplasty.

Infectious Etiologies

B. If an organism is identified, treat accordingly. If confocal microscopy results and scrapings are negative and there is no clinical improvement from empiric treatment, polymerase chain reaction (PCR) studies for viral etiology and corneal biopsy are indicated. Topical steroids may be used to help decrease the inflammatory response, if there is confirmation of microorganism eradication.

Manifestations of Systemic Disease

C. There are many systemic diseases that are associated with PUK. PUK may occur at any point during the course of the disease or may be the presenting manifestation. Along with PUK, systemic diseases are also associated with other ocular manifestations such as conjunctivitis, episcleritis, scleritis, and uveitis. Rheumatoid arthritis (RA) is the most common systemic disease associated with PUK, which tends to occur late in the disease course. RA with PUK is considered as a life-threatening disease that is associated with high mortality rate. PUK is commonly the presenting sign of Wegener granulomatosis, which has systemic manifestations, including respiratory symptoms, urinary tract involvement, and arthritis. Antineutrophil cytoplasmic antibody (ANCA) has a 99% sensitivity in patients with systemic disease. Relapsing polychondritis, diagnosed based on

history and findings of chondritis of the ears, nose, and larynx, has a prevalence of PUK of less than 10%. PUK seen in systemic lupus erythematosus is commonly secondary to keratoconjunctivitis sicca (KS). PUK associated with systemic disease is life threatening. Current management involves systemic corticosteroids with a cytotoxic agent during the active phase of the disease. Topical corticosteroids are not recommended in the setting of systemic disease because there is a risk of increase in corneal perforation from inhibition of collagen production. Specifically, initial treatment for RA with PUK is systemic corticosteroids and methotrexate. Wegener granulomatosis and polyarteritis nodosa, which are rapidly progressive life-threatening diseases, are initially treated with systemic corticosteroids and cyclophosphamide. In Wegener granulomatosis, response to therapy is reflected in cANCA level. In addition, resection of local perilimbal conjunctiva debulks the area of antibody-antigen complexes. Lubrication with preservative-free methylcellulose may help epithelial healing.

D. Rosacea with peripheral corneal neovascularization may lead to corneal ulceration and perforation, if left untreated. Therapy is based on severity of ocular involvement. With presence of ulceration, topical corticosteroids or cyclosporine may be beneficial along with oral doxycycline and lid hygiene.

Ocular manifestations of Stevens-Johnson syndrome and toxic epidermal necrolysis are characterized by inflammation of the entire ocular surface during the acute phase and keratinization in the chronic phase. Focus of acute management is to reduce inflammation and minimize symblepharon, keratinization, lid distortion, and corneal ulceration. Therapy involves frequent topical lubrication, topical corticosteroids, antibiotic drops, and sweeping of the fornices for symblepharon lysis and removal of membranes. Amniotic membrane transplantation over entire ocular surface may help to prevent complications.

Mucous membrane pemphigoid is a chronic subepithelial blistering disease that affects ocular, oropharyngeal, and anogenital mucous membranes and skin with progressive scar formation. Ocular manifestations include conjunctivitis, trichiasis, ankyloblepharon, and symblepharon. Corneal neovascularization, conjunctivalization, and opacification may cause severe vision loss. Tissue biopsy shows linear deposition of immunoreactants to heterogeneous antigens in the epithelial basement membrane zone. Negative biopsy cannot rule out diagnosis, so therapy should be initiated as long as biopsy has ruled out other disorders. Systemic immunotherapy with mycophenolate mofetil may control the inflammatory disease process. Surgical interventions may be required to correct ocular manifestations.

Local Insults

E. Correct eyelid and eyelash abnormalities to prevent deterioration of ocular surface integrity. Temporary tarsorrhaphy may assist healing. Chemical injuries require immediate copious irrigation. Use tear pH measurements to confirm clearance of irritant. Blepharitis may cause peripheral corneal inflammation and corneal thinning at the 2, 4, 8, and 10 o'clock positions. Treat with warm compress and topical antibiotics. Sutures or foreign bodies may cause corneal inflammation. Removal is curative.

F. KS has numerous etiologies including idiopathic, drug-induced tear hyposecretion, Sjögren syndrome, and collagen vascular diseases. Graft-versus-host disease (GVHD), associated with bone marrow transplantation, may have lacrimal gland failure, lymphocytic conjunctival infiltration, and goblet cell depletion. GVHD may benefit from systemic tacrolimus. Treat underlying condition and symptomatic therapy based on severity with lubricants, punctual occlusion, secretagogues, and topical and/or systemic anti-inflammatory agents (cyclosporine, corticosteroids, and tetracyclines).

Corneal graft rejection, characterized by keratic precipitates, an endothelial rejection line, stromal or epithelial edema with or without infiltrates, and anterior segment inflammatory signs, requires prompt aggressive management. Therapy consists of topical and systemic immune suppressions with corticosteroid and tacrolimus.

Symblepharon and corneal scarring require vigorous lubrication and mechanical treatment.

G. Phlyctenulosis is a small, white, painful nodule at the limbus with dilated conjunctival vessels. Often bilateral, it migrates centrally and may produce neovascularization. Topical corticosteroids, hygiene, and antibiotic ointments suppress this delayed hypersensitivity reaction to *Staphylococcus* antigen. Localized tuberculosis infection may also cause phlyctenulosis. Rare localized tuberculosis infection may present with phlyctenulosis. Positive tuberculin skin test or quantiferon gold and/or isolation of mycobacterial deoxyribonucleic acid from ocular fluids or tissue using PCR may contribute to diagnosis. The gold standard to establish the diagnosis is a positive culture from ocular tissue. Treatment involves standard tuberculosis therapy.

Idiopathic Etiologies

H. Mooren ulcer is painful and may be bilateral. It is characterized by an aggressive, grayish, overhanging advancing edge of an epithelial and stromal defect with vascularization of the ulcer base. Circumferential corneal involvement is observed in severe cases. Medical therapy is based on severity. Topical corticosteroids are successful in unilateral cases and with less than two quadrants of peripheral corneal involvement. More severe cases require oral and intravenous immune suppression with corticosteroids and immunomodulators (e.g. methotrextate). Conjunctival excision and superficial keratectomy may arrest progression.

I. Terrien marginal degeneration—a bilateral degeneration of the superior peripheral cornea, may show superficial vascularization with lipid deposits at the leading edge. Visual acuity will decrease as disease progresses. Corneal perforation is managed with keratoplasty.

Pellucid marginal degeneration is a nonvascularized, noninfiltrative inferior band of corneal thinning located 1–2 mm from the limbus. Corneal topography is utilized for early detection and to assess severity. Visual acuity deteriorates as condition progress. Visual acuity may be improved by nonsurgical methods (soft lenses, rigid gas permeable contact lenses, and other specialized lenses) and surgical methods (keratoplasty, intraocular lens, and collagen cross-linking). Acute complications include corneal hydrops and perforation.

Furrow degeneration is found peripheral to arcus senilis in elderly patients. No epithelial defect is present. This benign degeneration generally does not require treatment.

Dellen is corneal thinning at the limbus adjacent to a surface elevation, which creates poor spreading of the tear film with stromal desiccation under an intact epithelium. Lubrication and pressure patching will cure the defect.

BIBLIOGRAPHY

1. Amescua G, Miller D, Alfonso EC. What is causing the corneal ulcer? Management strategies for unresponsive corneal ulceration. Eye. 2012;26:228-36.
2. Ashar JN, Mathur A, Sangwan VS. Immunosuppression for Mooren's ulcer: evaluation of the stepladder approach—Topical, oral and intravenous immuno-suppressive agents. Br J Ophthalmol. 2013;97:1391-4.
3. Hsu M, Jayaram A, Verner R, et al. Indications and outcomes of amniotic membrane transplantation in the management of acute Stevens-Johnson syndrome and toxic epidermal necrolysis: a case-control study. Cornea. 2012;31:1394-402.
4. Jinabhai A, Radhakrishnan H, O'Donnell C. Pellucid corneal marginal degeneration: a review. Cont Lens Anterior Eye. 2011;34:56-63.
5. Ladas JG, Mondino BJ. Systemic disorders associated with peripheral corneal ulceration. Curr Opin Ophthalmol. 2000;11:468-71.
6. Moscovici BK, Holzchuh R, Chiacchio BB, et al. Clinical treatment of dry eye using 0.03% tacrolimus eye drops. Cornea. 2012;31:945-9.
7. Pflugfelder SC, Geerling G, Kinoshita S, et al. Management and therapy of dry eye disease: report of the Management and Therapy Subcommittee of the International Dry Eye Workshop (2007). Ocul Surf. 2007;5:163-78.
8. Srikumaran D, Akpek EK. Mucous membrane pemphigoid: recent advances. Curr Opin Ophthalmol. 2012;23:523-7.
9. Vieira ACC, Hofling-Lima AL, Mannis MJ. Ocular rosacea: a review. Arq Bras Oftalmol. 2012;75:363-9.
10. Wagoner MD, Kenyon KR, Foster CS. Management strategies in peripheral ulcerative keratitis. Int Ophthalmol Clin. 1986;26:147-57.
11. Yagci A. Update on peripheral ulcerative keratitis. Clin Ophthalmol. 2012;6:747-54.
12. Yeh S, Sen HN, Colyer M, et al. Update on ocular tuberculosis. Curr Opin Ophthalmol. 2012:23:551-6.

77

Central Corneal Ulcers

Ekta Kakkar, Kent L Anderson

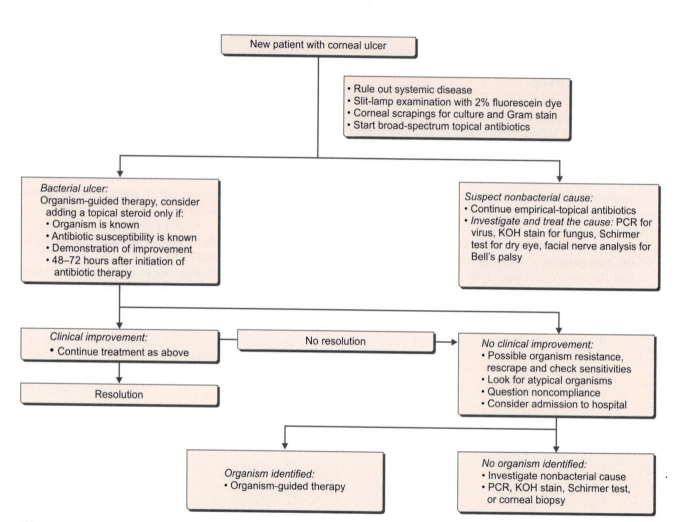

New patient with corneal ulcer

- Rule out systemic disease
- Slit-lamp examination with 2% fluorescein dye
- Corneal scrapings for culture and Gram stain
- Start broad-spectrum topical antibiotics

Bacterial ulcer:
Organism-guided therapy, consider adding a topical steroid only if:
- Organism is known
- Antibiotic susceptibility is known
- Demonstration of improvement
- 48–72 hours after initiation of antibiotic therapy

Suspect nonbacterial cause:
- Continue empirical-topical antibiotics
- *Investigate and treat the cause:* PCR for virus, KOH stain for fungus, Schirmer test for dry eye, facial nerve analysis for Bell's palsy

Clinical improvement:
- Continue treatment as above

No resolution

No clinical improvement:
- Possible organism resistance, rescrape and check sensitivities
- Look for atypical organisms
- Question noncompliance
- Consider admission to hospital

Resolution

Organism identified:
- Organism-guided therapy

No organism identified:
- Investigate nonbacterial cause
- PCR, KOH stain, Schirmer test, or corneal biopsy

Abbreviations: PCR: Polymerase chain reaction; KOH: Potassium hydroxide

The cornea, as the most anterior part of the eye, is exposed to the atmosphere and prone to injury. A corneal ulcer results from an epithelial defect that exposes the stroma to the environment leading to degradation. Superficial epithelial defects are repaired by the migration and division of adjacent epithelial cells, while larger ulcers require inflammatory cells from vessels to produce granulation tissue for healing.

SYMPTOMS

- Pain and foreign body sensation due to chemical effects of the toxins on exposed nerve endings
- Lacrimation
- Photophobia due to stimulation of the nerve endings
- Blurred vision due to corneal haze
- Redness due to congestion of corneal vessels

Table 77.1: Common causes and treatment of infectious keratitis

Type of infectious keratitis	Most common pathogens	Common treatment
• Bacterial (46%)		
– Gram positive (83%)	*Staphylococcus aureus, Staphylococcus epidermidis, Streptococcus pneumoniae*	Topical vancomycin, cefazolin, and/or fourth-generation fluoroquinolone
– Gram negative (17%)	*Pseudomonas spp., Serratia spp., Proteus spp.*	Topical tobramycin, ceftazidime, ceftriaxone, fourth-generation fluoroquinolone, and/or gentamicin
• Viral (28%)	Herpes (e.g. *herpes simplex virus*), varicella, adenovirus	*Herpes simplex virus* (HSV): Acyclovir, valacyclovir, and/or trifluridine
• Fungal (24%)	*Fusarium spp., Aspergillus spp., Fumigatus spp., Candida spp.*	Topical natamycin, amphotericin, and/or voriconazole
• Protozoan (2%)	*Acanthamoeba spp., Microsporidium spp., Onchocerca spp.*	Topical polyhexamethylene biguanide, chlorhexidine, diaminidines, aminoglycosides, and/or antifungal imidazoles/triazoles

Source: The corneal ulcer paper by Amescua et al.

SIGNS

- Swollen eyelids
- Marked blepharospasm
- Conjunctival hyperemia and ciliary congestion
- The ulcer starts as an epithelial defect with a grayish-white infiltrate that enlarges leading to stromal edema
- Pupil may be small due to the associated toxin-induced iritis
- Intraocular pressure may be elevated due to inflammation

CAUSES

Infection with bacteria, virus, fungus, or protozoa may cause a central corneal ulcer (Table 77.1). Noninfectious etiology include keratoconjunctivitis sicca, due to the lack of protective lysozyme and betalysin found in tears, decreased corneal sensation from neurotropic lesions, increased exposure in lagophthalmos or Bell palsy, chemical burns, and contact lens irritation.

DIAGNOSIS

For infectious keratitis, corneal scrapings are taken under topical anesthesia using a sterile instrument. Scrapings are taken from the edges and the base of the ulcer. The samples are microscopically examined using Gram and Giemsa stains, potassium hydroxide (KOH) preparation, and other specific media based on suspicion. Cultures should be grown for at least 7 days before declared negative, and susceptibility testing should be performed to guide therapy.

STAGES OF THE CORNEAL ULCER

- *Progressive infiltration:* Polymorphonuclear cells and lymphocytes infiltrate the corneal epithelium and may eventually lead to necrosis of the involved tissue.
- *Active ulceration:* Hyperemia of the corneal vessels leads to accumulation of purulent exudates. This also causes vascular congestion of the iris and ciliary body and iritis from absorption of toxins from the infection site. Exudate infiltration into the anterior chamber from the vessels of the iris and ciliary body may lead to hypopyon formation. Ulceration may progress further leading to corneal perforation.
- *Regression:* Induced by the host immune response, both humoral and cell mediated, and treatment. Leukocytes neutralize and phagocytose any infecting organism and necrotic cells. Digestion of the necrotic tissue may initially cause an enlargement of the ulcer along with a superficial vascularization that stimulates the host immune response. Normal corneal epithelium will then begin to grow over the edges of the ulcer.
- *Healing:* Corneal fibroblasts and endothelial cells of the new vessels lay granulation tissue underneath the epithelium. This causes thickening of the stroma and pushes the epithelium anteriorly. The degree of scarring may be variable. The ulcer is superficial, if it involves only the epithelial layer, but involvement

of Bowman membrane leads to a resulting scar called a nebula. If the ulcer involves up to one-third of the corneal stroma or more, the scar is called a macula or leukoma.

TREATMENT

Corneal ulcers should be cultured and treated empirically with a topical antibiotic with both gram-positive and gram-negative coverages. Systemic antibiotics are usually not needed but may be used in fulminant cases. Other nonbacterial infectious ulcers should be treated with broad-coverage topical antimicrobials directed at the specific inciting organism. One percent atropine or cyclopentolate drops should also be started to control pain from ciliary spasm and prevent development of posterior synechiae. Vitamins and non-steroidal anti-inflammatory drugs (NSAIDs) may be used to promote healing and anti-inflammatory effects. If the ulcer progresses despite therapy, search for a noninfectious cause. Cauterization or a contact lens may prevent further progression. A corneal biopsy may be needed, if no cause is identified. Penetrating keratoplasty may be performed if the ulcer is refractory to treatment and continues to progress with imminent perforation.

COMPLICATIONS

Ulcer may lead to corneal perforation due to a pressure tear in Descemet membrane or sloughing of the entire corneal epithelium if the offending organism is highly virulent. Toxic iridocyclitis may develop, if the toxins are absorbed into the anterior chamber. Fibrous exudates that block the angle of the anterior chamber may lead to secondary inflammatory glaucoma. Corneal scarring may lead to permanent visual impairment ranging from blurring to total blindness.

FOLLOW-UP

Daily follow-up of patients is recommended until a response to medical treatment is noted. Once there is an improvement in symptoms, the ulcer characteristics, and the anterior chamber reaction, treatment and follow-up may be tapered.

BIBLIOGRAPHY

1. Amescua G, Miller D, Alfonso EC. What is causing the corneal ulcer? Management strategies for unresponsive corneal ulceration. Eye. 2012;26:228-36.
2. Bourcier T, Thomas F, Borderie V, et al. Bacterial keratitis: Predisposing factors, clinical and microbiological review of 300 cases. Br J Ophthalmol. 2003;87:834-8.
3. Garg P, Rao GN. Corneal ulcer: Diagnosis and management. J Comm Eye Health. 1999;12:21-3.
4. Khurana AK. Comprehensive Ophthalmology, 4th Edition. New Delhi: New Age International Ltd, 2007.
5. Nijm LM. Seven clinical pearls for diagnosing and managing challenging corneal ulcers. Young Ophthalmologists (YO) Info. January 2010. Available at *http://www.aao.org/yo/newsletter/201001/article04.cfm*. [Accessed October 2013].

Corneal Endothelial Dystrophies

78

Lindsay T Davis

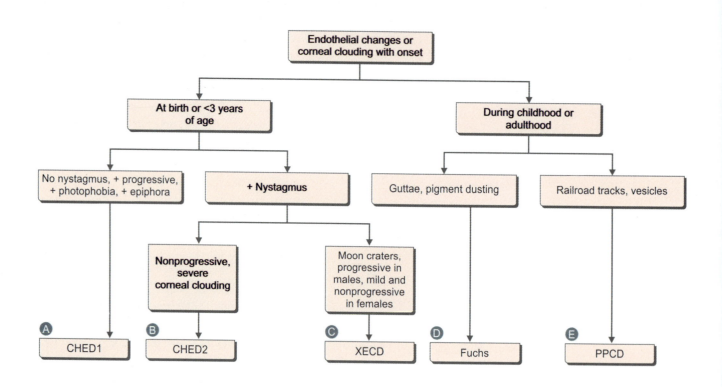

The word *dystrophy* comes from the Greek (*dys* = ill, abnormal and *trophe* = nourishment, growth) and was initially used to describe inherited pathology of muscles. The term corneal dystrophy traditionally implied a hereditary, bilateral, symmetric, and progressive condition. However, as more is known of the genetics, many conditions have proven to be sporadic, as in epithelial basement membrane dystrophy, or unilateral, as in the case of posterior polymorphous dystrophy.

Each dystrophy is categorized in the IC3D classification according to the evidence to support its existence. Category 1 (C1) is a corneal dystrophy with a mapped gene and specific mutations. Category 2 (C2) has been mapped to one or more chromosomal loci, but without identified genes. Category 3 (C3) is a dystrophy that has not been mapped to a locus.

Category 4 (C4) is either a previously documented or suspected new corneal dystrophy without convincing evidence of its existence as a distinct dystrophy.

A. *Congenital hereditary endothelial dystrophy 1 (CHED1) (C2):* This dystrophy is either congenital or begins in the first two years of life, with an autosomal dominant inheritance. Corneal clouding varies from diffuse haze to a milky-gray appearance and is often asymmetric. The cornea may be thickened with rare band keratopathy, causing blurred vision worse in the morning, photophobia, and epiphora. Nystagmus is not seen. Asymptomatic patients can have only peau d'orange endothelial changes with normal vision. Progression of disease occurs over 10 years. Thickening of the stroma and Descemet membrane with atrophic endothelial cells are noted, and keratin may replace parts of the endothelium. Treatment is surgical, by endothelial or penetrating keratoplasty.

B. *Congenital hereditary endothelial dystrophy 2 (CHED2) (C1):* Cases are autosomal recessive, noted at birth and stationary. Cases are often asymmetric, as in CHED1, but CHED2 is typically more common, with more severe corneal clouding, a more thickened cornea, rare band keratopathy, and possible intraocular pressure (IOP) elevation. This condition is characterized by blurred vision and is frequently associated with nystagmus. Tearing and photophobia are not present or are mild. Histology and treatment are similar to CHED1.

C. *X-linked endothelial corneal dystrophy (C2):* Cases are X-chromosomal dominant on Xq25 and seen at birth. Males have varying corneal clouding with possible nystagmus, as well as moon crater-like changes of the endothelium and band keratopathy. This is usually progressive. Females with the condition are often asymptomatic with only endothelial changes, which are nonprogressive. Histology in males shows loss of endothelial cells, thickening of Descemet membrane, and stromal disorganization. Bowman layer is thin, and granular material is deposited along the subepithelium.

D. *Fuchs corneal dystrophy:* This corneal dystrophy is classified as C1 for early-onset variant, and C2 or C3 in the typical adult-onset variant; it is also known as endoepithelial or endothelial corneal dystrophy. It is most commonly sporadic, but cases of autosomal dominance have been reported. Symptoms usually begin around the fourth decade, whereas the early variant can begin as soon as the first decade. These cases are progressive and cause vision that may wax and wane due to the edema. Patients may complain of vision that is worse in the morning, as well as photophobia, pain, and epiphora from bullae that have burst.

Characteristic features include beaten metal-like changes, or guttae, of the endothelium with possible pigment dusting. This is accompanied by stromal edema from endothelial pump dysfunction and can lead to epithelial bullae and bullous keratopathy. In chronic cases, subepithelial fibrosis and peripheral vascularization may be seen.

Histology reveals diffuse thickening of Descemet membrane and guttae, which are hyaline excrescences on Descemet membrane. Thinning, atrophy, or loss of endothelial cells are typically seen, as well as stromal thickening and disorganization. Confocal microscopy reveals pleomorphism and polymegathism of endothelial cells. Adult-onset Fuchs often reveals larger guttae than those seen in the early-onset variant. Pachymetry may also be used to follow the disease. Corneal thickness >640 μm, endothelial cell count <1000/mm^2, or epithelial edema suggest that the cornea may decompensate with intraocular surgery.

Sodium chloride drops and ointment are used as treatment to reduce corneal edema and pain. IOP lowering drops may also help with the edema. For epithelial damage, a bandage contact lens may be used, as well as anterior stromal puncture, amniotic membrane, or a conjunctival flap in advanced cases. Penetrating keratoplasty was previously the only option for end-stage disease, but this has largely been replaced by endothelial keratoplasty in recent years.

E. *Posterior polymorphous corneal dystrophy (PPCD or PPMD, Schlichting dystrophy) (C1 or C2):* This entity has an onset in early childhood, and inheritance is usually autosomal dominant, though isolated unilateral cases have been reported. In this condition, abnormal endothelial cells behave and appear like epithelial cells or fibroblasts. Epithelial and stromal edema, as well as secondary band keratopathy, may rarely occur due to the endothelial decompensation.

Twenty-five percent of patients have peripheral iridocorneal adhesions, and IOP is elevated in 15% of patients. Similar changes are seen in iridocorneal endothelial (ICE) syndrome, but ICE is unilateral and sporadic, with possible iris nevi or atrophy. Vision in PPCD is usually unaffected until stromal clouding occurs. Congenital cases may rarely have corneal clouding. Typical cases have stable endothelial signs, though possible progression of vesicles or thickening of Descemet membrane can occur with endothelial dysfunction.

Microscopy reveals thickening of Descemet membrane and endothelial polymegathism. Treatment is similar to that of Fuchs.

BIBLIOGRAPHY

1. Gottsch JD, Sundin OH, Liu SH, et al. Inheritance of a novel COL8A2 mutation defines a distinct early-onset subtype of Fuchs corneal dystrophy. Invest Ophthalmol Vis Sci. 2005; 46:1934-9.

2. Seitzman GD, Gottsch JD, Stark WJ. Cataract surgery in patients with Fuchs' corneal dystrophy: Expanding recommendations for cataract surgery without simultaneous keratoplasty. Ophthalmology. 2005;112: 441-6.

3. Terry MA. Endothelial keratoplasty: History, current state, and future directions. Cornea. 2006;25:873-8.

4. Weiss JS, Moller H, Lisch W, et al. The IC3D classification of the corneal dystrophies. Cornea. 2008;27(Suppl. 2): S1-42.

Corneal Edema

John Awad, Richard W Yee

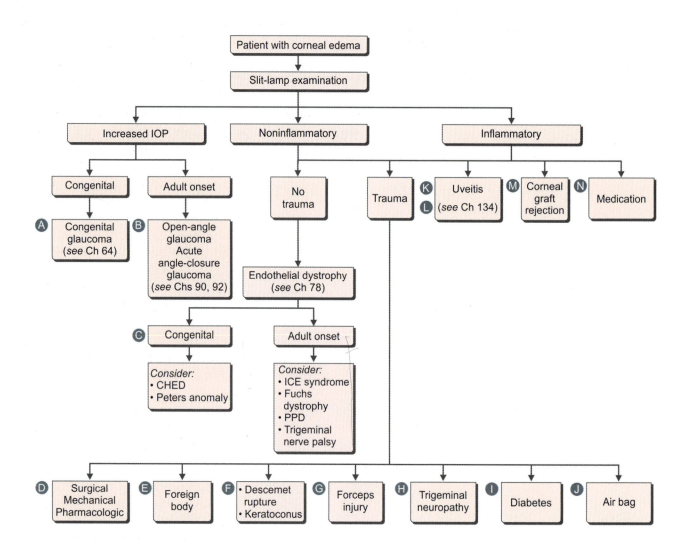

The cornea has three important layers: epithelium, stroma, and endothelium. Excess water in the epithelium or stroma results in corneal edema. Corneal water content depends on the equilibrium between forces driving water into the cornea and those pushing water out. The forces driving water into the cornea include the swelling pressure of the stroma and the intraocular pressure (IOP). The factors that keep the cornea from swelling are the barrier function and metabolic pump of the endothelium. Less important factors are the epithelial barrier and evaporation from the corneal surface. If any of these factors are not functional or damaged, corneal edema and increased corneal thickness can develop, with complaints of blurred vision most severe in the morning and improving as the day goes on. As the edema worsens, epithelial microcysts and bullae may form, leading to sharp, stabbing pain, photophobia, and redness. Prolonged edema can lead to scarring of Bowman membrane and stroma, as well as pannus and stromal vascularization.

Iris nerves. In
Chandler sx
Essential iris atrophy / 1° proliferative
endo disorder

Chapter 79   Corneal Edema   281

A. Increased IOP does not directly damage the endothelium but disrupts the balance of forces of transport across the cornea. Congenital glaucoma can be present and increase corneal thickness, corneal diameter, and produce horizontal linear tears of Descemet membrane.

B. Acute glaucoma can be diagnosed if there is epithelial edema, pain, closed chamber angles, and fixed middilated pupils. Usually, the pressure is > 60 mm Hg. The patient sees a halo around bright objects. Once the pressure is treated, the symptoms generally clear. However, untreated, increased pressure causes irreversible endothelial damage and chronic edema.

C. Endothelial dystrophies are hereditary diseases of the endothelium. Some are apparent at birth; others appear later in life. Peters anomaly is recognized by a bilateral central corneal leukoma, with edema in the affected areas, which is caused by defects in the posterior stroma, Descemet membrane, and endothelium. Congenital hereditary endothelial dystrophy can have two forms: dominant and recessive. The recessive is recognized at birth as a diffuse, bilaterally symmetric corneal edema and generally does not advance. The dominant form is not evident at birth. Edema develops in the first year and may advance in later life to severe edema, band keratopathy, and epithelial erosion. *Fuchs endothelial dystrophy* occurs later in life and can be diagnosed if corneal edema accompanied by many corneal guttae is seen posterior to Descemet membrane. Corneal guttae are focal, refractive collagen deposits. In posterior polymorphous dystrophy, several small lesions surrounded by faint halos or fewer large, blister-like lesions with dense halos are seen on Descemet membrane. Corneal guttae are not present. Iridocorneal endothelial syndrome is a spectrum of primary proliferative endothelial disorders, including iris nevus syndrome of Cogan-Reese, Chandler syndrome, and essential iris atrophy. These disorders are characterized by an attenuated endothelium, an extensive posterior collagenous layer, and development of an ectopic basement membrane over the iris. Although these diseases form a spectrum, they can be recognized individually. In iris nevus syndrome, iris stromal tissue herniates through the ectopic basement membrane. In Chandler syndrome, the posterior collagenous layer is associated with a diffuse corneal edema. Essential iris atrophy is characterized by a gray posterior collagenous layer, peripheral anterior synechiae, distorted pupil, and holes in the iris. Schnyder corneal dystrophy can occur in patients with hypercholesterolemia. Deposition of cholesterol in the cornea causes it to become cloudy, but, in most cases, the cornea does not swell.

D. The endothelium may be damaged during or after surgery. Intraoperative damage may be caused by corneal contact with surgical instruments or the intraocular lens or by toxic effects of intraocular drugs, preservatives, or irrigating solutions. Postoperative damage can be caused by intraocular hemorrhage, increased IOP, stripped Descemet membrane, and contact lens-induced hypoxia, as well as by corneal endothelial contact with vitreous, the intraocular lens, or its sutures. Postsurgical hypotony has also been observed to cause an imbalance in water transport into and out of the cornea resulting in edema. Brown-McLean syndrome, a peripheral edema of the cornea, is most common after intracapsular cataract extraction, though it can also occur after extracapsular extraction. Corneal haze is one of the more common complications in keratoconus patients treated with collagen cross-linking and may necessitate penetrating keratoplasty. A few cases of retained foreign bodies have been reported causing damage to corneal endothelium. Early diagnosis and removal of fragments may result in reversal of the damage.

E. Perforation of the cornea by a foreign body can cause endothelial damage and reduce cell count, producing corneal edema. Forceful contact of a foreign body with the cornea can cause a 0.5- to 0.1-mm diameter ringshaped opacity on the posterior corneal surface. These rings are caused by fibrin and leukocyte deposits in the corneal endothelium and disappear in a few days.

F. In patients with advanced keratoconus, Descemet membrane can break centrally. The aqueous humor can enter and cause edema. However, endothelial cells grow, and the wound soon heals so that the edema subsides within several months. All that persists is a small scar.

G. Breaks of Descemet membrane can occur at birth from forceps injury and typically appear vertically or in oblique orientation. Depending on the extent of injury, corneal edema may clear and recur later in life.

H. Sensorimotor trigeminal neuropathy, from surgical procedures, neoplasms, and other processes, can influence corneal hydration and result in corneal edema during exposure to low environmental temperatures. One case of corneal endothelial decompensation complicating Horner syndrome has been reported.

I. Diabetic keratopathy can occur following the undue stress of intraocular surgery or photocoagulation. Corneal endothelium of a diabetic exhibits abnormalities in cell morphology, so corneal edema tends to persist postoperatively.

J. Multiple reports have described cases of corneal decompensation after airbag trauma. Scanning electron microscopy reveals localized areas of complete endothelial destruction associated with areas of endothelium cell count <1000 cells/mm^2. Some persistent corneal edema may fail to resolve, requiring corneal transplantation.

K. Uveitis is inflammation of any part of the uveal tract of the eye, including the iris, ciliary body, and choroid. Inflammation of the iris and ciliary body, also called *anterior uveitis,* is usually painful and can cause visual impairment, sometimes blindness. Although the relationship is unclear, corneal edema often accompanies uveitis. Uveitis can be diagnosed if specular photo microscopy shows dark areas on the endothelium. These dark areas may be caused by keratic precipitates or localized endothelial edema. This damage is caused by invading microbes and by cells of the immune system. Corneal edema is secondary to the immunologic response. The edema typically is stromal and monocular. The organisms capable of eliciting this response include herpes simplex and herpes zoster viruses, some bacteria, and some fungi.

L. Along with herpes simplex and herpes zoster viruses, cytomegalovirus (CMV) has been identified as a possible culprit for corneal endotheliitis. CMV infection is especially prevalent in patients who develop endothelial keratic precipitates after undergoing penetrating keratoplasty. Keratic precipitates, Descemet membrane folds, and absence of vascularization of the donor are indicative of CMV infection in these patients. Ganciclovir has been shown to be an effective treatment in these cases.

M. After a corneal graft, lymphocytes may migrate to the endothelium and form a line that moves toward the center, destroying the endothelial cells in its path. By about 3 months after the graft, the line has disappeared and the damage is visible as many keratic precipitates and uniform graft edema.

N. Reversible corneal edema has been associated with keratitis during treatment with levodopa. Perfluorodecalin is a liquid used intraoperatively in retinal detachment surgery. Residual amounts may be retained in the anterior chamber in contact with the endothelium, causing corneal decompensation.

BIBLIOGRAPHY

1. Geggel HS, Griggs PB, Freeman MI. Irreversible bullous keratopathy after airbag trauma. CLAO J. 1996;22: 148-50.
2. Gokhale NS. Late corneal edema due to retained foldable lens fragment. Indian J Ophthalmol. 2009;57:230-1.
3. Gothard TW, Hardten DR, Lane SS, et al. Clinical findings in Brown-McLean syndrome. Am J Ophthalmol. 1993;115:729-37.
4. Hatton MP, Perez VL, Dohlman CH. Corneal oedema in ocular hypotony. Exp Eye Res. 2004;78:549-52.
5. Koizumi N, Suzuki T, Uno T, et al. Cytomegalovirus as an etiologic factor in corneal endotheliitis. Ophthalmology. 2008;115:292-7.
6. Levenson JE. Corneal edema: Cause and treatment. Surv Ophthalmol. 1976;20:190-204.
7. Nakamagoe K, Ohkashi N, Fujita T, et al. Keratitis and corneal edema associated with levodopa use—A case report. Rinsho Shinkeigaku. 1996;36:886-8.
8. Sharma A, Nottage JM, Mirchia K, et al. Persistent corneal edema after collagen cross-linking for keratoconus. Am J Ophthalmol. 2012;154:922-6.
9. Waring GO, Bourne NM, Edelhauser HF, et al. The corneal endothelium, normal and pathologic structure and function.Ophthalmology. 1982; 89:531-90.
10. Weiss JS, Khemichian AJ. Differential diagnosis of Schnyder corneal dystrophy. Dev Ophthalmol. 2011;48:67-96.
11. Wilbanks GA, Apel AJ, Jolly SS, et al. Perfluorodecalin corneal toxicity: Five case reports. Cornea. 1996;15: 329-34.
12. Zamir E, Chowers I, Banin E, et al. Neurotrophic corneal endothelial failure complicating acute Horner syndrome. Ophthalmology. 1999;106:1692-6.

Interstitial Keratitis

Elizabeth Shane, Richard W Yee

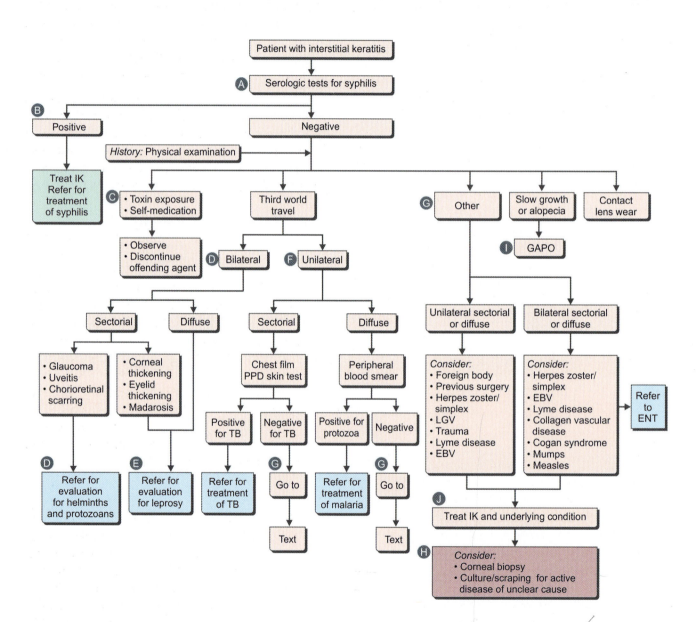

Active interstitial keratitis (IK) is any inflammation located in the corneal interstitial space or stroma. Symptoms included decreased vision, redness, pain, photophobia, and tearing. Superficial and deep stromal blood vessels and stromal edema can be seen diffusely or sectorially. Anterior chamber cells or flare may or may not be present. Inactive or old IK demonstrate deep corneal haze or scarring, lipid deposition, empty stromal blood vessels (ghost vessels), and corneal stromal thinning.

A. The approach to a patient with *active* IK should be to search for and treat associated systemic conditions, particularly syphilis, and to treat *active* inflammation of the anterior segment with topical steroids. In cases of *active* inflammation of uncertain cause not responding to steroids, consider cytologic examination on corneal biopsies. In patients with inactive IK, the goal is to ascertain whether a treatable systemic disease is involved.

B. Syphilis is by far the most common cause of IK (90% of cases). Therefore, serologic studies must be obtained. Distinguishing congenital from acquired syphilis is possible by history and physical examination. In congenital syphilis, ocular symptoms usually begin between the ages of 5 and 15 years. Patients present with bilateral red eye, photophobia, and decreasing vision. Other manifestations are pigmentary mottling of the fundus, Hutchinson teeth, mulberry molars, eighth nerve deafness, saber shins, frontal bossing, saddle nose, mental retardation, and tabes dorsalis. IK resulting from acquired syphilis usually occurs in an older age group, is unilateral, and does not have the associated physical findings. The evaluation of IK should, with few exceptions, always include laboratory testing for syphilis, taking care to exclude neurosyphilis by evaluation of the cerebrospinal fluid when indicated.

C. Numerous toxins and medications can result in IK. Toxic exposures range from acid and alkali burns to metal exposure (i.e. gold and arsenic).

D. In patients who live in or travel to developing countries, do not overlook syphilis. Once this cause has been ruled out, the differential diagnosis of bilateral IK in this setting includes helminths, protozoans, and *Mycobacterium leprae.* Onchocerciasis is caused by a helminth commonly found along rapid streams in equatorial Africa and parts of Central and South America. The microfilaria may be seen in the peripheral cornea, anterior chamber, and less often, the *vitre*ous. It causes a punctate keratitis, severe anterior uveitis, sclerosing keratitis, and chorioretinitis, as well as IK. Onchocerciasis is diagnosed by finding microfilaria in skin snips, nodules, body fluids, or the anterior chamber. The protozoa are uncommon culprits in IK. A diffuse bilateral IK has rarely been associated with *Trypanosoma gambiense*, which causes African sleeping sickness. When corneal involvement occurs, a mild iritis is common, but severe

necrosis and scarring of the cornea are rare. Along with the clinical picture of African sleeping sickness, the diagnosis can be made by demonstration of the parasite in serum or spinal fluid. The most common type of leishmaniasis to involve the eye is the American form, *Leishmania braziliensis.* A sectorial or nodular diffuse superficial interstitial process of the cornea may become vascularized, ulcerated, and opaque without prompt systemic therapy. Conjunctival manifestations include large ulcerative granulomas and trachoma-like follicles.

E. Leprosy, caused by *M. leprae,* usually creates a bilateral IK, either diffuse or sectorial. Ophthalmologic characteristics include nasolacrimal duct obstruction, ptosis, supraciliary ridge thickening, loss of eyebrows, lid thickening, madarosis, keratoconjunctivitis sicca, facial nerve dysfunction, and uncommonly, trigeminal nerve involvement. Cranial nerves III, IV, and VI are usually spared. Lepromatous leprosy causes a superficial punctate keratopathy with an avascular keratitis in the supertemporal quadrant. This is the most characteristic lesion of leprosy. "Beads on a string," or thickened corneal nerves, as well as limbal granulomas, scleritis, episcleritis, scleromalacia, and severe uveitis, may also occur. There are two forms of IK in leprosy. The first is caused by an autoimmune reaction that begins superiorly with occasional ghost vessels seen in middle to deep stroma. The second type is secondary to direct bacterial invasion and is characterized by inflammation, necrosis, and vascular invasion starting superiorly and superficially.

F. In the Third World, the most common causes of unilateral IK are tuberculosis (TB) and malaria. Unilateral IK caused by TB may appear similar to that of acquired syphilis. In addition to skin testing and a systemic work-up, some clinical clues help make this distinction. The ocular inflammatory attacks in TB are more common than in syphilis and are more likely to occur peripherally and sectorially. They usually spare the central cornea, and unlike the deep involvement of lues, this infiltration is seen mainly in the superficial and middle layers of the cornea. Also, vascularization occurs more superficially and later than in syphilitic infiltration. Malaria ocular involvement is uncommon and usually manifests a unilateral dendritic keratitis;

IK occurs less commonly as a superficial unilateral keratitis with little or no vascularization. The inflammatory process usually lasts several months and leaves residual scarring. The diagnosis is made by examination of serial thick blood smears.

G. Lyme disease, caused by *Borrelia burgdorferi*, may cause a bilateral diffuse IK. The lesions are multiple, focal, nebular opacities in the stroma. Corneal neovascularization, edema, and scarring, also occur. Systemic treatment may include tetracycline, 250 mg PO four times daily for 3 weeks. Lymphogranuloma venereum (LGV), caused by *Chlamydia trachomatis,* begins as a segmental IK of the upper third of the cornea and may spread, resulting in dense vascularization throughout. Herpes simplex virus type 1 and herpes zoster can cause unilateral stromal involvement. Epstein-Barr virus demonstrates both deep and superficial changes. The IK of mumps and measles usually resolves with time in the absence of intervention. However, severe cases of measles in underdeveloped countries may result in significant corneal scarring, secondary infection, and ocular perforation. Cogan syndrome is an ill-defined entity, causing nonsyphilitic IK and vestibuloauditory symptoms. Typically, young adults, after an upper respiratory tract infection, develop a bilateral subepithelial keratitis in the peripheral and posterior half of the cornea. Treatment with topical steroids usually prevents progression to IK. The systemic findings are varied, including cardiovascular, gastrointestinal, and central nervous systems. The hearing loss, unlike that of congenital syphilis, rapidly progresses toward deafness without steroid treatment. Infectious crystalline keratopathy is an invasion of the corneal stroma by microbial pathogens clinically characterized by crystal-like opacities. *Streptococcus viridans* is the most common pathogen recovered in culture, but other pathogens have been isolated, including *Haemophilus, Mycobacterium fortuitum, Pseudomonas* species, staphylococcal species, *Propionibacterium acnes,* and fungi. *Scedosporium apiospermum* is resistant to conventional antifungals. Voriconazole and surgical intervention is recommended for treatment. The lesions are needle-like, crystalline opacities with little or no inflammation. Also consider *Acanthamoeba* keratitis and microsporidial keratitis. IK is also associated with the initial phase of Wegener granulomatosis.

H. In cases of active IK of unclear cause, consider biopsy and/or culture to ascertain the diagnosis.

I. GAPO is the acronym for growth retardation, alopecia, pseudoanodontia, and optic atrophy. It is a very rare autosomal-recessive disease. There are only approximately 30 cases reported worldwide. GAPO has been found to include symptoms of bilateral idiopathic IK and hypothyroidism.

J. Contact lenses can alter the biochemistry of tear fluid causing the cornea to be susceptible to infections leading to IK.

BIBLIOGRAPHY

1. Fleiszig SM. The Glenn A. Fry award lecture 2005. The pathogenesis of contact lens-related keratitis. Optom Vis Sci. 2006;83:866-73.
2. Grant WM. Ocular complication of malaria. Arch Ophthalmol. 1946;35:48-54.
3. Kepez B, Hasanreisoglu M, Aktas Z, et al. Fungal keratitis secondary to Scedosporium apiospermum infection and successful treatment with surgical and medical intervention. Int Ophthalmol. 2013 [Epub ahead of print].
4. Kornmehl EW, Lesser RL, Jaros P, et al. Bilateral keratitis in Lyme disease. Ophthalmology. 1989;96:1194-7.
5. Lei S, Lyengarb S, Li S, et al. GAPO syndrome and interstitial keratitis. Clin Dysmorphol. 2010;19:79-81.
6. Maisler DM. Infectious crystalline keratopathy. Ophthalmol Clin North Am. 1994;7:577-82.
7. Roizenblatt J. Interstitial keratitis caused by American (mucocutaneous) leishmaniasis. Am J Ophthalmol. 1979;87: 175-9.
8. Spaide R, Nattis R, Lipka A, D'Amico R. Ocular findings in leprosy in the United States. Am J Ophthalmol. 1985;100:411-6.
9. Tabbara KF, Hyndiuk RA (Eds). Interstitial Keratitis. Infections of the Eye: Diagnosis and Management. Boston, MA: Little, Brown, 1986. pp. 601-12.
10. Tooker CW. Allergic phenomena in tuberculous keratitis. Arch Ophthalmol. 1929;2:540-4.

Corneal Neovascularization

Clinton Duncan, Daniel A Johnson

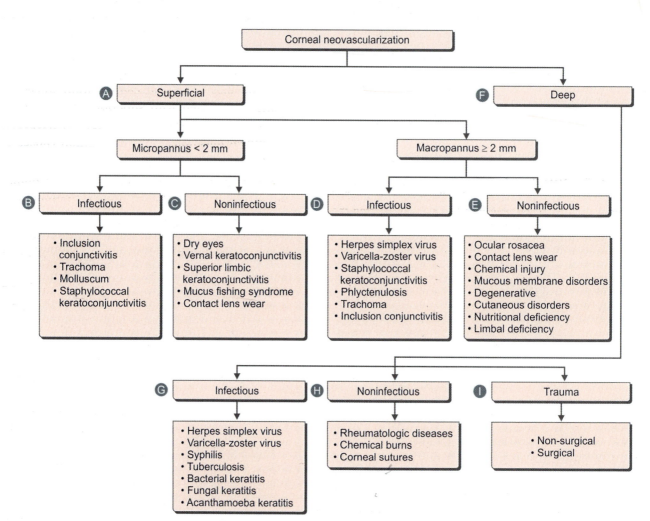

81

Adapted from: Brock RJ and Yee RW. Corneal Neovascularization. In: van Heuven WAJ, Zwaan J, (Eds). Decision Making in Ophthalmology, 1st edition.

Corneal transparency is critical for maintaining visual acuity. The normal cornea is avascular; however, disease, hypoxia, and injury (surgical and nonsurgical) can stimulate angiogenesis. While new vessel growth can aid in healing, it leads to a loss of both transparency and immunologic privilege. Corneal vascularization is induced when pro-angiogenic growth factors such as vascular endothelial growth factor (VEGF) overwhelm anti-angiogenic factors. This occurs primarily through one of three mechanisms:

inflammation, hypoxia, or loss of limbal barrier function. Corneal angiogenesis leads to a decrease in visual acuity from both the physical presence of vessels and from induced edema, lipid deposition, hemorrhage, and scarring. Corneal neovascularization is a strong risk factor for immune rejection after penetrating keratoplasty.

Topical steroids are the mainstay of treatment for corneal neovascularization. Argon laser photocoagulation, photodynamic therapy, ocular surface

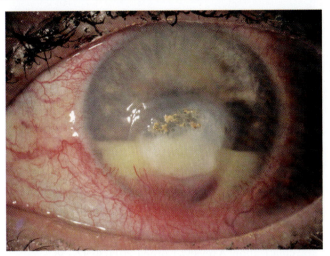

Fig. 81.1: Corneal pannus in a patient with a neurotrophic corneal ulcer and presumed herpes simplex virus (HSV). The patient had undergone trigeminal nerve ablation several months earlier. Note the inferior pannus, hypopyon admixed with hyphema, and cyanoacrylate glue that had been applied by a prior physician. The new blood vessels penetrated the deep cornea through tracts from exposed corneal sutures.

reconstruction, and anti-VEGF therapy have all been shown to have success, but each has its limitations.

A. Superficial neovascularization, or pannus, arises from the superficial marginal arcade (Fig. 81.1), which is formed from episcleral branches of the anterior ciliary arteries. Neovascularization extending less than 2 mm from the limbus is termed 'micropannus,' whereas that extending at least 2 mm from the limbus is termed 'macropannus.'

B. Infectious causes of micropannus are numerous and include chlamydial infections (trachoma and inclusion conjunctivitis), *Molluscum contagiosum*, staphylococcal/streptococcal keratoconjunctivitis, and phlyctenulosis. Patients should be examined for an associated follicular response and muco-purulent discharge for chlamydial infections. Small, elevated, umbilicated papules on eyelids can be found with molluscum infections.

C. The history and physical exam help differentiate common causes of noninfectious micropannus. Systemic conditions such as rheumatoid arthritis can lead to findings of micropannus on exam. Superiorly located micropannus may be caused by superior limbic keratoconjunctivitis and contact lens use. Atopic and vernal conjunctivitis may be found in children and young adults with allergies who have symptoms of itching and clear discharge. Other causes include mucus fishing syndrome and chronic dry eyes.

D. Common infectious causes of macropannus include herpes simplex virus keratitis, varicella-zoster virus keratitis, staphylococcal keratitis, phlyctenulosis, and trachoma. Clues to herpetic-related pannus include dendritic or geographic scars and decreased corneal sensitivity. Staphylococcal-associated pannus is often located inferiorly at the 4:00 and 8:00 locations. Pannus from trachoma is often associated with superior tarsal scarring, follicles, and/or Herbert pits. Tuberculosis, leprosy, and fungal infections are less common causes of infectious pannus.

E. Causes of noninfectious macropannus are numerous. Ocular rosacea often produces a pannus inferiorly; however, with disease progression, the entire circumference of the cornea may be involved. Pannus from contact lens wear is usually bilateral and can be found with soft or hard contact lenses. Conjunctival, corneal, or lid scarring can be found in eyes with a macropannus from toxic or chemical burns and mucous membrane disorders such as mucous membrane pemphigoid, scalded skin syndrome, and Stevens-Johnson syndrome. Other causes of limbal stem cell deficiency, both acquired (such as with significant ocular surface surgery) and congenital (such as aniridia keratopathy), can produce superficial neovascularization. Skin diseases such as psoriasis and ichthyosis have been associated with gross pannus. Nutritional deficiency (vitamin B, pellagra) and thyroid disorders (hypothyroid) can cause corneal pannus. Finally, a degenerative pannus caused by glaucoma, blind hypotensive eyes, or corneas with endothelial failure (Fuchs or bullous keratopathy) can occur.

F. Deep corneal vascularization (Fig. 81.2) generally runs in a single plane and arises from anastomoses of the anterior and posterior ciliary vessels. It can also extend from superficial vessels that follow suture tract into the cornea stroma.

G. Herpes simplex, varicella-zoster, syphilis, and infectious keratitis are common infectious causes of stromal vascularization. Less common causes in

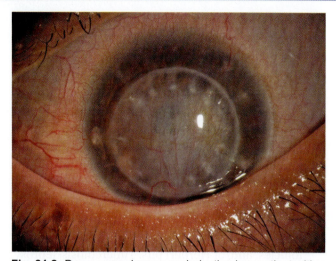

Fig. 81.2: Deep corneal neovascularization in a patient with a failed corneal transplant.

industrialized countries include malaria, onchocerciasis, and leishmaniasis. Tuberculosis, Epstein-Barr virus, and Lyme disease are other causes.

H. Rheumatologic diseases including rheumatoid arthritis, Behçet disease, polyarteritis nodosa, granulomatosis with polyangiitis (formerly Wegener granulomatosis), systemic lupus erythematosus, and others can lead to deep stromal vascularization. Hearing loss with stromal vascularization can be found with Cogan interstitial keratitis.

I. Trauma, both surgical and non-surgical, is an important cause of deep corneal vascularization. History and physical exam (corneal incisions, glaucoma filtering blebs) are important findings.

BIBLIOGRAPHY

1. Cursiefen C, Kruse FE. New aspects of angiogenesis in the cornea. Cornea and external eye disease. Essent Ophthalmol. 2006. pp. 83-99.
2. Gupta D, Illingworth C. Treatments for corneal neovascularization: A review. Cornea. 2011;30:927-38.
3. Maddula S, Davis DK, Maddula S, et al. Horizons in therapy for corneal angiogenesis. Ophthalmol. 2011;118:591-9.
4. Maguire MG, Stark WJ, Gottsch JD, et al. Risk factors for corneal graft failure and rejection in the collaborative corneal transplantation studies. Collaborative Corneal Transplantation Studies Research Group. Ophthalmology. 1994;101:1536-47.
5. Qazi Y, Maddula S, Ambati BK. Mediators of ocular angiogenesis. J Genet. 2009: 88:495-515.
6. Smolin G, Thoft RA. The Cornea. Boston, MA: Little, Brown; 2005. pp. 437-8.

82

Band Keratopathy

Abbie S Ornelas, Kent L Anderson

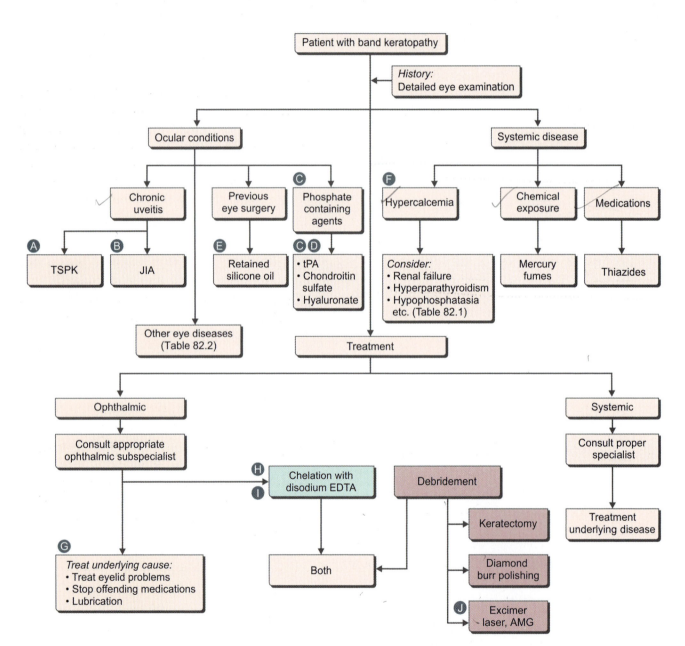

Abbreviations: AMG: Amniotic membrane graft transplantation; EDTA: Ethylenediaminetetraacetic acid; JIA: juvenile idiopathic arthritis; PTK: Phototherapeutic keratectomy; TSPK: Thygeson superficial punctate keratitis; tPA: tissue plasminogen activator

Band keratopathy is a chronic degenerative condition characterized by the deposition of gray to white opacities in the superficial layers of the cornea, most frequently in the interpalpebral zone with a band-like appearance running horizontally from the 3 to 9 o'clock position. Band keratopathy is the result of precipitation of mineral deposits on the corneal surface. These deposits are composed of calcium hydroxyapatite and noncrystalline forms of phosphate and carbonate salts of calcium. Patients will complain of decreased vision, ocular pain, foreign body sensation, and red eye. Examination will reveal decreased visual acuity and a whitish/gray plaque-like opacification extending across the cornea. Band keratopathy is typically a chronic, slowly progressive condition developing over months to years, although acute presentations (hour to days) have also been reported.

PATHOGENESIS

Serum and body fluids (e.g. tears and aqueous humor) contain calcium and phosphate in concentrations approaching their solubility product. Any slight increase in their concentration causes precipitation. Environmental changes in the corneal surface facilitate the precipitation of calcium. Dry eyes lead to increased tear osmolality as tear evaporation concentrates solutes and increases the tonicity, especially in the interpalpebral zone where the greatest cornea surface area exposed to ambient air occurs. The pH of the interpalpebral fissure is higher (i.e. more alkaline) than that of the rest of the ocular surface because of carbon dioxide released from the exposed zone. Elevation in surface pH out of the physiologic range changes the calcium solubility product and favors precipitation. Ocular inflammation causes temporary endothelial dysfunction leading to increased diffusion of aqueous into stroma, and when the endothelium recovers, the water is drawn out and the high concentrations of phosphate and calcium remain and tend to precipitate in the anterior superficial layers where the pH is more alkaline.

A. Thygeson superficial punctate keratitis (TSPK) is a chronic inflammatory condition that responds well to corticosteroids. Although generally no scarring occurs, rare cases of anterior scarring with band keratopathy have been reported.

B. Juvenile idiopathic arthritis (JIA) (previously named juvenile rheumatoid arthritis or JRA) is the most common rheumatologic condition associated with childhood uveitis in North America and has up to 20% incidence of uveitic development depending on subtype, and patients should be screened by an ophthalmologist. JIA patients with band keratopathy are also at risk for deprivation amblyopia.

C. Use of phosphate containing drops increases phosphate concentration in the cornea. Tissue plasminogen activator (tPA) has been described to treat significant postoperative inflammation after cataract extraction and/or penetrating keratoplasty; tPA contains a phosphate buffer that may acutely increase the phosphate concentration and precipitate. Phosphate and calcium from the fibrin clot may also diffuse into the stroma.

D. Chondroitin sulfate (4%) and sodium hyaluronate (3%) also contain a phosphate buffer.

E. Silicone oil, used in retina surgery, is generally removed after several weeks to months, but permanent silicone oil may be unavoidable in a small subgroup of patients. The main long-term silicone oil related complication observed when present in the eye for more than 12 months is band keratopathy.

F. Patients with end-stage renal dialysis (ESRD) may have associated hemodialysis effects, uremic states, elevations of the mineral (calcium phosphate) products, and fluctuations in intraocular pressure attributed to changes in serum osmolality or colloid osmotic pressure during hemodialysis, which may all result in deposition of band keratopathy. When the calcium phosphate product is elevated, calcium salts deposit in the tears.

Numerous systemic and ocular conditions may be accompanied by band keratopathy. They are listed in Tables 82.1 and 82.2, respectively.

TREATMENT

G. Treatment is aimed to improve visual acuity, lessen ocular discomfort, and reduce cosmetic deformity. Treatment consists of removing the calcium

Table 82.1: Systemic associations
• Systemic conditions associated with band keratopathy
– Hypercalcemia
- Renal failure
▪ ESRD
▪ Fanconi syndrome
- Hyperparathyroidism
- Excessive vitamin D
▪ Oral intake
▪ Osteoporosis
- Hypophosphatasia
- Sarcoidosis
- Multiple myeloma
- Milk-alkali syndrome
- Metastatic carcinoma to bone
– Paget disease
– JIA
– Discoid lupus
– Gout
– Tuberous sclerosis
– Norrie disease
– Proteus syndrome
– Chemicals/medications
- Thiazides
- Mercury fumes

Table 82.2: Ocular associations
• Ocular conditions associated with band keratopathy
– Corneal chemical burns
– Ocular medications
- Mercury-containing preservatives
- Phosphate-containing drops
– Severe dry eye and corneal exposure syndromes
– Spheroidal keratopathy
– Chronic persistent epithelial defects
– Intraocular inflammation
- TSPK
- Chronic uveitis
– Endothelial dysfunction
– Long-standing glaucoma
– Interstitial keratitis
– Prior surgeries
- Intraocular silicone oil
- Viscoelastics in phosphate buffer
- tPA
- Multiple ocular surgeries
- Toxic anterior segment syndrome
- Postoperative inflammation
- Phthisis bulbi
- Keratoprosthesis

deposits and to facilitate corneal healing. Before medical and surgical therapy are considered, it is important to first identify and treat any underlying systemic and/or ocular disorder. Any lid deformities should be addressed, phosphate-containing topical medications should be discontinued, and ocular lubrication therapy initiated.

H. Ethylenediaminetetraacetic acid (EDTA) chelation is cost-effective and straightforward and may be combined with a mechanical debridement method, that is, scraping, lamellar keratectomy, and/or diamond burr polishing.

I. There are two forms of EDTA available: disodium and calcium disodium. Only the disodium form is effective for band keratopathy as chelation therapy requires exchanging one mineral for another and therefore the calcium form would not be effective

as one would be exchanging calcium for calcium. In 2006, the availability of the disodium form was drastically restricted and not supplied by many pharmacies due to an US FDA advisory (Pharmacy 'Name Alert') where patients died when they were mistakenly given the disodium form instead of the calcium disodium form for 'chelation therapies' as both are called 'EDTA'. The disodium form was approved for patients with hypercalcemia and the calcium disodium form for severe lead poisoning. When given incorrectly (i.e. disodium form to treat lead poisoning), a fatal hypocalcemia would result. The calcium disodium was also becoming popular for 'chelation therapy' for patients with heart disease and removing 'toxic' heavy metals. Several deaths were reported when the disodium form was used in this setting. Pharmacies and manufacturers stopped distributing the disodium form to address the EDTA 'Name Alert' issue. Ocular treatment utilizes the disodium form for topical treatment only, and this form may need to be specially prepared by an approved compounding pharmacy. Special labeling is required when using the disodium form of EDTA for this topical application.

J.   If an excimer laser is available, phototherapeutic keratectomy can facilitate a smoother corneal plane. Adjunctive use of amniotic membrane transplantation may enhance epithelial healing.

BIBLIOGRAPHY

1. Angeles-Han S, Yeh S. Prevention and management of cataracts in children with juvenile idiopathic arthritis-associated uveitis. Curr Rheumatol Rep. 2012;14:142-9.

2. Beauchamp RA, Willis TM, Betz TG, et al. Deaths associated with hypocalcemia from chelation therapy—Texas, Pennsylvania, and Oregon, 2003–2005. MMWR Morb Mortal Wkly Rep. 2006;55:204-7.

3. Fintelmann RE, Vastine DW, Bloomer MM. Thygeson superficial punctate keratitis and scarring. Cornea. 2012; 31:1446-8.

4. Jhanji V, Rapuano CJ, Vajpayee RB. Corneal calcific band keratopathy. Curr Opin Ophthalmol. 2011;22:283-9.

5. Moisseiev E, Gal A, Addadi L, et al. Acute calcific band keratopathy: Cases report and literature review. J Cataract Refract Surg. 2013;39:292-4.

6. Morphis G, Irigoyen C, Eleuteri A, et al. Retrospective review of 50 eyes with long-term silicone oil tamponade for more than 12 months. Graefes Arch Clin Exp Ophthalmol. 2012;250:645-52.

7. Mullaem G, Rosner MH. Ocular problems in the patient with end-stage renal disease. Sem Dial. 2012;25:403-7.

83

Corneal Pigmentation

Mark L McDermott, Nitya Kumar, Richard W Yee

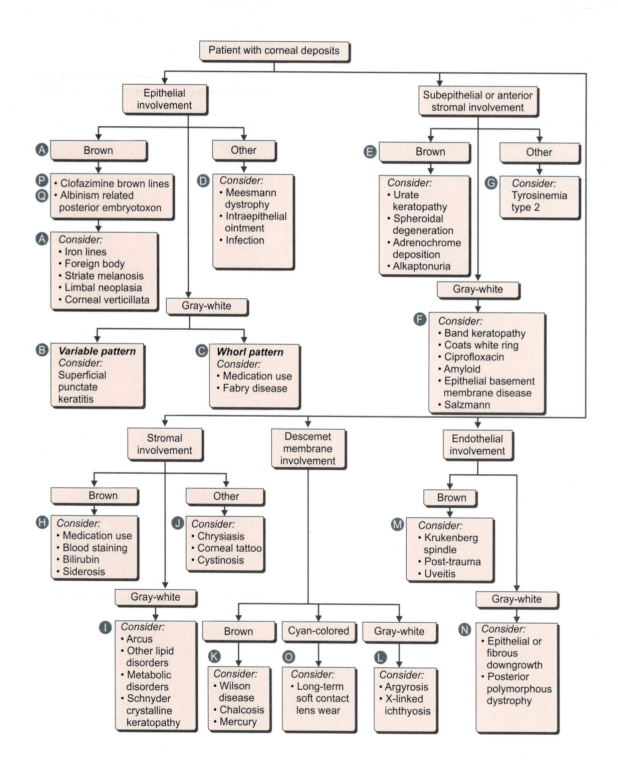

Corneal pigmentation may result from local or systemic processes. Pigmentation represents an abnormal deposition of a substance in the cornea, which manifests in an identifiable corneal opacity that may or may not be vision threatening. The two major characteristics of pigmentation, color and location, can be reliably determined by slit-lamp biomicroscopy. The location of a lesion is usually categorized by the most involved layer of the corneal anatomy, and color may vary by form and extent of involvement.

A. Brown pigmentation restricted to the corneal epithelium is most likely caused by iron or melanin deposition. Iron may be deposited in a variety of patterns reflecting different areas of tear distribution; for example, a horizontal line at the junction of the upper two-thirds and the lower one-third of the cornea (Hudson–Stahli Iine), a complete or partial ring at the base of the cone in keratoconus (Fleischer ring), an arclike deposition adjacent to a filtering bleb (Ferry line), or an arclike area adjacent to a pterygium (Stocker line). An iron line may form irregularity in any area of corneal surface, which disrupts tear distribution. Stellate iron lines may be seen in radial keratotomy, whereas central iron deposition may be seen in phototherapeutic keratectomy beds as either a central dot or surrounding central islands. Iron may also be deposited in a dense, rust-colored area where a ferruginous foreign body has been removed. In darkly pigmented patients, limbal conjunctival melanosis may result in injection of melanin pigment into the juxtalimbal corneal epithelium; the pigment then spreads onto the corneal surface in a whorl-1-like pattern, creating striate melanokeratitis. In a white adult patient with an acquired brown conjunctival plaque or nodule adjacent to the limbus, the adjacent corneal epithelium and stroma may be pigmented. In acquired melanosis, there is injection of melanin into the adjacent corneal epithelium, causing a whorl-like or plaque distribution. With an adjacent conjunctival-pigmented nodule, frank corneal stromal invasion by presumed malignant melanoma is possible. In more highly pigmented races, inflammation surrounding a squamous cell carcinoma may result in pigment deposition, rendering the lesion brown or black. This same pigment deposition may spread onto adjacent corneal areas. Drug-induced or metabolic verticillata may occasionally appear brown.

B. Gray-white epithelial opacities in a variety of distributions suggest superficial punctate keratitis (see Chapter 74).

C. Long-term use of amiodarone, chlorpromazine, chloroquine, tamoxifen, or indomethacin can cause epithelial deposits arranged in a whorl-like pattern usually centered on the inferior two-thirds of the cornea.

The deposits are bilateral, and gradually disappear with cessation of therapy. Amiodarone hydrochloride specifically results in corneal microdeposits in the majority of adults treated and can result in symptoms including visual halos or blurred vision in up to 10% of patients. Prolonged exposure to Amiodarone hydrochloride can sometimes result in a blue-gray pigmentation, but this is only of cosmetic significance. The appearance of the mentioned drugs is indistinguishable from that seen in X-linked α-galactosidase deficiency (Fabry disease). Fabry disease is an X-linked recessive inborn error of metabolism characterized by elevated urinary ceramide trihexoside levels. The cornea shows dust-like epithelial deposits in a whorl-like distribution. Vision is unaffected. Associated ocular findings include tortuous vessels in the conjunctiva and retina, as well as lens opacities. Systemic manifestation includes cutaneous angiokeratomas in a bathing suit distribution. Female carriers may be detected by a leukocyte α-galactosidase assay that shows levels to be reduced to 15-40% of normal.

D. Intraepithelial deposits may be found in Meesmann dystrophy consisting of 'peculiar' substance. Ophthalmic ointment used in the treatment of corneal abrasions and mucin may become temporarily trapped in intraepithelial cysts. Epithelial cysts may also be found in recurrent erosion syndromes, as well as in certain forms of acanthamoeba epithelitis and microsporidia infection.

E. Urate keratopathy may produce an orange-brown band keratopathy in addition to corneal crystals. Although more common in the conjunctiva, adrenochrome deposition from the use of topical epinephrine or, more uncommonly, dipivefrin may appear near the limbus as black subepithelial deposits. Spheroidal degeneration manifests as brown subepithelial nodules in the interpalpebral zone and may look similar to adrenochrome deposition. Alkaptonuria (ochronosis) is an autosomal-recessive disorder characterized by the absence of the enzyme homogentisic acid oxidase. The primary ocular manifestations are brown pigmentation of the sclera and episclera, especially at the insertions of the horizontal recti. In peripheral anterior corneal stroma, however, focal accumulations of light brown to black pinhead-size droplets may be seen. Vision is unaffected.

F. In degenerative diseases affecting the anterior segment (e.g., chronic iridocyclitis), calcium may accumulate, forming deposits in Bowman membrane. Initially, these deposits cause a peripheral ground-glass haze at the temporal and nasal horizontal meridian. With progression, the haze extends and becomes more opaque centrally. This may also result from the use of topical phosphate-containing medications. Other ocular medications (e.g. ciprofloxacin) may precipitate in chronic epithelial defects. Gelatinous deposits as found in Salzmann nodular degeneration and amyloid deposition may create grayish-blue subepithelial nodules. Excess basement membrane elements may accumulate in Reis-Buckler dystrophy and other basement membrane dystrophies.

G. In the rare amino acid disorder tyrosinemia type 2, caused by tyrosine aminotransferase deficiency, infants present with recurrent episodes of superficial central corneal ulceration. Characteristically, these ulcers assume stellate, pseudodendritic, or geographic patterns. With time, a central corneal opacity with thickening develops in the epithelium and subepithelial space. The corneal lesions may provide evidence for an early diagnosis. If the diagnosis is made early enough, dietary restriction of tyrosine results in resolution of the corneal opacities.

H. Long-term use of phenothiazine may result in deposition of yellow-white granules in the central corneal stroma at the level of Descemet membrane. A more common ocular finding is deposition of similar fine granules in a dendriform pattern beneath the anterior lens capsule. The most serious ocular finding is a bull's eye pigmentary maculopathy. Large hyphemas with elevated intraocular pressure refractory to treatment often result in deposition of hemoglobin and later hemosiderin in the corneal stroma. The pigmentation may appear rusty to greenish black to greenish yellow. Characteristically, bloodstaining is most dense centrally and clears from the peripheral cornea, closest to the limbal vasculature. Bilirubinemia may cause deposits in the deep corneal stroma, beginning in the periphery from the limbal circulation. Conjunctival involvement normally precedes corneal involvement. Siderosis from a retained intraocular foreign body or, less commonly, from hemochromatosis causes brown iron deposition in the posterior stroma.

I. With aging or in rare disorders affecting lipoprotein levels, cholesterol and phospholipids may accumulate in the peripheral corneal stroma. The accumulation begins superiorly and inferiorly and later spreads circumferentially. Vision is unaffected. Refer patients less than 40 years with corneal arcus formation for lipoprotein electrophoresis and fasting lipid profile; unilateral arcus may indicate contralateral ocular ischemic disease. Arcus senilis is a disease involving lipid deposition in the corneal stroma, with a clear zone of cornea separating the arcus border from the limbus. Schnyder corneal dystrophy is the accumulation of cholesterol in the corneal stroma, resulting in a gray-white haze with scattered crystals. Bilateral, diffuse, corneal clouding appearing to affect all layers in a child prompts an evaluation for metabolic storage diseases. Mucopolysaccharidoses I.H (Hurler), I.S (Scheie), I. HIS (Hurler-Scheie), IV-A (Morquio-classic),

IV-B (Morquio-like), VI-A (Maroteaux-Lamy), VI-B (Maroteaux-Lamy, mild form), and VII (glucuronidase deficiency) all have variable degrees of corneal clouding. Mucolipidoses (ML), ML I, ML I variant, ML II, ML III, ML IV, metachromatic leukodystrophy, mannosidosis, and fucosidosis have corneal clouding. The most severe clouding is seen in ML III and ML IV.

J. In an asymptomatic patient receiving gold salts for rheumatoid arthritis, yellow-brown granules possibly containing a metallic tint may be located in the cornea and conjunctiva, known as ocular chrysiasis. The deposition of gold is located in the posterior stroma and Descemet membrane and may disappear after cessation of therapy. Vision is unaffected. Various colored pigments can also be introduced intentionally into the stroma to hide corneal scars and decrease glare in patients with large iris defects. Stromal cystine crystals can be found in cystinosis (*see* Chapter 84).

K. Golden-brown, greenish-yellow, or blue-green pigmentation at the level of Descemet membrane in the corneal periphery is usually caused by copper deposition. Typically, the deposition begins as a superior arcus, later accumulates inferiorly, and then forms a complete ring involving the entire corneal periphery extending to the limbus. If there is accompanying neurologic and hepatic disease (Wilson disease), the ring is called a *Kayser-Fleischer ring*, a brown, green, or red band in the cortex beneath the anterior capsule (Sunflower cataract). However, patients with non-Wilsonian liver disease may have similar peripheral pigmented rings. Pigmentation resolves with chelation therapy. Intraocular copper foreign bodies with >85% copper content will cause chalcosis. Chalcosis is very similar in appearance to Wilson disease but is unilateral. Greenish-gray posterior stromal deposition of mercury can be found after long-term exposure to mercurial vapors. Both superficial and deep deposition can be found with old topical phenylmercurial nitrate medications. The inherited muscular dystrophy, myotonic dystrophy, results in multicolored opacities behind the anterior capsule (Christmas-tree cataract).

L. Long-term exposure to silver containing compounds may result in a gray-blue-green discoloration of Descemet membrane and deep stroma. Because silvercontaining eye drops are seldom used, cases of argyrosis in developed countries are usually related to industrial exposure to organic silver salts. X-linked ichthyosis may cause deep stromal gray-white opacities shaped as punctuation marks.

M. A fine dusting of brown pigment in a vertical spindle pattern on the endothelial surface—a Krukenberg spindle—is a characteristic feature of pigmentary dispersion syndrome. Accompanying findings include myopia, slit-like transillumination defects of the iris, and pigment dispersion upon mydriasis (*see* Chapter 26). Some patients have a secondary glaucoma. Intraocular surgery and blunt and penetrating trauma may result in iridocorneal touch, transferring pigment to the endothelium. Similarly, anterior uveitis and Fuchs dystrophy may result in endothelial pigment phagocytosis. Regarding Fuchs dystrophy, the patient experiences glare and blurred vision worst upon awakening, with symptoms rarely appearing before the age of 50 years.

N. Gray-white endothelial replacement may occur, extending from a site of surgical or traumatic ocular perforation, with epithelial or fibrous downgrowth. Prognosis is usually poor. Bilateral endothelial opacities consisting of vesicles and scalloping, sometimes associated with iris abnormalities, may be found in posterior polymorphous dystrophy. Unilateral findings may indicate iridocorneal endothelial syndrome.

O. At the Descemet membrane level, a mottled cyan-colored corneal opacity has been found in soft contact lens wearers. Located in the peripheral and mid-peripheral cornea, this opacity is likely associated with long-term contact lens wear.

P. Clofazimine may result in pigmentation of the conjunctiva and cornea, and fine brown lines resembling those of chloroquine keratopathy have been observed in psoriatic patients. These symptoms are reversible.

Q. Albinism can cause an inherited corneal dystrophy involving a noninflammatory bilateral opacity. In particular, 30% of ocular albinism 1 patients have normal skin but posterior embryotoxon, suggesting anterior segment dysgenesis, as well as fundus hypopigmentation.

BIBLIOGRAPHY

1. Arffa R, (Ed).Grayson's Diseases of the Cornea, 3rd Edition. St Louis, MA: Mosby; 1991. pp. 364-409.
2. Barraquer-Somers F, Chan CC, Green WR. Corneal epithelial iron deposition. Ophthalmology. 1983;90:729-34.
3. Duane TO, (Ed). Clinical Ophthalmology. Philadelphia, PA: Harper & Row; 1985.
4. Gerstenblith A, Rabinowitz M. The Wills Eye Manual, 6th Edition. Philadelphia, PA: Lippincott Williams & Wilkins; 2012.
5. Arffa RC. Grayson' Disease of the Cornea: 4th Edition. Mosby Year, St. Louis. 1997.
6. Krachmer JH, Mannis MJ, Holland EJ, (Eds). Cornea, 3rd Edition (Vol 1). St. Louis, MA: Mosby; 2010. pp. 299, 417-28,897-924.
7. Krueger RR, Tersi I, Seiler T. Corneal iron line associated with steep central islands after photorefractive keratectomy. J Refract Surg. 1997;13:401-3.
8. Spencer WH, (Ed). Ophthalmic Pathology: An Atlas and Text Book. Philadelphia, PA: WB Saunders; 1986. pp. 369-80.
9. Steinberg EB, Wilson LA, Waring GO Ill, et al. Stellate iron lines in the corneal epithelium after radial keratotomy. Am J Ophthalmol. 1984;98:416-21.

Corneal Crystals

84

Mark L McDermott, Lindsay T Davis

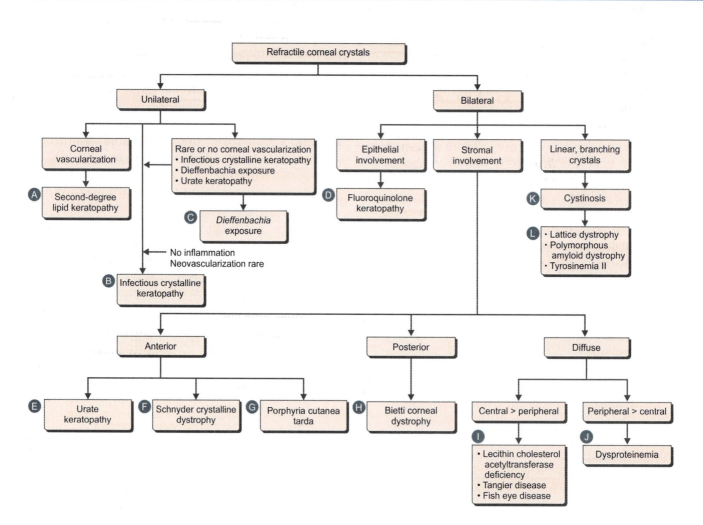

The discovery of crystals in the cornea may be expected, as in known cases of infantile cystinosis, or totally unexpected, as in cases of undiagnosed plasma cell dyscrasias. Careful attention to the location and distribution of the crystals is useful in considering diagnostic possibilities.

A. *Second-degree lipid keratopathy:* Accumulation of cholesterol and other lipids that leak from incompetent blood vessels leads to stromal neovascularization with unilateral, large, white crystals. This is usually discovered in corneas with a history of chronic corneal transplant rejection, infectious keratitis, or interstitial keratitis. Argon laser to the feeder vessels may be performed if the crystals involve the visual axis.

B. *Infectious crystalline keratopathy:* Patients with predisposing risk factors such as prior penetrating keratoplasty (PKP), history of topical or systemic steroid or other immunosuppression, or contact lens use may have unilateral, gray-white, branching accumulations of crystals, indicative of infectious crystalline keratopathy. This is most commonly caused by alpha hemolytic *Streptococcus* species (*S. viridans*), whose chains of bacteria appear crystalline, or by coagulase-negative *Staphylococcus*, *Acanthamoeba*, or fungi, whose branching hyphae may resemble crystals. Little to no inflammation is present, and neovascularization is not typically seen unless the disease is long standing. Diagnosis requires culture or biopsy. Treatment involves cessation of steroid and initiation of hourly fortified broad-spectrum antibiotics, or a fluoroquinolone alone if <3 mm in size, peripheral, and not associated with corneal thinning. It is thought that bacterial deposition of a biofilm confers a protective environment, requiring higher concentrations of antibiotic. If antibiotic therapy is not effective, lamellar keratectomy, neodymium-doped yttrium aluminum garnet (Nd:YAG) laser to disrupt the biofilm, or PKP is indicated.

C. *Dieffenbachia exposure:* A common houseplant of the species *Dieffenbachia* may eject high-speed, needlelike calcium oxalate crystals into the cornea and conjunctiva, creating a keratoconjunctivitis. Similar symptoms may be seen in the oral mucosa.

D. *Fluoroquinolone medications:* Fluoroquinolones, in particular ciprofloxacin, have been noted to cause diffuse corneal crystalline deposits. Diagnosis is made clinically in an eye treated with such medications and resolves without sequela after the medication is discontinued.

E. *Urate keratopathy:* Brown or yellow scintillating urate crystals in the interpalpebral epithelium extending to the limbus are typical of urate (gout) keratopathy. In some instances, crystals are found in the anterior corneal stroma. There is associated conjunctival hyperemia, which may be severe. These crystals may be irritating, causing erosions or vascularization. Simple epithelial debridement or phototherapeutic keratectomy (PTK) can result in substantial improvement in vision, though deposits may recur. The crystals may become confluent leading to a pigmented band keratopathy. The serum uric acid level is almost always elevated. Ocular manifestations may be improved with systemic gout treatment.

F. *Schnyder crystalline dystrophy:* Schnyder crystalline dystrophy, also called stromal crystalline dystrophy, is a rare autosomal-dominant disorder characterized by central accumulations of fine, polychromatic, randomly oriented, needlelike crystals at the level of Bowman layer and the anterior stroma. This was initially thought to be a stationary disease after childhood, but recent reports have demonstrated significant progression. Prominent arcus lipoides is characteristic of this dystrophy. Bilateral disciform central opacities may also be seen. The overlying epithelium is uninvolved, and the intervening areas of stroma are usually clear. The crystals consist of predominantly cholesterol esters and are strongly correlated with hypercholesterolemia. There is no definite association between ocular manifestations and the level of hyperlipidemia, but investigation should include a systemic work-up with a fasting lipid profile. Diagnosis may be facilitated by the discovery of cholesterol crystals on specular microscopy. PTK or PKP is indicated when sufficient clouding has occurred to incapacitate the patient visually, though crystals may recur. Tissue obtained at keratoplasty for suspected cases of this disorder should be submitted as frozen sections for neutral fat (oil red O) staining. Dietary treatment improves systemic lipid levels, but has no effect on corneal deposition.

G. *Porphyria cutanea tarda:* In rare instances, patients with porphyria cutanea tarda have displayed white-tan nonrefractile crystals in Bowman layer at the peripheral cornea. Other corneal changes include diffuse opacification of Bowman layer and the deep stromal lamellae. These findings are associated with high levels of urinary porphyrins.

H. *Bietti's corneal dystrophy:* Bietti crystalline dystrophy is a rare autosomal-recessive condition exhibiting crystals in the superficial stroma in a paralimbal distribution. In the cases described, there was an association with retinal crystals, fundus albipunctatus, and choroidal sclerosis. This progressive disorder may lead to nyctalopia or visual field loss secondary to retinal disease.

I. *Dyslipidemias:* In the autosomal-recessive disorder of lecithin cholesterol acetyltransferase (LCAT) deficiency, free plasma cholesterol and lecithin are elevated. Ocular findings include diffuse, fine, gray dots at all stromal levels, and a dense peripheral arcus. Occasionally, crystals are present at the level of Descemet membrane peripheral to the area of arcus formation. Vision is rarely affected, but the disease may result in nebular stromal haze. Tangier disease and fish-eye disease are also autosomal-recessive disorders that result in significantly reduced high-density lipoprotein (HDL) levels with findings similar to LCAT deficiency.

J. *Dysproteinemias:* Hypergammaglobulinemia states, including multiple myeloma, benign monoclonal gammopathy, cryoglobulinemia, Waldenström macroglobulinemia, dysproteinemia, and paraproteinemia are all associated with bilateral cornea opacities. These opacities consist of amorphous and crystallized immunoglobulin. Immunoglobulin crystals may appear as polychromatic, fine, punctate, or needlelike. They may be present in all levels and locations in the cornea. Noncrystalline corneal opacities have also been described, such as band keratopathy associated with hypercalcemia, or copper deposition in Descemet membrane. Associated findings include tortuosity of the conjunctival vasculature, conjunctival crystals, pars plana cysts, and hyperviscosity retinopathy.

K. *Cystinosis:* The presence of sparkling polychromatic crystals in the anterior corneal stroma of a photophobic child with growth retardation and renal failure is highly suggestive of type 1 (infantile) cystinosis. The disease results in intralysosomal accumulation of cystine and crystal formation in many locations, primarily the kidney and the eye. The corneal crystals are needle shaped with sharp edges, and are more concentrated in the peripheral corneal stroma, where they are present in both anterior and posterior stroma. They are less concentrated centrally and tend to lie more superficially in the stroma here. Recurrent erosions may occur secondary to the anterior location of some deposits.

Associated ocular findings include crystal formation in the conjunctiva, sclera, extraocular muscles, aqueous humor, and uvea. Conjunctival and corneal crystals are pathognomonic for cystinosis. A pigmentary retinopathy may precede crystal formation. In type 2 (juvenile) and type 3 (adult) cystinosis, the systemic manifestations are less severe, and in the adult form, corneal crystals may be the only finding. Biopsy specimens must be placed in absolute ethanol to prevent dissolution of the crystals, though invasive conjunctival biopsies are rarely necessary. Oral cysteamine stabilizes retinal frequency, but has little effect on corneal disease. Treatment involves oral cysteamine, which stabilizes renal function and decreases cystinotic retinal frequency, but typically has little effect on corneal disease. The use of topical cysteamine 0.5% has been proven safe and effective in dissolving corneal crystals and relieving eye pain. If conservative treatment fails, PKP is indicated, though cystine crystals may recur.

L. *Long crystalline keratopathies:* Long, linear branching refractile crystals are found in amyloid deposition in the form of lattice dystrophy and polymorphous amyloid dystrophy. The location of the branching filaments varies in lattice dystrophy types I–III, with type II having significant systemic manifestations including blepharochalasis, pendulous ears, and cranial, peripheral, and autonomic neuropathies. Tyrosinemia type II (Richner–Hanhart syndrome) may also exhibit long branching lines in the superficial stroma with pseudodendrites and superficial plaques. These may resemble herpetic dendrites; however, those in tyrosinemia do not stain with fluoroscein. This autosomal-recessive disorder is caused by a deficiency in tyrosine aminotransferase and causes painful skin blisters and variable central nervous system manifestations such as mental retardation, nystagmus, and epilepsy. Diagnosis is made with elevated tyrosine levels in the blood and urine and is treatable with a low tyrosine, low phenylalanine diet. Reduction in corneal opacities may occur with this treatment with subsequent improvement in vision.

BIBLIOGRAPHY

1. American Academy of Ophthalmology. Basic and clinical science course: External disease and cornea. San Francisco: American Academy of Ophthalmology, 2011;8:159-60, 268-85.
2. Arrfa R, (Ed). Grayson's Diseases of the Cornea, 3rd Edition. St Louis: Mosby, 1991. pp. 364-401.
3. Awwad ST, et al. Corneal intrastromal gatifloxacin crystal deposits after penetrating keratoplasty. Eye Contact Lens. 2004;30:169.
4. Jones NP, Postlethwaite RJ, Noble JL. Clearance of corneal crystals in nephropathic cystinosis by topical cysteamine 0.5%. Br J Ophthalmol. 1991;75:311-2.
5. Kaufman HE, Barron BA, McDonald MB, et al. The Cornea. New York: Churchill Livingstone, 1988. pp. 361-82.
6. Krachmer JH, Mannis MJ, Holland EJ. Cornea: Fundamentals, Diagnosis and Management, 3rd Edition. St Louis: Mosby, 2011.
7. Meisler DM, Langston RHS, Naab TJ, et al. Infectious crystalline keratopathy. Am J Ophthalmol. 1984;97:337-43.
8. Seet B, Chan WK, Ang CL. Crystalline keratopathy from *Dieffenbachia* plant sap. Br J Ophthalmol. 1995;79:98-9.
9. Spencer WH. Ophthalmic Pathology: A Textbook and Atlas. Philadelphia: WB Saunders, 1985. pp. 363-7.
10. Weisenthal RW, Krachmer JH, Folberg R, et al. Postkeratoplasty crystalline deposits mimicking bacterial infectious crystalline keratopathy. Am J Ophthalmol. 1988;105:70-4.

Corneal Epithelial Dystrophy

85

Maria Q Husain, Richard W Yee

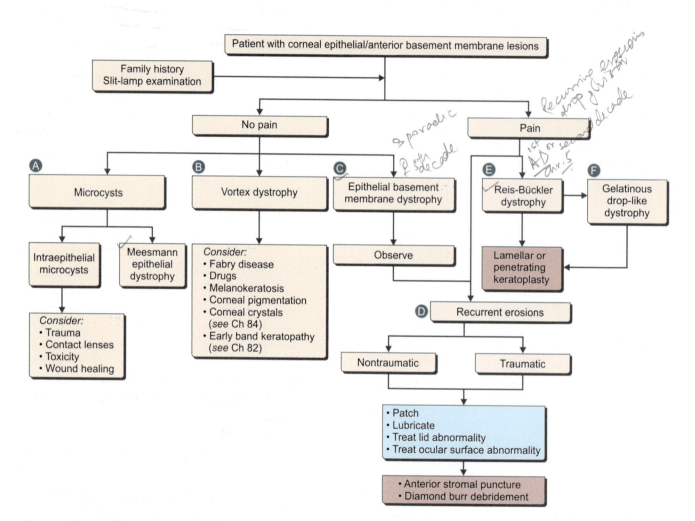

Corneal dystrophies are generally bilateral, symmetric, and inherited conditions without systemic associations or effects from the environment. They are usually slowly progressive and become more apparent with age. The epithelial dystrophies consist of abnormalities in the epithelium, basement membrane, and Bowman layer. Patient history, family history, and slit-lamp examination of the patient and the patient's immediate family members aid in the diagnosis, genetic pattern, and classification. It is well documented that some of the corneal dystrophies can occur spontaneously and be subsequently transmitted.

A. Intraepithelial microcysts can occur confluently or in isolated groups, either unilaterally or bilaterally, depending on the associated cause. They can be associated with localized areas of epithelial healing or recurrent erosions. Cystic spaces can occur in the epithelium with or without corneal edema. Typically, no staining occurs with fluorescein. Microcysts are nonspecific responses of the epithelium and occur with contact lens wear and long-term drug use. Typically, no symptoms occur unless there are actual epithelial erosions from the microcyst. Treatment consists of resolving the associated conditions. Meesmann epithelial dystrophy [autosomal dominant (AD), also called *Stocker-Holt dystrophy*] can have incomplete penetrance and is evident in the first few months of life. Most mutations are keratin 3 and 12 gene abnormalities. Patients are generally asymptomatic, demonstrating anterior epithelial cysts, which, on retro-illumination, appear as small, clear to gray-white punctate precipitates, mainly in the interpalpebral area. The cysts consist of degenerated epithelial cell products, "peculiar" substance on electron microscopy, which is PAS positive on light microscopy. Lisch epithelial corneal dystrophy (X-chromosomal dominant) presents with almost confluent microcysts as gray, band-shaped feathery opacities in a whorled pattern. Immunohistochemistry reveals scattered Ki67 staining. No treatment is necessary unless irritation or decreased vision occurs.

B. Vortex keratopathy, or *cornea verticillata*, presents with pigmented whorl-shaped lines in the epithelial and subepithelial tissues. These have been seen in Fabry disease, in toxic keratopathy, and in patients who are taking a variety of systemic medications such as amiodarone, chloroquine, hydroxychloroquine, indomethacin, phenothiazines, gentamicin, or tamoxifen. Striate melanokeratosis can also mimic vortex keratopathy. Melanotic cells growing from the limbus, particularly in African Americans, can also penetrate the central cornea as a response to a variety of noxious stimuli. Treatment is seldom necessary.

C. Anterior epithelial basement membrane dystrophy is also called *map-dot-fingerprint dystrophy, anterior basement membrane dystrophy,* and *Cogan microcystic dystrophy* (often sporadic but can be AD with incomplete expression). It is bilateral and epithelial, and is characterized by various patterns of dots, lines, and irregularities. It occurs more commonly in women after the fifth decade of life. Histopathologically, a thickened basement membrane extending into the epithelium, abnormal epithelial cells with microcysts, and fibrillar material between the basement membrane and the Bowman layer is seen. Most patients are asymptomatic. Common symptoms, when present, are blurring of vision and foreign body sensation.

Recurrent erosions can occur in about 10% of the patients, typically in the early mornings, when the patient awakens and experiences a sharp, stabbing pain. Treatment is necessary only when recurrent erosions occur.

D. Recurrent corneal erosions typically follow corneal trauma that involves the epithelium and the epithelial basement membrane. They can also occur with anterior basement membrane dystrophy. The disorder results from defects in the basement membrane healing, or failed or faulty production by the basement membrane. Symptoms can occur days to years after the injury. Treatment is aimed at encouraging re-epithelialization and at preventing recurrences. Acute erosions are treated with topical antibiotics, cycloplegic drops, and a pressure patch. Sometimes, 5% sodium chloride may help promote adherence of the epithelial cells to the underlying tissue to minimize epithelial edema. Lubricating ointments without preservatives are helpful, especially in patients with lagophthalmos. Treatment should continue to minimize recurrences and allow repair of the abnormal basement membrane. If recurrences persist, contact lenses may be helpful. Anterior stromal puncture has also been advocated in patients in whom other modes of therapy have failed. Debridement of abnormal epithelium may be effective occasionally when accompanied by the use of a diamond bur on the irregular surface of the anterior basement membrane. Phototherapeutic keratectomy into the anterior 2–4 μm of Bowman membrane can be effective for recurrent or central erosions.

E. Reis-Bückler dystrophy (AD) mainly affects the central Bowman membrane. Reis-Bückler dystrophy has also been reported to occur spontaneously, and is subsequently transmitted as a mutation on Chromosome 5. The dystrophy is bilaterally symmetric, and becomes evident in the first or second decade of life, with recurring erosions and decreased vision. Phenotypes can vary based on the history or erosions and effects of wound healing creating scar and variable slit-lamp findings. The coarse geographic opacities spare the peripheral 2 mm of the cornea. Slit-lamp examination demonstrates irregular epithelium with subepithelial fibrous tissue in the region of Bowman layer, with sparing of the posterior cornea. Histologically, a sheet-like connective tissue that has granular Masson trichrome-red deposits replaces the Bowman membrane. Electron-dense, rod-shaped bodies are present on transmission electron microscopy, distinguishing it from the curly fibers seen in Thiel-Behnke dystrophy. Thiel-Behnke dystrophy (AD) begins in the first or second decade of life. It is bilateral with reticular, or honeycomb-like opacities that spare the peripheral cornea. The genes for Thiel-Behnke dystrophy have been reported on Chromosomes 5 and 10. On light microscopy, thickened epithelium and replacement of the Bowman layer with a fibrocellular material in a wavy 'saw-toothed' pattern occurs. Treatment is similar to that for recurrent erosions. A lamellar keratoplasty or penetrating keratoplasty can be performed. Recurrence in the graft is common.

F. Patients with gelatinous drop-like dystrophy (autosomal recessive) present with photophobia, tearing, foreign body sensation, and impaired visual acuity in the first decade of life as a result of protuberant, opaque, subepithelial nodules that are located centrally and give the cornea a 'mulberry-like' irregular surface. Alternatively, symptoms may

stem from a band keratopathy-like appearance. Larger nodular lesions, or kumquat-like lesions, with stromal vascularization can occur. Amyloid deposits are present in subepithelial and stromal cells on light microscopy. Lamellar keratoplasty or penetrating keratoplasty can be performed; recurrences are common.

BIBLIOGRAPHY

1. Miller CA, Krachmer JH. Epithelial and stromal dystrophies. In: Kaufman H, Barron B, McDonald M, (Eds). The Cornea. Boston, MA: Butterworth-Heinemann; 1998.
2. Munier FL, Schorderet DF. Classification of corneal dystrophies on a molecular genetic basis. In: Reinhard T, Larkin F, (Eds). Cornea and External Eye Disease. Heidelberg, Germany: Springer; 2008.
3. Ramamurthi S, Rahman MQ, Dutton GN, et al. Pathogenesis, clinical features and management of recurrent corneal erosions. Eye. 2006;20:635-44.
4. Weiss JS, Møller HU, Lisch W, et al. The IC3D classification of the corneal dystrophies. Cornea. 2008; 27(Suppl 2):S6.
5. Zhao XC, Nakamura H, Subramanyam S, et al. Spontaneous and inheritable R555Q mutation in the *TGFBI/BIGH3* gene in two unrelated families exhibiting Bowman's layer corneal dystrophy. Ophthalmology. 2007;114:e39-e46.

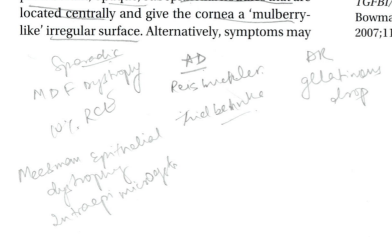

Sporadic
MDF dystrophy
w/c RCE

Meesman Epithelial dystrophy
Intraepi microcysts

AD
Reis-Bucklers.
Thiel-behnke.

AR
gelatinous drop

Corneal Stromal Dystrophy

Maria Q Husain, Richard W Yee

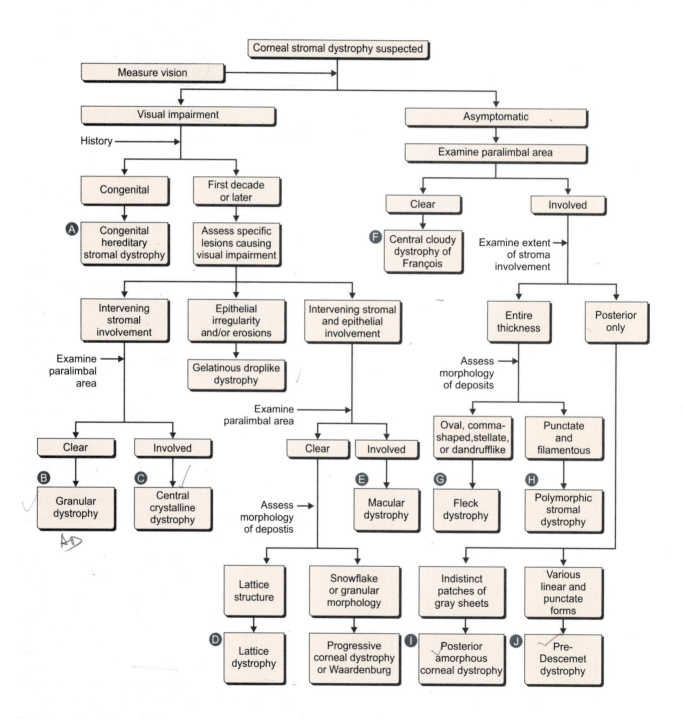

Corneal stromal dystrophies generally involve a genetically transmitted metabolic defect, which results in the deposition of an excessive amount of some metabolic product in the keratocytes. The accumulation of these deposits causes signs and symptoms ranging from essentially asymptomatic opacities to complete functional visual impairment. Characteristic histopathologic findings have led to further understanding. Accurately diagnosing a specific dystrophy early in its course better prepares both the physician and the patient to manage the condition as it progresses.

A. Present at birth, congenital hereditary stromal dystrophy [autosomal dominant (AD)] manifests with bilateral, symmetric, nonprogressive, and cloudy opacification of the stroma. The flaky or feathery opacities are most dense in the superficial central stroma, becoming progressively less dense in the peripheral regions. Epithelial and endothelial cells remain unaffected. The early visual impairment may result in nystagmus, esotropia, and amblyopia. Very early penetrating keratoplasty (PK) should be considered.

B. In granular dystrophy (AD) (Fig. 86.1), white-gray, bread-crumb-like opacities develop in the superficial central corneal stroma during the first decade of life. The opacities enlarge, coalesce, increase in number, and extend into the deeper stroma as the disease progresses, and these usually occur in the fourth or fifth decade of life. At that time, a diffuse ground-glass haze appears in the intervening stroma, resulting in the onset of visual impairment. A 2- to 3-mm area of peripheral cornea remains clear, and the epithelial erosions are rare but occur more often once the opacities coalesce. The opacities consist of a hyaline substance that is best seen on Masson trichrome staining, and are bilateral and symmetric. Corneal thickness remains stable. If visual acuity is affected, deep anterior lamellar keratoplasty (DALK) or PK have a good prognosis, but recurrence in the graft may occur several years later. Granular corneal dystrophy type 2 (Avellino dystrophy, AD) consists of deposits similar to those seen in granular and lattice dystrophies, both clinically and histologically. These patients have snowflake-like, stellate opacities in the superficial to mid stroma, and lattice lines deeper in the stroma. Anterior stromal haze increases with increasing age. Depending

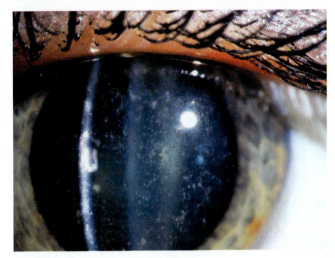

Fig. 86.1: Granular corneal dystrophy.

on the depth of the deposits, phototherapeutic keratectomy, lamellar keratoplasty, or PK can be performed. LASIK and LASEK are contraindicated as they may result in increased opacification.

C. In central stromal crystalline corneal dystrophy (also Schnyder corneal dystrophy, AD), minute polychromatic crystals, arranged in a discoid or ring configuration, appear in the central superficial stroma during the first year of life. Patients (80%) develop a limbal girdle and a dense corneal arcus by the third decade. Corneal sensation is decreased. Treatment is necessary in most patients over the age of 50 years as this reduces the photopic vision relatively more than the scotopic vision. PK is usually the treatment of choice; recurrences can occur in the graft. The crystals consist largely of cholesterol, which can be seen with Oil Red O staining. The disorder is often associated with hyperlipidemia and genu valgum. Therefore, serum cholesterol and triglyceride levels should be evaluated in these patients.

D. In lattice dystrophy (AD), a branched lattice network of refractile lines, white punctate opacities, and a diffuse central superficial stromal haze appear during the first and second decades of life. Recurrent, painful epithelial erosions also occur. Visual acuity deteriorates progressively through the fourth and fifth decades of life as central subepithelial opacities develop. The peripheral cornea remains clear, except in extreme cases. PK is often necessary, and recurrences of the disease within donor grafts are common. The opacities contain amyloid deposits that are best seen with Congo red staining. The lattice lines fluoresce under cobalt blue (365 nm) ultraviolet light in advanced cases. Lattice dystrophy type 2 (Meretoja syndrome, AD), associated with systemic amyloidosis, has mainly been described in Finnish patients, and has a more favorable visual outcome. Type 3 [autosomal recessive (AR)] and type 3A (AD) have also been described.

E. In macular dystrophy (AR), diffuse, central, superficial, stromal cloudiness develops during the first decade of life. During the second decade, this diffuse ground-glass opacification extends to involve the posterior and peripheral stroma as well. Focal, irregular, white opacities develop by the third decade and extend to the limbus. Later in the disease, irregularities of Descemet membrane and endothelium are evidenced by guttae. Painless epithelial erosions are common. Visual acuity is often significantly impaired by the fourth decade. Corneal thickness is reduced. Tinted contact lenses may reduce photophobia. PK or DALK are often necessary by 30 years of age. DALK may produce less postoperative complications. Recurrences with donor grafts are less common than in granular and lattice dystrophies. The primary defect is the accumulation of excess mucopolysaccharides (glycosaminoglycans), seen with Alcian blue staining in the keratocytes.

F. In central cloudy dystrophy of François (unknown genetics), small, indistinct, ovoid opacities, most dense posteriorly and restricted to the central third of the cornea are the classic findings. It is phenotypically similar to posterior crocodile shagreen. Visual acuity is rarely impaired, and the opacities are usually incidental findings.

G. Fleck dystrophy (AD) is a benign disorder in which discrete, flat, white, dandruff-like flecks are present throughout all the stromal layers, involving both the central and peripheral regions. These opacities may be congenital. This disorder has been associated with cortical lens opacities in certain families, and in others, decreased corneal sensation has been described. Visual acuity remains normal.

H. Polymorphic stromal 'dystrophy' (polymorphic amyloid degeneration) is a degenerative disorder featuring gray-white punctate and filamentous opacities involving the entire cornea. Its appearance can be similar to lattice dystrophy; however, the intervening stroma is clear, no corneal sensation is lost, and erosions do not occur. Onset is after 50 years of age, and visual acuity is spared.

I. In posterior amorphous dystrophy (AD), gray, sheetlike opacifications are present at various levels of the posterior stroma, and involve the entire width of the cornea. The opacities are noted during the first decade, and this is slowly progressive to nonprogressive. This dystrophy is associated with corneal thinning, flattening, and anterior iris abnormalities. It rarely impairs visual acuity significantly. Descemet membrane and the endothelium can be involved by the opacities.

J. Pre-Descemet dystrophy (genetics unknown) is thought to represent a degenerative process, and includes four clinical types. Onset occurs between the fourth and seventh decades of life. Focal, fine, gray opacities are located in the deep stroma and may have various shapes and distributions. Visual acuity is not affected.

BIBLIOGRAPHY

1. Cheng J, Qi X, Zhao J, et al. Comparison of penetrating keratoplasty and deep lamellar keratoplasty for macular corneal dystrophy and risk factors for recurrence. Ophthalmology. 2013;120:34-9.
2. Kim TI, Hong JP, Ha BJ, et al. Determination of treatment strategies for granular corneal dystrophy type 2 using Fourier-domain optical coherence tomography. Br J Ophthalmol. 2010;94:341-5.
3. Miller CA, Krachmer JH. Epithelial and stromal dystrophies. In: Kaufman H, Barron B, McDonald M, (Eds). The Cornea. Boston, MA: Butterworth-Heinemann, 1998.
4. Munier FL, Schorderet DF. Classification of corneal dystrophies on a molecular genetic basis. In: Reinhard T, Larkin F, (Eds). Cornea and External Eye Disease. Heidelberg, Germany: Springer, 2008.
5. Weiss JS, Møller HU, Lisch W, et al. The IC3D classification of the corneal dystrophies. Cornea. 2008; 27(Suppl 2):S6.

Macular A R   1st
                Alecian blue
                gAge..

Granular AD   Masson trichrome
                                Hyaline
Avellino type 2
    AD
      Superficial - Stellate
                         opacity

      deeper - lattic line

Lattice -.   congo red
                  Amyloid

         RCE
    onset 1 - 2nd decade

Corneal Hypesthesia

87

Gary L Legault, Mark L McDermott

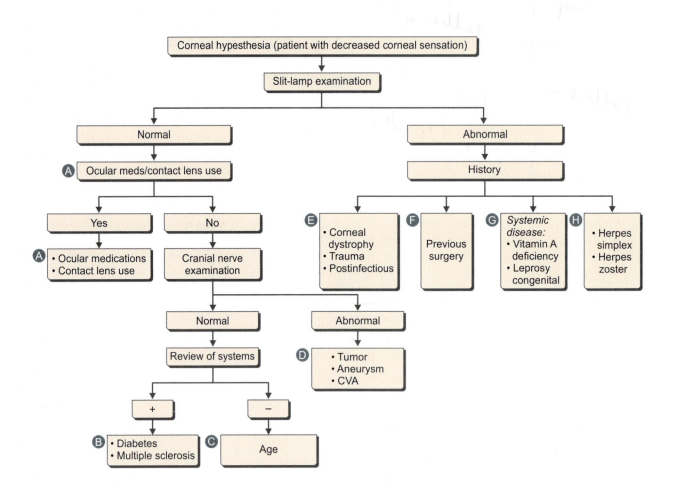

The ophthalmic division (V_1) of the cranial nerve V (CNV) provides the sensory innervation of the cornea. This division splits into three branches: lacrimal, frontal, and nasociliary. The nasociliary branch divides into long and short posterior ciliary nerves providing sensory innervation of the cornea, iris, and ciliary body, as well as motor innervation of the iris. Other portions of the nasociliary branch provide sensation to the conjunctiva, lacrimal drainage system, and skin of the nose. The long posterior ciliary nerves enter the cornea at the periphery and then travel radially, creating a plexus posterior to the Bowman's layer with branches extending anteriorly into the epithelium.

Corneal sensation is measured both qualitatively and quantitatively. The qualitative method is most commonly used and is typically performed using a cotton tip applicator rolled into a wisp. The quantitative method is performed using a handheld esthesiometer such as the Cochet–Bonnet shown in Figure 87.1. Sensation is measured in each quadrant of the cornea and compared with the fellow eye.

Adequate innervation of the cornea is critical in its maintenance and repair. The neurotrophic cornea is at risk of both infectious and noninfectious keratitis, as well as chronic epithelial defects and stromal lysis. Corneal hypesthesia has many systemic and local

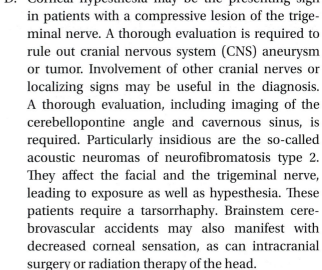

Fig. 87.1: Cochet-Bonnet handheld esthesiometer. A device used to quantitatively measure corneal sensation. (*Courtesy* of Dr. Joseph Zayac).

causes, making a detailed systemic and ophthalmic history critical in the diagnosis. Common etiologies in the differential include herpes simplex, herpes zoster, previous ocular surgery or trauma, topical medications, cerebellopontine-angle tumors, and dysautonomia.

A. Numerous ocular medications have been implicated in the loss of corneal sensation, most commonly: topical nonsteroidal antiinflammatory drugs (NSAIDs), beta-blockers, carbonic anhydrase inhibitors, and anesthetics. Beta-blockers impair corneal sensation by direct anesthetic action on the corneal nerves. Topical anesthetic use may lead to corneal hypesthesia or ulceration, and may mimic the appearance of infectious keratitis with infiltration and a chronic epithelial defect. Decreased corneal sensation is seen with long-term use of soft and gas permeable contact lens wear.

B. Diabetic patients develop hypesthesia with the severity often correlating with the duration as well as the type. Type 1 patients are at a higher risk than type 2 patients. Selective involvement of the portions of the trigeminal nerve will lead to isolated hypesthesia in patients with multiple sclerosis or myasthenia gravis.

C. Central corneal sensation is known to decrease, in the absence of other disease, with age. However, this rarely leads to clinical diseases and should be a diagnosis of exclusion. Exacerbating factors may include long-term environmental exposures to sun, wind, fumes, and other ocular irritants, which may contribute to desensitizing the cornea and ocular surface.

D. Corneal hypesthesia may be the presenting sign in patients with a compressive lesion of the trigeminal nerve. A thorough evaluation is required to rule out cranial nervous system (CNS) aneurysm or tumor. Involvement of other cranial nerves or localizing signs may be useful in the diagnosis. A thorough evaluation, including imaging of the cerebellopontine angle and cavernous sinus, is required. Particularly insidious are the so-called acoustic neuromas of neurofibromatosis type 2. They affect the facial and the trigeminal nerve, leading to exposure as well as hypesthesia. These patients require a tarsorrhaphy. Brainstem cerebrovascular accidents may also manifest with decreased corneal sensation, as can intracranial surgery or radiation therapy of the head.

E. Any corneal dystrophy with abnormal basement membrane disposition, such as lattice dystrophy and Reis–Buckler, can have decreased corneal sensation despite frequent painful erosions. In Fuchs endothelial dystrophy, decreased sensation develops following bullous keratopathy. Keratoconus will exhibit decreased sensation in areas of greatest thinning. Chronic corneal erosions may result in the loss of corneal sensation due to local trauma. In addition to trauma, local nerve damage can result from scarring secondary to acute and chronic infectious keratitis. An early presenting sign of *Acanthamoeba* can be corneal hypesthesia.

F. Any type of ocular surgery that interrupts the radial flow of sensory information from the cornea to the nasociliary nerve can result in corneal hypesthesia. Damage to the long ciliary nerves in panretinal photocoagulation may decrease corneal sensation. Keratoplasty, both penetrating and lamellar, results in early hypesthesia, with partial restoration of sensation after several years. Excimer photoablation and astigmatic keratotomy have been shown to reduce central corneal sensation, whereas radial incisions appear to preserve sensation. Sensation after laser-assisted in situ keratomileusis (LASIK) keratorefractive surgery appears to be greater than that after standard photorefractive keratectomy.

G. Many systemic diseases may include corneal hypesthesia with ocular involvement. Vitamin A deficiency may lead to keratoconjunctivitis sicca, conjunctival and corneal keratinization, epithelial defect, and stromal lysis. Leprosy results in large corneal nerves, scarring of the ocular adnexa, keratinization of the ocular surface, exposure, and corneal hypesthesia. Various types of hereditary sensory neuropathy and familial dysautonomia (Riley–Day syndrome) present with decreased corneal sensation at birth.

H. Herpetic disease is typically, but not exclusively, unilateral. The herpes viruses are neurotrophic, with most studies localizing their latency and reactivation to the trigeminal ganglion. Herpes simplex has the ability to manifest in many different forms. Initial infection commonly presents as a nonspecific conjunctivitis, with recurrences producing more profound symptoms of visual loss, pain, and keratitis. The loss of sensation in herpes simplex is characteristically more focal than with herpes zoster, and may result in metaherpetic or trophic ulcers. Herpes zoster virus (HZV) infection is more evident with the involvement and scarring of the adjacent structures supplied by the trigeminal ganglion in an acute setting. HZV corneal disease may precede, coincide with, or follow acute dermatologic disease by several weeks. Hypesthesia is often global, rather than focal, and may be severe, resulting in chronic epithelial defects and visual loss.

BIBLIOGRAPHY

1. Ben Osman N, Jeddi A, Sebai L, et al. The cornea of diabetics. J Fran Ophthalmol. 1995;18:120-3.
2. Campos M, Hertzog L, Garbus JJ, et al. Corneal sensitivity after photorefractive keratectomy. Am J Ophthalmol. 1992;114:51-4.
3. Glaser JS. Neuro-ophthalmology, 3rd Edition. Philadelphia, PA: Lippincott Williams and Wilkins; 1999. pp. 64-70.
4. Krachmer JH, Mannis M, Palay DA. Cornea. St Louis, MO: Mosby, 1996.
5. Lyne A. Corneal sensitivity after surgery. Trans Ophthalmol Soc UK. 1982;102:302-5.
6. Martin XY, Safran AB. Corneal hypoesthesia. Surv Ophthalmol. 1998;33:28-40.
7. Miller NR. Walsh and Hoyt's Clinical Neuro-ophthalmology, 4th Edition (Vol. 2). Baltimore, MD: Williams and Wilkins; 1985. p. 1056.
8. Myles WM, LaRoche GR. Congenital corneal anesthesia. Am J Ophthalmol. 1994;118:818-20.
9. Smolin G, Thoft RA, (Eds). The Cornea. New York, NY: Little, Brown; 1994. pp. 183-208, 490-2.
10. Van Buskirk EM. Corneal anesthesia after timolol maleate therapy. Am J Ophthalmol. 1979;88:739-43.

SECTION 5

Glaucoma and Intraocular Pressure Problems

Diagnosis of Glaucoma

Scott D Smith

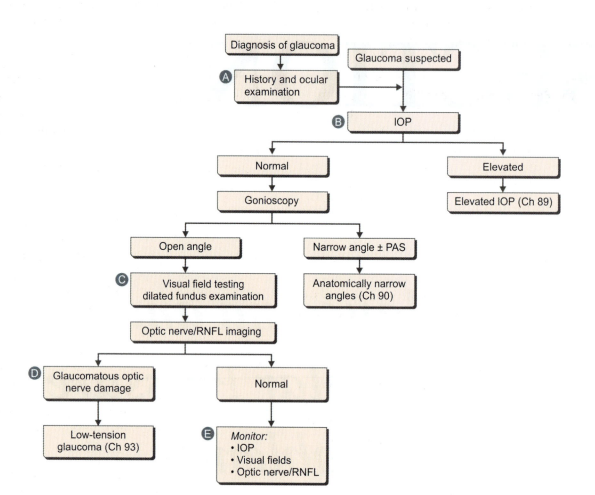

88

The diagnosis of glaucoma requires the identification of damage to the optic nerve in a characteristic, nerve fiber bundle pattern. If optic disc cupping and/or nerve fiber layer atrophy are moderate or advanced, corresponding visual field defects are present, and the diagnosis can be made with certainty. When the disease is less advanced, definitive diagnosis on a single examination is difficult because of the variability of the optic nerve appearance and intraocular pressure (IOP) in the normal population.

A. During the history and ophthalmic examination, factors that increase an individual's risk of having glaucomatous optic nerve damage should be identified. A family history of primary open-angle glaucoma (POAG), particularly in first-degree relatives, is associated with an increased risk of developing the disease. The prevalence of both POAG and primary angle-closure glaucoma (PACG) increases with age. POAG is about four times more common in individuals of African descent than in Caucasians. PACG appears to be more common in individuals of Asian descent. Diabetes and myopia appear to be associated with a greater risk of POAG. Episodic eye pain, redness, blurred vision, and/or seeing halos around lights should alert the clinician to possible intermittent angle closure. Gonioscopy must be performed to distinguish open from closed angles and to identify peripheral anterior synechiae.

B. Measurement of IOP is a poor method of glaucoma screening. Based on a single reading, as many as one-third of individuals with glaucoma have normal IOP, and many glaucoma patients consistently fall within the normal range. Furthermore, a substantial proportion of those with statistically elevated IOP may never experience optic nerve injury. Because of the variability in IOP over time and differences in susceptibility to pressure-related optic nerve damage within the population, a comprehensive ophthalmic examination is required to properly diagnose glaucoma. Although glaucoma may occur at any level of IOP, it is the primary target of current medical and surgical treatments.

C. When the anterior chamber angle is open and the IOP is normal, glaucoma may be suspected on the basis of the optic nerve appearance. Glaucomatous loss of optic nerve fibers leads to thinning of the neuroretinal rim, with a resultant increased size of the optic cup. Because normal eyes with small optic nerves tend to have a smaller cup/disc ratio, optic disc cupping should be considered in conjunction with the optic nerve size. In normally sized nerves, a cup/disc ratio of about 0.6 or greater may arouse suspicion of early glaucomatous damage. In eyes with small discs, glaucoma may be present with a much smaller cup/disc ratio. Imaging of the retinal nerve fiber layer (RNFL) by optical coherence tomography or scanning laser polarimetry may provide important clues to the presence of glaucomatous optic disc damage before changes in the optic disc or visual field are evident. Although damage from glaucoma may be diffuse, it is often asymmetric, both with respect to the upper and lower hemiretina within an eye and with respect to the contralateral eye. Therefore, the identification of vertical and/or contralateral asymmetry of the optic nerve and nerve fiber layer is important in evaluating cases of suspected glaucoma.

D. When glaucomatous optic nerve damage with visual field loss is present and the IOP is normal, intermittent IOP elevation should be considered as a part of the diagnostic evaluation. Visual field loss that does not correlate with glaucomatous optic nerve injury should prompt consideration of alternative diagnoses.

E. In the absence of definitive optic nerve or visual field abnormality, periodic clinical evaluation with serial optic nerve and/or RNFL imaging and visual field tests is required to confirm stability. Evidence of change in the optic disc or RNFL, the development of a visual field defect, or a rise in IOP should be considered in determining the need for treatment. The frequency of follow-up visits should be based on the level of suspicion for glaucoma. When multiple risk factors are present or when there is a risk of secondary open-angle glaucoma from pseudoexfoliation or pigment dispersion, closer follow-up may be advisable.

■BIBLIOGRAPHY

1. Airaksinen PJ, Tuulonen A, Werner EB. Clinical evaluation of the optic disc and retinal nerve fiber layer. In: Ritch R, Shields MB, Krupin T (Eds). The Glaucomas. St Louis, MO: Mosby; 1996. pp. 617-57.

2. Camejo L, Noecker RJ. Optic nerve imaging. In: Stamper RL, Lieberman MF, Drake MV, (Eds). Becker-Shaffer's Diagnosis and Therapy of the Glaucomas. Philadelphia, PA: Mosby Elsevier; 2009. pp. 171-87.

3. Tielsch JM, Katz J, Sommer A, et al. Family history and risk of primary open-angle glaucoma: The Baltimore eye survey. Arch Ophthalmol. 1994;112:69-73.

4. Tielsch JM, Sommer A, Katz J, et al. Racial variations in the prevalence of POAG: The Baltimore eye survey. JAMA. 1991;266:369-74.

5. Wilson MR, Martone JF. Epidemiology of chronic open-angle glaucoma. In: Ritch R, Shields MB, Krupin T (Eds). The Glaucomas. St. Louis, MO: Mosby; 1996. pp. 753-68.

Elevated Intraocular Pressure

89

Scott D Smith

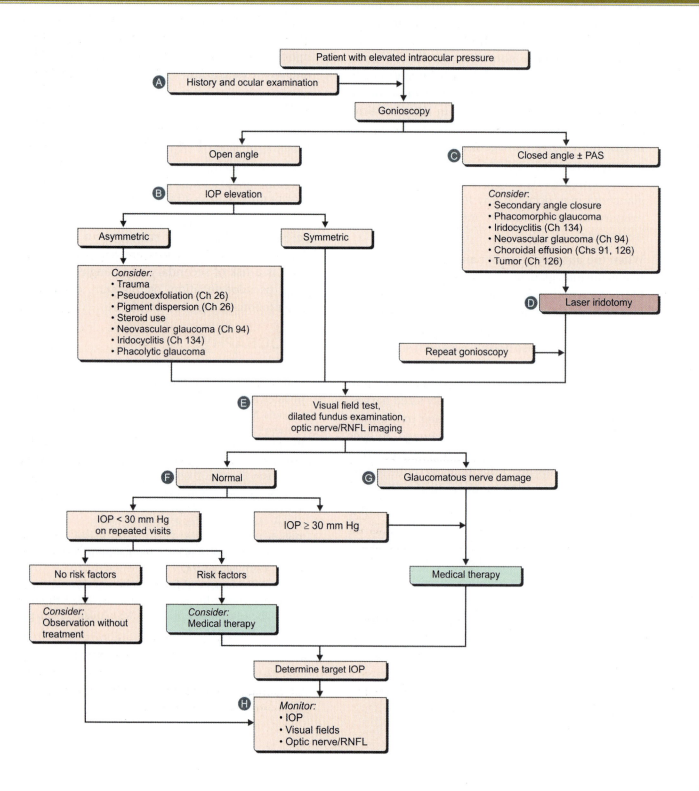

Elevated intraocular pressure (IOP) is an important risk factor for the development of glaucomatous optic nerve damage. Therefore, all patients with elevated IOP, traditionally defined as IOP ≥ 22 mmHg, require careful evaluation to determine the mechanism of IOP elevation and the presence and extent of optic nerve injury.

A. The first step in determining the mechanism of IOP elevation is a thorough history and slit-lamp examination. Patients may neglect reporting a distant history of ocular trauma or inflammation unless specifically questioned. Slit-lamp findings that provide evidence for secondary IOP elevation may be very subtle, and require careful observation by the clinician.

B. Primary open-angle glaucoma (POAG) is the most common form of glaucoma in the United States. In addition to the presence of an open anterior chamber angle on gonioscopy, the diagnosis of POAG requires the exclusion of any identifiable underlying cause for the IOP elevation. Asymmetry of IOP can be suggestive of the presence of a secondary form of glaucoma. However, unilateral or highly asymmetric IOP is occasionally seen in POAG and bilateral, symmetric secondary open-angle glaucoma is not uncommon. Therefore, the evaluation for secondary POAG should be equally thorough in all the patients regardless of the IOP symmetry.

C. In primary angle-closure glaucoma (PACG), a narrow or closed approach into the anterior chamber angle may make visualization of peripheral anterior synechiae (PAS) impossible until compression gonioscopy is performed. Before the diagnosis of PACG can be made, a different set of secondary causes of IOP elevation must be considered. Iridocyclitis and neovascular glaucoma can cause secondary open-angle or angle-closure glaucoma, depending on whether PAS have developed. In these cases, a wide approach into the anterior chamber angle may be present with a tent-shaped appearance of the PAS. Asymmetry of the angle approach in comparison with the contralateral eye can be suggestive of a posterior segment pathologic condition such as choroidal effusion (e.g. after panretinal photocoagulation) or tumor.

D. When pupillary block results in a narrow or closed anterior chamber angle, laser peripheral iridotomy is indicated. This procedure is required in all the cases of PACG. Repeat gonioscopy after laser treatment confirms the efficacy in opening the anterior chamber angle and permits the diagnosis of plateau iris syndrome (*see* Chapter 90). Laser iridotomy is also helpful when secondary pupillary block causes IOP elevation such as in phacomorphic glaucoma, or when iridocyclitis leads to pupillary seclusion and iris bombé. If secondary pupillary block is present, however, treatment must also be directed at the causative factor. For phacomorphic glaucoma, cataract extraction with or without combined filtration surgery is the definitive treatment. In uveitic glaucoma, treatment of the underlying inflammatory process is necessary.

E. Visual field testing and dilated fundus examination are required to determine whether IOP elevation has resulted in damage to the optic nerve. Optic nerve and/or retinal nerve fiber layer (RNFL) imaging are also useful in the identification of glaucomatous optic nerve damage. In cases of primary angle-closure, dilated fundus examination must not be performed until after laser iridotomy has been completed to prevent possible acute exacerbation of the increased IOP.

F. If no evidence of optic nerve damage is present, the level of IOP and the presence of risk factors for the future development of damage should be considered in determining the need for medical treatment. Because the risk of developing glaucoma increases dramatically when IOP exceeds 30 mm Hg, initiation of medical treatment in such cases is important. Initial glaucoma therapy usually consists of a topical prostaglandin analog, unless this class of medication is contraindicated. When the IOP is < 30 mm Hg, observation without treatment may be reasonable when risk factors for progression to glaucoma are absent. Factors to consider include the corneal thickness, a family history of glaucoma (especially blindness resulting from glaucoma), and the degree of suspicion of disc damage based on the cup/disc ratio and disc asymmetry. Social factors such as the patient's level of apprehension regarding untreated ocular hypertension and the likelihood of reliable follow-up must also be assessed. Elevated IOP from pseudoexfoliation or pigment dispersion may have an aggressive course with dramatic changes in IOP over a short time. Greater caution should be taken in following these patients without treatment.

G. Patients with glaucomatous optic nerve damage require medical therapy to lower the IOP to a level that is unlikely to lead to further damage. The level of IOP before the initiation of therapy should be used to help determine a target pressure below which further damage is unlikely. Advanced damage may lower the target pressure level even further, in which extensively damaged optic nerves may be more susceptible to injury. A significant reduction in IOP may follow laser iridotomy in patients with PACG, particularly when PAS formation has not been extensive. However, many patients will require the addition of medical therapy to reach an appropriate target pressure. The medical treatment of PACG differs from that of POAG, in which medications that act by increasing trabecular outflow facility (e.g. pilocarpine) are ineffective when extensive PAS are present. As a result, options for medical treatment of PACG with extensive PAS include prostaglandin analogs, β-blockers, α-2 agonists, and carbonic anhydrase inhibitors. For details of the management of POAG, *see* Chapters 96 and 101.

H. Once the target IOP is attained, visual fields and optic nerve status must be carefully monitored to rule out ongoing damage. If progressive damage occurs, a new, lower target pressure must be chosen, and the therapy must be adjusted accordingly.

BIBLIOGRAPHY

1. Camejo L, Noecker RJ. Optic nerve imaging. In: Stamper RL, Lieberman MF, Drake MV (Eds). Becker-Shaffer's Diagnosis and Therapy of the Glaucomas, 8th Edition. Philadelphia, PA: Mosby Elsevier; 2009. pp. 171-87.
2. McGalliard JN, Wishart PK. The effect of Nd: YAG iridotomy on IOP in hypertensive eyes with shallow anterior chambers. Eye. 1990;4:823-9.
3. Medical treatment of glaucoma: General principles. In: Stamper RL, Lieberman MF, Drake MV (Eds). Becker-Shaffer's Diagnosis and Therapy of the Glaucomas, 8th Edition. Philadelphia, PA: Mosby Elsevier; 2009. pp. 345-58.

Anatomically Narrow Angles

90

John M Parkinson, J Kevin McKinney, Manishi A Desai

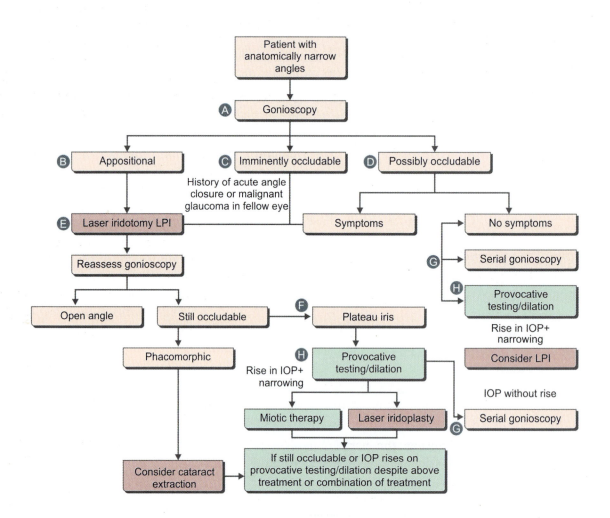

Relative pupillary block is the most common cause of anatomically narrow angles. Laser peripheral iridotomy (LPI) has been shown to be safe and effective for preventing angle-closure glaucoma caused by pupillary block. Because the visual sequelae of acute angle closure can be devastating and the risk of LPI is small, eyes with angles narrow enough to raise clinical suspicion of potential angle closure should receive a prophylactic LPI.

A. Attention to detail and experience in gonioscopy are necessary to accurately evaluate the angle configuration and thereby assess the potential for future angle closure. With proper training and practice, a general ophthalmologist should be able to perform gonioscopy with accuracy and skill. A four-mirror lens, such as a Zeiss or Posner lens, is best suited for evaluating the angle in this setting. During gonioscopy, the lens is held lightly against the cornea. Excessive pressure artificially widens the angle and is indicated by corneal striae. The room should be dark and the light beam should be narrow and small, avoiding direct illumination of the pupil, which would open the angle via pupillary miosis. If significant iris bombe (iris convexity indicative of relative pupillary block) is present, the mirror is rotated toward the observed angle or the patient is asked to look toward the mirror, allowing one to 'look over the hill' into the angle. The ability to accurately identify the trabecular meshwork (TM) in the presence of varying amounts of pigmentation is essential (e.g. pigment at Schwalbe's line may mimic the TM in a closed angle).

B. If the peripheral iris lies in direct contact with the posterior TM, appositional closure is present. Indentation gonioscopy with a four-mirror lens can often differentiate appositional closure from synechial angle closure. Peripheral anterior synechiae (PAS) can result from prolonged or intermittent appositional contact and may progress to extensive, irreversible angle closure. The presence of either apposition or synechiae implies the need for LPI.

C. An angle is imminently occludable if the angular separation between the TM and peripheral iris is <10°. Pharmacologic dilation of such eyes may precipitate acute angle closure and is usually deferred until an iridotomy has been performed.

D. Angles that are possibly occludable have a 10°–20° angle of separation between the peripheral iris and the TM, and the posterior (or pigmented TM) is visible in less than 180°–270° of the angle, though this definition may be too exclusionary. In this case, the decision to perform LPI is based on the presence of symptoms consistent with intermittent episodes of angle closure (e.g. colored halos around lights, blurred or misty vision, ocular redness and discomfort), as well as the individual's social situation (e.g. the ability to identify and report symptoms of angle closure, and to readily access medical care). Other relative indications for iridotomy include individuals with possibly occludable angles who require frequent dilation

(e.g. diabetic patients) or who take systemic medications that might provoke acute angle closure (e.g. tricyclic antidepressants, some cold preparations).

E. An iridotomy is proven to be patent by direct visualization of lens capsule or a black void posterior to the iris plane. Transillumination alone is insufficient to prove patency. Gonioscopy should be repeated after laser iridotomy to determine the effectiveness of the treatment. If the narrow angle configuration was caused by relative pupillary block, and the LPI is of adequate size and patency, a relatively flat iris configuration and an open angle should be found.

F. Up to one-third of the angles without PAS remain narrow after LPI, because of either plateau iris configuration or a relatively crowded anterior segment (e.g. a large lens). With plateau iris anteriorly located, ciliary processes hold the peripheral iris forward, creating a narrow angle in the face of a flat iris configuration. With a crowded anterior segment, the iris assumes a convex configuration as it drapes over the lens curvature. Once an appropriate plan has been instituted (i.e. observation, miotics, or iridoplasty), gonioscopy should be repeated after pharmacologic dilation to rule out appositional angle closure. If appositional angle closure persists despite treatments or combination of treatments thereof, the physician should consider lens extraction.

G. Because narrow angles tend to become narrower with age (as a result of increasing lens size), continued gonioscopy is indicated if iridotomy is deferred or if the angle remains narrow after iridotomy. Eyes with coexistent pseudoexfoliation are especially prone to this phenomenon.

H. In the absence of other indications for LPI, some specialists would recommend provocative testing to further determine the susceptibility to angle closure (dark room testing or pharmacologic). Although such tests may be reassuring to the patient and physician, their sensitivity, specificity, and predictive power are uncertain. If such a test is performed, gonioscopic evidence of angle closure must accompany a rise in intraocular pressure before the test can be considered positive.

BIBLIOGRAPHY

1. Alward WLM. Color Atlas of Gonioscopy. London, UK: Wolfe, 1994.
2. Foster P, He M, Liebmann J. Epidemiology, Classification, and mechanism. In: Weinreb RN, Friedman DS (Eds). Angle Closure and Angle Closure Glaucoma: Reports and Consensus Statement (Consensus 3). The Hague, The Netherlands: Kugler Publications, 2006. pp. 1-20.
3. Moster MR, Schwartz LW, Spaeth GL, et al. Laser iridectomy: A controlled study comparing argon and neodymium: YAG. Ophthalmology. 1986;93:20-4.
4. Ritch R, Lowe RF. Angle closure glaucoma: Clinical types. In: Ritch R, Shields MB, Krupin T (Eds). The Glaucomas. St. Louis, MO: Mosby, 1996. pp. 821-40.
5. Ritch R, Lowe RF. Angle closure glaucoma: Therapeutic overview. In: Ritch R, Shields MB, Krupin T (Eds). The Glaucomas. St Louis, MO: Mosby, 1996. pp. 1521-31.
6. Savage J. Primary angle closure. In: Zimmerman TJ, Kooner KS (Eds). New York, NY: Thieme Medical Publishers, Inc; 2001. pp. 81-106.

Acutely Elevated Intraocular Pressure

91

Scott D Smith, John M Parkinson

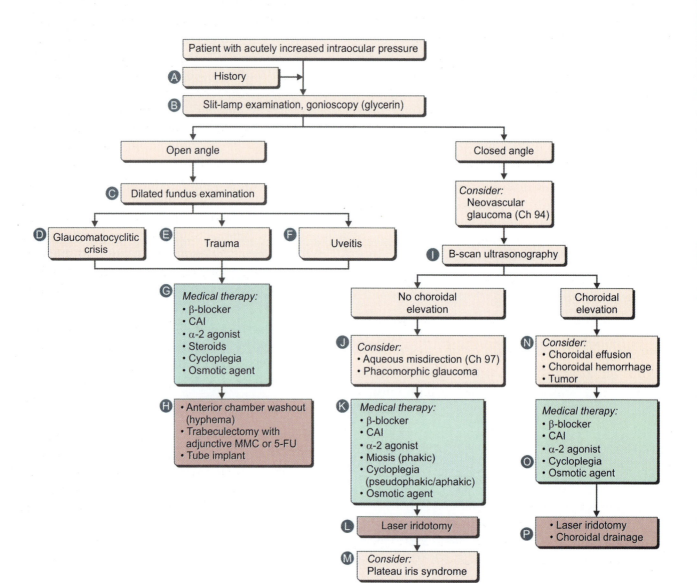

A. A complete medical and ocular history may provide clues about the cause of acutely elevated intraocular pressure (IOP). Special attention should be given to the history of ocular trauma, inflammation, and previous episodes of elevated IOP. History of systemic vascular disease such as diabetes mellitus that might result in anterior segment neovascularization should be determined. The nature and timing of the current ophthalmic condition should be described, including any symptoms of visual loss, blurred vision, halos around lights, pain, redness, or photophobia.

B. When secondary corneal edema is present, slit-lamp examination and gonioscopy are facilitated by the application of topical glycerin. If the view is limited even with the use of glycerin, a narrow angle in the opposite eye helps to confirm angle-closure caused by pupillary block in the affected eye. Asymmetry of the anterior chamber angles should suggest another cause of angle-closure. Careful examination of the iris and anterior chamber angle for the presence of iris neovascularization is required to distinguish neovascular glaucoma from other causes of acute IOP elevation. IOP elevation caused by neovascular glaucoma is generally accompanied by partial or complete synechial angle-closure, and requires prompt management of the cause of the anterior segment neovascularization (*see* Chapter 94).

C. A dilated fundus examination is performed in cases of open-angle glaucoma to identify abnormalities of the posterior segment and to evaluate the optic nerve. Although more commonly associated with chronic, asymptomatic elevation of IOP, acute IOP elevation may also occur in pigmentary or pseudoexfoliation glaucoma.

D. Glaucomatocyclitic crisis occurs in young-to-middle-aged adults with symptoms of mild unilateral ocular irritation and blurred vision. IOP in the range of 40-60 mmHg is usually associated with mild ocular inflammation (ciliary injection with trace anterior chamber cells and flare, and fine keratic precipitates). Posterior and peripheral anterior synechiae are notably absent in this syndrome. Episodes are self-limited (lasting several hours to several weeks) and variably recurrent.

E. Trauma may result in acutely elevated IOP by direct damage to outflow structures or by occlusion of these structures with erythrocytes, inflammatory cells, pigment, fibrin, and other debris. In cases of hyphema in African-Americans, a sickle cell preparation should be obtained to identify patients at risk for prolonged pressure elevation because of the obstruction of outflow by sickled erythrocytes.

F. Elevated IOP in uveitis results from direct inflammatory involvement of the trabecular meshwork and obstruction of outflow by inflammatory cells and fibrin. Progressive synechial angle-closure caused by the contraction of inflammatory membranes or precipitates in the angle may also occur.

G. Medical therapy in each condition is directed primarily at aqueous humor suppression. Effective medications include topical β-blockers, α-2 agonists, and carbonic anhydrase inhibitors (CAIs). Systemic CAIs may be more effective in treating acute IOP elevation than the topical drugs in this class, but they are contraindicated in patients with sickle cell disease. Hyperosmotic agents can also be used for the temporary control of IOP when the initial response to other medications is inadequate. Prostaglandins and parasympathomimetic agents may increase ocular inflammation and should be avoided. Topical steroids are used in all three conditions to reduce ocular inflammation, but prolonged use may be associated with a subsequent steroid-induced rise in IOP. Short-acting cycloplegic agents help relieve the symptoms of ciliary spasm, and may help in preventing posterior synechiae by ensuring pupillary mobility. Long-acting cycloplegic agents may help reduce rebleeding in traumatic hyphema by immobilizing the iris.

H. Most cases of acutely elevated IOP resulting from these conditions can be successfully managed medically. When necessary, traditional filtration surgery is most successful after acute inflammation is medically controlled. In cases of imminent corneal blood staining, previous optic nerve damage, or impending retinal vascular occlusion, early surgical intervention may be necessary. Adjunctive mitomycin-C or 5-fluorouracil can improve the success of trabeculectomy in patients with inflammatory glaucoma. Glaucoma drainage implant surgery may be considered in the setting of active inflammation, when conjunctival scarring is present, or when previous trabeculectomy has failed.

I. Ultrasonography effectively rules out uncommon secondary causes of acute angle-closure. If ultrasonography is not available, an anatomically narrow angle in the fellow eye supports the diagnosis of simple pupillary block as the mechanism of angle-closure. A dilated fundus examination should be performed after the angle-closure is adequately treated to rule out abnormalities of the posterior segment.

J. The presence of high IOP with a shallow axial anterior chamber, particularly in patients with a history of prior ocular surgery or peripheral iridotomy, suggests aqueous misdirection. An extremely narrow anterior chamber angle in the presence of mature cataract and a normal posterior segment on ultrasound suggests phacomorphic glaucoma. Definitive therapy requires cataract extraction with or without combined trabeculectomy, depending on the chronicity of IOP elevation. Before surgery, medical therapy is required to attempt to lower the IOP and reduce ocular inflammation. Laser iridotomy can relieve angle-closure before definitive surgery, and is performed because an element of pupillary block may also be present.

K. In the absence of choroidal abnormality, medical therapy is directed at reducing IOP, corneal edema, and iris ischemia. Aqueous humor suppressants, including β-blockers, CAIs, and α-2 agonists, are used initially. Prostaglandin analogues may be less useful in the setting of acute IOP elevation, as they have a slower onset of IOP reduction, and may promote ocular inflammation. Hyperosmotic agents are useful in patients with extremely high IOP or when the initial response to other medications is inadequate. In phakic eyes, several doses of 1 or 2% pilocarpine may effectively break an attack of acute angle-closure but may be more effective after aqueous suppression has begun to lower IOP and iris ischemia has decreased. In aphakic or pseudophakic eyes without an iridectomy, pupillary block may be relieved by pupillary dilation and cycloplegia.

L. When acute IOP elevation is caused by pupillary block, laser peripheral iridotomy should be performed. If possible, this should be delayed until medical treatment has reduced the IOP and corneal edema has cleared. In cases refractory to medical treatment, topical glycerin may be helpful in clearing the cornea long enough to permit laser iridotomy. Emergent filtration surgery is rarely required in the treatment of primary angle-closure glaucoma.

M. Recurrent acute angle-closure after laser iridotomy suggests the presence of plateau iris syndrome, which can be confirmed by gonioscopy. Such patients may need to continue 1 or 2% pilocarpine to reduce the risk of recurrent episodes until they receive more definitive therapy. *See* Chapter 90 for additional therapeutic considerations.

N. Choroidal elevation or thickening on ultrasonography suggests choroidal effusion, choroidal hemorrhage, or tumor. Choroidal effusion may be primary (idiopathic) or secondary to posterior scleritis, central retinal vein occlusion, scleral buckling procedures, panretinal photocoagulation, or may occur as a complication of topiramate use.

O. Medical therapy consists of aqueous humor suppression with maximal cycloplegia to allow posterior rotation of the ciliary body, lens, and iris.

P. Surgical intervention is indicated in cases of persistently flat anterior chamber, corneal decompensation, refractory pressure elevation, or 'kissing choroidals'. When some degree of pupillary block also exists, a laser iridotomy may re-establish anterior aqueous flow. Drainage of choroidal effusion or blood (in the absence of intraocular tumor) is a definitive therapy.

▌BIBLIOGRAPHY

1. Larsson LI. Intraocular pressure 24 hours after a single-dose administration of latanoprost 0.005% in healthy volunteers: A randomized, double-masked, placebo controlled cross-over single center study. Acta Ophthalmol Scand. 2001;79:567-71.
2. Maus TL, Larsson L, Mclaren JW, et al. Comparison of dorzolamide and acetazolamide as suppressors of aqueous humor flow in humans. Arch Ophthalmol. 1997;115:45-9.
3. Raitta C, Vannas A. Glaucomatocyclitic crisis. Arch Ophthalmol. 1977;95:608-12.
4. Ritch R, Lowe RF. Angle-closure glaucoma: Clinical types. In: Ritch R, Shields MB, Krupin T (Eds). The Glaucomas. St. Louis, MO: Mosby; 1996. pp. 821-40.
5. Stamper RL, Lieberman MF, Drake MV (Eds). Becker-Shaffer's Diagnosis and Therapy of the Glaucomas. 8th Edition. Philadelphia, PA: Mosby Elsevier; 2009. pp. 359-431.
6. Walsh JB, Muldoon TO. Glaucoma associated with retinal and vitreoretinal disorders. In: Ritch R, Shields MB, Krupin T (Eds). The Glaucomas. St. Louis, MO: Mosby; 1996. pp. 1055-71.

Primary Open-Angle Glaucoma

92

Scott D Smith, Roy Whitaker Jr

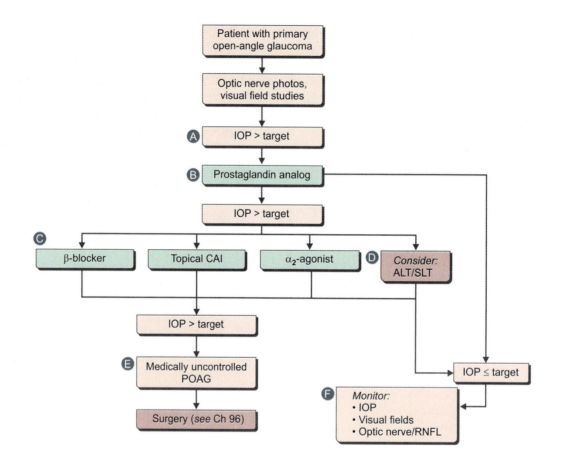

After the diagnosis of primary open-angle glaucoma (POAG) is established, medical therapy should be instituted to prevent progressive visual loss. The lowest dosage that achieves an intraocular pressure (IOP) level that prevents progressive damage to the optic nerve and nerve fiber layer is desirable because lower dosages are less likely to cause medication side effects. All medications used to treat glaucoma are potentially harmful; therefore, the practitioner treating glaucoma should fully understand the pharmacology and side effects of these medications.

The availability of different classes of glaucoma medication is important as drugs with different mechanisms of IOP lowering may have an additive effect. In addition, the effect of a drug may decrease with time, leading to a need to substitute different therapies. Different medications or medical combinations work for different patients; therefore, the therapy must be individualized.

A. The level of IOP before the initiation of therapy should be used to help determine a target pressure below which further damage is unlikely. Advanced damage may result in a need to set a very low-target pressure level, as the extensively damaged optic nerves may be more susceptible to injury.

B. Topical prostaglandin analogues (latanoprost, travoprost, and bimatoprost) have been shown to be the most effective class of medication for reducing IOP. Their efficacy and the convenience of once daily dosing have led to these drugs being preferred for initial medical therapy in POAG patients without a contraindication to their use. These drugs reduce IOP by increasing uveoscleral outflow, a mechanism that differs from any other class of glaucoma medication. The principal side-effects of these drugs include iris color change in patients with light irides, periocular skin pigmentation, and ocular redness and irritation. In addition, there have been reported associations between prostaglandin analogues and reactivation of uveitis and exacerbation of macular edema. Ineffective drugs should be discontinued in favor of alternative treatments, thereby avoiding the potential adverse effects resulting from unnecessary medications.

C. When prostaglandin analogues are effective but the IOP reduction is insufficient to reach the target IOP, combinations of medications may be used to treat the patient successfully. Several nonselective β-blockers are available in the United States. These drugs are contraindicated in patients with greater than first-degree heart block and bronchospastic disorders, and should be used cautiously in patients with diabetes and congestive heart failure. Because of its intrinsic sympathomimetic activity, carteolol may be less likely to cause bradycardia and has a less detrimental effect on serum lipid profiles than other β-blockers. Betaxolol, a selective $β_1$-adrenergic antagonist, is associated with fewer pulmonary side effects than the nonselective β-blockers but should still be avoided in patients with bronchospastic disorders. Their efficacy in reducing IOP during sleep appears to be less than that of other glaucoma medications. Although oral carbonic anhydrase inhibitors (CAIs) are effective in reducing IOP, systemic side-effects often limit their usefulness in the treatment of glaucoma. The topical CAIs, dorzolamide and brinzolamide, appear to have minimal systemic effects, and have largely replaced their oral counterparts for long-term treatment. Brimonidine is an $α_2$-adrenergic agonist that can be effective in reducing IOP. Its long-term usefulness can be limited by allergies. It has also been associated with central nervous system depression in some patients, and should be used with caution in young children.

D. Argon laser trabeculoplasty and selective laser trabeculoplasty have traditionally been reserved for the treatment of medically uncontrolled open-angle glaucoma. Studies evaluating these procedures as alternatives to medical therapy for the initial treatment of POAG have shown them to be nearly 50% effective in controlling IOP without the need for medications for at least 2 years. While most clinicians recommend medications as first-line therapy for POAG, some consider using laser trabeculoplasty early in the course of the disease, particularly for individuals with significant medication side-effects or when compliance is inadequate.

E. When glaucoma is progressive despite the use of maximally tolerated medical therapy and laser trabeculoplasty, glaucoma surgery is indicated. Glaucoma surgery has traditionally been reserved for patients failing medical and laser therapy because its complications may lead to significant ocular morbidity. Newer minimally invasive glaucoma procedures have been introduced that may reduce the risk of complications, and may be appropriate for use earlier in the course of the disease.

F. Once the target IOP is achieved, monitoring of visual fields and optic nerve status is required to ensure that the IOP reduction is sufficient to prevent glaucoma progression. Optic nerve and retinal nerve fiber layer imaging are useful adjuncts to the clinical examination to verify stability. If progressive damage occurs in spite of patient adherence to recommended therapy, a lower target IOP should be set with a corresponding advancement of therapy.

BIBLIOGRAPHY

1. Samples JR, Singh K, Lin SC, et al. Laser trabeculoplasty for open-angle glaucoma: A report by the American Academy of Ophthalmology. Ophthalmology. 2011;118:2296-302.
2. Stamper RL, Lieberman MF, Drake MV, (Eds). Becker-Shaffer's Diagnosis and Therapy of the Glaucomas, 8th Edition. Philadelphia, PA: Mosby Elsevier, 2009. pp. 359-431.

Low-Tension (Normal-Tension) Glaucoma

93

Alvaro PC Lupinacci, Peter A Netland

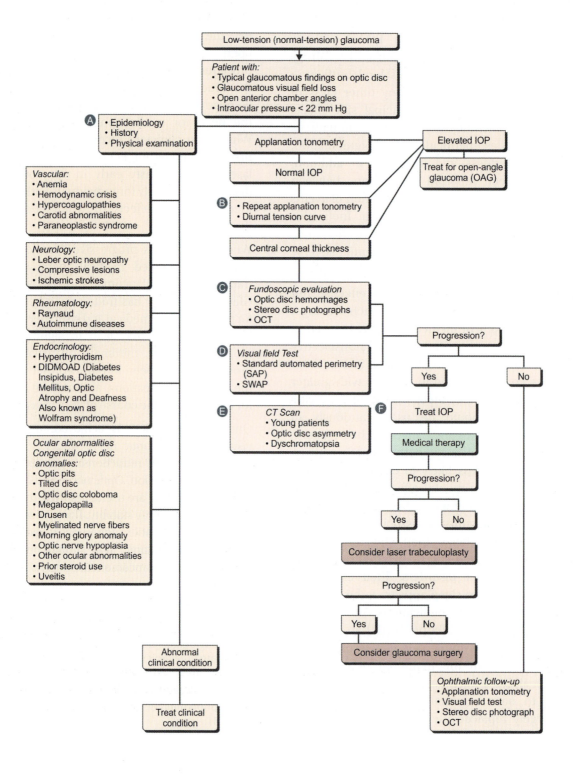

Low-tension glaucoma (also known as "normal-tension glaucoma") is characterized by glaucomatous optic nerve cupping, visual field defects, open anterior chamber angles, and the absence of elevated intraocular pressure (IOP). The absence of elevated IOP usually is IOP below 22 mm Hg for all recorded measurements of the IOP. Because thinner-than-average central corneal thickness may lead to underestimation of IOP, central corneal thickness should be considered for accurate IOP measurements. The diagnosis is less certain in the absence of demonstrable progressive optic nerve changes or visual field loss over time. Low-tension glaucoma occurs primarily in the elderly with onset usually in the sixth or seventh decade of life, being more common in females and Japanese descendants. This entity is a relatively common disorder, present in one-fifth to one-half of all open-angle glaucoma patients.

Low-tension glaucoma is a diagnosis of exclusion based on the history and the clinical findings. The evaluation of a patient with low-tension glaucoma should include a careful history and a complete ophthalmic examination including IOP determination, gonioscopy, visual fields, dilated fundoscopic examination, and disc photographs.

A. The history should include inquiries about migraine, Raynaud, cancer, toxic exposures such as methanol or ethambutol, hemodynamic crisis, or abnormalities of blood pressure. Previous elevations of IOP may occur in glaucoma associated with corticosteroid use, uveitis, or trauma. The past and present medication list is also relevant because systemic beta-blockers and calcium channel blockers may mask elevated IOP. In select patients, a general physical examination may be performed to evaluate systemic diseases including neurologic, endocrine and vascular abnormalities, including carotid artery abnormalities. A 24-hour blood pressure evaluation may show nocturnal lowering of blood pressure and/or heart rate. Vascular stiffness and ocular perfusion pressure are two other significant diagnostic aspects.

B. IOP measurements less than 22 mm Hg have been considered normal, but intermittent elevations of IOP may not be detected. Thus, IOP should be measured on more than one occasion and at different times of the day in an attempt to detect fluctuations. Diurnal variations of IOP can occur, and these may be exaggerated in glaucoma patients. Thin central corneal thickness may mask an elevated IOP. Mean central corneal thickness on normal population is approximately 537 µm. Transient elevations of IOP may be found in intermittent angle-closure glaucoma, glaucomatocyclitic crisis, and glaucoma associated with uveitis.

C. In the ocular examination, the finding of optic disc hemorrhage should be noted. A higher prevalence of optic disc hemorrhages has been reported in patients with low-tension glaucoma compared with those with open-angle glaucoma. Some non-glaucoma conditions may also resemble low-tension glaucoma, such as congenital abnormalities, Leber hereditary optic neuropathy, ocular ischemic syndrome, and compressive lesions of the optic nerve.

D. Patients with a normal visual field, normal IOP, and an optic disc that appears suspicious for glaucoma should be observed without treatment. Because glaucoma may develop in the future, stereo disc photographs and/or other optic nerve imaging devices are useful to document progressive changes of the optic nerve head contour. Earlier visual field defects can be detected with the short wavelength automated perimetry test (SWAP). Optical coherence tomography (OCT) of the retinal or retinal nerve fiber layer thickness should be evaluated. The visual field test should be repeated at regular intervals.

E. If visual field testing reveals glaucomatous loss, the diagnosis is most likely glaucoma. Deep central visual field defects are characteristic of groups of patients with low-tension glaucoma, although individual patients may not manifest this finding. In patients under evaluation for low-tension glaucoma, laboratory and imaging studies may be useful to identify other causes of visual field loss and optic nerve damage. Although not recommended for patients with typical clinical findings of low-tension glaucoma, CT scanning can identify patients with compressive lesions of the optic nerve. Patients younger than 50 years suspected of having low-tension glaucoma, with optic nerve atrophy and normal intraocular pressure, should be considered for a CT scan. Also, a CT scan should be obtained in any patient with significant asymmetry of the optic nerve heads, optic nerve head pallor, pain, or dyschromatopsia. Visual field results that are not characteristic for glaucoma, such as temporal field loss or field loss respecting the vertical meridian, should prompt neurological evaluation.

F. Patients with low-tension glaucoma who have progressive visual field loss should be treated with lower IOP to a level that prevents progression. This may require medical, laser, or surgical therapy. The use of therapy in low-tension glaucoma is controversial, but most treatment strategies for low-tension glaucoma center around the assumption that IOP should be reduced by at least 30% in patients. Thus, the target IOP for patients with low-tension glaucoma is usually in the low teens. Treatment with systemic calcium channel blockers and/or topical brimonidine may be considered because of available neuroprotective evidence. Surgical treatment of low-tension glaucoma is usually reserved for those patients whose progression of disease is well documented despite conventional medical and even laser therapies. Trabeculectomy with antifibrosis agents has become a popular surgical therapy for progressive low-tension glaucoma, because this procedure achieves low mean IOP and has a low complication rate. Despite conventional medical and surgical therapies, patients with low-tension glaucoma may continue to demonstrate intractable progression of their disease.

BIBLIOGRAPHY

1. Anderson DR, Drance SM. The effectiveness of intraocular pressure reduction in the treatment of normal-tension glaucoma. Collaborative Normal-Tension Glaucoma Study Group. Am J Ophthalmol. 1998;126:498-505.
2. Copt RP, Thomas R, Mermoud A. Corneal thickness in ocular hypertension, primary open-angle glaucoma, and normal tension glaucoma. Arch Ophthalmol. 1999;117:14-6.
3. De Moraes CG, Liebmann JM, Greenfield DS, et al. Risk factors for visual field progression in the low-tension glaucoma treatment study. Am J Ophthalmol. 2012;154:702-11.
4. Firat PG, Doganay S, Demirel EE, et al. Comparison of ganglion cell and retinal fiber layer thickness in primary open-angle glaucoma and normal-tension glaucoma with spectral-domain OCT. Graefes Arch Clin Exp Ophthalmol. 2013;251:831-8.
5. Meyer JH, Brandi-Dohrn J, Funk J. Twenty four-hour blood pressure monitoring in normal-tension glaucoma. Br J Ophthalmol. 1996;80:864-7.
6. Mroczkowska S, Benavente-Perez A, Negi A, et al. Primary open-angle glaucoma vs normal-tension glaucoma: The vascular perspective. JAMA Ophthalmol. 2013;131:36-43.
7. Netland PA. Low-tension glaucoma. Mediguide Ophthalmol. 1997;7:1-6.

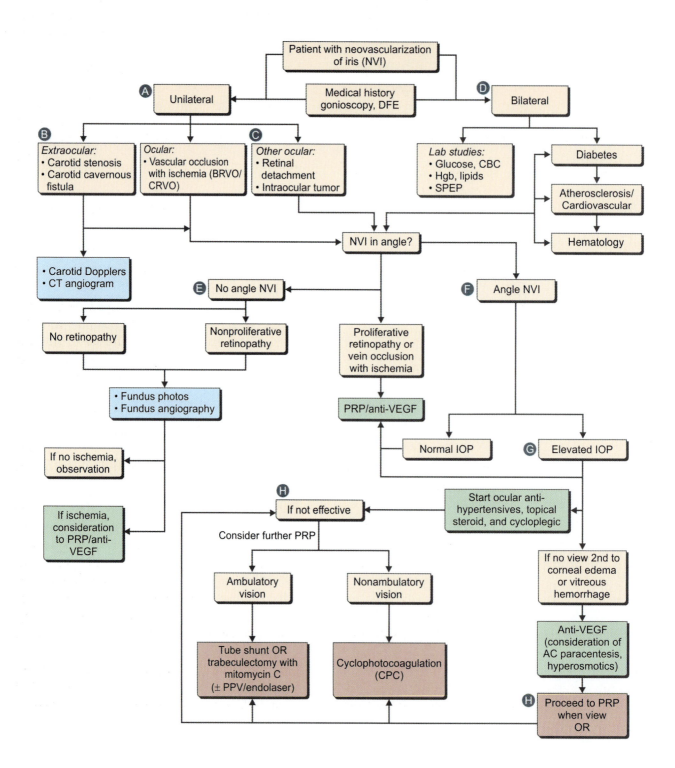

The presence of abnormal vessels on or within the iris is called neovascularization of the iris (NVI) or rubeosis iridis. In lightly pigmented irides, normal iris vessels are sometimes visible and can be clearly distinguished from NVI because normal vessels radiate from the pupillary margin and do not extend into the anterior chamber angle. With iris fluorescein angiography, normal vessels do not leak. Because NVI is generally caused by ocular ischemia, local and systemic conditions that may result in ischemia should be sought.

A. When NVI is present, gonioscopy is required to determine whether neovascularization involves the anterior chamber angle. A dilated fundus examination after gonioscopy often identifies the causes of ocular ischemia. Once the cause of ocular ischemia is identified, appropriate treatment can be initiated.

B. If the fundus examination is normal, extraocular causes of ischemia should be considered and the carotid arteries and heart should be evaluated. The presence of a carotid bruit is an important clue to the presence of carotid stenosis. However, the absence of a bruit does not rule out carotid stenosis because the low-flow state of high-grade stenosis may not produce an audible bruit. Therefore, appropriate referral for carotid noninvasive studies should be obtained regardless of the results of carotid auscultation. Laboratory studies are needed to rule out diabetes, hyperviscosity syndromes, and other hematologic disorders.

C. Fundus examination is important in excluding retinal detachment, malignant melanoma or other intraocular tumors, and retinal vascular diseases such as central or branch retinal vein occlusion. Central and branch retinal artery occlusion rarely cause NVI because they tend to produce tissue anoxia rather than hypoxia.

D. When bilateral NVI is present, systemic causes can be suspected. However, symmetric involvement of the eyes can often be seen, and unilateral involvement is often seen even when a systemic cause is present. If a patient has no known systemic disease that can account for the ocular findings, appropriate laboratory tests should be ordered. When common conditions such as diabetes have

been ruled out, further tests such as a complete blood count (CBC), serum lipid studies, and hemoglobin and protein electrophoresis (i.e. to rule out conditions noted in part B.) should be obtained.

E. When gonioscopy shows an open angle with no vessels, the results of dilated fundus examination determine the appropriate treatment. In diabetic patients without retinopathy or with mild nonproliferative retinopathy, fluorescein angiography may reveal areas of retinal ischemia not visualized clinically. If retinal ischemia is absent, other potential causes of NVI (as noted in B.) should be considered. Careful observation with an initial follow-up after several weeks is needed to prevent undetected progression to neovascular glaucoma. When proliferative diabetic retinopathy or retinal vascular occlusion are present, prompt panretinal photocoagulation (PRP) is required along with the administration of an antiendothelial vascular growth factor (anti-VEGF) agent. Regression of NVI on follow-up examination confirms that photocoagulation has been adequate.

F. When gonioscopy shows an open angle with neovascularization, urgent PRP and an anti-VEGF are indicated in an effort to prevent progressive synechial angle closure. Medical treatment with aqueous suppressants may be required. Effective medications include topical beta-blockers, alpha2-adrenergic agents, topical or systemic carbonic anhydrase inhibitors, but prostaglandins analogs can also be effective. If inflammation or hyphema exists, topical steroids and cycloplegics should be added to the treatment regimen.

G. When synechial angle closure has already developed, the intraocular pressure (IOP) is usually elevated and corneal edema is often present, limiting the ability to perform adequate PRP. Medical therapy (as noted in F.) is often effective. However, hyperosmotic agents may be needed to adequately reduce IOP and improve corneal clarity. In order to lower IOP urgently, anterior chamber paracentesis with a 30-gauge needle can also be considered. Anti-VEGF agents are required in these cases where corneal edema limits placement of PRP. The anti-VEGF agents often induce rapid regression of neovascularization, decreasing the IOP and corneal edema and facilitating the visualization for PRP. If visualization remains poor, secondary to the corneal edema or vitreous hemorrhage, surgical intervention or peripheral retinocryopexy need to be considered.

H. Because neovascular glaucoma can often be refractory and present in the setting of high morbidity, the appropriate surgical intervention will be influenced by the potential for recovery of useful vision, optic nerve cupping, and retinal examination. When visual potential is limited, laser cyclophotocoagulation may be preferable over filtration surgery. The success of trabeculectomy for neovascular glaucoma is substantially lower than that for most other glaucoma subtypes. As a result, adjunctive mitomycin-C is often necessary to increase the probability of a successful outcome. Because of the substantial risk of hyphema after surgery and the limited success even when antimetabolites are used, anti-VEGF agents are often given prior to surgery and preference is given to tube implant surgery. With either procedure, the risk of choroidal effusion and shallow anterior chamber are higher than usual when PRP has been recently performed or when ocular inflammation is present at the time of surgery. As a result, it is preferable to delay surgery by 3–4 weeks unless unacceptable IOP elevation persists despite medical therapy. When vitreous hemorrhage is present, vitrectomy with endolaser to the retina and ciliary processes can be effective in aphakic or pseudophakic eyes. Early recognition of NVI is important so that the development of synechial angle closure and subsequent neovascular glaucoma can be prevented.

BIBLIOGRAPHY

1. Ciftci S, Sakalar YB, Unlu K, et al. Intravitreal bevacizumab combined with panretinal photocoagulation in the treatment of open angle neovascular glaucoma. Eur J Ophthalmol. 2009; 19:1028-33.
2. Ehlers JP, Spirn MJ, Lam A, et al. Combination intravitreal bevacizumab/panretinal photocoagulation versus panretinal photocoagulation alone in the treatment of neovascular glaucoma. Retina. 2008;28:696-702.
3. Leszczynski R, Domanksi R, Forminksa-Kapuscik M, et al. Contact transscleral cyclophotocoagulation in the treatment of neovascular glaucoma: A five-year follow-up. Med Sci Monit. 2009;15:BR84-7.
4. Olmos LC, Lee RK. Medical and surgical management treatment of neovascular glaucoma. Int Ophthalmol Clin. 2011; 51:27-36.
5. Park UC, Park KH, Kim DM, et al. Ahmed glaucoma valve implantation for neovascular glaucoma after vitrectomy for proliferative diabetic retinopathy. J Glaucoma; Vol. 7 2011. pp. 433-8.
6. Saito Y, Higashide T, Takeda H, et al. Beneficial effects of preoperative intravitreal bevacizumab on trabeculectomy outcomes in neovascular glaucoma. Acta Ophthalmologica. 2010;88:96-102.
7. Takihara Y, Inatani M, Fukushima M, et al. Trabeculectomy with mitomycin-C for neovascular glaucoma: Prognostic factors for surgical failure. Am J Ophthalmol. 2009;147:912-8.
8. Takihara Y, Inatani M, Kawaji T, et al. Combined intravitreal bevacizumab and trabeculectomy with mitomycin-C versus trabeculectomy with mitomycin-C alone for neovascular glaucoma. J Glaucoma. 2011;20:196-201.

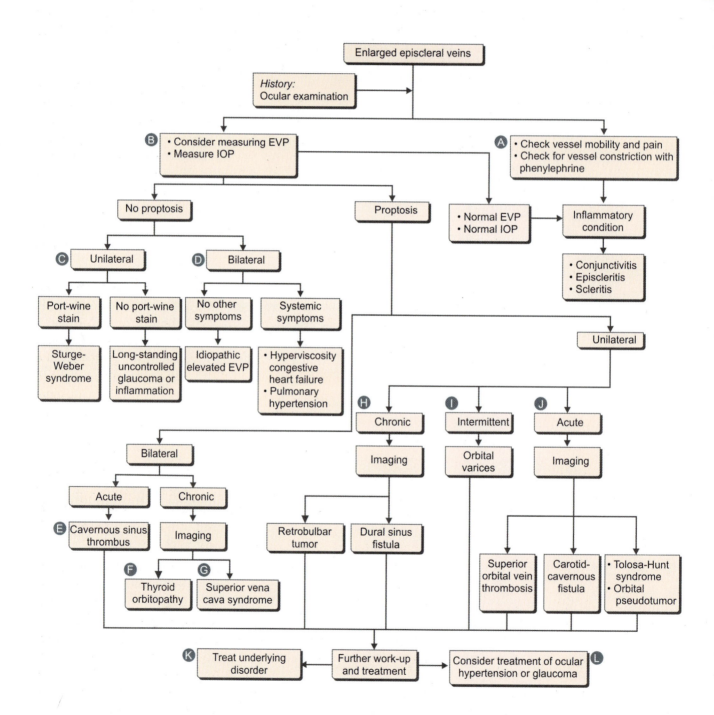

Enlarged episcleral veins may result from a variety of ocular and nonocular conditions. The cause of this entity can be divided into three etiologies: (i) obstruction of venous outflow, (ii) arteriovenous fistulas, and (iii) idiopathic elevated episcleral venous pressure (EVP). Depending on the etiology, these patients may also have chemosis, proptosis, orbital bruits, and/or pulsations in conjunction with engorged episcleral veins. It may also be possible to see refluxed blood in Schlemm canal under gonioscopy. In addition to a complete ophthalmic examination and careful history, a clinician should consider additional tests to help diagnose the cause of enlarged episcleral veins. These may include imaging such as ultrasound, orbital magnetic resonance imaging (MRI) or computed tomography (CT), or angiography. Thyroid studies may also be considered. In addition to potentially dangerous or fatal underlying etiologies of enlarged episcleral veins, the clinician must be aware that elevated EVP can also lead to open-angle glaucoma. Indirect effects of elevated EVP may cause other forms of glaucoma. If elevated EVP involves the vortex vein system, resultant choroidal congestion and detachment may cause angle closure, which may be managed with cycloplegia and hyperosmotic agents. Venous obstruction may lead to ocular ischemia or a central retinal vein occlusion with subsequent neovascular glaucoma. Severe orbital congestion may raise the intraocular pressure (IOP) through compression of the globe.

A. Enlarged episcleral veins should be differentiated from other causes of redness in the sclera or conjunctiva, such as conjunctivitis, scleritis, or episcleritis. While conjunctival vessels are freely movable with a cotton-tipped applicator and blanch with topical epinephrine, deeper episcleral vessels have neither of these characteristics. While scleritis is often painful, enlarged episcleral veins typically are asymptomatic.

B. Aqueous humor exits the eye through the trabecular meshwork, Schlemm canal, and episcleral veins. Thus, elevated EVP will present an obstruction to outflow and raise IOP. Normal EVP is 8–10 mm Hg. The IOP increases approximately 1 mm Hg for every mm Hg above normal EVP. While commercial venomanometers are available for measuring EVP directly, they are not commonly used in clinical practice. It is much more common and more convenient to use IOP as a surrogate measurement. If IOP is normal, attention should again be directed at possible inflammatory conditions mimicking elevated EVP. If IOP or EVP are elevated, one should next examine for proptosis.

C. The differential for patients with unilateral enlarged episcleral veins without proptosis is relatively small. The patient should be carefully examined for a port-wine stain, which indicates Sturge-Weber syndrome. This is a sporadic phakomatosis. In addition to skin findings, the fundus should be carefully checked for choroidal hemangiomas. About 30% of the patients with Sturge-Weber syndrome develop glaucoma. Of these, roughly 60% are diagnosed shortly after birth and are thought to result from an abnormality of the anterior chamber angle. The remainder are diagnosed later in childhood and are caused by elevated EVP due to episcleral hemangiomas with arteriovenous fistulas.

D. If a patient has bilateral enlarged episcleral veins without proptosis, a work-up for systemic abnormalities such as hyperviscosity syndromes, pulmonary hypertension, or congestive heart failure should be considered. Idiopathic elevated EVP is a diagnosis of exclusion and a rare cause of enlarged episcleral veins. Cases can be congenital or spontaneous. Patients usually present in the second or third decade of life. The symptoms are usually bilateral, but can be very asymmetric.

E. An infectious cavernous sinus thrombosis may present with acute, bilateral proptosis and enlarged episcleral veins. Treatment is with systemic antibiotics in conjunction with a neurologist and/or an infectious disease specialist.

F. Thyroid orbitopathy causes enlarged episcleral veins and a chronic, bilateral proptosis that may be asymmetric. This condition may cause inflammation in any of the periocular tissues, and thus causes venous congestion and elevated EVP. A small but significant subset of these patients develop open-angle glaucoma, which is bilateral in 95% of the cases. Over 90% of the patients are hyperthyroid at presentation. Patients may have diplopia and eye motility dysfunction, optic nerve involvement, or exposure keratopathy. They may need orbital decompression, strabismus surgery, and ptosis surgery in certain circumstances. Referral to an endocrinologist should be considered.

G. Superior vena cava syndrome also causes enlarged episcleral veins and a chronic, bilateral proptosis. It can be distinguished from thyroid orbitopathy by imaging studies. Causes include aortic aneurysms, mediastinal masses, hilar adenopathy, and intrathoracic goiter. Signs are typically bilateral and may be associated with exophthalmos, edema, cyanosis of the face and neck (pumpkin head appearance), and dilated veins of the upper body.

H. A chronic, unilateral proptosis associated with enlarged episcleral veins is most likely caused by an orbital mass lesion or a low-flow dural sinus fistula. These two entities can be distinguished from one another by imaging. Elevated IOP occurs in 60–70% of the patients with a dural sinus fistula. Physical findings in dural sinus fistulas tend to be more subtle than in carotid-cavernous fistulas; sometimes only the dilated episcleral vessels distinguish this from primary open-angle glaucoma. Dural sinus fistulas are more commonly spontaneous, most often in middle-aged to elderly women. Up to 50% of fistulas will close spontaneously or after angiography, with normalization of the IOP within days to weeks.

I. An intermittent, unilateral proptosis associated with enlarged episcleral veins is characteristic of an orbital varix, a vascular tumor that can change size frequently, usually with bending over or the Valsalva maneuver. Glaucoma is not common because the elevated EVP is intermittent. Treatment depends on the extent and damage of the varix.

J. An acute, unilateral proptosis associated with enlarged episcleral veins is an emergency and should be imaged accordingly. One possibility is that of a carotid-cavernous sinus fistula, which most commonly occurs after trauma. Findings begin acutely and include pulsating exophthalmos, bruit over the globe, conjunctival chemosis, restriction of motility, and evidence of ocular ischemia. Findings usually occur on the same side as the fistula, but may be bilateral or alternating. Angiography is

considered the most useful imaging modality to describe the lesion. These patients should be treated in conjunction with a neurosurgeon. Other causes of acute, unilateral proptosis associated with enlarged episcleral veins are superior orbital vein thrombosis and idiopathic orbital inflammation (orbital pseudotumor), including the Tolosa-Hunt variation. Idiopathic orbital inflammation causes a thyroid-like inflammation of the orbital tissues, but is distinguished by its painfulness and the involvement of the muscle tendons, which thyroid inflammation spares.

K. Initial therapy of enlarged episcleral veins is often directed toward eliminating the cause of the elevated EVP. This is especially true for thyroid ophthalmopathy, superior vena cava syndrome, retrobulbar tumors, and cavernous sinus thrombosis.

L. Treatment of glaucoma or ocular hypertension associated with EVP should begin with medical therapy. Laser trabeculoplasty is not indicated. If surgery is needed, extreme care should be taken to minimize the risk of uveal effusion and choroidal hemorrhages. Surgical techniques may include intracameral viscoelastic injection at the time of surgery, tying off the tube of a drainage implant, creation of a prophylactic sclerotomy, placement of moderately tight scleral flap sutures, and delayed suture lysis. Glaucoma drainage implants are thought to be somewhat safer than trabeculectomy in this clinical scenario.

BIBLIOGRAPHY

1. Greenfield D. Glaucoma associated with elevated episcleral venous pressure. J Glaucoma. 2000;9:190-4.
2. Higginbotham E. Glaucoma associated with increased episcleral venous pressure. In: Albert DM, Jakobiec FA (Eds). Principles and Practice of Ophthalmology. Philadelphia, PA: WB Saunders; 1994. pp. 1467-79.
3. Keizer R. Carotid-cavernous and orbital arteriovenous fistulas: Ocular features, diagnostic and hemodynamic considerations in relation to visual impairment and morbidity. Orbit. 2003; 22:121-42.
4. Sit A, McLaren J. Measurement of episcleral venous pressure. Exp Eye Res. 2011;93:291-8.
5. Watson P. Diseases of the sclera and episclera. In: Tasman W, Jaeger EA (Eds). Duane's Clinical Ophthalmology. Philadelphia, PA: Lippincott-Raven; 1995. pp. 1-45.

Surgical Treatment of Medically Uncontrolled Primary Open-Angle Glaucoma

96

Scott D Smith, John M Parkinson

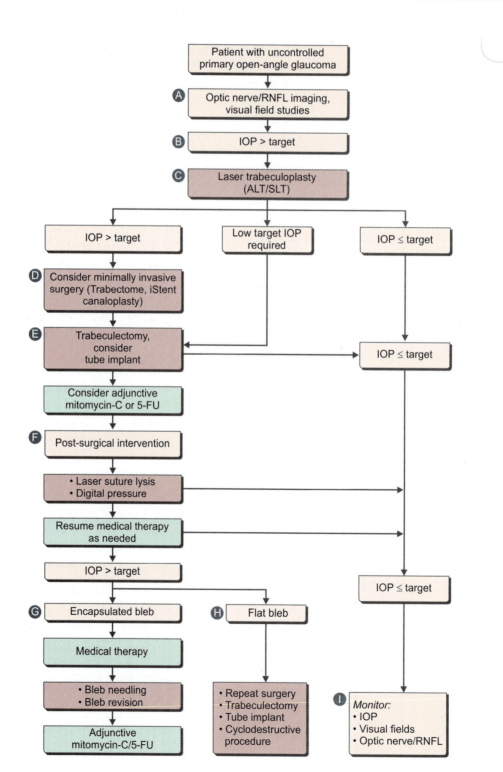

Patient with uncontrolled primary open-angle glaucoma

A — Optic nerve/RNFL imaging, visual field studies

B — IOP > target

C — Laser trabeculoplasty (ALT/SLT)

- IOP > target
- Low target IOP required
- IOP ≤ target

D — Consider minimally invasive surgery (Trabectome, iStent canaloplasty)

E — Trabeculectomy, consider tube implant

IOP ≤ target

Consider adjunctive mitomycin-C or 5-FU

F — Post-surgical intervention

- Laser suture lysis
- Digital pressure

Resume medical therapy as needed

IOP > target

IOP ≤ target

G — Encapsulated bleb

H — Flat bleb

Medical therapy

- Bleb needling
- Bleb revision

- Repeat surgery
- Trabeculectomy
- Tube implant
- Cyclodestructive procedure

I — *Monitor:*
- IOP
- Visual fields
- Optic nerve/RNFL

Adjunctive mitomycin-C/5-FU

A. Primary open-angle glaucoma is considered to be medically uncontrolled when progressive optic nerve damage or visual field loss occurs despite maximum tolerated medical therapy. It may also be considered medically uncontrolled when glaucoma progression is considered likely based upon the level of intraocular pressure. Examination of the optic nerve should include the evaluation of contour changes, as well as the changes in vessel position, disc color, and retinal nerve fiber layer (RNFL). Progressive visual field deterioration must be differentiated from change due to other causes (e.g. cataract and retinal pathology) and from test-retest variability. SWAP (short-wavelength automated perimetry/blue-yellow perimetry) and frequency doubling technology perimetry may detect field loss or progression several years before standard automated perimetry.

B. Knowledge of intraocular pressure (IOP) levels before initiation of therapy helps to determine a target pressure below which further damage is unlikely. The target pressure should be adjusted lower in view of younger patient age, more advanced degree of glaucomatous damage or signs of progressive damage (disc or RNFL changes, disc hemorrhage, or progressive visual field loss).

C. Because of their low complication rate compared with traditional filtering surgery, argon laser trabeculoplasty (ALT) or selective laser trabeculoplasty (SLT) may be considered as the first step in surgical therapy. SLT has the potential advantage over ALT of the absence of photocoagulative damage to the trabecular meshwork, offering the potential for retreatment. Following ALT or SLT, IOP should be monitored to determine the efficacy in achieving the target pressure. The maximal treatment effect may not be observed for several weeks after the procedure. Topical α_2-agonists should be used before and immediately after laser trabeculoplasty to reduce the incidence of post-laser IOP spikes. When the IOP is greater than the expected efficacy of laser trabeculoplasty, it may be appropriate to proceed directly to filtering surgery.

D. Due to the risk of complications of trabeculectomy and glaucoma implant surgery, alternative procedures have been introduced that may reduce these risks. These procedures include viscocanalostomy, nonpenetrating deep sclerectomy, canaloplasty, Trabectome, and iStent micro-bypass shunt. In general, their efficacy appears to be somewhat less than what can be achieved by other surgical approaches, making them best suited to patients who do not require an extremely low target IOP.

E. The decision to use adjunctive mitomycin-C is based on the risk of failure of standard filtering surgery and on the desired target pressure. When conjunctival scarring is present from previous ocular surgery, trabeculectomy without an adjunctive antimetabolite has already failed or a postoperative IOP <10–12 mm Hg is desired, adjunctive mitomycin-C use is generally necessary. Careful consideration of the potential benefit of mitomycin-C is required for each patient, given the evidence of an increased risk of persistent hypotony, cataract, and late bleb leak, particularly when higher dosages are used. Lower concentrations of mitomycin-C (0.2–0.25 mg/mL) and shorter application times (1–3 min) have reduced the incidence of postoperative complications. Adjunctive 5-fluorouracil (5-FU) may not be as effective as mitomycin-C, requires multiple postoperative injections, and can lead to corneal epithelial toxicity. However, the dosage can be tailored to the individual patient based on the postoperative inflammatory response, and the risks of hypotony and other complications may be less than with mitomycin. Studies have demonstrated similar efficacy and complication rates between glaucoma implant surgery and trabeculectomy, leading to the consideration of glaucoma implants as an option for initial surgery.

F. Procedures to reduce elevated IOP after glaucoma filtration surgery are most effective when performed within the first few weeks of surgery. Slit-lamp examination and gonioscopy help to determine the cause of diminished outflow. Internal obstruction of the sclerostomy with pigment or membranes, can be treated with argon or yttrium aluminum garnet (YAG) laser. If outflow is restricted externally, laser lysis of trabeculectomy flap sutures combined with digital pressure, steroids, or adjunctive 5-FU can be beneficial. If elevated IOP persists, resumption of medical therapy is required.

G. Encapsulation of the filtering bleb often responds to conservative treatment, including aqueous suppression and digital massage. When these measures fail to result in an adequate level of IOP control, bleb needling to incise the tissue surrounding the trabeculectomy flap may give good long-term results. Adjunctive 5-FU after bleb needling may increase the probability of success. Surgical revision of an encapsulated bleb is occasionally necessary when the IOP remains uncontrolled or in cases of secondary dellen unresponsive to medical therapy.

H. If a scarred, flat bleb results from primary surgery, a second filtering operation should be performed in an unoperated quadrant using adjunctive mitomycin-C, or a glaucoma drainage implant should be placed. Because of the potential complications of visual loss and phthisis, cyclodestructive procedures such as laser trans-scleral cyclophotocoagulation have traditionally been reserved when other surgical options have failed. Endoscopic laser cyclophotocoagulation may be safer than the trans-scleral procedure, and may be a reasonable alternative for the treatment of eyes earlier in the course of disease.

I. If the target IOP is attained after surgical intervention, visual fields and optic nerve status must be carefully monitored to rule out ongoing damage. If progressive damage occurs, a new, lower target pressure must be chosen and the therapy must be adjusted accordingly.

BIBLIOGRAPHY

1. Francis BA, Singh K, Lin SC, et al. Novel glaucoma procedures: A report by the American Academy of Ophthalmology. Ophthalmology. 2011;118:1466-80.
2. Gedde SJ, Singh K, Schiffman JC, et al. The tube versus trabeculectomy study: Interpretation of results and application to clinical practice. Curr Opin Ophthalmol. 2012;23:118-26.
3. Ishida K. Update on results and complications of cyclophotocoagulation. Curr Opin Ophthalmol. 2013; 24:102-10.
4. Robin AL, Ramakrishnan R, Bhatnagar R, et al. A long-term dose-response study of mitomycin in glaucoma filtration surgery. Arch Ophthalmol. 1997;115: 969-74.
5. Samples JR, Singh K, Lin SC, et al. Laser trabeculoplasty for open-angle glaucoma: A report by the American Academy of Ophthalmology. Ophthalmology. 2011;118: 2296-302.
6. Shingleton BJ, Richter CU, Dharma SK. Long-term efficacy of argon laser trabeculoplasty: A 10 year follow-up study. Ophthalmology. 1993;100:1324-9.
7. Stamper RL, Lieberman MF, Drake MV, (Eds). Becker-Shaffer's Diagnosis and Therapy of the Glaucomas, 8th Edition. Philadelphia, PA: Mosby Elsevier; 2009. pp. 508-48.

Shallow Anterior Chamber After Glaucoma Surgery

J Kevin McKinney, Roy Whitaker Jr, Kundandeep S Nagi

97

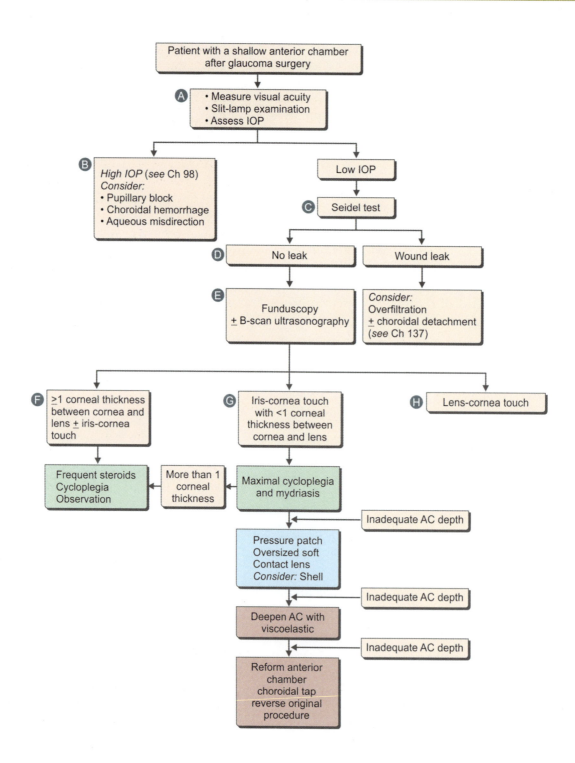

Glaucoma filtration surgery is designed to lower the intraocular pressure (IOP) to a level that prevents progressive visual loss by creating an alternate drainage pathway for the escape of aqueous humor from the anterior chamber (AC). A shallow or flat AC in the early postoperative course implies either excessive escape of aqueous humor from overfiltration or a wound leak, or posterior pressure on the lens-iris diaphragm from pupillary block, aqueous misdirection, or choroidal hemorrhage. Postoperative shallow chambers, after trabeculectomy, are less common with the use of adjunctive antimetabolites such as 5-fluorouracil (5-FU) and mitomycin-C because a tighter scleral flap closure is necessary to prevent postoperative hypotony. Recognition of the cause underlying a shallow AC and timely institution of appropriate management are essential for preserving postoperative IOP control and visual function.

A.   The AC depth may be unstable for several days after filtration surgery. Both the patient and the examiner must avoid excessive pressure on the globe to prevent flattening of the AC. IOP measurement is critical in determining the cause of a shallow AC but must be performed and interpreted with caution. In a very soft eye, applanation IOP is notoriously difficult to measure but can be obtained with accuracy, if performed gently with the applanation dial initially set to <10 mm Hg. Folds in Descemet membrane are a useful slit-lamp indicator of a potentially low IOP. With a flat AC, IOP measurements may be spurious as a result of applanation of the lens or intraocular lens. Cautious tactile assessment of the IOP is useful in this situation. A careful ocular examination should be performed daily until intraocular conditions stabilize.

B.   Iris bombé with a relatively deeper central AC, in the absence of a patent iridectomy, implies the presence of pupillary block. The AC tends to be diffusely shallow with choroidal hemorrhage and aqueous misdirection (see Chapter 98 for details of evaluation and management of elevated IOP with a shallow AC).

C.   When a shallow AC and a low IOP are present, a wound or bleb leak should be excluded by application of topical fluorescein (moistened strip or 2% solution) to the wound and bleb under illumination with a cobalt blue light (Seidel test). A stream of bright yellowgreen fluid against the dark background indicates a leak. Such leaks are more common if adjunctive antimetabolites have been used (see Chapter 100 for management of wound leaks).

D.   With a low IOP, careful funduscopy and/or B-scan ultrasonography should be used to determine the presence, extent, and nature of choroidal detachment. Although serous choroidal detachment most often results from hypotony, it may also perpetuate hypotony and AC shallowing because of the detachment of the ciliary body with aqueous hyposecretion.

E.   With a low IOP and no evidence of a wound leak, overfiltration, with or without choroidal detachment, is the most likely cause for a shallow AC. A shallow chamber from overfiltration may be diagnosed by placing a pressure patch for 10–20 minutes or by applying gentle pressure over the scleral flap with a moistened cotton-tipped applicator for 1–2 minutes: deepening of the AC indicates overfiltration. Management varies with the central depth of the AC and the presence or absence of lens-cornea touch.

F.   Although prolonged iris-cornea touch may cause some endothelial cell loss and peripheral anterior synechiae (PAS) formation, conservative measures are usually adequate until spontaneous deepening occurs, as long as the lens-cornea touch is absent. Inflammation should be suppressed with frequent steroids, and adequate cycloplegia (atropine) should be maintained to encourage posterior rotation of the ciliary body and to hinder PAS formation.

G.   A central AC depth of less than one corneal thickness runs the risk of intermittent lens-cornea touch and therefore warrants additional efforts to deepen the AC. Maximal cycloplegia (atropine) and mydriasis (phenylephrine) are indicated and may be initiated as a "burst" of one drop every 5 minutes for three doses. If the AC deepens to one corneal thickness or greater, careful observation is continued. If no effect is observed, various methods of tamponading filtration may be tried. A properly applied pressure patch (particularly a "torpedo" patch) is usually sufficient to deepen the chamber. If the AC shallows again with observation, the patch may be replaced daily for several days until the AC remains deep spontaneously. An oversized soft contact lens may provide sufficient tamponade in some eyes, whereas others may require placement of a Simmons glaucoma shell or symblepharon ring. These devices should be used only by those with skills and experience in their proper placement and management because significant side effects (discomfort, corneal epithelial defects, corneal edema) may occur with their use. Some specialists would recommend the use of hyperosmotic to shrink the vitreous at this point. Caution should be used because these agents carry some risk of potentiating the hypotony and its attendant complications. If the AC remains so shallow that the lens almost touches the cornea, one should proceed to the measures outlined for lens-cornea touch.

H. Lens-cornea touch mandates immediate intervention because of the high-risk of corneal decompensation and cataract formation. A cycloplegic/mydriatic "burst" may be given followed by a temporary pressure patch for a few hours, but continued conservative management is indicated only if the chamber deepens to one corneal thickness or greater. A completely flat chamber after a glaucoma drainage tube implant is a special situation that may also damage the cornea and lens; it seldom responds to conservative measures and usually requires surgical intervention. Deepening of the AC with viscoelastic through a pre-existing or new paracentesis track can cause permanent deepening but may require repeated injections. This may be performed at the slit-lamp with instillation of appropriate broad-spectrum antibiotics or 5% povidone-iodine drops before the injection. For a more definitive approach, the patient is returned to the operating room so that the AC can be reformed with saline or viscoelastic, and so that the choroidals can be drained. Occasionally, this procedure must be repeated. If all of the aforementioned measures fail, the original procedure may need to be revised with resuturing of a scleral flap or ligation of a drainage implant tube (using an absorbable suture). Cycloplegia and patching may still prove to be useful for persistent or recurrent AC shallowing after these procedures.

BIBLIOGRAPHY

1. Cioffi GA. Postoperative flat anterior chamber. In: Roy FH (Ed). Master Techniques in Ophthalmic Surgery. Baltimore, MD: Williams & Wilkins; 1995. pp. 37-45.
2. Fourman S. Management of lens-cornea touch after filtering surgery for Glaucoma. Ophthalmology. 1990;97:424-8.
3. Liebermann JM, Ritch R. Complications of glaucoma filtering surgery. In: Ritch R, Shields MB, Krupin T (Eds). The Glaucomas. St. Louis, MO: Mosby; 1996. pp. 1703-36.
4. Simmons RJ, Kimbrough RL. Shell tamponade in filtering surgery for glaucoma. Ophthalmic Surg. 1979;10:17-34.
5. Stewart WC, Shields MD. Management of anterior chamber depth after trabeculectomy. Am J Ophthalmol. 1988;106:41-4.

High Intraocular Pressure After Glaucoma Filtration Surgery

98

John M Parkinson, J Kevin McKinney, Kundandeep S Nagi

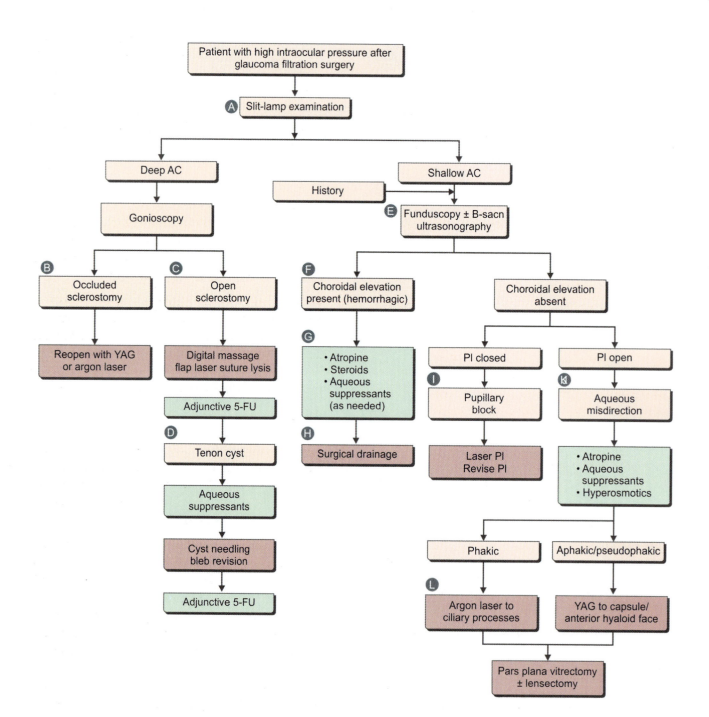

A. Careful slit-lamp examination is essential in differentiating the causes of elevated intraocular pressure (IOP) after glaucoma filtration surgery. Most commonly, elevated postoperative pressure is associated with a deep anterior chamber (AC) and only mild-to-moderate discomfort. Bleb appearance can be helpful but must be interpreted in light of the other findings. A flat bleb indicates internal or external obstruction of filtration, but an elevated bleb does not rule out partial obstruction.

B. Despite open angles by gonioscopy, the internal sclerostomy may be occluded by iris, iris pigment epithelium, blood, fibrin, or viscoelastic or transparent membranes (inflammatory, proliferative, or residual Descemet membrane). The Argon or Neodymium: Yttrium Aluminium Garnet (YAG) laser can be used to reopen the internal sclerostomy. Blood and fibrin clots that occlude the internal sclerostomy often resorb spontaneously. If available, fibrinolytic agents such as tissue plasminogen activator or streptokinase may be injected intracamerally to dissolve the clot.

C. In the presence of a patent internal sclerostomy, external factors are responsible for elevated pressure. Within the first few postoperative days, ocular digital pressure may break fibrinous adhesions between the scleral bed and trabeculectomy flap to restore adequate outflow. If elevated IOP persists, serial laser suture lysis (Argon, Krypton, or diode) of trabeculectomy flap sutures can be performed using a handheld contact lens to compress the overlying conjunctiva. If significant external scarring is likely, supplemental injections of 5-fluorouracil (5-FU) are considered.

D. In the early postoperative period, encapsulation of the filtering bleb (a Tenon 'cyst') may respond to the measures outlined in Section C. Failing this, pharmacologic aqueous suppression and intermittent digital massage will often soften the cyst. Refractory IOP elevation may require needling of the cyst with supplemental 5-FU or revision of the bleb.

E. In the presence of a shallow AC, funduscopy and B-scan ultrasonography are used to determine the presence, extent, and nature (serous or hemorrhagic) of choroidal elevation. High-resolution ultrasound biomicropscopy may be helpful in visualizing peripheral annular choroidal detachments.

F. The presence of choroidal elevation in the face of elevated IOP and shallow or flat AC usually implies a hemorrhagic cause. In such cases, a history of sudden, severe eye pain is usually obtained.

G. Initial treatment includes maximum cycloplegia (atropine), frequent topical and possibly systemic steroids, and aqueous suppression, if the IOP is elevated (β-blocker, carbonic anhydrase inhibitor, and/or α-agonist), treat underlying systemic problems (uncontrolled hypertension or bleeding diatheses).

H. After consultation with a vitreoretinal subspecialist, surgical drainage may be performed after waiting 7 to 10 days to allow the clot to liquefy. Indications of surgical drainage include massive choroidal detachment with decreased visual acuity, corneal decompensation, persistently flat AC, and elevated IOP unresponsive to medical therapy.

I. In the absence of choroidal separation, pupillary block should be ruled out by ensuring the patency of the peripheral iridectomy (PI). In aphakic and pseudophakic eyes, posterior loculation of aqueous may occur despite a patent iridectomy, and another laser PI in the affected quadrant(s) may be curative.

J. A centrally shallow or flat AC, in the presence of a patent iridectomy and elevated or normal IOP, implies posterior misdirection of aqueous into the vitreous (malignant glaucoma). This may occur as a result of ciliary-lenticular apposition (ciliary block), or may represent the misdirection of aqueous behind an intact anterior vitreous face.

K. Medical therapy includes maximal cycloplegia (atropine) and pupillary dilation (phenylephrine), aqueous suppressant therapy (see Section F), and hyperosmotic therapy (glycerin, mannitol, or isosorbide). Approximately 50% of the cases resolve within 3 to 5 days of medical therapy. The patient is monitored for electrolyte imbalance and dehydration. Indications of earlier surgical intervention include a persistently flat AC, corneal decompensation, cataract development in phakic eyes, and uncontrolled IOP (depending on the optic nerve status).

L. In patients who do not respond to medical therapy, laser treatment is often effective. In phakic eyes, the Argon laser can be applied gonioscopically through the PI or pupil to shrink visible ciliary processes, thus breaking the ciliolenticular block. Because of its high success rate in aphakic and pseudophakic eyes, laser treatment may be attempted before a trial of medical therapy in such eyes. In aphakic eyes, YAG laser disruption of the anterior hyaloid face may promote normal anterior flow of the aqueous. YAG capsulotomy/hyaloidotomy is often successful in pseudophakic eyes, and is best performed beyond the edge of the optic. In refractory cases, pars plana vitrectomy with disruption of the anterior hyaloid is indicated, and lensectomy may be necessary in phakic eyes.

BIBLIOGRAPHY

1. Lundy DC, Sidoti P, Winarko T, et al. Intracameral tissue plasminogen activator after glaucoma surgery. Ophthalmology. 1996;103:274-82.
2. Pederson JE, Smith SG. Surgical management of encapsulated filtering blebs. Ophthalmology. 1985;92:955-8.
3. Simmons RJ, Maestre FA. Malignant glaucoma. In: Ritch R, Shields MB, Krupin T (Eds). The Glaucomas. St Louis, MO: Mosby, 1996. pp. 841-55.
4. Stamper RL. Elevated intraocular pressure after filtering surgery. In: Roy FH (Ed). Master Techniques in Ophthalmic Surgery. Baltimore, MD: Williams & Wilkins, 1995. pp. 629-38.

The Glaucoma Patient with Cataract

99

John W Boyle IV, Peter A Netland

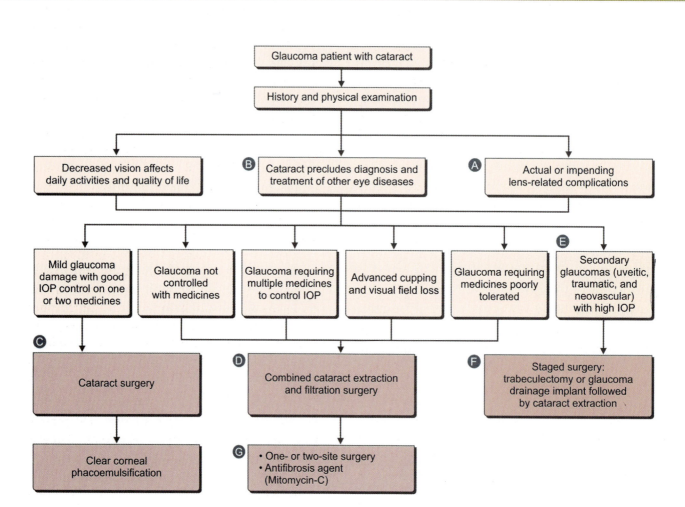

Glaucoma patient with cataract

History and physical examination

Decreased vision affects daily activities and quality of life

Ⓑ Cataract precludes diagnosis and treatment of other eye diseases

Ⓐ Actual or impending lens-related complications

Mild glaucoma damage with good IOP control on one or two medicines

Glaucoma not controlled with medicines

Glaucoma requiring multiple medicines to control IOP

Advanced cupping and visual field loss

Glaucoma requiring medicines poorly tolerated

Ⓔ Secondary glaucomas (uveitic, traumatic, and neovascular) with high IOP

Ⓒ Cataract surgery

Ⓓ Combined cataract extraction and filtration surgery

Ⓕ Staged surgery: trabeculectomy or glaucoma drainage implant followed by cataract extraction

Clear corneal phacoemulsification

Ⓖ • One- or two-site surgery
• Antifibrosis agent (Mitomycin-C)

The two most common causes of vision loss in the elderly are cataracts and glaucoma. Cataract is the leading cause of reversible blindness in the world, and glaucoma is the leading cause of age-related irreversible vision loss. Because of the aging population, cataract and glaucoma frequently coexist in the same individual. The presence of cataracts can complicate the decision-making process for the surgical management of the glaucoma patient. In patients with well-controlled intraocular pressure (IOP) or early glaucoma, cataract surgery alone may be effective. In patients with advanced glaucoma or poor control of IOP, combining trabeculectomy with cataract extraction and intraocular lens implantation in one operation may be the preferred option. Combining cataract surgery with newer surgical techniques, such as iStent (a trabecular microbypass shunt), trabectome (ab interno trabeculotomy), or endoscopic cyclophotocoagulation (ECP) may be appropriate for patients with mild to moderate glaucoma because these techniques avoid many of the complications associated with trabeculectomies.

A. The evaluation of a patient with glaucoma and cataract should include a careful history and a complete ophthalmic examination. The history includes questions about the onset and time course of vision loss, an assessment of visual function and impact of daily living, and a review of current medications, previous ocular history, and past ocular surgery. Compliance to treatment and any adverse effects to local or systemic glaucoma medications should also be ascertained in the history. The examination includes assessment of the best corrected vision, with optimal refraction. Visual acuity testing in high- and low-contrast settings may be performed, as well as potential acuity testing. IOP measurement, optic nerve head and retinal nerve fiber analysis, and visual field testing are obtained. The surgeon's view into the eye should correspond to the patient's symptoms. In patients whom media opacity due to cataract precludes examination of the fundus, ultrasonography may be required. Assessment of the pupil size after dilation may help the surgeon plan for intraoperative management of a small pupil.

B. In the glaucoma patient with a cataractous lens, there are several indications of cataract surgery. Firstly, cataract extraction is indicated when decreased visual acuity affects a patient's quality of life and causes limitation of the patient's ability to function in daily activities, including employment, reading, writing, driving, or recreation. Secondly, surgery may benefit the patient when cataract precludes diagnosis and/or treatment of other eye diseases, such as diabetic retinopathy. Thirdly, cataract extraction is necessary when there are actual or impending complications of lens-induced ocular diseases, such as phacolytic and phacomorphic glaucoma. Combined cataract extraction and filtering surgery is indicated when there is a visually significant cataract and the glaucoma is not controlled with medications or laser trabeculoplasty, there is advanced optic nerve cupping and visual field loss, or the patient is taking maximal tolerated medical therapy.

C. Patients with visually significant cataracts and mild glaucoma damage with good IOP control on one or two glaucoma medications may be treated with cataract surgery alone. In addition, patients who have angle-closure glaucoma will often benefit from cataract surgery alone.

Cataract surgery alone is technically simpler and is associated with fewer complications as compared with combined cataract extraction and glaucoma filtration procedures. Surgeons should take into account the possible need for glaucoma surgery in the future. Therefore, clear cornea temporal phacoemulsification cataract surgery (PECE) is preferred over extracapsular cataract extraction (ECCE) since it avoids manipulating the conjunctiva and inducing conjunctival scarring, which would preclude filtration surgery later. When a limbal peritomy is performed, incisions should ideally be restricted to one quadrant to preserve areas for possible subsequent filtration surgery. In patients with dense cataracts, intraoperative assessment of the optic nerve may be necessary to determine whether the eye has minimal optic nerve damage and may be treated with cataract surgery alone, or has extensive optic nerve damage and should be treated with combined cataract and filtration surgery. Cataract extraction after both PECE and ECCE usually results in an IOP decrease of 2–4 mm Hg at 1–2 years follow-up. Patients with mild glaucoma controlled on one or two medicines may benefit from combined cataract surgery with ECP, iStent, or Trabectome tool. These procedures are performed through the cataract incision to avoid manipulation of the conjunctiva and allow for faster visual recovery.

D. Patients with cataract and borderline IOP control, with moderate to advanced glaucoma damage, benefit from a combined cataract extraction and filtration procedure. The indications for a combined procedure include a visually significant cataract requiring extraction with the following: Glaucoma uncontrolled with medicines or after laser trabeculoplasty, glaucoma requiring multiple medications to control IOP, glaucoma controlled with medicines poorly tolerated by the patient, or advanced cupping and visual field loss. Patients undergoing combined glaucoma and cataract operations have better long-term IOP control compared to the patients undergoing cataract surgery alone. In addition, combined surgery may avoid the risk of an early postoperative increase in IOP. Postoperative elevation of IOP may occur after cataract extraction alone, and may further damage the already compromised optic nerve in patients with moderate to advanced glaucoma. However, long-term IOP control after a combined surgery is slightly worse than trabeculectomy alone. Several surgical approaches may be considered today in combination with cataract and glaucoma surgery. For years, phacoemulsification performed through the standard trabeculectomy flap has been the most widely accepted approach. Two-site surgery with a clear corneal cataract incision temporally and a standard trabeculectomy flap superiorly, may provide slightly lower IOP than one-site surgery. IOP is also further lowered by small-incision phacoemulsification than by nuclear expression in combined procedures. The antifibrosis agent, mitomycin-C, has been shown to improve the success of combined cataract and filtration surgery. Combining phacoemulsification and the EX-PRESS glaucoma filtration device placed under a partial thickness scleral flap is an alternative to a combined standard trabeculectomy and phacoemulsification. Advantages of this procedure include a more stable anterior chamber with a lessened risk of hypotony, and a quicker visual recovery without the need for a peripheral iridotomy. Another option is combined cataract surgery with canaloplasty, which involves circumferential viscodilation and tensioning of Schlemm's canal using a microcatheter (iScience) and suture.

E. A combined surgery should be avoided in situations when there is an emergent need to reduce the IOP. Patients with visually significant cataracts and secondary refractory glaucomas such as uveitic, traumatic, or neovascular glaucoma should have a staged surgery, that is, filtration surgery first followed by cataract extraction because of the increased risk of postoperative complications. Staged surgery should also be considered for patients with very advanced glaucoma and cataract who require a very low-target IOP. Cataract surgery decreases bleb function, on average, in patients with functioning filters. Patients may require an increased number of glaucoma medications postoperatively to control IOP. Injections of 5-FU and/or bleb needling at the time of or after surgery may improve bleb function. Patients with mild glaucoma well controlled on one or two medicines are treated, usually with cataract surgery alone. Glaucoma drainage implants are indicated in patients with refractory glaucomas in which filtration surgery has failed or has a high likelihood for failure. Combined cataract surgery and drainage implant surgery has been shown to achieve successful control of IOP in the majority of the treated patients.

F. Small pupils and exfoliation syndrome are commonly encountered in glaucoma patients. Adequate pupil size enhances visualization and reduces the incidence of intraoperative complications during cataract extraction. A decreasing pupil size during surgery has been shown to be a significant risk factor for vitreous loss. Stretch pupilloplasty, to gently stretch the iris sphincter, will often yield a suitable pupillary aperture. Small iris sphincterotomies with subsequent stretching of the sphincter is another useful option. Iris hook retractors (Mackool, de Juan) can be helpful, particularly in enlarging very small pupils to an adequate size to perform phacoemulsification. Various elegant iris suturing techniques have been described, but these often require considerable efforts and operating time. The Graether pupil expander, Beehler pupil dilator, Oasis iris expander, and Malyugin ring are devices that can be placed in the eye during surgery to expand the pupil. Sector or keyhole iridectomy is not optimal for several reasons: the pupil is cosmetically deformed, aspiration of the cut ends of iris may interfere with phacoemulsification, and visualization often remains poor in the area away from the sector iridectomy. Pseudoexfoliation syndrome also poses unique challenges during cataract surgery. In addition to poor pupillary dilation, patients with pseudoexfoliation syndrome have weak zonules, which increase the risk of capsular rupture, vitreous loss, and lens dislocation. Capsular tension rings may be used during phacoemulsification to improve capsular support.

G. Patients with significant amounts of astigmatism, undergoing cataract surgery, benefit from astigmatism correction or toric lens implantation. However, these lenses should be used with caution in patients undergoing combined cataract and filtration surgery. The toric lens may shift position when used in combined surgery because of potential anterior chamber shallowing. Patients with pseudoexfoliation or prior trauma may also show greater variation in lens position if zonular support of the capsular bag has been disrupted. Patients who have mild to moderate glaucoma and elect to have a toric lens may benefit from a staged procedure. Multifocal lens such as the Restor or TECNIS® lens may be inappropriate for patients with moderate to severe glaucoma since these diffractive lens split the light and may aggravate visual field defects.

Patients undergoing glaucoma filtration surgery are at a significantly increased risk of developing cataract. Multiple glaucoma clinical trials have documented this increased risk. The Collaborative Initial Glaucoma Treatment Study found that patients treated with surgical therapy had twice the incidence of cataract compared with patients treated with medical therapy. In the Advanced Glaucoma Intervention Study, patients treated with trabeculectomy had an increased risk of cataract compared with patients treated with laser trabeculoplasty. The Collaborative Normal-Tension Glaucoma Study found that 38% of the patients treated medically or surgically developed cataracts compared with 14% of the patients who were not treated. Young patients after filtration surgery may require cataract surgery after trabeculectomy. Patients treated medically for glaucoma also have an increased risk of cataract formation. The Ocular Hypertension Treatment Study observed that the patients treated with glaucoma medications had a slightly higher incidence of cataract surgery compared with the control group. The Barbados Eye Study found a threefold increased risk of lens opacity in patients treated with topical medicines. In summary, both surgical and (to a lesser extent) medical therapy of glaucoma increase the risk of cataract formation. Other factors that may increase cataract formation after filtration surgery include corticosteroid use and a flat anterior chamber postoperatively. Cataract progression occurs more commonly after full thickness filtration surgery, compared with trabeculectomy. Little is known about cataract progression after nonpenetrating glaucoma surgeries.

Cataracts and glaucomas frequently coexist in patients, and this common clinical problem will only confront physicians more frequently with the increasing age of the population. Surgical options include cataract surgery alone, combined surgery, or staged surgery. Management of both should be individualized for each patient to maximize the surgical success for these two common causes of vision loss.

BIBLIOGRAPHY

1. Advanced Glaucoma Intervention Study (AGIS) Investigators. The Advanced Glaucoma Intervention Study: 8. Risk of cataract formation after trabeculectomy. Arch Ophthalmol. 2001;119:1771-9.
2. Collaborative Normal-Tension Glaucoma Study Group. Comparison of glaucomatous progression between untreated patients with normal-tension glaucoma and patients with therapeutically reduced intraocular pressures. Am J Ophthalmol. 1998;126:487-97.
3. Friedman DS, Jampel HD, Lubomski, et al. Surgical strategies for coexisting glaucoma and cataract: An evidenced-based update. Ophthalmology. 2002;109:1902-13.
4. Hoffman KB, Feldman RM, Budenz DL, et al. Combined cataract extraction and Baerveldt glaucoma drainage implant: Indications and outcomes. Ophthalmology. 2002;109:1916-20.
5. Jampel HD, Friedman DS, Lubomski, et al. Effect of technique on intraocular pressure after combined cataract and glaucoma surgery: An evidenced-based review. Ophthalmology. 2002;109:2215-24.
6. Kanner EM, Netland PA, Sarkisian SR, et al. Ex-PRESS miniature glaucoma device implanted under a sclera flap alone or combined with phacoemulsification cataract surgery. J Glaucoma. 2009;18:488-91.
7. Kass MA, Heuer DK, Higginbotham EJ, et al. The ocular hypertension treatment study: A randomized trial determines that topical ocular hypertensive medication delays or prevents the onset of primary open-angle glaucoma. Arch Ophthalmol. 2002;120:701-13.
8. Lee RK, Gedde SJ. Surgical management of coexisting cataract and glaucoma. Int Ophthalmol Clin. 2004;44:151-66.
9. Lewis RA, von Wolff K, Tetz M, et al. Canaloplasty: Three-year results of circumferential viscodilation and tensioning of Schlemm canal using a microcatheter to treat open-angle glaucoma. J Cataract Refract Surg. 2011;37:682-90.
10. Lichter PR, Musch DC, Gillespie BW, et al. Interim clinical outcomes in the collaborative initial glaucoma treatment study comparing initial treatment randomized to medications or surgery. Ophthalmology. 2001;108:1943-53.
11. Rebolleda G, Munoz-Negrete FJ. Phacoemulsification in eyes with functioning filtering blebs: A prospective study. Ophthalmology. 2002;109:2248-55.

100

Ocular Hypotony

John Ryan McManus, J Kevin McKinney, Peter A Netland

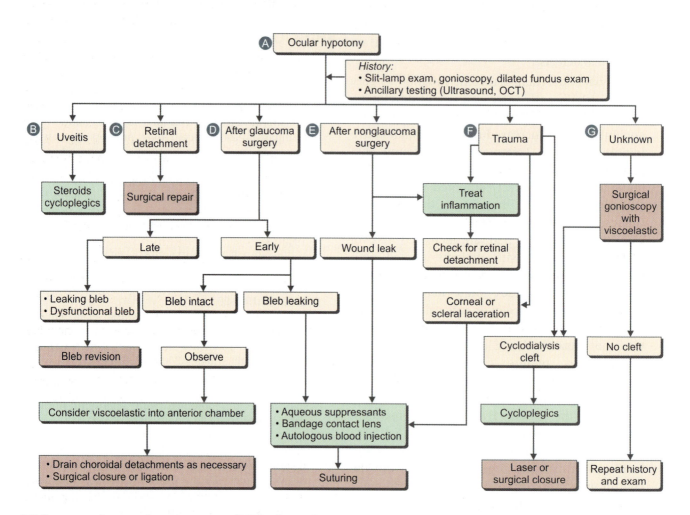

While any intraocular pressure (IOP) less than 6.5 mm Hg is considered ocular hypotony, visual sequelae are most common with an IOP less than 4 mm Hg. These sequelae include corneal folds, choroidal detachment, and hemorrhage, optic nerve swelling, hypotony maculopathy, cataract, and phthisis bulbi. Timely diagnosis and treatment of ocular hypotony are critical for the restoration and preservation of vision.

A. A detailed history is essential in determining the cause of ocular hypotony. Any recent or distant history of ocular surgery or trauma should be elucidated. A detailed medication list should be obtained, carefully noting the use of topical or systemic ocular hypotensive medications. Symptoms of uveitis (decreased vision, photophobia, and ocular pain) and retinal detachment (flashing lights, floaters, or curtain-like field loss) should be sought.

B. Uveitis may be associated with high or low IOP. It can cause hypotony by decreasing the aqueous production or increasing the uveoscleral outflow. Treatment of the hypotony is aimed at inflammation control, typically with topical, periocular, or even systemic steroids. Systemic steroid-sparing agents are also used. Cycloplegic agents reduce discomfort from ciliary spasm and aim to prevent formation of posterior synechiae.

C. Retinal detachments are often associated with ocular hypotony and must be excluded in any case of unexplained low IOP. The exact mechanism by which retinal detachments lower IOP is undetermined but may involve decreased aqueous production, increased uveoscleral outflow, or posterior flow of fluid through the retinal break and across the retinal pigment epithelium. The extent of the detachment does not correlate with the degree of hypotony. Surgical repair of the detachment is the treatment of choice. Cyclitic membrane may also be associated with hypotony, presumably due to reduced aqueous production.

D. Ocular hypotony is commonly encountered after glaucoma surgery. If the surgery is in the distant past, one can suspect overfiltration, hyposecretion of aqueous, or leaking bleb. If a leak is discovered, a bleb revision or autologous blood injection should be considered. Bleb leaks can also occur in the early postoperative period. Early bleb leaks can be treated with suturing, aqueous suppressants, pressure patching, or bandage contact lenses. Decreasing the frequency of topical steroids may promote healing of the wound. If the bleb is intact and elevated, overfiltration is the probable cause of hypotony. Depending on the particular circumstances, overfiltration may be treated with observation, filling of the anterior chamber with viscoelastic, or drainage of any serous or hemorrhagic choroidal detachment that may be present. Rapid lowering of IOP after glaucoma surgery may be associated with decompression retinopathy, manifested with mostly mid-peripheral retinal hemorrhages.

E. Ocular hypotony after nonfiltering intraocular surgery can also occur. The most common cause is wound leakage. Any incisions should be checked with fluorescein under a cobalt-blue light. A wound leak beneath the intact conjunctiva may produce an inadvertent filtering bleb, as suggested by subconjunctival fluid and conjunctival microcysts. Small wound leaks can be treated conservatively with pressure patches, bandage contact lenses, aqueous suppressants, or cyanoacrylate glue. Larger leaks may require surgical revision. Hypotony may also occur after intraocular surgery due to inflammation or an inadvertent cyclodialysis cleft created during the procedure.

F. There are two common causes of hypotony in eyes with a recent history of trauma. First, visible or hidden corneal or scleral lacerations may be leaking. Second, a cyclodialysis cleft may be present. Most clefts can be identified by gonioscopy, but anterior segment ultrasound or optical coherence tomography may be necessary to identify the cleft. The size of the cleft does not correlate with the IOP. Cycloplegic agents are the first-line medical therapy and are effective in closing many clefts. Persistent cases can be treated with laser photocoagulation to the cleft. In refractory cases, direct suturing (cyclopexy) is often successful. A modified capsular tension ring may be used to tamponade and close the cleft. Closure of the cleft may be associated with a dramatic increase in the IOP that lasts days to weeks. Posterior wounds such as scleral rupture after blunt ocular trauma and inadvertent scleral perforation from retrobulbar needles should be kept in mind as less common causes of hypotony.

G. If no cause of hypotony can be identified, surgical exploration of the eye can be considered. Many "idiopathic" cases of chronic hypotony are caused by occult cyclodialysis clefts. These may be obscured by peripheral anterior synechiae. Detection of the cleft can be improved by gonioscopy after deepening of the anterior chamber with a viscoelastic agent. Other causes of hypotony may be determined during surgical exploration, including occult bleb leak or fistula and other causes.

BIBLIOGRAPHY

1. Allingham RR, Damji K, Freedman S, et al. Shields' Textbook of Glaucoma. Philadelphia, PA: Lippincott Williams & Wilikins, 2005. pp. 371-86.
2. Ioannidis AS, Barton K. Cyclodialysis cleft: causes and repair. Curr Opin Ophthalmol. 2010;21:150-4.
3. Lupinacci APC, Netland PA. Bleb-related problems after glaucoma filtering surgery. Contemp Ophthalmol. 2008;7:1-8.
4. Moster MR, Azuara-Blanco A. Incisional therapies: compli-cations of glaucoma surgery. In: Schacknow PN, Samples JR (Eds). The Glaucoma Book. New York, NY: Springer, 2010. pp. 841-69.
5. Pederson JE. Ocular hypotony. The Glaucomas. Ritch R, Shields MB, Krupin T (Eds). St Louis, MO: Mosby, 1996. pp. 1737-44.
6. Yuen NSY, Hui SP, Woo DCF. New method of surgical repair for 360-degree cyclodialysis. J Cataract Refract Surg. 2006;32:13-7.

101

Medical Therapy of Glaucoma

Kevin Gamett, Johan Zwaan, Peter A Netland

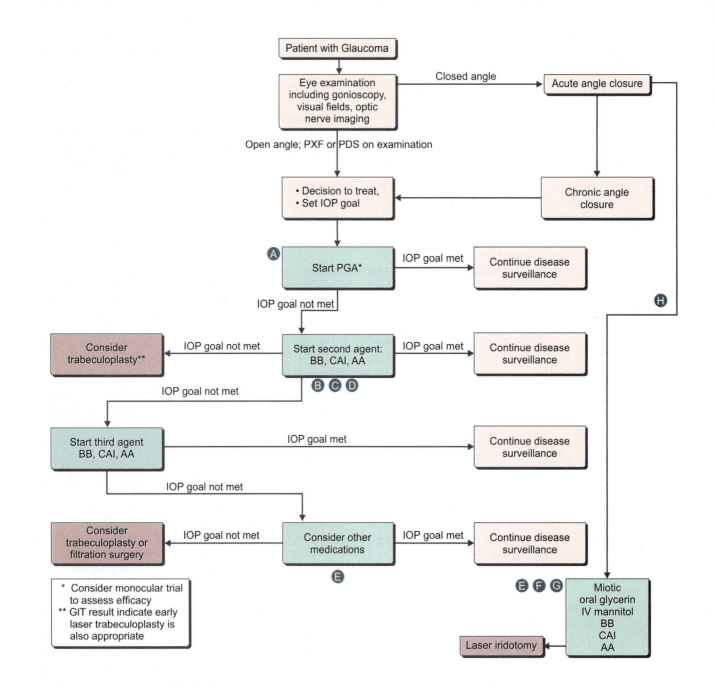

* Consider monocular trial to assess efficacy
** GIT result indicate early laser trabeculoplasty is also appropriate

When it is determined that a patient has glaucoma and needs medical therapy to lower intraocular pressure (IOP), a target IOP is chosen for clinical management. If the target IOP is reached with appropriate medical therapy, continued monitoring of the visual field and optic nerve appearance is performed to ensure that the optic nerve pathology is not progressing. If the visual field or the optic nerve appearance continues to worsen despite having reached the patient's target IOP, a lower target IOP must be set and additional medical or surgical therapy should be undertaken until the progression is halted. The algorithm described in this chapter pertains to primary open-angle glaucoma (POAG). Section H briefly discusses medical therapy for glaucomas other than POAG.

A. *Prostaglandin analogs:* Prostaglandins are first-line agents due to their efficacy, infrequent systemic side effects, and simple once daily dosing. Latanoprost, travaprost, bimatoprost, tafluprost, and unoprostone are available for clinical use. They decrease IOP approximately 30% by increasing the uveoscleral and conventional outflow. Side effects include conjunctival hyperemia, ocular allergy, iris color change, eyelash changes, and skin pigmentation. Uveitis and cystoid macular edema have also been described. Prostaglandins are effective and indicated for POAG, pseudoexfoliation glaucoma, pigmentary glaucoma, and chronic angle-closure glaucoma. Uveitic patients should be treated with caution, but stable patients with well-controlled inflammation can be treated safely.

B. *Beta-blockers:* Beta-blockers (BBs) remain one of the most commonly used classes of IOP-lowering topical medications. They act by decreasing the aqueous production with an approximate IOP decrease of 20–30%. Systemic side effects include bronchospasm, bradycardia, arrhythmia, worsening of congestive heart failure, depression, and fatigue. Local side effects include corneal anesthesia, ocular allergy, discomfort upon instillation, and decreased tear production. Betaxolol is selective for B1 receptors, which may have the advantage of exhibiting fewer pulmonary side effects. BBs have been indicated for all types of glaucoma and they are available in a variety of formulations and combination drops.

C. *Adrenergic agents:* Alpha-selective agonists (AAs) include clonidine, brimonidine, and apraclonidine. These medications decrease aqueous production, increase trabecular outflow, decrease episcleral venous pressure, and provide theoretical neuroprotection. Brimonidine is primarily used for long-term therapy, whereas apraclonidine use is often limited to brief use before and after procedures. A 20–30% decrease in IOP can be expected. Side effects include ocular allergy, dry mouth, and lethargy. AAs must be avoided in young children due to possible central nervous system and respiratory depression.

Nonselective agonists include epinephrine and dipivefrin. Both are now rarely used due to their lower efficacy and intolerable side-effect profile, which includes tachycardia, arrhythmia, hypertension, palpitation, anxiety, local irritation, allergic blepharoconjunctivitis, cystoid macular edema, and corneal or conjunctival adenochrome deposits.

D. *Carbonic anhydrase inhibitors:* Carbonic anhydrase inhibitors may decrease aqueous production when >90% of the carbonic anhydrase in ciliary epithelium is blocked. CAIs can be administered topically, orally, or intravenously. Dorzolamide and brinzolamide are the topical medications commonly used, either alone or in combination drops. Side effects of these topical medications include bitter taste, transient blurred vision, and punctate keratopathy. Caution is advised in patients with sulfa allergies due to potential cross-reactivity. Oral and intravenous (IV) CAIs are discussed later in the chapter.

E. *Miotics:* Parasympathomimetics are the oldest class of medical glaucoma therapies. Although they are more rarely used today, they may still be effective and appropriate in certain clinical situations.

Pilocarpine is a direct acting agent, which acts by the contraction of the longitudinal ciliary muscle, causing increased trabecular outflow. It may simultaneously decrease the uveoscleral outflow. It can cause a paradoxical angle closure due to the forward movement of the lens-iris diaphragm, which can lead to pupillary block. It breaks down the blood-aqueous barrier, so its use in uveitic patients or postoperatively should be limited. It is often poorly tolerated due to the decreased vision (induced myopia), miosis, headache, retinal detachment, epiphora, and cataract formation.

Echothiophate is a cholinesterase inhibitor. It has a higher incidence of systemic side effects, including diarrhea, abdominal cramps, bronchospasm, and enuresis. These symptoms may persist for 6 weeks due to the irreversible action of the drug on the enzyme.

F. *Oral agents:* Acetazolamide or methazolamide can be given when topical therapy fails or in the case of an acute pressure increase. Onset of action occurs at 1 hour and its peak action at 2–4 hours. Systemic side effects include paresthesias, fatigue, lack of libido, anorexia, weight loss, mental depression, sulfa cross-reactivity, abdominal discomfort, and an unpleasant metallic taste. Patients often do not tolerate acetazolamide or methazolamide for a long-term, so it is most commonly used as a temporizing measure before a more permanent IOP reduction strategy is employed.

Oral glycerin is a hyperosmotic agent that exhibits its effects by dehydrating the vitreous via an osmotic gradient. Onset is rapid, with the onset of action occurring approximately 20–30 minutes after oral administration. Its use is limited by the systemic side effects, including nausea, vomiting, hyperglycemia, renal failure, and headaches. Specifically, it should be used cautiously in diabetics and cardiac patients due to the risks associated with fluid shifts and hyperglycemia.

G. *Intravenous agents:* IV acetazolamide has an onset of action of approximately 2 minutes and has its peak effect at 15 minutes. The systemic side effects are the same as for oral acetazolamide.

Intravenous mannitol depletes the vitreous fluid through an osmotic gradient, similar to oral glycerin. Side effects include fluid retention, hyperglycemia, nausea, vomiting, electrolyte disturbance, and renal failure. Specifically, it must be used cautiously in cardiac patients where it can worsen congestive heart failure and in diabetics where it can precipitate ketoacidosis.

H. *Other causes of glaucoma:* Aside from POAG, there are many entities that also cause elevated IOP with subsequent damage to the optic nerve. Initial evaluation may reveal pseudoexfoliation or pigment dispersion syndrome. Both follow the same algorithm as POAG for medical therapy. Laser trabeculoplasty may be especially effective due to the increased trabecular meshwork pigmentation.

Gonioscopy may reveal either chronic or an acutely closed angle with or without neovascularization. With chronic angle-closure glaucoma, similar medical therapy can be employed as POAG. In acute angle closure, oral and topical medications may be used while preparing to perform a laser iridotomy. Pilocarpine may break the angle closure by bringing the pupil down and relieving the iridolenticular apposition. Osmotic drugs may be helpful when there is marked elevation of IOP.

BIBLIOGRAPHY

1. Glaucoma medical therapy: Principles and management, 2nd Edition. Netland PA (Ed). New York, NY: Oxford University Press, 2008.
2. Konstas AGP, Kozobolis VP, Tersis I, et al. The efficacy and safety of the timolol/dorzolamide fixed combination vs latanoprost in exfoliation glaucoma. Eye. 2003;17:41-6.
3. Lichter PR, Musch DC, Medzihradsky F, et al. Intraocular pressure effects of carbonic anhydrase inhibitors in primary open-angle glaucoma. Am J Ophthalmol. 1989;107:11-7.
4. Netland PA, Landry T, Sullivan EK, et al. Travaprost compared with latanoprost and timolol in patients with open-angle glaucoma or ocular hypertension. Am J Ophthalmol. 2001; 132:472-84.
5. Shields MD, Ritch R, Krupin TK. Classifications and mechanisms of the glaucomas. In: Ritch R, Shields MB, Krupin T (Eds). The Glaucomas. St Louis, MO: CV Mosby; 1996.

Uveitis-Associated Glaucoma

101A

John Ryan McManus, Ashvini K Reddy, Peter A Netland

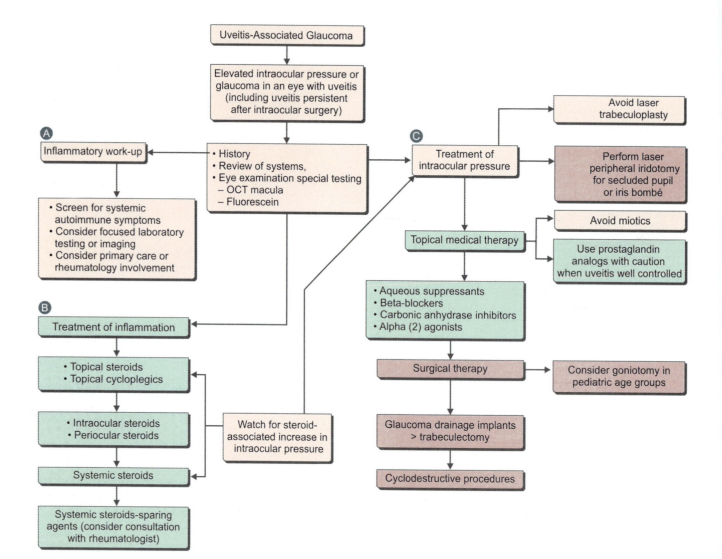

INTRODUCTION

Intraocular inflammation can be associated with elevated, normal, or low intraocular pressure. High intraocular pressure can also lead to a secondary, uveitic glaucoma. The mechanism of increased intraocular pressure in acute uveitis is thought to be direct inhibition of aqueous drainage at the level of the trabecular meshwork. In more chronic cases, the anterior chamber angle can be closed by anterior synechiae. The management of uveitic glaucoma is threefold: a clinician should seek to identify the cause of inflammation, treat the inflammation, and lower the intraocular pressure to limit glaucomatous damage.

A. Identify Cause of Inflammation

The differential of systemic autoimmune diseases associated with uveitis is broad, and 50% of cases are idiopathic. Sometimes, intraocular surgery or trauma can cause a chronic uveitis in an eye that is prone to inflammation. It is important for a clinician to take a complete history and perform a detailed review of symptoms to identify an etiology. The eye examination should carefully note the findings in anterior and posterior segments related to stigmata of inflammation as these may also provide clues as to the etiology. Gonioscopy and a careful examination of anterior chamber should be performed before dilation. Dilation often makes the rest of the examination more comfortable for the patient, as cycloplegic agents reduce the ciliary spasm associated with uveitis. A careful fundus examination should be performed looking for signs of inflammation in the vitreous, retina, retinal pigment epithelium, retinal blood vessels, and choroid. If macular edema is suspected, ocular coherence tomography should be performed. Fluorescein angiography can be helpful in the evaluation of retinal vascular leakage, macular leakage, and disc edema. Indocyanine green angiography and fundus autofluoresence may be indicated in the evaluation of the choroid and retina.

These results should prompt a focused work-up for possible causes of uveitis, which may include ancillary laboratory testing, imaging studies, and consultation with a rheumatologist or other specialist. If a cause of uveitis can be identified, treatment regimens can be tailored much more effectively.

B. Treatment of Inflammation

The mainstay of treatment for uveitis and the inflammatory component of uveitic glaucoma are topical steroids. In some uveitides, like Posner-Schlossman syndrome, steroids alone can reduce the intraocular pressure. In others, like Fuchs Heterochromic Iridocylitis, steroids have little effect on the inflammation or the intraocular pressure. Nonetheless, topical steroids remain first-line therapy for most cases. Patients with uveitis may also receive local steroid therapy with Sub-Tenon injections, intravitreal triamcinolone, or implants containing dexamethasone or fluocinolone acetonide. Steroid therapy of any kind can lead to elevation of intraocular pressure, which can complicate management. It is sometimes difficult to tell whether intraocular pressure rise is due to inflammation, the use of steroids, or a mixed mechanism.

Topical cycloplegic agents are also used frequently during the initial therapy period. These agents reduce pain from ciliary spasm as well as prevent posterior synechiae formation. Shorter-acting cycloplegic agents dosed more frequently are preferred, as a small amount of iris movement can prevent synechiae from forming in the dilated position. In mild cases or in cases with a significant steroid-induced intraocular pressure rise, non-steroidal anti-inflammatory drugs can also play a role.

Systemic prednisone may be necessary when inflammation is severe or bilateral. Uveitis that is refractory to systemic steroids or requires greater than 10 mg of oral prednisone daily may require steroid-sparing agents such as antimetabolites or biologics. Because of the side-effect profile and the risk of infection with these drugs, most ophthalmologists utilize them in consultation with or under the supervision of a rheumatologist or other specialist.

C. Treatment of Intraocular Pressure

The mainstay of treatment of uveitic glaucoma is aqueous suppression with beta-blockers, carbonic anhydrase inhibitors, and alpha-agonists. Miotics increase the permeability of the blood-aqueous barrier and increase flare in the anterior chamber. In addition, they create a fixed, miotic pupil and increase the risk of synechiae and a secluded pupil. For that reason, they are relatively contraindicated. Prostaglandin analogues are also known to have proinflammatory characteristics and increase the risk of cystoid macular edema. However, they are also very effective in lowering intraocular pressure by increasing uveoscleral outflow in eyes with poor trabecular drainage secondary to inflammation. These agents should be used with caution and primarily in eyes with well-controlled uveitis.

Laser trabeculoplasty is generally deferred in uveitic glaucoma, as it may incite more damage to the trabecular meshwork and is not effective at lowering intraocular pressure. Laser peripheral iridotomy, however, is indicated in cases of pupil seclusion causing iris bombé with elevated pressures.

When medical therapy fails to control the intraocular pressure, surgery is indicated. Trabeculectomy, with or without antifibrotic agents, has a worse prognosis than in primary open-angle glaucoma. It is thought that the inflammatory cells and proteins in the aqueous increase the risk of scarring and failure of the bleb. Glaucoma drainage implants have better success in uveitic glaucoma and are generally preferred. Microincision or minimally invasive glaucoma surgery procedures are under investigation for their clinical role in uveitic glaucomas. In children, uvetic glaucoma has been successfully treated with goniotomy. Cyclodestructive procedures, including diode cyclophotocoagulation, also have a role in the treatment of uveitic glaucoma. Although reasonable success has been reported with the use of cyclophotocoagulation as a primary glaucoma procedure in uveitic glaucoma, this technique is generally performed as an adjunctive procedure when the intraocular pressure remains elevated after glaucoma drainage implant surgery. Cyclodestructive procedures may put patients with chronic inflammation at risk of ciliary body shutdown and chronic hypotony and should be performed with caution.

BIBLIOGRAPHY

1. Da Mata A, Burk SE, Netland PA, et al. Management of uveitic glaucoma with Ahmed glaucoma valve implantation. Ophthalmology. 1999;106:2168-72.
2. Freedman SF, Rodriguez-Rosa RE, Rojas MC, et al. Goniotomy for glaucoma secondary to chronic childhood uvetis. Am J Ophthalmol. 2002;133:617-21.
3. Iwao K, Inatani M, Seto T, et al. Long-term outcomes and prognostic factors for trabeculectomy with mitomycin C in eyes with uveitic glaucoma: A retrospective cohort study. J Glaucoma. 2012. [EPub. In press].
4. Netland PA, Denton NC. Uveitic glaucoma. Contemp Ophthalmol. 2006;5:1-8.
5. Radhakrishnan S, Cunningham ET, Iwach A. "Inflammatory Disease and Glaucoma." In: Schacknow PN, Samples JR (Eds). The Glaucoma Book. New York, NY: Springer; 2010. pp. 527-43.
6. Schlote T, Derse M, Zierhut M. Transscleral diode laser cyclophotocoagulation for the treatment of refractory glaucoma secondary to inflammatory eye diseases. Br J Ophthalmol. 2000;84:999-1003.

SECTION 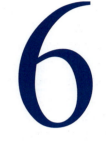 6

Lens Disorders

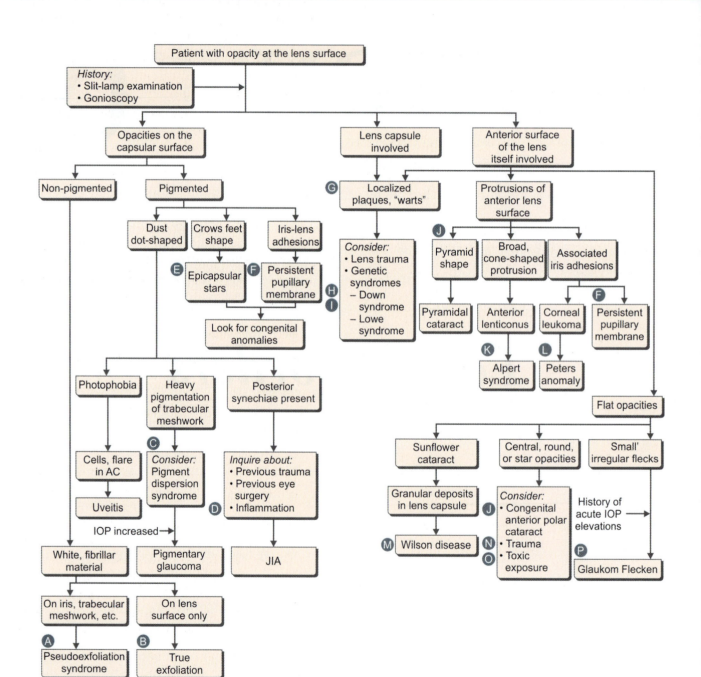

Opacities associated with the anterior lens surface may be caused by abnormalities of the lens capsule and epithelium, by irregularities in the most superficial anterior cortex or by abnormal deposits on the anterior lens capsule. Visual acuity is affected less than in posterior lens opacities because the lesions are further removed from the macula, and are generally smaller and lead to less irregularity of the lens surface.

A. White, flaky material is found on the lens capsule, iris, trabecular meshwork, lens zonules, and anterior vitreous face in pseudoexfoliation syndrome. Typically, the material is best seen as a disc of dandruff-like material on the anterior lens capsule after the pupil has been dilated. The disc is surrounded by a clear zone, which is followed by fibrillar white material on the peripheral lens surface and the zonules. The syndrome is rarely seen before the age of 50 years and doubles in prevalence for every decade after this. The nature of the white material and its origin are unclear (Chapter 26).

B. True exfoliation of the lens capsule is rare and is usually caused by infrared radiation. It was commonly seen in glass blowers. It is caused by delamination of the anterior lens capsule, resulting in a very thin membrane with a free edge floating in the aqueous.

C. Pigmentary dispersion syndrome results from the release of melanosomes from the posterior iris epithelium, which rubs against the lens zonules when the iris has a concave configuration within a deep anterior chamber (AC). Thus, the syndrome is primarily seen under conditions leading to a concave iris (i.e. myopia, male sex). Both of these factors lead to a deep AC. The pigment granules accumulate in the trabecular meshwork, increasing the risk for glaucoma, and on the corneal endothelium and lens capsule (Chapter 26).

D. Posterior synechiae may be the first indication of the presence of juvenile idiopathic arthritis. Asymptomatic, chronic, nongranulomatous iridocyclitis may precede the onset of arthritis. Acute febrile and polyarticular forms of arthritis are generally not associated with eye findings. However, the pauciarticular types carry a much higher risk for the development of iritis, up to 20%. Because the onset is insidious, significant ocular damage may be caused before the disease is diagnosed. In addition to pigment deposits on the lens capsule and posterior synechiae, band keratopathy and cataracts are common complications.

E. Epicapsular stars are minimal remnants of the embryonic pupillary membrane. These stellate clusters of epithelial cells in the shape of bird tracks have no clinical significance.

F. Remnants of the pupillary membrane are commonly adherent to the anterior capsule in small areas. At the adhesion site, a small anterior lens opacity is often present. Neither the cataract nor the membrane is progressive, and unless they are in the visual axis, they do not interfere with vision.

G. In some inherited syndromes or after localized trauma to the epithelium, groups of anterior lens epithelial cells take on a fibroblast-like configuration. They get arranged in whorls and produce abnormal amounts of capsular materials, interspersed between and around the cells. Sometimes, the lens capsule becomes duplicated or the plaques may protrude from the anterior lens surface. These plaques are an example of true metaplasia of lens epithelial cells into myofibroblasts.

H. Trisomy 21 may be associated with cataract formation, which usually develops later in childhood rather than in infancy. The capsule is often thickened and shows the anomalies discussed in Section G.

I. Children with Lowe syndrome often have cataracts, in which the lens is reduced to a relatively thin disc with epithelial cells both anteriorly and posteriorly. Anterior plaques are usually present. The face has a characteristic appearance with frontal bossing and chubby cheeks. The syndrome is associated with mental retardation, hypotonia, and aminoaciduria. Glaucoma and anterior segment dysgenesis are common. Inheritance is X-linked, and the carriers may be detected by the presence of punctate lens opacities in the peripheral cortex.

J. Pyramidal cataracts are small pyramids of lens tissue protruding into the AC. They are considered remnants of the embryonic lens stalk, which connects the lens rudiment with the surface epithelium. Anterior polar cataracts are small and located in the center of the anterior capsule and may have a similar origin as the pyramidal cataracts. Either type is generally not progressive and causes little visual disturbance. There are exceptions to this, and in some reports, as many as 30% of the patients developed amblyopia or other visual problems. Periodic follow-up is therefore recommended.

K. Alport syndrome is a nephropathy with progressive hematuria and is often associated with sensorineural deafness and anterior lenticonus. It is usually an X-linked dominant trait but in some cases appears to be autosomal recessive. The molecular defect in the X-linked form has been identified as an abnormality of the common subunit of collagen IV (COL4A5), which is found in the glomerular basement membrane.

L. In the most severe forms of Peters anomaly, the lens can be broadly adherent to the cornea. More commonly, a stalk-shaped adhesion is present or a pyramidal cataract is found as a remnant of the corneolenticular connection. Although the lens anomalies are variable, Peters syndrome always has a central corneal leukoma with abnormal or absent endothelium and adhesions between the edge of the leukoma and the peripupillary iris.

M. An inherited absence or low level of the copper-transporting serum protein, ceruloplasmin (Wilson disease), leads to high tissue levels of copper. The effects of the abnormal copper levels become visible in young adults. Basal ganglia degeneration in the central nervous system causes tremors and choreoathetosis. Liver cirrhosis occurs, and renal involvement results in aminoaciduria. Brownish-green copper deposits may be seen in the peripheral Descemet membrane, particularly at 6 and 12 o'clock (Kayser–Fleischer ring). The subcapsular sunflower cataract is highly characteristic but not always present.

N. Localized trauma to the anterior lens epithelium may lead to a localized repair process, which results in plaque formation at the lens surface (see Section G).

O. A variety of drug exposures may lead to opacities in the anterior superficial lens cortex. Best known for this complication are chlorpromazine and anticholinesterases.

P. Periods of elevation of intraocular pressure by acute angle closure may cause focal necrosis of lens epithelial cells. These form irregular subcapsular lens opacities, first consisting of necrotic epithelium and later of fibroblast-like repair tissue. These 'Giaukom Flecken' can be subtle and require careful slit-lamp examination of the anterior lens. Their presence necessitates a work-up for occludable AC angles.

▌BIBLIOGRAPHY

1. Cashwell LF Jr, Holleman IL, Weaver RG, et al. Idiopathic true exfoliation of the lens capsule. Ophthalmology. 1989;96:348-50.
2. Cibis GW, Waeltermann JM, Whitcraft CT, et al. Lenticular opacities in carriers of Lowe's syndrome. Ophthalmology. 1986;93:1041-5.
3. Foster CS, Barrett F. Cataract development and cataract surgery in patients with juvenile rheumatoid arthritis-associated iridocyclitis. Ophthalmology. 1993;100:809-17.
4. Jaafar MS, Robb RM. Congenital anterior polar cataracts: A review of 63 cases. Ophthalmology. 1984;91:249-54.
5. Knebelmann B, Breillat C, Forestier L, et al. Spectrum of mutations in the COL4A5 collagen gene in X-Linked AIport syndrome. Am J Hum Genet. 1996;59:1221-32.
6. Lipman RM, Tripathi BL, Tripathi RC. Cataracts induced by microwave and ionizing radiation. Surv Ophthalmol. 1988; 33:200-10.
7. Richter CU, Richardson TM, Grant WM. Pigmentary dispersion syndrome and pigmentary glaucoma: A prospective study of the natural history. Arch Ophthalmol. 1986;104:211-7.
8. Wheeler DT, Mullaney PB, Awad A, et al. Pyramidal anterior polar cataracts. Ophthalmol. 1999;106:2362-7.

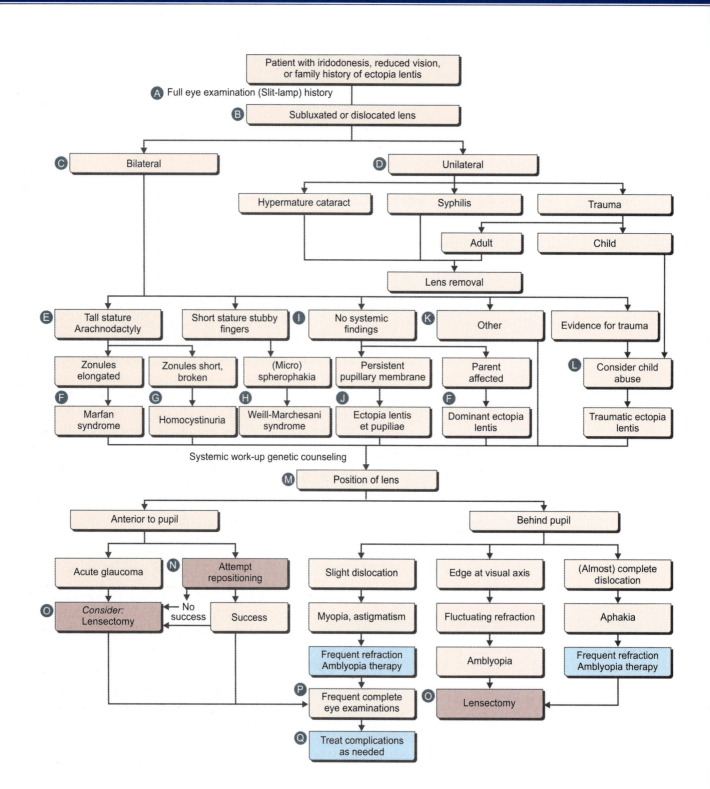

In many patients, eye complaints are the presenting symptoms of ectopia lentis. This obligates the ophthalmologist not only to evaluate and treat the ectopia lentis by itself but also to initiate the work-up or make the necessary referrals to diagnose the systemic disease underlying the ocular manifestation. In a small group of patients, the dislocation of the lens is secondary to eye abnormalities or to systemic diseases that are *severe* enough to allow a diagnosis well before the ectopia lentis is discovered. The emphasis in this chapter is on patients whose presenting problem is ectopia lentis.

A. Reduced vision is the presenting symptom in many patients for several reasons. Fluctuations in refraction may be caused by small changes in the lens position or by image formation through different parts of the lens. Myopic astigmatism is the rule in patients with moderately subluxated lenses, whereas an aphakic correction is needed when the lens is (almost) totally dislocated. Particularly challenging are the lenses that are halfway dislocated, thus bringing the edge close to the visual axis. Changes from aphakia to high myopia may occur, and monocular diplopia is not uncommon. In a child, this situation is highly amblyopigenic, another cause for reduced vision. Finally, accommodation is hampered, disturbing the switch from distance to near vision.

B. Slit-lamp examination is the best way to diagnose ectopia lentis. A subluxated lens, although, not in its normal position, remains within the pupillary space. A dislocated lens is away from the pupillary space. The lens may be dislocated anteriorly, which carries the risk of acute glaucoma and corneal decompensation, or posteriorly into the vitreous.

C. Bilaterally dislocated lenses almost always indicate a genetic disorder or a congenital eye abnormality. They often are congenital but may be acquired and progressive. Most are present in children.

D. A unilateral dislocated lens usually indicates an acquired problem and may occur at any age.

E. Although tallness and arachnodactyly are thought to be typical for Marfan syndrome, they are also present in homocystinuria.

F. Marfan syndrome is the most common cause of pediatric ectopia lentis. High myopia, a tendency for retinal detachments, and cataracts may also be found. Cardiac anomalies are the most important systemic findings (i.e. a dilated aortic root, aortic aneurysms, mitral valve prolapse). Thus, always obtain cardiologic consultation. Kyphoscoliosis and chest deformities are typical. There is a wide variation in expression. The diagnosis is not always easy. Inheritance is autosomal dominant, and Marfan syndrome may be genetically heterogeneous. Mutations in the *fibrillin* gene are responsible for the various manifestations of Marfan syndrome. The variations in patients with different severity of phenotypes may result from differences in the mutations or in the level of mutant protein being expressed. Autosomal-dominant ectopia lentis has also been linked to a fibrillin abnormality. The dislocation of the lens in these syndromes is probably congenital and is stable in > 90% of the patients.

G. Homocystinuria, an autosomal-recessive disease, is often not diagnosed until later in childhood, when psychomotor retardation and failure to thrive are present. Dislocation of the lens may not be present early and is typically progressive. A urine nitroprussid test is a good screening test, although it can be falsely negative. If a diagnosis of homocystinuria is suspected, serum and urinary aminoacids (homocystine levels) should be studied, ideally after a loading dose of methionine. The underlying cause in most patients is a deficiency of cystathionine-13-synthetase. Pyridoxine is a cofactor of this enzyme, and about half of the patients benefit from large doses of this vitamin B_6. Patients are at risk of thromboembolic episodes, which can be lethal and can be provoked by surgery. Thus, eye surgery should not be undertaken lightly and requires special precautions (IV hydration, compressive stockings, or preoperative aspirin).

H. Patients with Weill-Marchesani syndrome have a spherical lens, which tends to dislocate anteriorly, giving pupillary block glaucoma and acute *severe* pain.

I. Isolated ectopia lentis is a diagnosis of exclusion, which should be made only after a systemic work-up. A work-up should be performed in all the patients with ectopia lentis.

J. Ectopia lentis et pupillae is characterized by the dislocation of the lens and pupil in opposite directions. Corectopia may be absent or hardly noticeable. In my experience, these patients almost always have remnants of persistent pupillary membranes, which may play a role in the pathogenesis of the dislocation. Myopia is not only lenticular but also axial. The cornea may be enlarged and the iris may be translucent. Inheritance is autosomal recessive.

K. Several rare disorders and some ocular anomalies can be associated with ectopia lentis. The primary diagnosis is usually well established and ectopia lentis is a secondary finding in most of these patients. Several disorders are listed in Table 103.1.

L. Unilateral lens dislocation in a child almost always results from trauma. Even in bilateral cases, trauma may be the cause. Consider the possibility of child abuse, most certainly when there is evidence for unusual trauma (e.g. many bruises, burns, and multiple fractures). Up to 40% of nonaccidental injuries in children may involve the eyes.

M. The position of the lens gives some indication about the cause of ectopia lentis but is not pathognomonic. Usually, the lens is displaced upward and temporally in Marfan syndrome, downward in homocystinuria. A position in the anterior chamber is typical for homocystinuria and Weill-Marchesani syndrome but not exclusively so.

N. If the lens is anteriorly dislocated, attempt should be made first to reposition it posteriorly by

Table 103.1: Disorders sometimes associated with ectopia lentis

Ocular disorders	Systemic disorders
Megalocornea	Hyperlysinemia
Congenital glaucoma	Sulfite oxidase deficiency
Aniridia	Scleroderma
Rieger syndrome	Sturge-Weber syndrome
Retinitis pigmentosa	Ehlers-Danlos syndrome Craniofacial disorders

dilating the pupil, placing the patient in a supine position, and pressing on the cornea. Even if this is successful, one should consider lensectomy to prevent further episodes. Alternatively, long-term treatment with miotics is useful.

O. The decision to remove a dislocated lens must be individualized; it may often be unnecessary. Minor subluxations and complete dislocations can be treated with refractive corrections. A posteriorly dislocated lens needs to be removed only if it causes complications, such as lens-induced uveitis. Surgery should be undertaken in children with fluctuating refraction, who are at risk of amblyopia. Closed lensectomy and anterior vitrectomy with vitreous cutting instruments, either through the limbus or through the pars plana/plicata, is the technique of choice. Occasionally, intracapsular delivery, extracapsular methods, or aspiration can be appropriate, but one should be prepared to deal with the vitreous loss that almost always accompanies these methods.

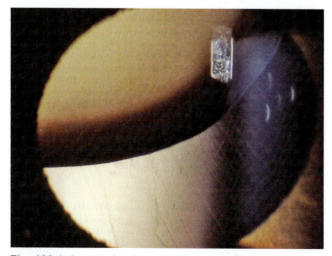

Fig. 103.1: Lens in Marfan syndrome, dislocated upward and outward.

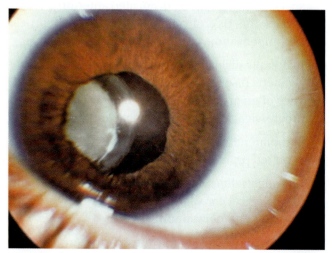

Fig. 103.2: Cataractous lens in homocystinuria typically dislocated downward and inward.

P. Frequent follow-up is essential in all children with ectopia lentis to adjust refractive corrections, provide amblyopia therapy as required, and check for the many possible complications.

Q. Glaucoma, lens-induced uveitis, cystic retinal degeneration, peripheral retinal tears, retinal dialysis, and retinal detachment can all accompany ectopia lentis, whether lens removal has taken place or not. They need to be diagnosed and treated promptly.

BIBLIOGRAPHY

1. Goldberg MF. Clinical manifestations of ectopia lentis et pupillae in 16 patients. Ophthalmology. 1988;95:1080-8.
2. Gray JR, Davies SJ. Marfan syndrome. J Med Genet. 1996;33: 403-8.
3. Halpert M, BenEzra D. Surgery of the hereditary subluxated lens in children. Ophthalmology. 1996;103: 681-6.
4. Maumenee IH. The eye in Marfan syndrome. Trans Am Ophthalmol Soc. 1981;79:684-733.
5. Michalski A, Leonard J, Taylor D. The eye and inherited metabolic disease. J R Soc Med. 1988;81:286-90.
6. Nelson LB, Maumenee IH. Ectopia lentis. In: Rennie WA, (Ed). Goldberg's Genetic and Metabolic Eye Diseases. Boston, MA: Little, Brown, 1986.
7. Tongue AC. The ophthalmologist's role in diagnosing child abuse. Ophthalmology. 1991;98:1009-10.

104

Pain After Cataract Surgery

Kristin Story Held, Irene M Lee

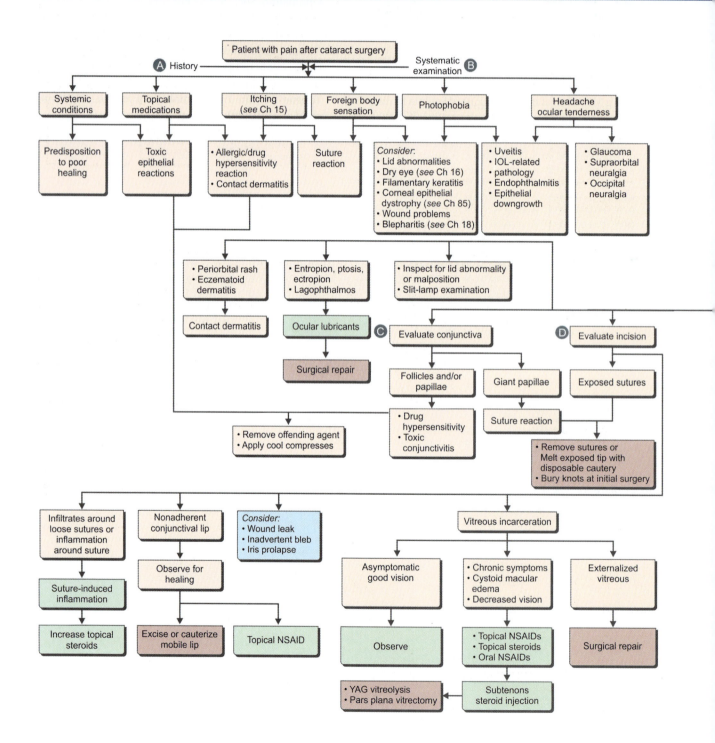

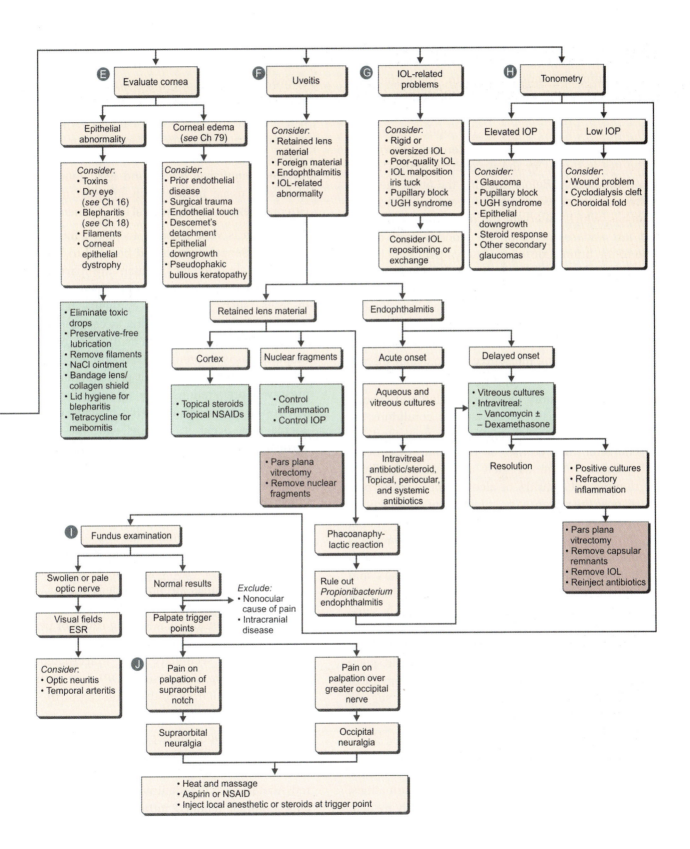

Pain after cataract surgery can be produced by a broad-spectrum of causes: some obvious, easily curable, and benign; others obscure, difficult to manage, and potentially devastating. The conjunctiva, cornea, and iris are exquisitely sensitive to pain. The extraocular muscles, sclera, choroid, and optic nerve sheath require a stronger stimulus to produce pain, usually with extraocular movements. The optic nerve itself and the retina are pain free. The sensory innervation of the eye is served by the nasociliary branch of the ophthalmic nerve. Before entering the orbit, the ophthalmic nerve gives off several recurrent meningeal branches, which innervate the dura of the tentorium and falx and segments of the blood vessels at the base of the brain. Consequently, eye pain may be the referred pain from an intracranial abnormality. Patient history, pupillary response, visual fields, and associated neurologic signs and symptoms are important in differentiating ocular diseases from nonocular causes. Thorough patient history and physical examination are the key in identifying the source of the ocular discomfort and the initiation of appropriate therapy.

A. The patient history must be detailed and specifically address associated systemic conditions, all systemic and topical medications used, and the character and course of the pain. Underlying systemic conditions such as diabetes mellitus, rheumatoid arthritis, or alcohol abuse might predispose the patient to poor healing or delayed postoperative complications. History of ocular trauma should be obtained. Any topical preparations used, such as preserved topical steroid or antibiotic preparations, are potential offenders and should not be overlooked. Nature of the pain should be reviewed in detail. Foreign-body sensation that is present immediately, can postoperatively suggest an exposed suture or another foreign body, whereas a relatively asymptomatic postoperative course followed by the development of pain, photophobia, and redness might suggest epithelial downgrowth or the delayed onset of endophthalmitis.

B. A complete, systematic approach to examination begins with the examination of the lids and ocular adnexa for structural or functional abnormalities, which can then be medically or surgically treated. A thorough slit-lamp examination and funduscopic examination should follow.

C. Conjunctiva, including upper lid eversion, should be thoroughly inspected to look for giant papillae associated with suture reactions. Rose Bengal staining suggests keratitis sicca or toxic conjunctivitis.

D. The surgical wound can be a great source of persistent ocular discomfort after cataract surgery. The incision is carefully inspected for loose or exposed sutures; suture-induced inflammation; a rolled, mobile conjunctival lip; wound leak; inadvertent bleb; and tissue incarceration. If uveal tissue or vitreous is externalized, surgical repair is necessary.

E. The cornea is very sensitive to pain. Fluorescein and Rose Bengal dyes should be used to look for epithelial abnormalities, which are particularly problematic in patients with underlying epithelial diseases, such as corneal epithelial basement membrane dystrophy, keratitis sicca, blepharitis, and systemic disorders, such as diabetes mellitus. Preparations used preoperatively, intraoperatively, and postoperatively, especially gentamicin and any preserved preparations such as topical steroids, can result in corneal epithelial toxicity. Corneal edema may occur in patients with pre-existing corneal endothelial disease such as Fuchs dystrophy, or prior intraocular surgery. Corneal edema may also be a result of surgical insult by either direct mechanical trauma, such as Descemet detachment, or endothelial touch with surgical instruments or the intraocular lens, or may be a result of toxic agents injected into the eye, including miotics and viscoelastics, particularly if reusable cannulas are not properly rinsed with detergents. Pseudophakic bullous keratopathy is occasionally seen and is a leading cause of penetrating keratoplasty in the United States. Corneal edema may be secondary to or exacerbated by increased intraocular pressure (IOP). Late corneal edema may result from epithelial downgrowth.

F. Mild intraocular inflammation after cataract surgery is common and expected. When inflammation is severe enough to cause significant pain, other causes of inflammation should be considered. Acute causes of inflammation include retained lens material, retained intraocular foreign body, incarcerated uvea or vitreous, IOL chafing, or acute endophthalmitis. Toxic anterior segment syndrome

(TASS) is an acute cause of sterile intraocular inflammation accompanied by corneal edema that is infrequently associated with pain. Potential causes of TASS include IOL polishing compounds, detergent residue on IOL's or instruments, intraocular medications or ointments, and denatured viscoelastics.

When suspected, acute endophthalmitis requires immediate diagnosis and treatment. Risk factors for endophthalmitis include capsular rupture, longer operative time, diabetics, advanced age, presence of a bleb, a leaking wound, and uveal/vitreal incarceration. Suspected cases require immediate diagnostic aqueous and vitreous cultures, and intravitreal antibiotics [Vancomycin (1 mg/0.1 mL) with Amikacin (400 mg/0.1 mL) or Ceftazidime (2 mg/0.1 mL)]. Gram stain, Giemsa stain, and aerobic and anaerobic cultures should be obtained, and held for 14 days. The endophthalmitis vitrectomy study (EVS) demonstrated that patients who present with initial vision of light perception had improved outcomes if immediate diagnostic and therapeutic vitrectomy was performed. There was no difference in the outcome between vitrectomy and vitreous tap in patients who were presented with initial visual acuity of hand motions or better. Subconjunctival or topical antibiotics can be used as an adjunct to intravitreal therapy. The EVS showed no difference in visual outcome with or without systemic antibiotics. Steroids are controversial. In the EVS, steroids were given subconjunctivally, topically, and orally since steroids can modulate associated vigorous inflammation.

Delayed causes of inflammation include delayed-onset endophthalmitis caused by less virulent organisms such as *Propionibacterium* species, *Staphylococcus epidermidis,* and fungi. It has a more favorable prognosis than acute-onset endophthalmitis; however, aggressive diagnostic and therapeutic measures are essential. Fungal cases require intravitreal amphotericin B (5 mg/0.1 mL) or voriconazole (50-100 mg/0.1 mL). Refractory cases may require repeated vitrectomy, intravitreal antibiotics, removal of capsular remnants, and IOL removal or exchange.

G. Problems related to the type, size, and position of the IOL may lead to ocular pain. Rigid anterior chamber IOLs cause ocular pain that increases with pressure applied to the eye, especially if vertically oriented or oversized. Rough, sharp edges on the lenses or malpositioned lenses may lead to chafing of the iris and uveitis-glaucoma-hyphema (UGH) syndrome. Pupillary block or iris tuck may occur from a poorly positioned lens. The IOL position with the patient's head should be evaluated in various positions to look for movement and contact with corneal endothelium or iris. Macular edema and corneal edema may occur even months or years postoperatively, especially in patients with iris—plane or closed-loop IOLs. IOL repositioning or exchange should be considered in these cases.

H. Increased lOP is a potential source of pain. Glaucoma is common in the postoperative course and is responsible for the largest number of eyes enucleated after cataract surgery. All the causes of secondary glaucoma, including pupillary block, aqueous misdirection syndrome, peripheral anterior synechiae formation, epithelial or fibrous downgrowth, hemolytic glaucoma, and inflammatory glaucoma should be considered. In acute cases, the lOP may be elevated by retained sodium hyaluronate or excessively tight wound closure. Lower lOP is associated with wound leak, cyclodialysis cleft, ciliary body shutdown from vigorous inflammation, or choroidal folds.

I. A pale or swollen nerve on funduscopic examination suggests optic neuritis. Patients may complain of photophobia and pain with eye movement, and exhibit blurred vision, decreased color vision, afferent pupillary defect, and visual field abnormalities. Temporal arteritis must be excluded in the elderly population. Sedimentation rate (ESR) and C-reactive protein (CRP) must be obtained, and the patient should be treated accordingly. Suprachoroidal hemorrhage presents with sudden onset of severe pain, shallow anterior chamber, and detached, dark choroid on examination. Treatment consists of control of lOP, inflammation, and pain control. A persistently flat anterior chamber and large or kissing choroidal detachments require surgical intervention.

J. Finally, once one has excluded an ocular cause of the pain, nonocular causes of pain can be considered, such as migraine, cluster headache, or sinusitis. Occipital neuralgia is referred pain from the occipital region, and is diagnosed by reproducing the pain with palpation of the greater occipital nerve in the region of the posterior insertion of the sternocleidomastoid on the mastoid process. Occasionally, herpes zoster ophthalmicus can present with ocular or periocular pain before the characteristic papulovesicular rash appears.

BIBLIOGRAPHY

1. Brady SE, Cohen FJ, Fischer DH. Diagnosis and treatment of chronic postoperative bacterial endophthalmitis. Ophthalamic Surg. 1988;19:580-4.
2. Endophthalmitis vitrectomy study group. Results of the endophthalmitis vitrectomy. Arch Ophthalmol. 1995;113:1479-96.
3. Fastenberg OM, Schwartz PL, Golub BM. Management of dislocated nuclear fragments after phacoemulsification. Am J OphthalmoI.1991;112:535-9.
4. Fong OS, Topping TM. Postoperative endophthalmitis. In: Steinert RF, (Ed). Cataract surgery: Technique, complications, and management. Philadelphia, PA: WB Saunders; 1995. pp. 426-33.
5. Fox GM, Joondeph BC, Flynn HW, et al. Delayed-onset pseudophakic endophthalmitis. Am J Ophthalmol. 1991;112:163-73.
6. Jaffe NS, Jaffe MS, Jaffe GF. Cataract surgery and its complications, 6th edition. St Louis, MO: Mosby; 1997.
7. Kohrman SO, Warfield CA. Eye pain: Ocular and nonocular causes. Hosp Pract (Off). 1987;11:33-50.
8. Olk RI, Bohigian GM. The management of endophthalmitis: Diagnostic and therapeutic guidelines including the use of vitrectomy. Ophthalmic Surg. 1987;18:262-7.
9. Rishi R, Doshi J, Arevalo F, et al. Evaluating exaggerated, prolonged, or delayed postoperative intraocular inflammation. Am J Ophthalmol. 2010;150:295-304.
9. Stern GA, Engel HM, Driebe WT. The treatment of postoperative endophthalmitis: Results of differing approaches to treatment. Ophthalmology. 1989;96:62-6.
10. Zambrano W, Flynn HW, Pflugfelder SC, et al. Management options for *Propionibacterium acnes* endophthalmitis. Ophthalmology. 1989;96:1100-05.

Poor Vision After Cataract Surgery

105

Sonya Dhar

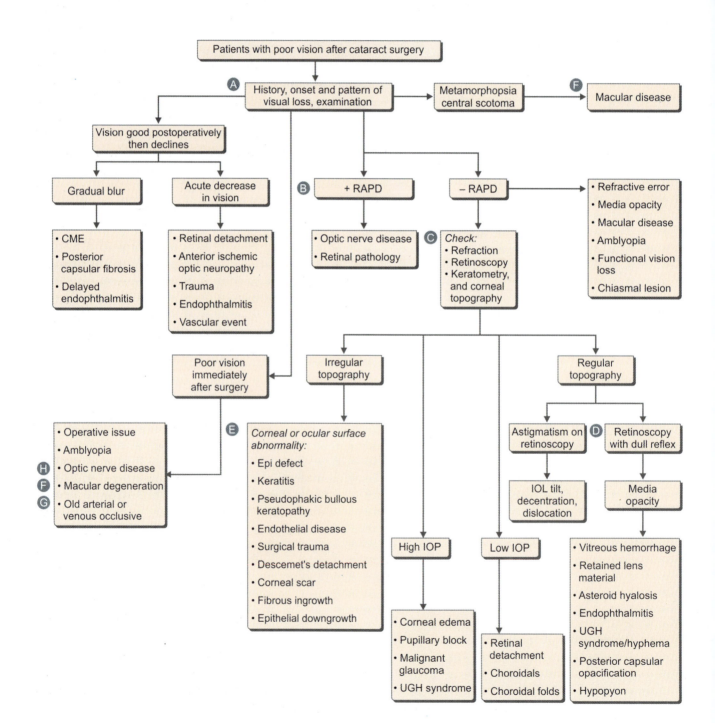

Patients with poor vision after cataract surgery

A — History, onset and pattern of visual loss, examination

Metamorphopsia central scotoma → F — Macular disease

Vision good postoperatively then declines

- Gradual blur
  - CME
  - Posterior capsular fibrosis
  - Delayed endophthalmitis

- Acute decrease in vision
  - Retinal detachment
  - Anterior ischemic optic neuropathy
  - Trauma
  - Endophthalmitis
  - Vascular event

B — + RAPD
- Optic nerve disease
- Retinal pathology

− RAPD

C — Check:
- Refraction
- Retinoscopy
- Keratometry, and corneal topography

- Refractive error
- Media opacity
- Macular disease
- Amblyopia
- Functional vision loss
- Chiasmal lesion

Poor vision immediately after surgery

- Operative issue
- Amblyopia
- H — Optic nerve disease
- F — Macular degeneration
- G — Old arterial or venous occlusive

E — Corneal or ocular surface abnormality:
- Epi defect
- Keratitis
- Pseudophakic bullous keratopathy
- Endothelial disease
- Surgical trauma
- Descemet's detachment
- Corneal scar
- Fibrous ingrowth
- Epithelial downgrowth

Irregular topography

Regular topography

Astigmatism on retinoscopy
- IOL tilt, decentration, dislocation

D — Retinoscopy with dull reflex
- Media opacity

High IOP
- Corneal edema
- Pupillary block
- Malignant glaucoma
- UGH syndrome

Low IOP
- Retinal detachment
- Choroidals
- Choroidal folds

- Vitreous hemorrhage
- Retained lens material
- Asteroid hyalosis
- Endophthalmitis
- UGH syndrome/hyphema
- Posterior capsular opacification
- Hypopyon

Cataract surgery is one of the most common surgeries performed in the United States. Patients usually complain of a gradual worsening of vision in one or both eyes, and difficulty participating in their activities of daily living, such as driving and reading. Unexpected or poor outcomes after cataract surgery can be disappointing for the patient and their family, as well as the cataract surgeon. In order to minimize the unexpected outcomes, it is imperative to obtain a detailed history and to perform a thorough physical examination preoperatively. This allows the surgeon to identify pre-existing ocular issues that may limit the postoperative visual prognosis and/or complicate the surgery. The surgeon can then adequately prepare for the surgery and the expected outcomes. It is particularly important to identify history of amblyopia, ocular disease, glaucoma, stroke, toxic systemic medications, scotomas, metamorphopsias, and other issues that may be suggestive of visual decline from disease other than cataracts. One must always obtain information regarding the vision prior to the cataract developing, and any history of visual decline over time. Rapid vision loss may indicate a condition other than cataracts, for example.

In evaluating a patient preoperatively, it is helpful to look closely at the fellow eye for clues that may indicate bilateral ocular disease. Ultrasonography should be performed if there is no view of the fundus. Once necessary information is gathered from a detailed history and examination, the patient should be counseled appropriately regarding realistic expectations for postoperative vision. Patients having a good understanding of their expected visual potential may help avoid undue postoperative disappointment and unwanted surprises. When confronted with a patient with unexpected poor vision after uncomplicated cataract surgery, the surgeon must expediently and effectively pursue a definitive diagnosis so that treatable conditions can be managed early and appropriately, whereas untreatable conditions will not be subjected to fruitless therapeutic endeavors.

A. A detailed history of the visual loss provides clues to the diagnosis. Old photographs may show strabismus in a patient whose visual loss suggests amblyopia. A four-base-out prism test or Worth-4-dot test might be useful. Characterization of the chronology and pattern of the visual loss provides clues to the diagnosis as well. At what point after cataract surgery did the vision start to decline? Was the loss of vision sudden or gradual? A thorough ocular examination should follow.

B. A thorough ocular examination begins with the swinging flashlight test to detect a Marcus Gunn pupil. This is most commonly seen with optic nerve lesions. Retinal lesions occasionally produce this finding, but it is much less marked. An eye with 20/40 vision because of optic neuritis is likely to show a more pronounced afferent pupillary defect than an eye with 20/400 vision from a retinal lesion. In the presence of a Marcus Gunn pupil, bilateral formal visual fields should be obtained and the optic nerve and macula should be carefully evaluated. In the absence of a Marcus Gunn pupil, the decreased vision could be caused by refractive error, macular lesions, media opacities, amblyopia, chiasmal lesions, or functional visual loss.

C. Keratometry and corneal topography are extremely useful in revealing irregular astigmatism, which is caused by ocular surface or corneal abnormalities, and high astigmatism, which is important in determining the proper refraction. They are helpful in determining if the refraction is stable, allowing one to assess one's wound closure technique and to detect wound healing problems. For example, a sudden shift in the axis of astigmatism may indicate an alteration of the wound, possibly from suture breakage or ocular trauma. One should then evaluate the wound for leakage or an inadvertent bleb. Keratometry readings help one fine-tune the axis and amount of cylinder. Disparity between keratometry readings and retinoscopy may indicate intraocular lens (IOL) tilt or decentration. IOL tilt may be secondary to zonular weakness, asymmetric capsular phimosis, or asymmetric haptic positioning. A hard contact lens is useful in evaluating decreased vision from irregular astigmatism. Incorrect axial length and keratometry readings preoperatively may lead to incorrect IOL power or incorrect axis of implantation for toric IOLs. Combining keratometry, topography, and retinoscopy allows one to solve most refractive problems.

D. Retinoscopy provides crucial information about the cause of decreased vision. An abnormal 'scissoring' streak indicates an astigmatic or corneal problem, whereas a dull streak indicates a media opacity anterior to the retina. A media opacity is an abnormality that impairs transmission of light to the retina. The abnormality is easily identified by slit-lamp examination. A hyphema could be related to iris trauma, IOL chafing, or spill over from a vitreous hemorrhage. A vitreous hemorrhage may indicate globe rupture, retinal break, or detachment. A normal crisp streak in the face of poor vision may indicate an issue with the retina, optic nerve, or central visual pathways.

E. The cornea is a common source of poor vision after cataract surgery. Careful preoperative evaluation of the cornea is essential. Specular microscopy in select cases is important in developing a surgical strategy for those patients with endothelial disease. Intraoperatively, great care should be taken to avoid damaging the cornea both mechanically and with injection of toxic substances. Prolonged use of phaco power and intraocular irrigation may also damage the cornea. Corneal decompensation from corneal edema, ocular surface disease, and Descemet membrane detachments may occur. Postoperatively, vitreous, nuclear fragments, or foreign bodies adherent to the posterior aspect of the cornea may need to be removed. Intraocular pressure control will minimize the stress on the endothelial cells. Topical medications should be minimized in the face of epithelial erosion, especially in diabetic patients and in patients with underlying corneal epithelial dystrophy or dry eye syndrome. A high index of suspicion for acute endophthalmitis should be maintained, if there is a hypopyon or vitreous opacity, and for late postoperative endophthalmitis in cases of persistent uveitis. The key to effective therapy is rapid intervention with vitreous culture and injection of intravitreal antibiotics. In severe cases of endophthalmitis, the patient may require additional pars plana vitrectomy.

F. Biomicroscopic examination of the posterior pole is essential. Many retinal causes of decreased vision can be diagnosed by their characteristic clinical appearance. Patients with macular abnormalities often complain of central scotomas and metamorphopsias. Amsler grid testing is useful in these cases. Cystoid macular edema (CME) is one of the most common causes of decreased vision after cataract surgery. In cases of pseudophakic CME (Irvine-Gass syndrome), the vision is good immediately postoperatively but then declines after 6–10 weeks. CME is more common after surgical complications such as vitreous incarceration, iris prolapse, and vitreous loss. Fundus examination reveals loss of the foveal depression and retinal edema. At times, retinal exam may appear unremarkable. If the history suggests CME but the classic clinical findings are not obvious, fluorescein angiography (FA) is indicated and is diagnostic. FA classically shows leakage from perifoveal capillaries in a petaloid pattern on late phases. Optical coherence tomography may be helpful to demonstrate cystic spaces as well as to document central macular thickness over time. CME occurs angiographically in 5–16% of patients and clinically in 0.8–3.5% after extracapsular cataract extraction and posterior chamber IOL implantation with an intact posterior capsule. Many cases resolve spontaneously within 6 months. Treatment is recommended for clinically apparent cases that cause decreased vision. In these cases, it is imperative to rule out vitreous incarceration, IOL chafing, and persistent uveitis. The first line of treatment for CME is topical steroids and non-steroidal antiinflammatory drugs (NSAIDs). If these are ineffective, sub-Tenon or intravitreal triamcinolone should be considered. Depending on the scenario, yttrium aluminium garnet (YAG) laser vitreolysis or vitrectomy for vitreous incarceration, or IOL repositioning or exchange, may be needed.

'Dry' age-related macular degeneration (AMD) is characterized by drusen, pigment clumping, and geographic atrophy. This may be poorly seen preoperatively if a dense cataract is present but postoperatively it is more easily appreciated. FA shows characteristic transmission defects. 'Wet' AMD has additional features of hemorrhage, exudates, retinal elevation, or a grayish subretinal, choroidal neovascular membrane. FA is diagnostic and localizes the source of leakage to guide laser treatment. Anti-vascular endothelial growth factor treatment is usually indicated for cases of 'wet' AMD.

Macular pucker is often seen in people over 50 years old and is a common cause of failure to achieve optimal vision after cataract surgery. The epiretinal membrane may be surgically removed if the vision is worse than 20/50 or the patient has significant metamorphopsia. Evidence of photic maculopathy may be seen in up to 7% of patients after extracapsular cataract surgery with posterior chamber IOL implantation. Patients may report an oval-shaped central scotoma that correlates with a macular lesion. Minimizing exposure to microscope illumination intraoperatively and using a microscope filter may reduce the incidence of photopic maculopathy.

G. Similar to macular lesions, many retinal vascular diseases can be diagnosed on clinical appearance and history. However, FA is useful in more subtle cases. Retinal vascular occlusions, such as central retinal artery or vein occlusion may also occur.

H. The appearance of the optic nerve is the key in evaluating patients with poor vision. Decreased vision and visual field defects (nerve fiber bundle defects) may result from optic nerve damage or visual pathway issues. If optic atrophy is present, check the visual field in the other eye. Postoperative anterior ischemic optic neuropathy can present with disc edema and hemorrhage or atrophy. An erythrocyte sedimentation rate (ESR) and c-reactive protein (CRP) are used to exclude temporal arteritis. Traumatic optic neuropathy or retrobulbar hemorrhage may result from retrobulbar or peribulbar anesthetic block. CT scanning and MRI may be indicated.

BIBLIOGRAPHY

1. Cionni RJ, Osher RH. Intraoperative complications of phacoemulsification surgery. In: Steinert RF, (Ed). Cataract Surgery: Techniques, Complications, and Management. Philadelphia, PA: WB Saunders; 1995. pp. 325-439.
2. Henderson BA, Kim JY, Ament CS, et al. Clinical pseudophakic cystoid macular edema. Risk factors for development and duration after treatment. J Cataract Refract Surg. 2007;33:1550-8.
3. Jaffe NS, Jaffe MS, Jaffe GF. Cataract Surgery and Its Complications, 6th Edition. St. Louis, MO: Mosby; 1997.
4. Ruiz RS, Saatci OA. Visual outcome in pseudophakic eyes with clinical cystoid macular edema. Ophthalmic Surg. 1991;22:190-5.
5. Stark WJ, Terry AC, Maunenee AE. Anterior Segment Surgery: IOLs, Lasers, and Refractive Keratoplasty. Baltimore, MD: Williams & Wilkins; 1987.

Shallow Anterior Chamber After Cataract Surgery

106

Sonya Dhar

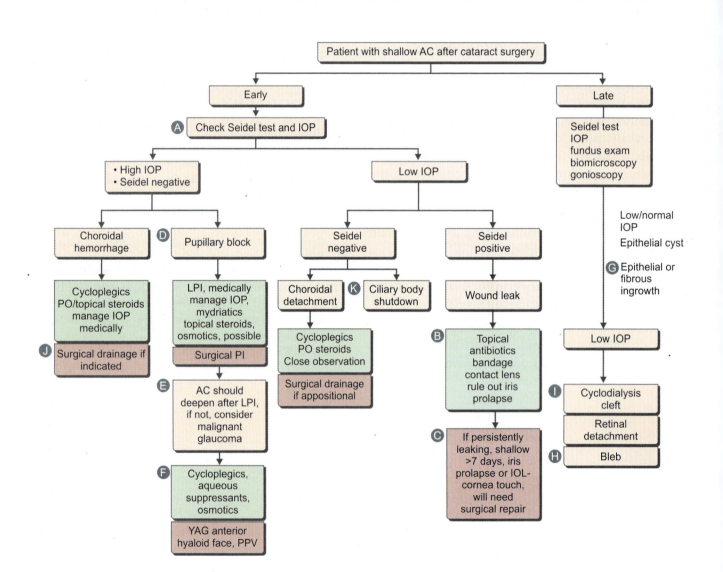

A flat or shallow anterior chamber (AC) after cataract surgery is cause for great concern. Fortunately, this complication occurs less often because of the use of phacoemulsification techniques and smaller wound sizes. The most common causes of shallow AC are wound leak, pupillary block, or a combination of the two. Serous choroidal detachment (choroidals) may occur simultaneously or secondary to low intraocular pressure (IOP). Most cases of shallowing of the anterior chamber occur within the first few weeks postoperatively. Proper diagnosis and treatment are imperative because permanent sequelae may occur after 5–7 days of a shallow AC. Complications include chronic angle-closure glaucoma secondary to peripheral anterior synechia, glaucoma secondary to pupillary block, hypotony from choroidal detachment, inflammation, or corneal decompensation from iridocorneal or IOL–cornea touch. Fortunately, the AC usually reforms spontaneously after medical treatment, and surgery is rarely needed.

A. The Seidel test is used to reveal an area of wound leak. Two percent fluorescein sodium solution should be placed over the wound while observing the area with a slit lamp and a cobalt blue filter. The dark-orange fluorescein turns bright green and fluoresces if it is diluted by leaking aqueous. If the AC is completely flat, there may not be enough aqueous to leak. In this situation, external pressure to provoke the leak should be cautiously applied. If a flat AC persists, it may be reformed with balanced salt solution (BSS) in the operating room, where the Seidel test may be repeated and definitive repair undertaken.

B. Wound leak, the most common cause of a flat AC, may be caused by poor wound apposition secondary to incarceration of vitreous, capsule, or iris in the wound; excess cautery; poor wound construction and closure; or postoperative trauma, emesis, or increased IOP. Most cases occur within 3 weeks postoperatively and resolve with conservative measures. Throughout the observation period, topical antibiotics must be applied. Often, a bandage contact lens is placed. Wound leaks are best prevented by creating self-sealing beveled incisions, properly placing 10-0 nylon corneal suture, avoiding excess cautery and incarceration of tissue into the wound, utilizing postoperative eye shields, and controlling IOP and nausea.

C. Iris prolapse is evidence of a potential wound leak. Iris incarceration may result in poor wound healing, excess astigmatism, epithelial or fibrous ingrowth, striate keratopathy, iridocyclitis, and cystoid macular edema or endophthalmitis. If the iris is externalized and the prolapse is progressive, it must be repaired promptly. A prolapsed iris rapidly becomes necrotic and strongly adherent to the wound, Tenon capsule and conjunctiva. If prolapse is recognized early (<48 h), the iris may be swept

from the wound and repositioned. Otherwise, the tissue must be dissected from the wound edge and excised before wound revision is undertaken.

D. Pupillary block results when there are adhesions between the iris and the vitreous face, retained lens material, or the intraocular lens (IOL). The normal flow of aqueous from the posterior chamber through the pupil is obstructed, so the aqueous does not reach the AC. A pressure gradient builds up between the anterior and posterior chambers, which causes the peripheral iris to bow forward and occlude the angle. This ultimately leads to decreased outflow of aqueous from the angle, shallowing of the AC, and usually elevated IOP. The IOP is high when no wound leak is present, but may be normal or low if a leak is present. In some cases, the wound leak is the inciting event for shallowing of the AC; subsequently, inflammation, adhesions, occlusion of the pupil, and peripheral synechiae occur. In other cases, the pupillary block occurs first, and the wound leak develops in the setting of a fresh incision and significantly elevated IOP. Initial treatment includes a peripheral iridotomy (PI), if the corneal clarity is sufficient. The argon and/or Neodymium: Yttrium Aluminum Gornet laser (Nd: YAG) laser is used to create the PI. If a laser PI is unsuccessful or if the AC is too shallow (risk of corneal endothelial damage with laser), steps are taken to increase cornea clarity by lowering the IOP with topical and systemic medications. At times, topical glycerin may need to be used to increase corneal clarity. If a PI is successfully completed, the pressure gradient between the anterior and posterior chambers will equalize, and the peripheral iris bowing will resolve, opening the angle. Resolution of the pupillary block results in immediate deepening of the AC. Additional PI's may be placed to ensure maintenance of patency.

Topical corticosteroids are used to decrease the associated inflammation and prevent adhesions. Osmotic agents may dehydrate the vitreous and retract the anterior hyaloid face from the iris. In some cases, a surgical PI may be indicated. Permanent synechial closure of the angle may necessitate glaucoma-filtering surgery. If the AC fails to deepen immediately following the creation of a PI, the diagnosis of malignant glaucoma should be considered.

A flat AC in the presence of IOL–cornea touch, particularly an anterior chamber intraocular lens (ACIOL), is an emergency that requires immediate correction to minimize the corneal damage. If pupillary block occurs with an ACIOL in place, it is imperative to determine whether a patent PI is present, and if not, to create PI immediately.

E. Malignant glaucoma is a rare but potentially disastrous complication of cataract surgery. The ciliary body is anteriorly rotated, causing the aqueous to be diverted posteriorly towards the vitreous. This leads to an increase in posterior volume that forces the anterior vitreous forward. A flat AC and high IOP ensue. The response to mydriatics is limited, and the AC fails to reform after patent PI. Medical treatment, including cycloplegics, aqueous suppressants and osmotic agents, may decrease the posterior aqueous diversion and IOP. If medical treatment fails, surgical/laser intervention is necessary. The anterior hyaloid face may be disrupted with a YAG laser. If this is not successful, an anterior vitrectomy must be performed and is curative.

F. After 5–7 days of medical management, a flat AC may need definitive surgical repair. Because wound leak, pupillary block, and choroidal detachment may occur together, adequate surgical repair of an aphakic or pseudophakic flat AC eliminates all possible causes. In the operating room, the AC is filled with BSS and any areas of possible leak are identified and resutured. Incarcerated tissue must be removed by appropriate means. Large choroidal detachments are drained, and the AC is reformed. Rarely, the anterior hyaloid face must be incised and/or anterior vitrectomy performed in the face of malignant glaucoma.

G. A shallow AC in the late postoperative period may be related to epithelial or fibrous invasion. Careful examination, including biomicroscopy, Seidel test, gonioscopy, fundus examination, and ultrasonography, identifies the cause in most cases. Epithelial downgrowth should be considered in all cases. If the Seidel test is positive, the wound leak must be definitively repaired with great care to treat any fistula or incarcerated tissue. True epithelial downgrowth carries a guarded prognosis. The patient complains of tearing, photophobia, and pain after a relatively normal immediate postoperative course. Epithelium may be seen on the posterior cornea as an irregularly shaped advancing line. Photocoagulation of the epithelium on the iris turns it into a fluffy white material. Specular microscopy may be useful. Treatment is usually difficult. This complication is best avoided by achieving meticulous wound closure, correct placement of suture depth, and minimal corneal endothelial trauma. Fibrous ingrowth tends to be self-limited. The leading edge looks frayed in contrast to that of epithelial downgrowth. The treatment involves treating only the sequelae, such as glaucoma.

H. If an inadvertent-filtering bleb is present but Seidel testing of the wound and bleb is negative, the patient may be observed while using topical antibiotic coverage. Of inadvertent-filtering blebs, 80% spontaneously disappear within 4 months. Beyond 6 months, the bleb should be closed to prevent endophthalmitis, particularly if the bleb is thin walled or a contact lens is to be worn. Laser photocoagulation or cryotherapy may be applied to the bleb to initiate an inflammatory response with subsequent bleb closure after 1–8 weeks. The bleb may be surgically closed as well. If the filtering bleb is the intentional outcome of a prior glaucoma-filtering procedure, referral to a glaucoma specialist may be necessary.

I. If a wound leak or filtering bleb is not detected on examination, in the setting of persistent ocular hypotony, gonioscopy should be performed to rule out a cyclodialysis cleft. If the chamber is not deep enough, the AC should be reformed and gonioscopy should be repeated. A suspected cleft may also be diagnosed after injecting fluorescein solution into the AC and retrieving this fluorescein in the suprachoroidal fluid. Attempts should be made to close the cleft using either laser photocoagulation, cryotherapy, partial-thickness diathermy, or through-and-through sutures to secure the detached ciliary body to the overlying sclera.

J. An acute or delayed choroidal detachment/effusion, in the absence of a wound leak, may occasionally present an issue and is usually associated with normal or low IOP. The differential diagnosis would include retinal detachment and intraocular tumor. Clinical examination and ultrasonography aid in the diagnosis. Medical treatment is similar to that used for other forms of shallow AC. In addition, systemic corticosteroids may result in more rapid resolution of the choroidal detachment by decreasing the associated ocular inflammation. Small choroidals can often be observed closely. Larger choroidals, such as kissing (touching) choroidals, may need to be surgically drained.

A suprachoroidal hemorrhage is caused by rupture of the short posterior ciliary vessels, with subsequent collection of blood in the supra-choroidal space. They are often associated with high IOP and pain, and usually occur intraoperatively or in the early postoperative period. Dark fluid is seen on funduscopic exam and ultrasonography may be useful. Most suprachoroidal hemorrhages resolve within 6 weeks. Topical and oral steroids are usually necessary, as is medical management of IOP. Hemorrhages may need to be drained

if there is a persistently flat AC or retinal apposition (kissing choroidals).

K. Ciliary body shutdown may occur, and is usually associated with low IOP. It tends to occur in the early postoperative period and usually resolves over time, often with the aid of topical steroids that minimize inflammation.

BIBLIOGRAPHY

1. Bauer B. Argon laser photocoagulation of cyclodialysis clefts after cataract surgery. Acta Ophthalmol Scand. 1995;73:283-4.
2. Cionni RJ, Osher RH. Intraoperative complications of phacoemulsification surgery. In: Steinert RF (Ed). Cataract Surgery: Technique, Complications, and Management. Philadelphia, PA: WB Saunders; 1995. pp. 325-439.
3. Gimbel HV, Sun R, DeBroff BM. Recognition and management of internal wound gape. J Cataract Refract Surg. 1995;21:121-4.
4. Jaffe NS, Jaffe MS, Jaffe GF. Cataract Surgery and Its Complications, 6th Edition. St Louis, MO: Mosby; 1997.
5. Menapace R. Delayed iris prolapse with unsutured 5.1 mm clear corneal incisions. J Cataract Refract Surg. 1995;21:353-7.

Diplopia After Cataract Surgery

107

Johan Zwaan

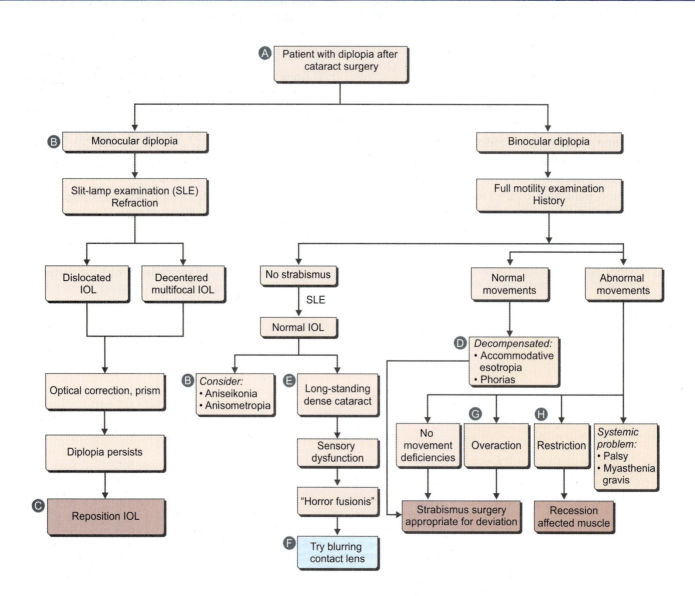

Diplopia may still happen after cataract surgery, but the incidence has decreased over the last two decades, even though it has not disappeared. The lower occurrence probably is related to the changes in the anesthesia for cataract extraction. The remaining cases are mostly due to sensory and strabismus problems.

A. Retrobulbar or peribulbar injections and infusion of the local anesthetic under Tenon capsule may be associated with postoperative ocular misalignment and diplopia due to direct toxic effects on the extraocular muscles and their nerves. No such problems, as expected, have been seen with topical or general anesthesia. Interestingly, one study of about 7,000 cataract patients, half of which received peribulbar anesthetic with hyaluronidase and half did not, strongly suggested that the enzyme use significantly reduced the incidence of postoperative diplopia (0, versus 27 in the control group). This probably is caused by the lower concentrations of anesthetic near the muscles, as the enzyme allows an easier diffusion away from the muscle.

B. If the diplopia is still present with one eye closed, it is probably due to a refractive problem such as a dislocated intraocular lens implant (IOL) or to decentration of a multifocal IOL. Aniseikonia or anisometropia may also be responsible.

C. The choice of technique for repositioning the IOL depends largely on the status of the posterior lens capsule.

D. A careful history and full eye examination may reveal that the patient had a childhood esotropia for which plus lenses were worn and that there is a weakness of binocularity. The patient may also have been prescribed prism glasses for a phoria.

E. Long-standing obscuration of the vision in one eye, for instance, by a dense cataract, may lead to the impossibility to fuse. After cataract extraction has removed the optical obstacle, if the patient cannot suppress the image, intractable diplopia may be the result.

F. If diplopia cannot be controlled, one solution is to blur or patch one eye, effectively making the patient monocular. While most patients do not like the idea of a patch, a high-plus or high-minus contact lens may be more acceptable.

G. After the damage of an extraocular muscle from the local anesthetic, the muscle appears underactive, or paretic. This results in an overaction of the opposing muscle. If, for instance, the inferior rectus, which is the muscle most often involved, is damaged, one would expect the eye to be hypertropic. When, over the next weeks, the muscle becomes scarred, the opposite is true. Thus, it is advisable to wait several weeks for the situation to stabilize, before planning on strabismus surgery.

H. Once the muscle motility has become restricted, a recession is the right choice of surgery.

BIBLIOGRAPHY

1. Capo H. Diplopia after cataract surgery. Semin Ophthalmol. 1999;14:62-4.
2. Costa PG, Debert I, Passos LB, et al. Persistent diplopia and strabismus after cataract surgery under local anesthesia. Binoc Vis Strabismus Q. 2006;21:155-8.
3. Golnik KC, West CE, Kay E, et al. Incidence of ocular misalignment and diplopia after uneventful cataract surgery. J Cataract Refract Surg. 2000;26:1205-9.
4. Gunton KB, Armstrong B. Diplopia in adult patients following cataract extraction. Curr Opin Ophthalmol. 2010;21:541-4.
5. Hamada S, Devys JM, Xuan TH, et al. Role of hyaluronidase in diplopia after peribulbar anesthesia for cataract surgery. Ophthalmology. 2005;112:879-82.
6. Koide R, Honda M, Kora Y, et al. Diplopia after cataract surgery. J Cataract Refract Surg. 2000;26:1198-204.
7. Zwaan J. Strabismus induced by radial keratotomy. Mil Med. 1996;161:630-1.

SECTION 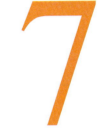 7

Retinal and Vitreous Disorders

Retinal Imaging (Imaging in Ophthalmology)

108

Gelareh Abedi

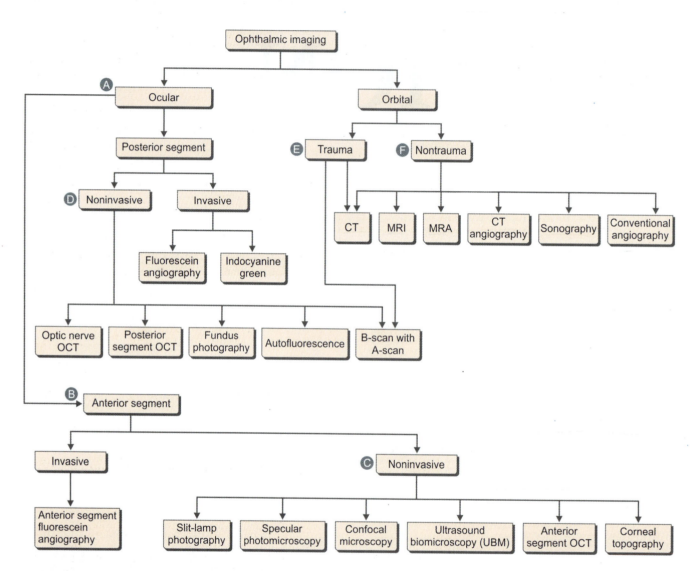

Ophthalmic imaging techniques are broad and some are rapidly becoming a routine part of ophthalmic examination. When used in conjunction with clinical examination, they can provide invaluable information. Imaging techniques are constantly evolving and it is important for the ordering physician to know the capabilities and limitations of each diagnosis test.

A. Ocular imaging modalities vary based on the anatomical location (anterior segment versus posterior segment) and type (invasive versus noninvasive). Images are used to document the presence of pathology, follow progression, aid in diagnosis, and assess the effectiveness of a treatment plan.

B. Anterior segment fluorescein angiography is used to study the circulation of the bulbar conjunctiva, episcleral, scleral, and iris vessels, and it is particularly useful in detecting iris neovascularization as in ischemic diseases, and areas of vascular nonperfusion as in necrotizing scleritis.

C. External eye photography is done with a slit lamp and has a magnification ratio of 1:1. The images are mainly used for the permanent documentation of a pathology seen externally. Specular photomicroscopy and confocal microscopy focus on the cellular level of cornea. Specular photomicroscopy allows the visualization of the corneal endothelium and specific quantification such as cell density and variation. Confocal microscopy images cell layers of the cornea despite edema and scarring, and can be extremely useful in diagnosing infectious entities such as amebic keratitis. Anterior segment OCT (optical coherence tomography) uses high-frequency ultrasound and can detect anterior chamber (AC) foreign body, ciliary body tumor, allows the measurement of AC depth and iris anatomy, evaluates the extent of trauma, and determines the lens position. Ultrasound biomicroscopy also qualitatively classifies the anterior segment features. Corneal topography maps the curvature of cornea in addition to several other parameters such as pupil size and location, presence of regular or irregular astigmatism, and stimulates keratometry.

D. Fundus photography, posterior segment/optic nerve OCT, B-scan ultrasound, and fundus autofluorescence are all noninvasive imaging techniques of posterior segment and optic nerve. Similar to slit-lamp photography, fundus photography allows for the permanent documentation of pathology in the posterior segment. Stereophotography documents the optic nerve head. Posterior segment OCT has evolved considerably and the newer versions of OCT devices allow for greater, faster, and higher resolution imaging of the retina layers, retinal pigment epithelium (RPE), and the choroid. Optic nerve OCT detects nerve fiber layer loss and is used in conjunction with several other tests. Fundus autofluorescence detects the changes in RPE and photoreceptors that are otherwise undetectable in routine imaging. B-scan ultrasound is quite useful when direct visualization of the intraocular content is difficult or impossible. It is also a diagnostic tool in clinically visible pathology such as choroidal tumors.

E. Imaging in traumatic cases is quite important not only to identify the extent of the injury, but also to detect the presence of an intraocular foreign body (IOFB). Computed tomography (CT) scan is the most utilized test in assessing open globes. B-scan should be used with caution in traumatic cases and the examiner should avoid placing pressure on a possibly open globe.

F. Computed tomography (CT) is an X-ray-based technique that assigns values to the tissues based on their coefficient of X-ray absorption, and orbit provides an excellent environment due to the high contrast between orbital fat and the globe. CT outlines the shape, location, extent, and character of the orbital lesions and helps in differential diagnosis. It is also excellent for the detection of orbital bone fractures. A three-dimensional CT enables the surgeon to view the three-dimensional projections of the bony orbital wall. Magnetic resonance imaging can be done with and without gadolinium and gives better soft tissue details. It should not be used if IOFB is suspected. Orbital sonography is used to detect size, shape, and position of the normal or abnormal tissues. B-scan (two-dimensional images) and A-scan (one-dimensional) can be helpful in distinguishing the degrees of disease activity. Vascular imaging has been possible with techniques such as MRA, CT angiography, and conventional CT. They are best for the detection of arteriovenous malformations, aneurysms, and arteriovenous fistulas. A radiologist and/or neuroradiologist should be consulted while ordering specific test to get the most benefit.

▌BIBLIOGRAPHY

1. Buerger DE, Biesman BS. Orbital imaging: A comparison of computed tomography and magnetic resonance imaging. Ophthalmol Clin North Am. 1998;11:381-410.
2. Cavanagh HD, Petroll WM, Jester JV. Confocal microscopy. In: Krachmer JH, Mannis MJ, Holland EJ, (Eds). Cornea, 2nd Edition (Vol. 1). Philadelphia, PA: Elsevier/Mosby; 2005. pp. 283-97.
3. Corbetter MC, O'Brart DPS, Rosen E, et al. Corneal Topography: Principle and Applications. London, UK: BMJ Books; 1999.
4. Goins KM, Wagoner MD. Imaging the anterior segment. Focal points: Clinical modules for ophthalmologists. San Francisco, CA: American Academy of Ophthalmology; 2009, module 11.

Macular Bull's Eye

109

Gelareh Abedi, Joseph M Harrison

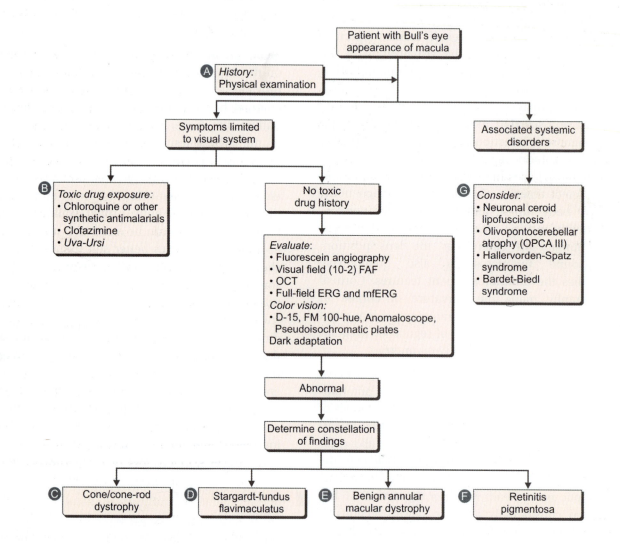

Macular bull's eye is an ophthalmoscopic pattern of a more pigmented area in the center of the fovea surrounded by a partial or full ring of depigmented retinal pigment epithelium (RPE), which is seen as an early or late manifestation of a variety of disorders. (Fig. 109.1) Complaints of blurry vision, difficulty with reading (because of paracentrally decreased sensitivity), or decreased visual acuity generally precede discovery of the bull's eye lesion. The history and physical examination should determine whether the following are present: day blindness, congenital infections, central nervous system (CNS) symptoms, extra digits on hands or feet (or an incision on hands and/or feet where a previous digit was), history of *[handwritten annotations in top margin: "→ Flying Saucer (preservation of subfoveal outer retinal layers/loss of photoR, Perifoveal ellipsoid band → ONL atrophy"]*

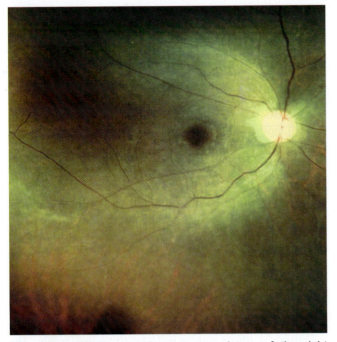

Fig. 109.1: Fundus autofluorescence picture of the right eye in a patient with Bull's eye maculopathy secondary to hydroxychloroquine toxicity. The mfERG was diffusely reduced throughout the central 45 degrees. Photo taken by Carrie A. Cooke.

medication with synthetic antimalarials, acquired nystagmus, photophobia, or problems with night or color vision.

A. Bull's eye maculopathy has a wide differential diagnosis and requires a careful history taking. In some of these disorders, detection of these lesions on a routine ophthalmic examination can be challenging in the early stages of the maculopathy. There are several imaging modalities that can assist in the early detection. These include noninvasive tests such as spectral domain optical coherence tomography (SD-OCT) and fundus autofluorescence (FAF) and invasive tests such as fluorescein angiography. SD-OCT gives a clear view of the inner segment/outer segment (IS/OS) junction of the photoreceptors; IS/OS junction lack of integrity is seen in variety of maculopathies. FAF is noninvasive imaging of lipofuscin fluorescence induced by ultraviolet light. In the absence of RPE and its accompanying lipofuscin, the area appears dark. In the fovea, FAF is naturally decreased due to absorption by lutein and zeaxanthin, and in the parafoveal region, FAF is higher. Any retinal pathology that can influence the amount of autofluorescence within the RPE (such as lipofuscin concentration) or over the RPE can affect the signal; therefore, it is important to correlate these findings with mfERG, SD-OCT, and Humphrey visual field (HVF 10-2). Fluorescein angiography reveals a window defect associated with RPE atrophy.

B. Chloroquine, hydroxychloroquine (HCQ), and other synthetic antimalarials bind to melanin in the RPE and choroid. A paracentral scotoma demonstrable with HVF 10-2 perimetry and increased macular dazzle occur early in the toxicity. Later, there may be complaints of blurred and decreased vision as the lesion spreads inward. A frequent later manifestation is a type 3 (blue-yellow or tritan) color vision defect on the Farnsworth–Munsell 100-hue (FM 100-hue) test of color vision. The bull's eye lesion is also a later development. There is a cumulative effect, which sometimes leads to deterioration despite discontinuation because the medication, chloroquine, is excreted very slowly. Rare advanced retinopathy can cause a tapetoretinal fundus appearance with constricted visual fields and equal loss of the cone and rod electroretinogram (ERG), ending in an unrecordable ERG and flat electrooculogram. The revised American Academy of Ophthalmology (AAO) guidelines consider mfERG, SD-OCT, and FAF more sensitive than HVF. Even in advanced cases, the final dark-adapted threshold tends to be normal. On SD-OCT, loss of the perifoveal IS/OS junction with intact outer retina directly under the fovea creates the 'flying saucer' sign that has been seen in HCQ toxicity cases. Clofazimine and Uva ursi both cause bull's eye lesions. Clofazimine is a phenazine dye used to treat dapsone-resistant leprosy and Uva ursi (bearberry), an herbal supplement to treat urinary bladder infection is a known inhibitor of melanin synthesis and contains hydroquinone.

C. Cone or cone-rod degeneration is a photoreceptor degeneration, presenting with photophobia, decreased visual acuity, acquired nystagmus, poor color vision (even though visual acuity may be 20/40–20/60), normal peripheral visual fields, decreased cone ERG and preserved rod ERG, elevated or absent cone threshold, and normal final rod threshold during dark adaptation. The color vision defect is usually type 1 (red-green or protan-deutan) on the FM 100-hue test. Fluorescein angiography often shows bull's eye lesions not visible ophthalmoscopically, with widespread RPE defects. In the more common autosomal-dominant form, the bull's eye pattern remains stable, with later development of pigment clumping and midperipheral and peripheral pigmentation. The autosomal-recessive form may have a paramacular 'crown' of Stargardt-like flecks. Often, there is a small central atrophic spot in the foveolar pigmented island, which progresses peripherally to complete foveolar atrophy. Vision is usually decreased. If foveal function is retained, color vision may be normal or there may be a type 3 defect that progresses to a type 2 defect (red-green and blue-yellow defect) with loss of the preserved central island and occasionally to complete achromatopsia. Night vision is normal in the early stages. The cone ERG is almost always abnormal, but the rod ERG is normal in the early stages. This ERG pattern is diagnostic and is the defining characteristic of cone degeneration. With progression, there is a slightly elevated final dark-adapted threshold (less than a factor of 100) and depressed or absent rod ERG.

D. In Stargardt–fundus flavimaculatus, there is a widespread retinal pigment epitheliopathy with engorgement of cells by lipofuscin. It is usually autosomal recessive, causing a central maculopathy with early complaints of decreased vision. Classically, there is a type 1 color vision defect (red green), some loss of cone ERG amplitude, a prolonged cone-rod break on dark adaptation, and central visual field defects. Early in the disease, there is macular mottling and broadening of the foveal reflex. Often, a small region of atrophy develops in the center of the central pigmented island. This may progress to the atrophic 'beaten bronze' macula. One form is without flecks (feathery soft yellow or gray deposits in the RPE), although flecks are a part of the classic description. These generally develop after the central maculopathy and may be seen as a crown surrounding the macula or may

be more widespread in the posterior pole beyond the arcades and nasal to the disc. Unlike drusen, the fresh flecks do not fluoresce. With time, the RPE cells die, leaving window defects. Fluorescein angiography may show a faint bull's eye or the dark choroid sign because of RPE blocking (vermilion fundus on ophthalmoscopy), which occurs in 50–80% of the cases early in the disease, even though ophthalmoscopically, the defect appears limited to the posterior pole. FAF is emerging as a noninvasive test to detect and follow the patients. The autofluorescence signal is generally depressed. There can be a reticular pattern of flecks and atrophic pigment patches or even 'bone spicule' pigmentation and localized 'punched-out' areas. A type 1 color vision defect is a classic finding seen in 50% of the cases with macular involvement. In about 8% of the cases, there is a type 3 color vision defect, when foveolar fixation is preserved. In 37%, there is no or only a mild color vision defect. The final dark-adapted threshold is normal or slightly elevated.

E. In the original description of the benign concentric annular macular dystrophy with bull's eye lesions (autosomal dominant), there was unusually good visual acuity (20/25 or better), even in the oldest patients. With 10 years follow-up, some of these patients complained of deterioration of day and night vision, and color vision. The fundus abnormalities progressed with involvement of the periphery, including bone spicule pigmentation in some. Rod and cone ERGs were equally involved.

F. Bull's eye lesions are also seen in 30–40% of the patients with retinitis pigmentosa, a rod-cone photoreceptor degeneration, which is sporadic in about half the cases or inherited by any of the genetic patterns. Patients complain of problems with night vision and have an elevated final dark-adapted threshold (greater than a factor of 100). They also have constricted visual fields or an expanding midperipheral ring scotoma, photophobia, selectively more decreased rod ERG, a delayed cone ERG, and a type 3 color vision defect. The ERG is absent or too small to be recorded by standard techniques in 70% of patients. Classically, there are attenuated arterioles, midperipheral pigment clumping and depigmentation, bone spicule pigmentation, and waxy-appearing discs. In the early stage of the disease, the fundus signs may only be a blond or mottled appearance.

G. Bull's eye lesions are also seen in syndromes-neuronal ceroid lipofuscinosis (Jansky–Bielchowsky and Vogt–Spielmeyer), olivopontocerebellar atrophy with retinal dystrophy [OPCA III or spinocerabellar ataxia type 7(SCA7)] (autosomal dominant), Hallervorden–Spatz, and Bardet–Biedl–and rarely in fucosidosis and methylmalonic aciduria. The latter two are diagnosed by enzyme assays and urinalysis, respectively. Fucosidosis is rare and includes prominent facial and skeletal abnormalities. In neuronal storage diseases associated with bull's eye lesions (Jansky–Bielchowsky, Vogt–Spielmeyer, fucosidosis and methylmalonic aciduria, and Bardet–Biedl syndrome—all autosomal recessive), the ERG is either unrecordable or very subnormal in children. Bardet–Biedl syndrome also includes polydactyly, obesity, and renal disorders. Neuronal ceroid lipofuscinosis can be distinguished from the other conditions with CNS symptoms by the finding of curvilinear or fingerprint inclusion bodies in ultrastructural examination of conjunctival biopsies and peripheral blood lymphocytes. OPCA III involves cerebellar symptoms, such as ataxia, whereas Hallervorden–Spatz syndrome includes deterioration of voluntary movements and increased involuntary movements and muscle rigidity. The macula is hyperpigmented in Hallervorden–Spatz syndrome and may have a fine granular pigmentation in OPCA III.

BIBLIOGRAPHY

1. Aleman TS, et al. Spinocerebellar Ataxia 7 (SCA7) shows a cone-rod dystrophy phenotype. Exp Eye Res. 2002;74:737-45.
2. Batemen R, Lange GE, Maumenee IH. Genetic metabolic disorders associated with retinal dystrophies. In: Ryan S, (Ed). Retina (Vol. 1). St. Louis, MO: Mosby, 1989. pp. 421-45.
3. Blacharski PA. Fundus flavimaculatus. In: Newsome DA, (Ed). Retinal dystrophies and degenerations. New York, NY: Raven, 1988. pp. 135-9.
4. Chen E, Brown DM, Benz MS, et al. Spectral domain optical coherence tomography as an effective screening test for hydroxychloroquine retinopathy (the flying saucer sign). Clin Ophthalmol. 2010;4:1151-8.
5. Deutman AF. Macular dystrophies. In: Ryan S (Ed). Retina. (Vol. 2). St Louis, MO: Mosby; 1989. pp. 243-98.
6. Gass DM. Stereoscopic atlas of macular diseases: Diagnosis and treatment, Third edition (Vols. 1 and 2). St. Louis, MO: Mosby;1987.
7. Krill AE. Hereditary retinal and choroidal diseases (Vol. 2). Clinical characteristics. Philadelphia: Harper & Row. 1977.
8. Marmor MF, et al. Revised recommendations on screening for chloroquine and hydroxychloroquine retinopathy. Ophthalmology. 2011;118:415-22.
9. Schmitz-Valckenberg S, Holz FG, Bird AC, et al. Fundus autofluorescence imaging: Review and perspectives. Retina. 2008;28:385-409.
10. Weleber RG, Eisner A. Cone degeneration (Bull's-eye dystrophies) and color vision defects. In: Newsome DA (Ed). Retinal dystrophies and degenerations. New York, NY: Raven; 1988. pp. 233.
11. Weleber RG. Retinitis pigmentosa and allied disorders. In: Ryan S (Ed). Retina (Vol. 1). St. Louis, MO: Mosby; 1989. pp. 299-420.

Macular Star

110

Gelareh Abedi

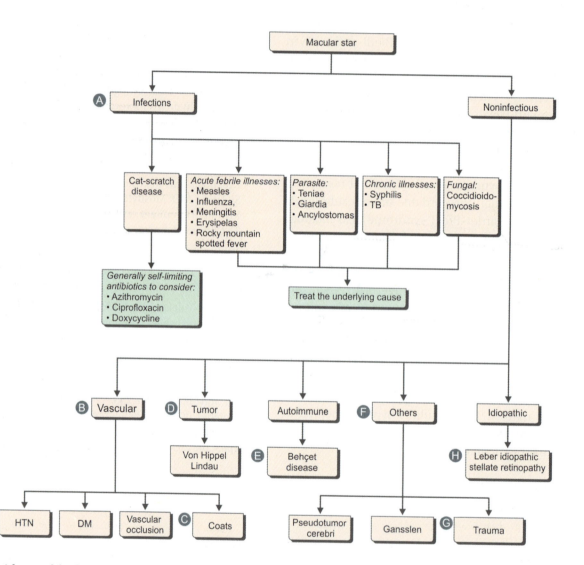

Lipid residues of leakage from capillaries form hard exudates. In Henle's layer, these exudates can present in a star-like formation known as macular star. Any event that compromises capillaries in the macula region and leads to the leakage potentially forms a macular star. Cat-scratch disease, acute febrile illnesses (measles, influenza, meningitis, erysipelas, Rocky Mountain spotted fever), chronic infections (tuberculosis and syphilis), fungal (coccidioidomycosis), and parasites (teniae, Giardia, Ancylostoma) are among the infectious causes. Noninfectious illnesses include any occlusion of a vascular entity supplying the macula, retinal periphlebitis, hypertension, diabetes, Coats disease, Behçet disease, ocular or cerebral trauma, papillitis, papilledema, and Gansslen syndrome.

A. Retinal vasculitis and eventual leakage occurs in the setting of many infections. The most commonly known is cat-scratch disease caused by *Bartonella henselae* following a scratch or bite from a cat. The classic manifestation includes regional lymphadenopathy and flu-like symptoms that can last from weeks to several months. In addition to macular star formation, as many as 2/3 of patients present with optic disc edema. It is generally a self-limiting disease; however, antibiotics such as azithromycin and doxycycline have been used with unclear benefits. Other manifestations of the same syndrome are Parinaud oculoglandular syndrome (with granulomatous conjunctivitis and swellings of lymph nodes near the ear), optic neuritis (also called neuroretinitis), bacillary angiomatosis and bacillary peliosis (both seen in HIV and immunocompromised patients), and acute meningitis.

B. Hypertension and diabetes are the most common vascular entities with capillary leakage. In severe hypertension, optic nerve swelling is noted; therefore, checking a patient's blood pressure (BP) is crucial, and, if high, may require hospitalization for lowering BP.

C. Coats is a nonhereditary congenital eye disease that is typically unilateral and affects young boys. Hallmark of Coats disease is retinal telangiectasia and it presents with massive hard exudates secondary to leakage and hemorrhages. In moderate to severe disease, serous retinal detachments are seen. Laser and cryotherapy can be used in early stages to treat the telangiectatic vessels. In the later stages of disease, total retinal detachment occurs and permanent blindness is unavoidable.

D. Retinal capillary hemangiomas are fed by large arterioles and drained by even larger veins. When left untreated, they can gradually grow, leak serous fluid and bleed. They can present by themselves or be a part of series of findings including cerebellar/spinal cord hemangioblastoma, renal cell carcinoma, pheochromocytoma, and visceral cysts. The retinal hemangiomas may be in the periphery and difficult to detect. Therefore, a careful periodic examination of peripheral retina is important.

E. Behçet disease is an immune-mediated systemic disease with recurrent oral and genital ulcers, visceral system, and ocular involvements. Though anterior and posterior uveitis and retinal vasculitis are common ocular presentations, macular star formation has also been reported and should be considered as a possible manifestation.

F. Several miscellaneous conditions have macular star as part of their presentation. History and physical examination can aid in diagnosis. Pseudotumor cerebri (idiopathic intracranial hypertension) is typically seen in overweight females with an elevated opening pressure on lumbar puncture (LP) and otherwise normal brain scan. Patients present with headache, nausea, vomiting, tinnitus, diplopia, and other visual symptoms. Lowering central nervous system pressure by either LP, medication (diamox), and surgery (intracranial shunt) can alleviate symptoms.

G. Gansslen syndrome (also known as Familial Hemolytic Icterus) is a rare autosomal-dominant inheritance that occurs mainly in Caucasians with ocular and systemic manifestations. Dilated retinal vessels, hemorrhages, and hard exudates, including the formation of a macular star, have been reported.

H. Leber idiopathic stellate retinopathy presents with optic disc swelling and macular hard exudates. First described by Leber in 1916, the four features include: unilaterality, stellate macular exudates, spontaneous resolution, and unknown etiology. Therefore, prior to diagnosing the patient with this condition, all other etiologies must be ruled out.

BIBLIOGRAPHY

1. Carroll DM, Franklin RM. Leber's idiopathic stellate retinopathy. Am J Ophthalmol. 1982;93:96-101.
2. Ghauri RR, Lee A. Optic disk edema with a macular star. Surv Ophthalmol. 1998;43:270-4.
3. Paul-Chan RV, Lee TC, Chaganti RK. Macular star associated with Behcet disease. Retina. 2006;26:468-70.
4. Rolain JM, Brouqui P, Koehler JE, et al. Recommendations for treatment of human infections caused by Bartonella species. Antimicrob Agents Chemother. 2004;48:1921-33.

Macular Cherry-Red Spot

Armand Daccache, Amir Mohsenin, Elizabeth Yang

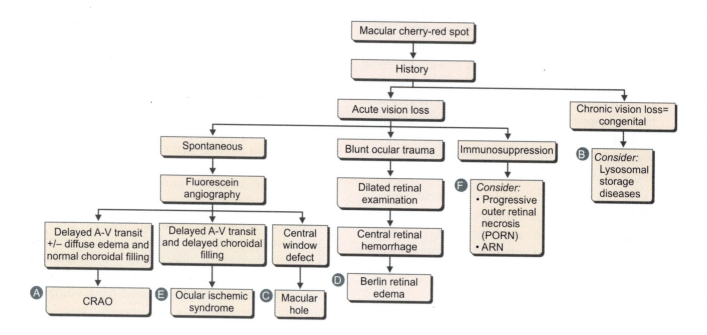

111

A macular cherry-red spot describes the fundus appearance of the choroidal vasculature as seen through a normal transparent fovea surrounded by a whitened posterior retina. This appearance can arise from different disease mechanisms including vascular disease, metabolic derangements, trauma, or infection.

A. A central retinal artery occlusion (CRAO) is the most common cause of an acute cherry-red spot in adults. A CRAO is typically present in patients over 60 years of age and is slightly more common in males. It is characterized by sudden-onset, painless vision loss that usually occurs over seconds from a loss of blood supply to the inner retina. It is most commonly caused by emboli, cardiac anomalies or valvular defects, atherosclerotic disease, vasculitidies including temporal arteritis, hypercoagulable states, vasospasm, or dissecting aneurysms. On examination, a relative afferent pupillary defect will be present. The posterior retina becomes a pale, opaque white due to inner retinal edema and ischemic retinal necrosis. The fovea, however, maintains its transparency as it is partially nourished by the underlying choriocapillaris. The posterior pole becomes the most opaque because of the high density of the nerve fiber layer and retinal ganglion cells. On fluorescein angiography, there may be a delay in retinal arterial filling, but the most common finding is a delay in arteriovenous transit time. Choroidal filling is usually normal.

B. Macular cherry-red spots in children or infants are most commonly a result of metabolic disease. Diseases that result in accumulation of storage material such as glycolipids or sphingolipids cause this fundus appearance when the materials accumulate in the cellular layers of the macula. The cherry-red spot appearance is due to the fovea being spared from lipid accumulation due to it being devoid of ganglion cells and being the thinnest part of the retina. The classic associations are with Tay-Sachs disease (GM2 Gangliosidosis type 1) or Sandhoff disease (type 2), in which ganglioside accumulation leads to hepatosplenomegaly, hypotonia, and neuroregression. Niemann-Pick disease (GM1 Gangliosidosis) is suggested in infants who develop interstitial pneumonia and neurologic deterioration as well as ophthalmoplegia. Many other lysosomal storage diseases, including sialidosis, Fabry disease, Hunter syndrome, and galactosialidosis, are all potential causes for the presence of a macular cherry-red spot in a child.

C. Macular holes can also mimic cherry-red spots due to the absence of the central retinal layers. The pathogenesis of idiopathic macular holes is thought to be from antero-posterior traction from the vitreous, causing a posterior hyaloid detachment from the fovea and subsequent foveolar dehiscence. While the surrounding retina is usually normal, the underlying retinal pigment epithelium and choroid can be clearly seen through the retinal defect creating the cherry-red appearance. Symptoms include a gradual loss or blurring of central vision and metamorphopsia. On slit-lamp examination, a Watzke sign may be elicited where the patient can appreciate a break in a light beam directed over the hole. Optical coherence tomography (OCT) will show a full thickness disruption of the retinal layers with a perifoveal area of intraretinal fluid. Fluorescein angiography will demonstrate a window defect that gradually fades, possibly surrounded by partial blockage of fluorescence if subretinal fluid is present around the macular hole.

D. Berlin edema (commotio retinae) is caused by blunt trauma to the globe and results in whitening of the posterior pole from disruption of the photoreceptor—pigment epithelium complex. The cherry-red spot is most evident when the contusion extends into the posterior pole and may be accompanied by retinal hemorrhages. Visual acuity is typically decreased, but there can be complete visual recovery as the commotio retinae resolves. On OCT, there may be apparent thickening of the outer retina that correlates with histopathologic photoreceptor outer segment disruption and retinal pigment epithelium damage. Fluorescein angiogram may show blocked fluorescence of the macula.

E. Ocular ischemic syndrome is a collection of findings that occurs after chronic, severe arterial hypoperfusion of the eye, most commonly due to high-grade carotid stenosis, ophthalmic artery stenosis, Takayasu syndrome, temporal arteritis, or vasospasm. It is characterized by the classic triad of mid-peripheral dot and blot retinal hemorrhages, dilated veins, and iris neovascularization. Along with vision loss and periorbital pain, anterior chamber inflammation and evidence of posterior segment ischemia, including a cherry-red spot, is often present. On fluorescein angiography, there is an increase in arteriovenous transit time and delayed choroidal filling.

F. Progressive outer retinal necrosis (PORN) is a disease entity caused by the varicella zoster virus in immunocompromised patients. Typical manifestations include multifocal, deep, whitish retinal lesions that can present initially in the parafoveal region and cause a cherry-red spot appearance, although the entire retina can be quickly involved in the following days. PORN can often lead to rhegmatogenous retinal detachments, and the prognosis is generally poor. Acute retinal necrosis (ARN) occurs in immunocompetent individuals and is distinguished from PORN in that it usually involves the entire thickness of the retina, begins circumferentially in the periphery, and is accompanied by occlusive arteritis and severe inflammation.

BIBLIOGRAPHY

1. De Graeve C, Van de Sompel W, Claes C. Ocular ischemic syndrome: two case reports of bilateral involvement. Bull Soc Belge Ophtalmol. 1999;273:69-74.
2. Gentile RC, Landa G, Pons ME, et al. Macular hole formation, progression, and surgical repair: case series of serial optical coherence tomography and time lapse morphing video study. BMC Ophthalmol. 2010;10:24.
3. Matri LE, Chebil A, Kort F, et al. Optical coherence tomographic findings in Berlin's edema. J Ophthalmic Vis Res. 2010;5:127-9.
4. Suvarna JC, Hajela SA. Cherry-red spot. J Postgrad Med. 2008;54:54-7.
5. Yiu G, Young LH. Progressive outer retinal necrosis presenting as cherry-red spot. Ocul Immunol Inflamm. 2012;20:384-6.

Crystals in the Fundus

Gelareh Abedi

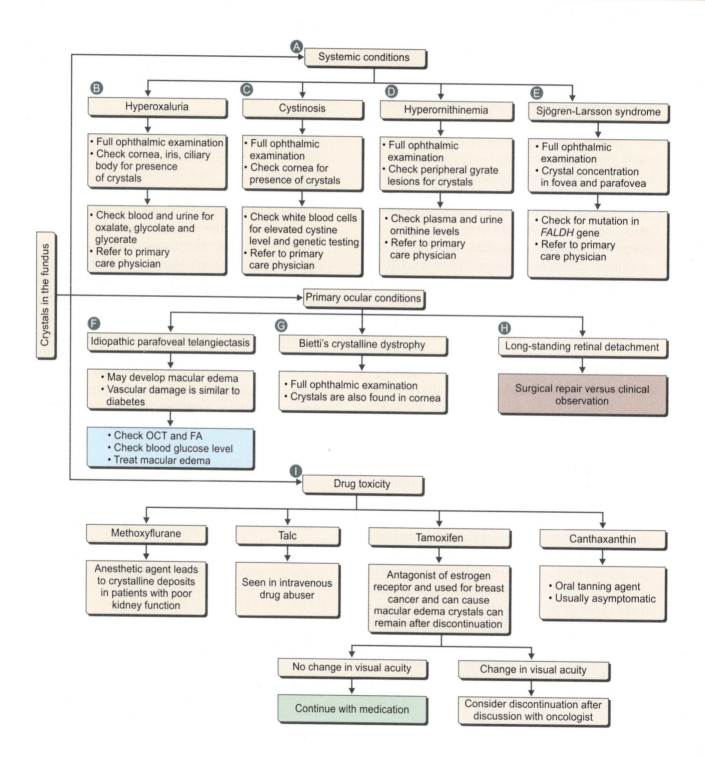

112

Crystals in the retina are intraretinal refractile bodies. Also known as "crystalline retinopathy," crystals are caused by a variety of conditions such as systemic diseases, primary ocular conditions, and drug toxicity and they can be completely benign or lead to decreased visual acuity. Careful examination of the retina is essential since hard exudates and calcific drusen may resemble crystals.

A. A variety of systemic conditions lead to crystalline formation and their presence in the retina should initiate a systemic work-up. These include hyperoxaluria leading to oxalosis, cystinosis, hyperornithinemia, and Sjögren–Larsson syndrome.

B. The first signs of hyperoxaluria appear anytime from infancy to early adulthood and vary from mild to severe. A complete ophthalmic examination is recommended and crystals can be present in cornea, iris, and ciliary body in addition to the retina. If suspected, blood and urine tests for oxalate and a prompt referral to pediatrician are recommended.

C. Cystinosis is an autosomal-recessive lysosomal storage disease with an abnormal accumulation of cystine. Three distinct types include nephropathic, juvenile and ocular, and the symptoms are first seen at about 3–18 months of age. Diagnosis can be achieved by genetic testing and measuring elevated white blood cell cystine content. Corneal cystine crystals are present in all patients after the age of 1 year.

D. Hyperornithinemia is a systemic disease where there is a deficiency in ornithine aminotransferase (OAT). Although ocular involvement is the most clinically significant manifestation, other organs such as brain and liver can be affected as well. OAT deficiency causes gyrate atrophy in the retina, and crystals can be seen in the demarcation lines of peripheral gyrate lesions in some patients.

E. Sjögren–Larsson syndrome is an autosomal-recessive neurocutaneous disorder present at birth. It presents with ichthyosis, spastic paraplegia, and mental retardation. Ophthalmic manifestations include crystals in the retina that appear as superficial yellow white dots in the fovea and parafovea and sparing foveola. There is also mottled hyperpigmentation in the macula. If suspected, referral to a primary care physician is recommended.

F. Idiopathic parafoveal telangiectasis refers to a group of retinal disorders that are characterized by telangiectatic alterations and variable aneurysmal dilation of the juxtafoveolar capillary network in one or both eyes. Visual decrease is secondary to macular edema and exudates and treatments, including laser and anti-VEGF injections, have variable results.

G. Bietti crystalline dystrophy presents with a mild to moderate decrease in visual acuity, nyctalopia, and paracentral scotoma. It is a slowly progressive disease and intraretinal crystalline deposits are most numerous in the posterior pole. In addition, multiple areas of geographic atrophy and loss of choriocapillaries are seen. In addition to retina crystals, there are paralimbal, conjunctival, or corneal crystals as well.

H. Long-standing retinal detachment leads to superficial yellowish crystals in the area of the detached retina. In addition to the primary ocular disorders mentioned, West African Crystalline Retinopathy, autosomal-dominant crystalline dystrophy, and retinal arterial emboli are other disorders where crystals can be seen.

I. Several drugs can lead to crystal formation in the retina. These include methoxyflurane, talc, tamoxifen, and canthaxanthin. Crystals are generally asymptomatic and can resolve; however, some can lead to macular edema and decreased visual acuity. In addition to the above, intravitreal injection of triamcinolone can also lead to persistent crystals in the retina and posterior hyaloids.

BIBLIOGRAPHY

1. Fielder AR, Garner A, Chambers TL. Ophthalmic manifestations of primary oxalosis. Br J Ophthalmol. 1980;64:782-8.
2. Nadim F, Walid H, Adib J. The differential diagnosis of crystals in the retina. Int Ophthalmol. 2001;24:113-21.
3. Rossi S, Testa F, Li A, et al. Clinical and genetic features in Italian Bietti crystalline dystrophy patients. Br J Ophthalmol. 2013;97:174-9.
4. Srikantia N, Mukesh S, Krishnaswamy M. Crystalline maculopathy: A rare complication of tamoxifen therapy. J Cancer Res Ther. 2010;6:313-5.
5. Zarifa R, Shaikh S, Kester E. Persistence of triamcinolone crystals after intra-vitreal injection: Benign crystalline hyaloidopathy. Indian J Ophthalmol. 2013;61:182-3.

113

Retained Lens Fragments

Lina Marouf, Gelareh Abedi, Timothy P Cleland

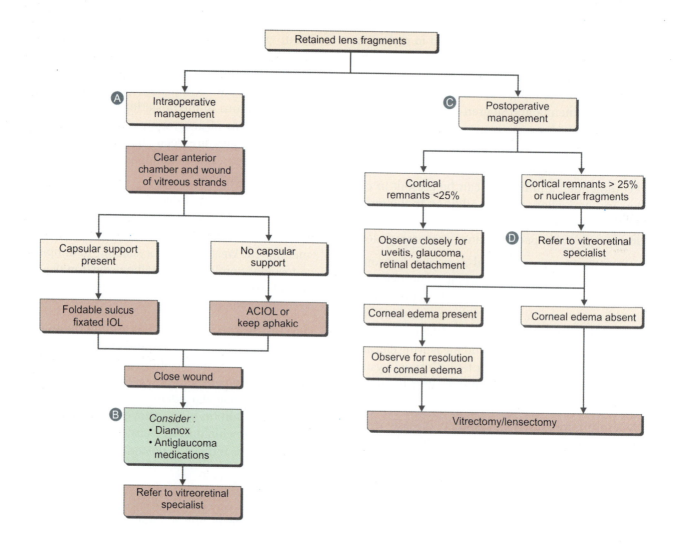

The most common causes of retained lens fragments are a hard nucleus, pseudoexfoliation of the lens capsule, previous vitrectomy, and less surgical experience.

A cataract surgeon has a 3% chance per year of getting sued in relation to cataract surgery. The most common complications related to cataract surgery resulting in a lawsuit in ascending order are: endophthalmitis followed by retinal complications and finally intraocular lens problems: such as wrong intraocular lens implant (IOL) power, size and dislocation of lens fragments.

The incidence of dislocation of lens fragments varies between 0.3 % and 1.1%. Studies have shown that the incidence of dislocation of the lens fragment decreases between the second and third year of residency. The incidence is also less in a private practice setting in comparison to a residency training setting.

The most common complications of retained lens fragments are uveitis, glaucoma, cystoid macular edema, and retinal detachment. The incidence of retinal detachment varies between 5% and 21% after dislocation of the lens fragment. Therefore, a dilated fundus examination with scleral depression is important postoperatively.

A. When a surgeon experiences rupture of the posterior capsule and dislocation of the lens fragment, it is very important not to be aggressive in performing a posterior vitrectomy and not to go after the dislocated lens fragments. This will minimize the development of corneal edema, which would impair visualization of the posterior segment, should vitrectomy be necessary. The most appropriate management would be to clear the anterior chamber and wound of any vitreous strands. In the presence of good capsular support, a foldable one-piece intraocular lens can be inserted. Toric, restore, and silicon lenses should be avoided. In the absence of adequate capsular support, the patient should be left aphakic or an anterior chamber lens should be inserted.

B. Postoperatively, in addition to the usual eyedrops, Diamox 500 mg PO, antiglaucoma drops and referral to a vitreoretinal specialist should be considered.

C. Postoperative management depends on the size of the retained lens fragments. Cortical remnants of less than 25% in size may be tolerated in the eye; however, the patient should be monitored closely for signs of glaucoma or uveitis. Cortical remnants greater than 25% in size and nuclear fragments will usually require surgical removal. Referral to a vitreoretinal specialist is important. The timing of vitrectomy depends on the presence or absence of corneal edema.

D. A retrospective chart review comparing early vitrectomy (within the first 14 days after cataract surgery) to late vitrectomy (performed after 2 weeks of cataract surgery) for retained lens fragment after phacoemulsification showed that there was no significant difference in the patients' final visual acuity between the two groups. There was a trend, however, toward a higher rate of cystoid macular edema in patients with retained lens material when delayed lensectomy/vitrectomy was performed.

Dislocation of lens fragments occurs even with a skilled surgeon. It is a side effect rather than a complication of cataract extraction.

In order to decrease the chance of litigation and further retinal complications, the choice of a qualified vitreoretinal surgeon who will defuse the patients' fears, and provide a good surgical outcome is of utmost importance.

▌BIBLIOGRAPHY

1. Abedi G, Cleland T, Marouf L. Management of retained lens fragments after phacoemulsification: Comparing visual outcomes of early pars plana lensectomy versus lake pars plana lensectomy. ARVO. 2012.
2. Fuller D. MedicoLegal issues from complications of cataract surgery. Retina Subspecialty Day; 1998. pp. 193-5.

Subretinal Neovascular Membranes

Juan E Rubio Jr, Lina Marouf, Bailey L Lee

114

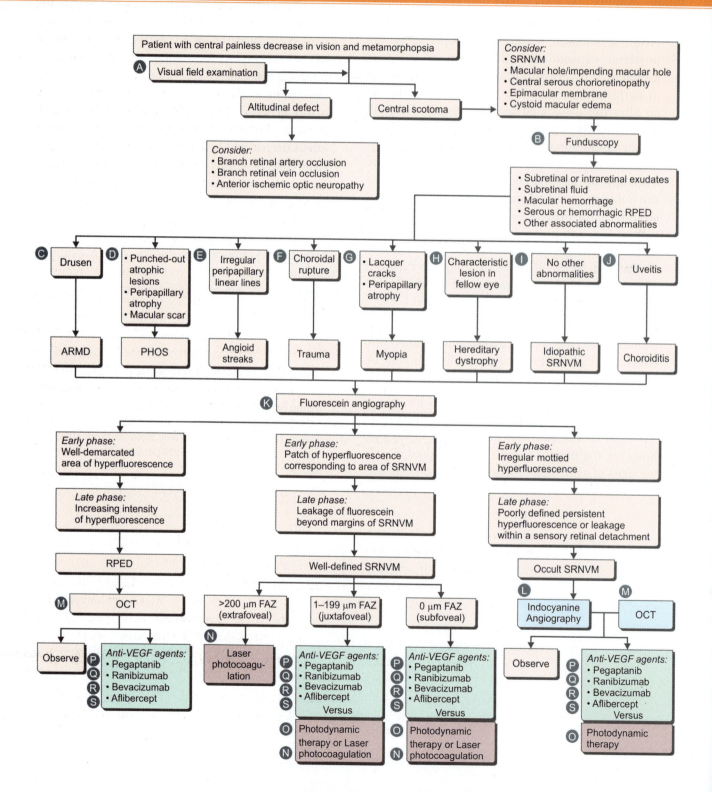

Subretinal neovascular membrane (SRNVM) refers to the growth of choroidal vessels through Bruch's membrane into the subretinal pigment epithelial space or the subretinal space. Any disease process that affects the integrity of the retinal pigment epithelium-Bruch membrane-choriocapillaris complex, can be associated with a SRNVM. Patients with SRNVMs usually present with the sudden onset of painless decrease in central vision and metamorphopsia.

A. Visual field testing is important in assessing a patient with metamorphopsia and decreased central vision. The central 20 degrees of the visual field can be assessed with an Amsler grid. A central scotoma may denote macular, optic nerve, or cortical abnormality; however, metamorphopsia indicates macular disease.

B. A detailed dilated fundus examination is performed with a contact lens biomicroscopy and indirect ophthalmoscopy. Signs of subretinal neovascular proliferation include macular hemorrhages, serous macular detachment, serous or hemorrhagic retinal pigment epithelial detachment (RPED), and macular exudates. Funduscopic findings in the same or fellow eye may help establish the cause of a SRNVM.

C. Age-related macular degeneration (AMD) is the leading cause of central visual loss in the United States in people >50 years of age. Signs of AMD include macular drusen, retinal pigment epithelial changes, atrophic changes, serous and hemorrhagic RPEDs, choroidal neovascularization (CNV), subretinal fibrosis, and disciform scars. The disease presents in two forms: the nonexudative or "dry" form affects most patients; the exudative or "wet" form is responsible for severe visual loss in affected eyes. There is no known therapy for the dry form of AMD. The Age-Related Eye Disease Study (AREDS) showed a reduction in dry AMD progression in patients taking zinc, beta-carotene, vitamin C, and vitamin E.

D. Subretinal neovascular membrane (SRNVM) secondary to ocular histoplasmosis syndrome (OHS) usually occurs in healthy persons (20–50 years old). The classically described triad of the disease includes peripheral punched-out atrophic lesions (histo spots), peripapillary chorioretinal scarring, and macular scars.

E. Angioid streaks are linear dehiscences in Bruch membrane. Clinically, they are irregular, jagged lines that vary from reddish orange to dark red. They typically extend from the peripapillary area to the peripheral fundus. The disease is usually bilateral. Choroidal vessels may grow the through breaks in Bruch membrane into the subretinal pigment epithelial space, resulting in serous and hemorrhagic RPED. The visual prognosis in such eyes is usually poor. Of patients with angioid streaks, 50% have associated systemic abnormalities, the most common being Paget disease, sickle cell hemoglobinopathy, Ehlers–Danlos syndrome, and pseudoxanthoma elasticum.

F. Trauma to the eye can rupture Bruch membrane and the choroidal layers. This is known clinically as choroidal rupture. SRNVM may arise at the site of rupture months to years after the injury, resulting in decreased vision.

G. The progressive thinning of the choroidal and retinal layers in pathologic myopia can result in peripapillary chorioretinal atrophy, geographic areas of chorioretinal atrophy, and linear breaks in Bruch membrane called lacquer cracks. SRNVM can grow through these foci, resulting in decreased central vision.

H. Several hereditary macular dystrophies and inflammatory retinal diseases are associated with SRNVMs. Each exhibits a characteristic funduscopic lesion in the fellow eye, denoting the cause of the SRNVM.

I. In the absence of drusen and chorioretinal abnormalities, young patients with SRNVM are classified as having idiopathic SRNVM.

J. Posterior segment uveitis can lead to choroidal inflammation and the development of SRNVM. Examples include multifocal choroiditis, punctate inner choroidopathy, toxoplasmosis retinochorioiditis, multiple evanescent white-dot syndrome, and serpiginous choroiditis.

K. Fluorescein angiography (FA) is useful in determining not only the lesion location, type, and size, but also whether the SRNVM is active (and not just a scar tissue). FA can also help define the margins of an SRNVM and its proximity to the foveal avascular zone (FAZ). SRNVM, accordingly, can be categorized into predominantly classic (well defined) CNV, minimally classic (<50% classic) CNV, or occult (poorly defined) CNV. SRNVM can also be classified as extrafoveal (200–2,500 µm from the center of the fovea), juxtafoveal (<199 µm), or subfoveal SRNVM. A characteristic angiographic finding of a predominantly classic (well defined) SRNVM is the early hyperfluorescence in the area of CNV with late leakage.

L. Indocyanine green angiography (ICG) can be a useful adjunct in visualizing SRNVMs that are occult CNV by fluorescein angiography, or those SRNVMs with overlying hemorrhage. Focal areas of leakage or well-defined plaques visualized with ICG have been treated with involution of SRNVM.

M. High-resolution images obtained with optical coherence tomography (OCT) are useful in the evaluation of SRNVM. OCT can identify intraretinal fluid, subretinal fluid, and RPEDs. OCT may be used to characterize SRNVM lesion and aid in treatment decision.

N. Initial treatment for SRNVM was originally restricted to laser photocoagulation, which is a "hot laser" treatment that effectively seals the SRNVM. The Macular Photocoagulation Study (MPS) demonstrated the value of laser photocoagulation in patients with *subfoveal* SRNVM secondary to wet AMD, and in those with well-defined *extrafoveal* and *juxtafoveal* SRNVM secondary to wet AMD, OHS, and idiopathic SRNVM. For eligible patients with SRNVM, laser treatment reduced the risk of severe visual loss, but it did not restore or improve vision. Laser treatment is still a proven treatment option for nonsubfoveal SRNVM in wet AMD, with best results for *extrafoveal* SRNVM. Patients with *extrafoveal* or *juxtafoveal* SRNVM secondary to OHS, angioid streaks, pathologic myopia, or idiopathic causes should also be considered for laser treatment. After laser therapy, patients should be re-examined at frequent intervals, and fluorescein angiography should be performed after the treatment to confirm the complete occlusion of SRNVM and to detect recurrence.

O. Photodynamic therapy (PDT) consists of an intravenous infusion of FDA-approved photosensitizing dye, verteporfin (Visudyne®), followed by a nondestructive "cold laser" application to activate the dye and seal the SRNVM. PDT decreases or delays vision loss, but does not improve vision. *Subfoveal* classic SRNVM in wet AMD responds best to PDT, but small occult or minimally classic *subfoveal* SRNVM in wet AMD may also respond. PDT should also be considered for the treatment of *subfoveal* SRNVM secondary to OHS, angioid streaks, pathologic myopia, or idiopathic causes. PDT is usually performed every 3 months for 1–2 years.

P. Pegaptanib (Macugen®) was the first FDA-approved anti-VEGF aptamer, approved for all *subfoveal* SRNVM subtypes in wet AMD, and injected intravitreally every 6 weeks for 1–2 years. Macugen® was shown to be more effective than PDT in treating SRNVM, and to reduce the probability of developing severe vision loss. However, like PDT, it only delayed vision loss but did not prevent it. Macugen® can be considered for the treatment of *subfoveal* SRNVM in wet AMD (better for early, smaller lesions), OHS, angioid streaks, pathologic myopia, or idiopathic causes. Macugen® is not used very often since more effective treatments for SRNVM are now available.

Q. Ranibizumab (Lucentis®) is an anti-VEGF antibody fragment, injected intravitreally at 1–3 months' intervals and is FDA approved for all *subfoveal* SRNVM subtypes in wet AMD. In phase III clinical trials, Lucentis®, unlike other treatments, was shown to improve visual acuity by as much as three or more Snellen lines in 30–40% of the eyes in 1 year. Subsequently, Lucentis® was able to prevent further vision loss: about 95% of the patients maintained their baseline vision while on treatment. Furthermore, up to 40% of the patients treated with Lucentis® achieved vision of 20/40 or better. Lucentis® acts against the growth of SRNVM in wet AMD and is injected into the eye on a monthly basis for best results. Lucentis® should be considered as a primary treatment for *subfoveal* SRNVM due to wet AMD, OHS, angioid streaks, pathologic myopia, or idiopathic causes.

R. Bevacizumab (Avastin®) is a full-length anti-VEGF antibody from which Lucentis® is derived. Although FDA approved for colon cancer, off-label use as an intravitreal injection has been shown to be beneficial for the treatment of SRNVM in wet AMD. The advantages of Avastin® are lower cost and longer half-life (allowing for 6-weekly dosing, rather than 4-weekly as for Lucentis®). Use of Avastin® for wet AMD has become very common with some ophthalmologists choosing it exclusively, while others treat with Lucentis® and then switch to Avastin®. Recently, the National Eye Institute released the results of a study comparing Avastin® to Lucentis® (Comparison of AMD Treatment Trial or CATT). Individuals in the study were given Lucentis®, either monthly or as needed, or Avastin®, either monthly or as needed. It concluded that Lucentis® and Avastin® are essentially equal in effectiveness and safety. Depending on how often the treatment is received, Lucentis® was somewhat more effective and safer. Avastin®, rather than Lucentis®, may be considered as the primary treatment for *subfoveal* SRNVM due to wet AMD, OHS, angioid streaks, pathologic myopia, or idiopathic causes.

S. Aflibercept (VEGF–TRAP or Eylea®) is the newest treatment available for SRNVM in wet AMD. Unlike Lucentis®, which is an antibody (Fab) fragment against VEGF, Eylea® is a soluble receptor for VEGF. Eylea® has a higher binding affinity than Lucentis®, which may improve its efficacy and/or duration of effect. Eylea® also blocks platelet-derived growth factor (in addition to all isoforms of VEGF), which may provide some additional antiangiogenic properties. Eylea® injected every other month was shown to be comparable to Lucentis®, when injected monthly. The possible benefit of Eylea® is the potentially fewer number of treatments needed to halt or slow the progression of SRNVM. The recommendation for Eylea® is the treatment every 4 weeks for the first 3 months, followed by the treatment every 8 weeks. Mispelled Eylea® may be helpful in patients with *subfoveal* SRNVM due to wet AMD, OHS, angioid streaks, pathologic myopia, or idiopathic causes that do not completely respond to either Lucentis® or Avastin®.

T. Initial enthusiasm for submacular surgery in treating subfoveal SRNVM was tempered by the poor visual results in patients with AMD. Better visual outcomes were seen in younger patients with POHS or idiopathic SRNVMs. This may be because of the location of SRNVM (primarily sub-RPE versus subretinal) and the status of the retinal epithelium (older patients in AMD versus younger patients in POHS). Even with submacular surgery, there is a risk of recurrence comparable with laser photocoagulation. Submacular surgery can still be considered as a treatment option for *subfoveal* SRNVM due to OHS or idiopathic causes.

U. All patients at risk of SRNVM should be taught to monitor their vision with an Amsler grid, and to see an ophthalmologist as soon as new symptoms develop. Low-vision rehabilitation for patients with bilateral visual loss is essential.

BIBLIOGRAPHY

1. Age-Related Eye Disease Study Research Group. A randomized, placebo-controlled, clinical trial of high dose supplementation with vitamin C and E, beta carotene, and zinc for age-related macular degeneration and vision loss: AREDS report no. 8. Arch Ophthalmol. 2001;119:1417-36.
2. Antoszyk AN, Tuomi L, Chung CY, et al. Ranibizumab combined with verteporfin photodynamic therapy in neovascular age-related macular degeneration (FOCUS): Year 2 results. Am J Ophthalmol. 2008;145: 862-74.
3. Brown DM, Kaiser PK, Michels M, et al. Ranibizumab versus verteporfin for neovascular age-related macular degeneration. N Engl J Med. 2006;355:1432-44.
4. Gragoudas ES, Adamis AP, Cunningham ET Jr., et al. Pegaptanib for neovascular age-related macular degeneration. N Engl J Med. 2004;351:2805-16.
5. Heier JS, Brown DM, Chong V, et al. Intravitreal aflibercept (VEGF trap-eye) in wet age-related macular degeneration. Ophthalmology. 2012;119:2537-48.
6. Laser photocoagulation of subfoveal neovascular lesions in age-related macular degeneration: Results of a randomized clinical trial. Arch Ophthalmol. 1991;109:1220-31.
7. Macular Photocoagulation Study Group. Argon laser photocoagulation for neovascular maculopathy: Five-year results from randomized clinical trials. Arch Ophthalmol. 1991; 109:1109-14.

8. Macular Photocoagulation Study Group. Krypton laser photocoagulation for neovascular lesions of ocular histoplasmosis: Results of a randomized clinical trial. Arch Ophthalmol. 1987;105:1499-507.

9. Macular Photocoagulation Study Group. Krypton laser photocoagulation for idiopathic neovascular lesions: Results of a randomized clinical trial. Arch Ophthalmol. 1990;108:832-37.

10. Macular Photocoagulation Study Group. Krypton laser photocoagulation for neovascular lesions of age-related macular degeneration: Results of a randomized clinical trial. Arch OphthaimoI. 1990;108:816-24.

11. Martin DF, Maguire MG, Ying GS, et al. Ranibizumab and bevacizumab for neovascular age-related macular degeneration. N Engl J Med. 2011;364:1897-908.

12. Regillo CO, Brown DM, Abraham P, et al. Randomized, double-masked, sham-controlled trial of ranibizumab for neovascular age-related macular degeneration: PIER Study year 1. Am J Ophthalmol. 2008;145:239-48.

13. Rosenfeld PJ, Brown DM, Heier JS, et al. Ranibizumab for neovascular age-related macular degeneration. N Engl J Med. 2006;355:1419-31.

14. Thomas MA, Dickinson JD, Melberg NS, et al. Visual results after surgical removal of subfoveal choroidal neovascular membranes. Ophthalmology. 1994;101:1384-96.

15. Treatment of age-related macular degeneration with photodynamic therapy [TAP Study Group]. Photodynamic therapy of subfoveal choroidal neovascularization in age-related macular degeneration with verteporfin: One-year results of 2 randomized clinical trials-TAP report. Arch Ophthalmol. 1999;117:1329-45.

Ron A Adelman, Aaron J Parnes

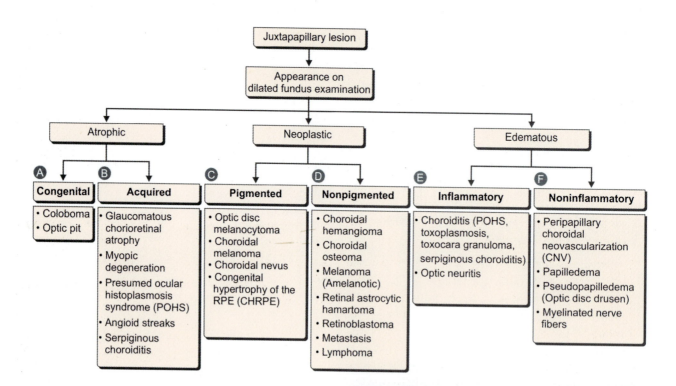

Juxtapapillary lesion

↓

Appearance on dilated fundus examination

Atrophic | Neoplastic | Edematous

A **Congenital**
- Coloboma
- Optic pit

B **Acquired**
- Glaucomatous chorioretinal atrophy
- Myopic degeneration
- Presumed ocular histoplasmosis syndrome (POHS)
- Angioid streaks
- Serpiginous choroiditis

C **Pigmented**
- Optic disc melanocytoma
- Choroidal melanoma
- Choroidal nevus
- Congenital hypertrophy of the RPE (CHRPE)

D **Nonpigmented**
- Choroidal hemangioma
- Choroidal osteoma
- Melanoma (Amelanotic)
- Retinal astrocytic hamartoma
- Retinoblastoma
- Metastasis
- Lymphoma

E **Inflammatory**
- Choroiditis (POHS, toxoplasmosis, toxocara granuloma, serpiginous choroiditis)
- Optic neuritis

F **Noninflammatory**
- Peripapillary choroidal neovascularization (CNV)
- Papilledema
- Pseudopapilledema (Optic disc drusen)
- Myelinated nerve fibers

Juxtapapillary lesions can be broadly classified on the basis of appearance:

- Atrophic
- Neoplastic
- Edematous

A. An optic disc coloboma results from incomplete closure of the embryonic fissure, appearing as sharply demarcated loss of Bruch membrane with overlying retinal atrophy (Fig. 115.1). Optic pits appear as dark-gray depressions, usually in the temporal portion of the optic nerve. Serous macular detachments may develop in 40–50% of these cases.

B. Common causes of acquired, atrophic juxtapapillary lesions include glaucomatous chorioretinal atrophy, myopic degeneration, and presumed ocular histoplasmosis syndrome (POHS). Glaucomatous

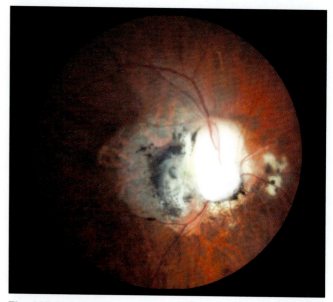

Fig. 115.1: Coloboma.

juxtapapillary changes include chorioretinal atrophy involving the temporal disc margin that can be more advanced in the more severely affected eye. In individuals with high myopia, lacunar atrophy or a scleral crescent may be present both surrounding the optic nerve and in isolated patches involving the posterior pole (Fig. 115.2). Juxtapapillary atrophy in POHS is frequently associated with scattered mid-peripheral 'punched-out' chorioretinal lesions (*see* Chapter 114). Angioid streaks are lacunar crack-like dehiscences, representing breaks in Bruch membrane radiating outward from the optic nerve. Near the optic nerve they may be interconnected circumferentially. Serpiginous choroiditis is an uncommon, focal recurring inflammatory process that affects primarily the choriocapillaris and retinal pigment epithelium (RPE). It begins in the peripapillary region and spreads over months to years in a serpiginous fashion outward to involve the peripheral retina and macula.

C. Neoplastic juxtapapillary lesions are best separated by the presence of dark pigmentation. Optic disc melanocytoma is a benign, but ominous appearing, pigmented tumor that is commonly jet-black with fibrillated margins adjacent to or over the optic nerve (Fig. 115.3). Choroidal melanomas arising in the peripapillary region may extend anteriorly over the optic nerve head, but do not insinuate into the nerve fiber layer. Classic ophthalmoscopic findings include a mottled gray or yellow-white colored 'collar button' tumor with associated exudative retinal detachment. There is often intrinsic pigmentation with orange lipofuscin. Fluorescein angiography reveals hot spots and an intrinsic circulation, but this is not diagnostic. Echography typically demonstrates solid consistency (inability to indent), medium to low reflectivity, and internal blood flow (*see* Chapter 127). In contrast to melanoma, benign choroidal nevi usually are flat or minimally elevated, are asymptomatic, have no associated orange pigmentation or subretinal fluid, and may display overlying drusen. While not usually seen in a juxtapapillary location, congenital hypertrophy of the RPE (CHRPE) is flat, darkly pigmented, and has a distinct margin.

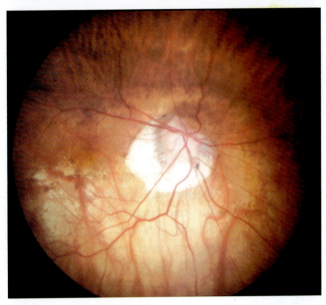

Fig. 115.2: Scleral crescent.

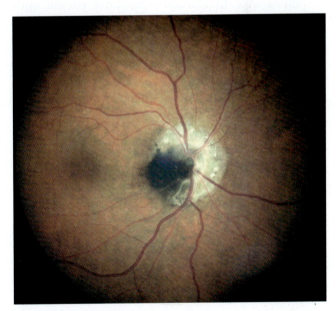

Fig. 115.3: Melanocytoma.

D. Choroidal hemangioma is a vascular lesion typically located near and temporal to the optic disc. They usually are orange-red or orange-yellow in color. Their early mottled pattern on fluorescein angiography and highly reflective echographic appearance are helpful in distinguishing this lesion from an amelanotic melanoma. Choroidal osteoma appears as a yellow-white choroidal lesion typically in the juxtapapillary region. Variability in color occurs secondary to thinning, depigmentation, or hyperplasia of the RPE. The tumor is usually oval with well-defined scalloped margins. The retinal vasculature and the optic nerve are unaffected. Ocular echography is most helpful in making the diagnosis because of the bony content, which causes acoustic shadowing. Astrocytic hamartoma typically occurs at or near the optic nerve showing a yellow-gray or pink-gray color. Fluorescein angiography demonstrates a diffuse capillary network. Metastasis and intraocular lymphoma can have a juxtapapillary location; however, in many cases, multiple lesions are seen elsewhere in the fundus.

E. Inflammatory and infectious conditions of the choroid are often associated with an elevated appearance. In addition to optic disc edema, optic neuritis or papilledema can result in the edematous appearance of the juxtapapillary nerve fiber layer.

F. Peripapillary choroidal neovascularization results in retinal edema and hemorrhage adjacent to the optic disc. Pseudopapilledema or optic disc drusen are 70% bilateral and appear as opalescent autofluorescent 'rocks' (Fig. 115.4). Myelinated optic nerve fibers may be mistaken for edema and look like glossy white patches within the nerve fiber layer, feathering out peripherally like the end of a paintbrush (Fig. 115.5).

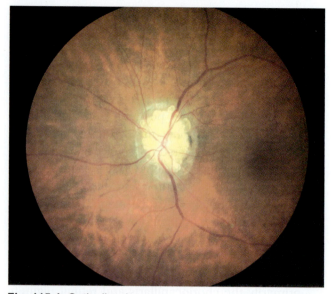

Fig. 115.4: Optic disc drusen.

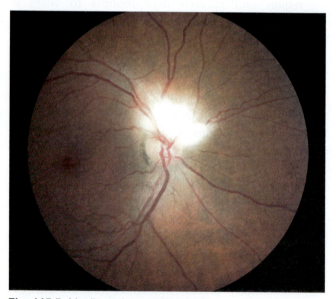

Fig. 115.5: Myelinated nerve fiber layer.

BIBLIOGRAPHY

1. Dutton GN. Congenital disorders of the optic nerve: excavations and hypoplasia. Eye (Lond). 2004;18: 1038-48.
2. Georgalas I, Ladas I, Georgopoulos G, et al. Optic disc pit: a review. Graefes Arch Clin Exp Ophthalmol. 2011;249:1113-22.
3. Lam BL, Morais CG Jr, Pasol J. Drusen of the optic disc. Curr Neurol Neurosci Rep. 2008;8:404-8.
4. Mashayekhi A, Shields CL. Circumscribed choroidal hemangioma. Curr Opin Ophthalmol. 2003;14:142-9.
5. Prasad AG, Van Gelder RN. Presumed ocular histoplasmosis syndrome. Curr Opin Ophthalmol. 2005;16:364-8.
6. Shields CL, Demirci H, Materin MA. Clinical factors in the identification of small choroidal melanoma. Can J Ophthalmol. 2004;39:351-7.
7. Shields JA, Demirci H, Mashayekhi A. Melanocytoma of the optic disk: A review. Surv Ophthalmol. 2006;51:93-104.
8. Shields JA, Federman JL, Tomer TL, et al. Angioid streaks 1. Ophthalmoscopic variations and diagnostic problems. Br J Ophthalmol. 1975;59:257-66.

Choroidal Folds

Farhan F Malik, Deeba Husain

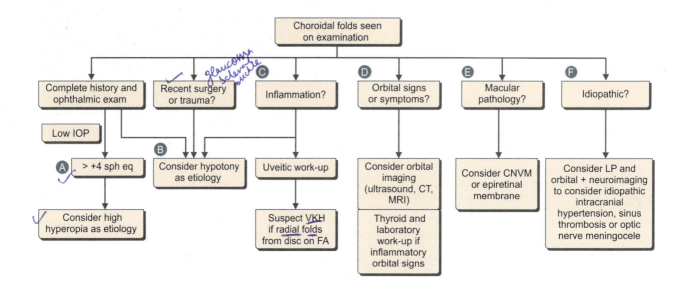

Choroidal folds may be apparent on fundoscopy, and this finding should warrant a complete history and ophthalmologic examination, with particular attention to refraction, tonometry, and orbital findings.

Patients with choroidal folds may be asymptomatic or complain of blurred vision or metamorphopsia as a direct result of the folds. Choroidal folds appear as striae of the posterior fundus that are often aligned horizontally and parallel, but sometimes are present as vertical, oblique, concentric, or radial lines (Fig. 116.1A). These are usually seen posterior to the equator and often temporal to the macula. The crests of the folds are a hypopigmented yellow due to the stretching of RPE with relatively hyperpigmented and more congested troughs. Fluorescein angiography reveals hyperfluorescent peaks and relatively hypofluorescent valleys of the folds, which correlate with the relative density and ease of transmission through the pigment epithelium (Fig. 116.1B). Optical coherence tomography (OCT) reveals changes in the RPE (retinal

pigment epithelium)–Bruch complex and inner layers of the choroid, which can translate into involvement of folds in the neurosensory retina (Fig. 116.1C). Histopathologically, Bruch membrane and RPE show wave-like corrugations, and the choriocapillaris is congested.

The etiopathogenesis and the management of the choroidal folds include the following:

A. High degrees of hyperopia usually indicate small eyes that may have increased choroidal congestion, resulting in choroidal folds.

B. Recent ocular surgery, especially glaucoma procedures, can lead to hypotony maculopathy that can manifest as retinochoroidal folds on fundus examination or OCT. Patients with scleral buckle can also have folds posterior to the area of buckle indentation.

C. Any moderate-to-severe intraocular inflammation can result in choroidal folds, and should prompt an ancillary work-up. B-scan should be done if posterior

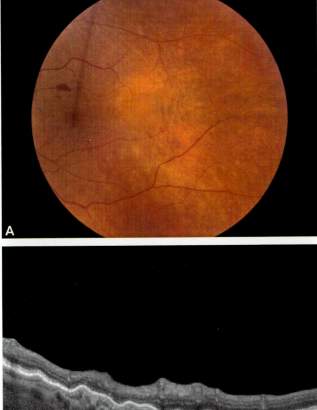

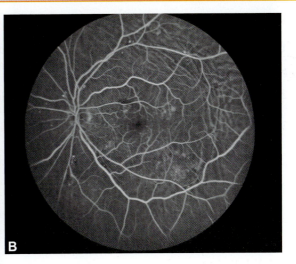

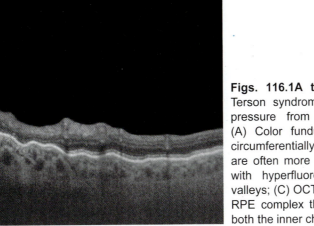

Figs. 116.1A to C: Bilateral choroidal folds in a Terson syndrome patient with elevated intracranial pressure from a traumatic subdural hematoma. (A) Color fundus photograph shows extramacular circumferentially oriented striae; (B) Choroidal folds are often more apparent on fluorescein angiography with hyperfluorescent peaks and hypofluorescent valleys; (C) OCT demonstrates corrugations of Bruch-RPE complex that translates into combined folds of both the inner choroid and neurosensory retina.

scleritis is suspected. Also, Vogt–Koyanagi-Harada disease, in particular, can manifest with radial folds emanating from the disc, apparent on fluorescein angiography in 12% of the patients.

D. A retrobulbar/orbital mass from choroidal hemangioma, orbital metastases, meningioma, thyroid associated orbitopathy, orbital inflammatory syndrome, and so on are important considerations in the differential diagnosis, and any orbital symptoms or signs, such as lid retraction, proptosis, decreased retropulsion or restricted ocular motility, or abnormal exophthalmometry, should prompt the consideration of orbital imaging, such as sonography, CT, or MRI, as well as laboratory work-up that may include thyroid panel, inflammatory, and infectious markers.

E. In patients with decreased visual acuity, epiretinal membrane or disciform scar from choroidal neovascular membrane (CNVM) may be seen on macular examination.

F. Recent research suggests that choroidal folds previously labeled as idiopathic can often be explained by elevated intracranial pressure from sinus thrombosis, meningocele, or idiopathic intracranial hypertension. For this reason, the clinician may consider orbital and neuroimaging and lumbar puncture with opening pressure prior to calling an idiopathic case. Long-term spaceflight is an esoteric cause of choroidal folds in a syndrome that also consists of papilledema and flattening of the posterior globe, which may be related to relative intracranial hypertension in zero gravity.

BIBLIOGRAPHY

1. Griebel SR, Kosmorsky GS. Choroidal folds associated with increased intracranial pressure. Am J Ophthalmol. 2000; 129:513-6.
2. Kalina RE, Mills RP. Acquired hyperopia with choroidal folds. Ophthalmology. 1980;87:44-50.
3. Kroll AJ, Norton EWD. Regression of choroidal folds. Am Acad Ophthalmol Otolaryngol. 1970;74:515-25.
4. Mader TH, Gibson CR, Pass AF, et al. Optic disc edema, globe flattening, choroidal folds, and hyperopic shifts observed in astronauts after long-duration space flight. Ophthalmology. 2011;118:2058-69.
5. Newell FW. Choroidal folds. Am J Ophthalmol. 1975;75:930-42.
6. Wu W, Wen F, Huang S, et al. Choroidal folds in Vogt-Koyanagi-Harada disease. Am J Ophthalmol. 2007;143:900-1.

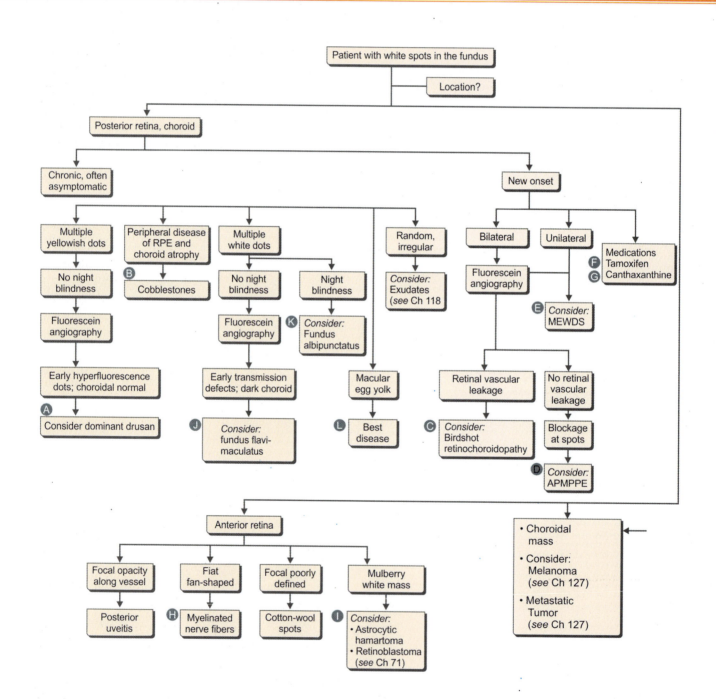

The etiology of white spots in the fundus can be numerous. In general, they fall into the following categories: (1) Degenerative, (2) Inflammatory, (3) Toxic, and (4) Hereditary.

DEGENERATIVE

A. Drusen appear as round, discrete, sharply defined yellowish clusters predominantly in the posterior pole. They are often round, can appear hard or soft around the borders, and can be small (<65 microns), medium (65–125 microns), or large (>125 microns). Fluorescein angiography can stain drusen and often reveal more numerous deposits than seen on ophthalmoscopy. Drusen can be found in the macula, optic nerve, and retinal periphery.

B. Cobblestones are round areas of retinal pigment epithelial and choroidal atrophy that appear in the far periphery of the retina. They often appear round and present in linear clusters. They are visually insignificant.

INFLAMMATORY

C. Birdshot retinochoroidopathy typically presents in middle-aged women in their 5th and 6th decade of life. It is most often seen bilaterally. Eyes have a quiet anterior chamber with vitreous cellular inflammation without pars planitis. Deep, circular cream-colored lesions, each most often less than a disc area in size, are present in the posterior pole. Other common examination findings include cystoid macular edema and optic nerve edema. Fluorescein angiography is helpful in delineating the degree of retinal vascular leakage and associated macular edema. This disorder has a strong association with HLA-A29 positivity.

D. Acute posterior multifocal placoid pigment epitheliopathy (APMPPE) is an inflammatory syndrome of unknown etiology, which manifests as multiple plaquelike lesions, posterior to the equator, at the level of the retinal pigment epithelium (RPE). It is associated with temporary vision loss. APMPPE typically presents as sudden vision blurring in men or women in their 30s, often preceded with a recent viral illness. Fluorescein angiography demonstrates

initial blockage at the lesions with late staining. The clinical course is self-limited and often results in spontaneous improvement, with visual acuity returning to normal. There is often residual RPE stippling in areas of previously affected lesions.

E. Multiple evanescent white dot syndrome is another idiopathic inflammatory syndrome that typically presents unilaterally in young women as a sudden drop in visual acuity. Clinically, multiple small discrete white dots at the level of the RPE are present in the posterior pole to the midperiphery with a "grainy" appearance. There is an average 7-week course. Visual improvement to 20/20 to 20/40 acuity typically occurs. The lesions gradually fade.

TOXIC

F. *Tamoxifen:* The use of tamoxifen in excess of 90 g for treatment of breast carcinoma may produce white refractile deposits in the inner retinal layers with loss of central vision and macular edema. Deposition of calcium oxalate in oxalosis may be limited to the eye or part of a diffuse process. Yellow-white crystalline deposits are found in the posterior pole and midperiphery.

G. *Canthaxanthine:* Long-term use of oral canthaxanthine as a tanning aid may lead to symmetric distribution of yellow flecks in the macula.

HEREDITARY/CONGENITAL

H. Myelinated nerve fibers may appear as a discrete fan-shaped spot. Although usually about one disc diameter, they may be large enough to cover an entire quadrant. The peripheral edge appears like the end of a paintbrush. Large bundles of myelinated nerve fibers running with the vascular arcades may be associated with high myopia, strabismus, and dense amblyopia.

I. Astrocytic hamartoma typically presents as a large white calcified mulberry mass or flat translucent noncalcified lesion. Most occur at or near the optic nerve. Fluorescein angiography demonstrates a rich capillary network. It can occur spontaneously without systemic association or can be seen in hereditary phakomatoses, specifically associated with tuberous sclerosis or neurofibromatosis.

J. Fundus flavimaculatus, or Stargardt disease, is a bilateral, progressive RPE disorder typically presenting in the second or third decade of life. It can cause blurring of central vision. Retinal findings range from diffuse soft yellow-gray pigment epithelial flecks without macular findings to atrophic macular findings without flecks. The electroretinogram (ERG) is typically mildly reduced, and electroculographic (EOG) ratios are abnormal in 75–80% of patients. Fluorescein angiography is extremely helpful in making the diagnosis as a result of the typical blocked choroidal fluorescence, or "dark choroid", due to a build up of lipofuscin.

K. Fundus albipunctatus is a recessive stationary nightblinding condition with small, discrete, raised, uniform white dots, ranging from the posterior pole to the entire retina. The dots do not appear in clusters, and fluorescein angiography shows a mottled pattern of the pigment epithelium. In contrast to drusen, the dots do not hyperfluorescence in the later phases of the fluorescein angiogram. The visual acuity is typically minimally affected.

L. Best vitelliform is an autosomal-dominant dystrophy of the RPE initially presenting with a distinctive "egg yolk" appearance in the macula. It typically occurs between the ages of 4 and 10 years. More than 75% of patients maintain better than 20/40 acuity. Only Best vitelliform and butterfly dystrophy share the trait of a normal ERG with an abnormal EOG light-to-dark ratio.

BIBLIOGRAPHY

1. Carr RE. Fundus flavimaculatus. Arch Ophthalmol. 1965; 74:163-8.
2. Cleasby GW, Fung WE, Shelker WB. Astrocytoma of the retina. Am J Ophthalmol. 1967;64:633-7.
3. Cortin P, Corriveau LA, Rousseau A, et al. Canthaxanthine retinopathy. J Ophthalmic Photogr. 1983;6:68.
4. Damato BE, Nanjiani M, Foulds WS. Acute posterior multifocal placoid pigment epitheliopathy. A follow-up study. Trans Ophthalmol Soc UK. 1983;103:517-22.
5. Deutman AF, Jansen LMAA. Dominantly inherited drusen of Bruch's membrane. Br J Ophthalmol. 1970;54:373-82.
6. Fuerst Dl, Tessler HH, Fishman GA. Birdshot retinochoroidopathy. Arch Ophthalmol. 1984;102:214-9.
7. Gass JDNI. Acute posterior multifocal placoid pigment epitheliopathy. Arch Ophthalmol. 1968;80:177-85.
8. Kaiser-Kupfer Ml, Kupfer C, Rodrigues MM. Tamoxifen retinopathy: A clinicopathologic report. Ophthalmology. 1981; 88:89-93.
9. Meredith TA, Wright JD, Gammon JA, et al. Ocular involvement in primary hyperoxaluria. Arch Ophthalmol. 1984;102:584-7.
10. Mohler CW, Fine SL. Long-term evaluation of patients with Best's disease vitelliform dystrophy. Ophthalmology. 1981;88: 688-92.
11. Newsome DA (Ed). Retinal Dystrophies and Degeneration. New York: Raven, 1988.
12. Ryan SI, Maumenee AE. Birdshot retinochoroidopathy. Am J Ophthalmol. 1980;89:31-45.

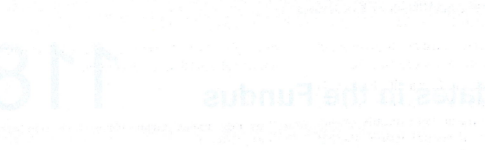

Nisha Warrier, Steven Ness

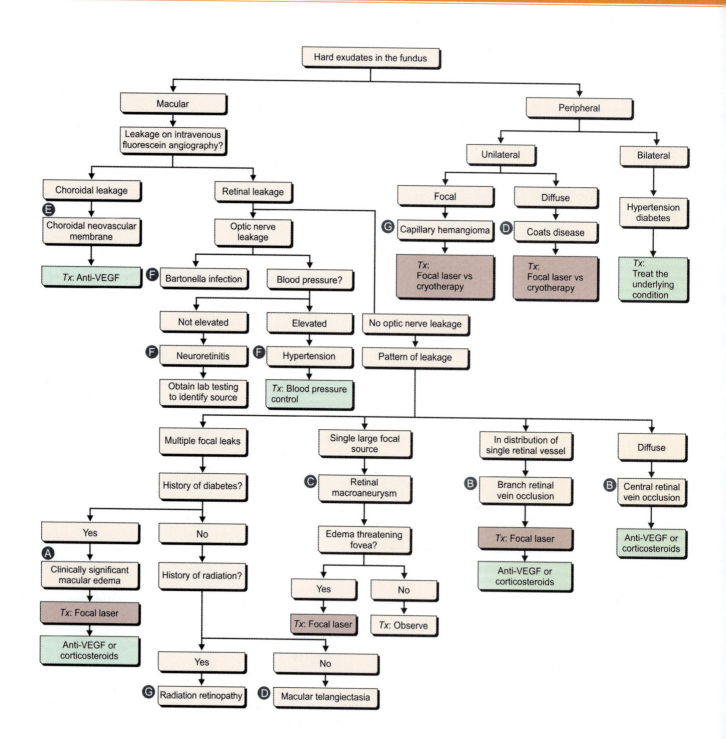

Retinal hard exudates are yellow or whitish specks with distinct margins. On clinical ophthalmoscopic examination, they appear shiny or waxy and have a variety of patterns including individual dots, patches, confluent clumps, or circinate rings. Rarely, hard exudates can be confused with drusen or intravascular plaques. As opposed to the outer plexiform layer location of hard exudates, drusen are found deeper in the retinal pigment epithelium/Bruch membrane complex, and plaques are located within the retinal vessels. When clinical examination is equivocal, optical coherence tomography (OCT) can be helpful in distinguishing between these entities.

Hard exudates result when increased vascular permeability allows for the leakage of lipoprotein and serous fluid from the retinal vessels. When fluid resorbs, lipid precipitates are left behind in the outer plexiform (Henle) layer of the retina. Histologically, the vertically oriented Müller fibers restrain the lateral spread of exudate, accounting for the punctate appearance seen on clinical examination. However, in cases with extensive exudation, they can erupt into the subretinal space.

Hard exudates can be seen in a number of conditions:

A. Hard exudates in association with intraretinal fluid (clinically significant macular edema) represent the primary cause of vision loss in nonproliferative diabetic retinopathy. The Early Treatment of Diabetic Retinopathy Study (ETDRS) established the role of focal laser treatment for clinically significant macular edema (CSME), but more recent studies indicate that intravitreal anti-vascular endothelial growth factor (anti-VEGF) medications may have additional visual benefit.

B. Retinal vein occlusions present with exudation, hemorrhage, and edema in the distribution of a single retinal venule (branch retinal vein occlusion), or diffusely through the fundus (central retinal vein occlusion). When fluorescein angiography shows macular edema with intact macular perfusion, treatment options include focal laser, intravitreal corticosteroids, and intravitreal anti-VEGF.

C. Retinal artery macroaneurysms are focal dilations of retinal arterioles, usually occurring within the first three orders of arterial bifurcation. While in most cases macroaneurysms involute spontaneously, exudation or hemorrhage may require focal laser treatment to prevent vision loss.

D. Coats disease is a rare spontaneous condition associated with telangiectatic and aneurysmal retinal vessels. It is generally unilateral, involves primarily the temporal retina, and is most commonly seen in males. Presentation can vary from localized peripheral asymptomatic leakage to massive subretinal exudation, with resulting serous retinal detachment (Figs. 118.1 and 118.2).

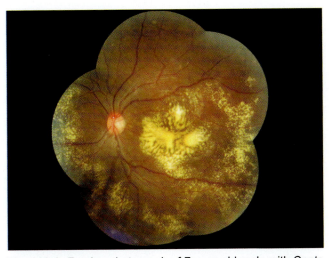

Fig. 118.1: Fundus photograph of 7-year-old male with Coats disease and extensive macular and peripheral hard exudates.

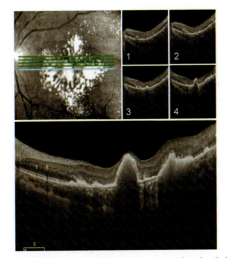

Fig. 118.2: OCT of same patient demonstrating both intra- and subretinal exudation.

Telangiectatic and aneurysmal vessels, limited to the posterior pole, likely represent macular telangiectasia, as opposed to Coats disease.

E. Choroidal neovascular membranes (CNVM) of any cause can present with exudates, hemorrhage, and intra- or subretinal fluid. While age-related macular degeneration remains the most common etiology of CNVM, conditions including pathologic myopia, idiopathic polypoid choroidal vasculopathy, angioid streaks, presumed ocular histoplasmosis, and chorioretinitis should be kept in the differential. Intravitreal anti-VEGF medications are the current gold standard treatment for CNVM.

F. Exudates in the pattern of a macular star, in association with optic nerve edema, can be seen in cases of severe hypertensive retinopathy or neuroretinitis (most commonly due to Bartonella).

G. Rare causes of hard exudates in the fundus include radiation retinopathy and retinal capillary hemangioma.

BIBLIOGRAPHY

1. Adam RS, Kertes PJ, Lam WC. Observation on the management of Coats' disease: Less is more. Br J Ophthalmol. 2000;91: 303-6.
2. Aiello LP, Avery RL, Arrigg PG, et al. Vascular endothelial growth factor in ocular fluid of patients with diabetic retinopathy and other retinal disorders. N Engl J Med. 1994;331:1480-7.
3. Cheung N, Mitchell P, Wong TY. Diabetic retinopathy. The Lancet. 2010;376:124-36.
4. Diabetic Retinopathy Clinical Research Network, Elman MJ, Aiello LP, et al. Randomized trial evaluating ranibizumab plus prompt or deferred laser or triamcinolone plus prompt laser for diabetic macular edema. Ophthalmology. 2010;117:1067-77.
5. Grover D, Li TJ, Chong CC. Intravitreal steroids for macular edema in diabetes. Cochrane Database Syst Rev. 2008;CD005656.54.
6. Rabena MD, Pieramici DJ, Castellarin AA, et al. Intravitreal bevacizumab (avastin) in the treatment of macular edema secondary to branch retinal vein occlusion. Retina. 2007;27:419-25.

119

Black Spots in the Fundus

Vasiliki Poulaki, Sotiria Palioura

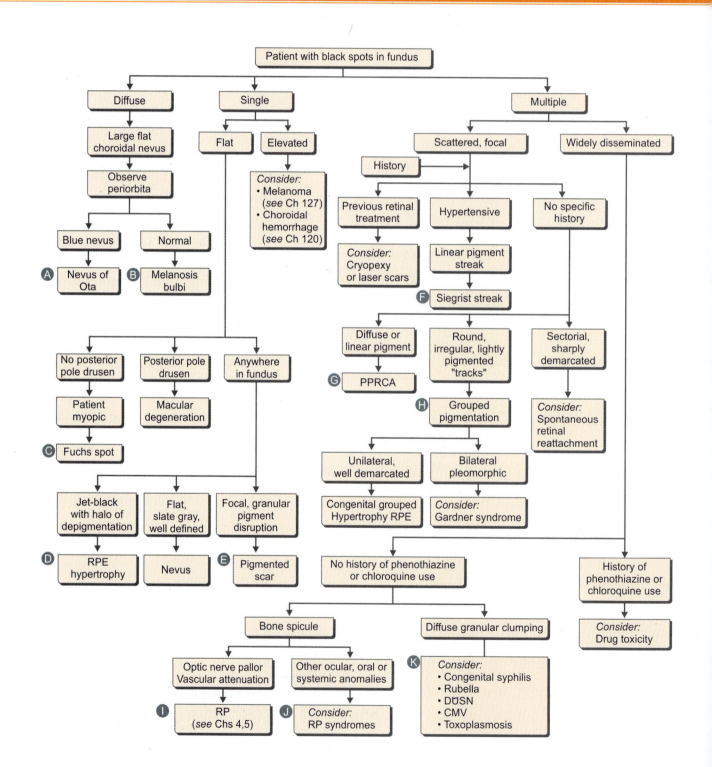

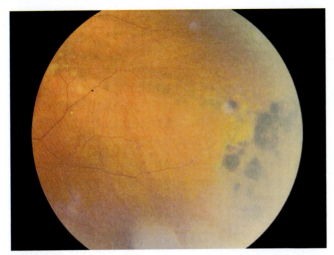

Fig. 119.1: Fundus photograph of a CHRPE showing a flat black well-defined lesion with atrophic spots (lacunae).

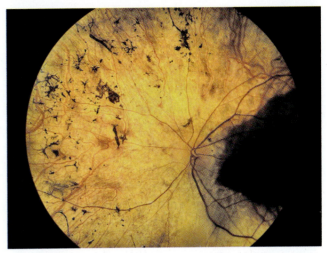

Fig. 119.3: Fundus photograph of a patient with end-stage RP showing extensive retinal atrophy sparing the macula, with RPE granularity and migration, bone spicules and attenuation of the retinal vessels.

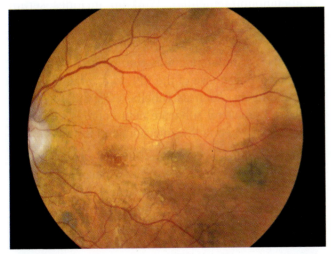

Fig. 119.2: Fundus photograph of a choroidal nevus showing a heavily pigmented choroidal lesion with overlying drusen without associated orange pigment or subretinal fluid.

A. Congenital melanocytosis is characterized by localized epithelial pigment flecks or diffuse subepithelial conjunctival pigment that can involve the sclera and uvea (ocular melanocytosis or melanosis bulbi). It is generally unilateral and found in African Americans and Asians. Diffuse uveal involvement can cause iris heterochromia. When present in Caucasians, it can rarely undergo malignant transformation.

Ocular melanocytosis associated with a blue nevus of the skin in the distribution of the ophthalmic and maxillary divisions of the trigeminal nerve (nevus of Ota), or the shoulder area (nevus of Ito) comprises oculodermal melanocytosis. It is usually unilateral and diagnosis is based on the typical clinical appearance of a slate-gray discoloration of the sclera, and increased pigmentation of the periorbital skin and uveal tract. Though there is no increased risk of malignant transformation in the lids and ocular surface, there is a higher risk of uveal melanoma (1:400), particularly in Caucasians. Thus, periodic dilated fundoscopic examination is indicated.

B. A Fuchs spot is a pigmented scar in the macula caused by a nearly punctate macular hemorrhage (hemorrhagic lesion of Foerster) due to fine subretinal neovascularization. It is often present in both eyes of patients with high myopia and it results in a scotoma. The lesion persists with minimal subsequent change.

C. The typical unifocal congenital hypertrophy of the retinal pigment epithelium (CHRPE) is a flat or minimally elevated, dark brown or black, well-defined lesion with one or more atrophic spots (lacunae) and a hypopigmented border (Fig. 119.1). Lesions may enlarge over several years and very rarely do they undergo malignant change.

D. Reactive hyperplasia of the retinal pigment epithelium occurs in response to trauma, inflammation, or hemorrhage. The lesions are typically small, but when large, they can be mistaken for choroidal melanoma.

E. Linear configurations of pigmentation along choroidal arteries form Siegrist streaks and are chronic manifestations of severe hypertensive choroidopathy.

F. Pigmented paravenous retinochoroidal atrophy is characterized by pigment epithelial and choroidal atrophy, often with intraretinal bone spicule pigmentary changes along the distribution of the retinal veins. It is a rare disorder that may represent an acquired response pattern to an infectious or inflammatory disease rather than a genetic dystrophy. The disease is slowly progressive with respect to loss of peripheral retinal function.

G. Grouped pigmentation of the retina, also called *bear tracks* or typical multifocal CHRPE, is a benign condition characterized by multiple retinal pigment epithelial lesions clustered in one region of the fundus. Retinal function and electrophysiology are normal. Multiple small bilateral CHRPE-type lesions can be seen in association with familial adenomatous polyposis or Gardner syndrome (dominantly inherited polyposis of the colon).

H. Choroidal nevus is a benign neoplasm of the choroidal melanocytes that occurs in 5%–10% of the population. It appears as a flat slate-gray choroidal lesion with overlying drusen, and without associated orange pigment (Fig. 119.2). Rarely, they can be amelanotic. Nevi can be associated with compression of the choriocapillaris and secondary RPE/photoreceptor degeneration, or with choroidal neovascularization and serous detachment and therefore cause visual disturbance. The risk of nevi converting to malignant melanoma is low, with estimates varying between one in 4,800 to one in 8,800.

I. Retinitis pigmentosa (RP) and the related rod-cone and cone-rod dystrophies are a group of inherited disorders characterized by progressive visual dysfunction due to photoreceptor death. Visual impairment is usually manifested as night blindness, visual field constriction, and in some cases, central field loss. The classic appearance includes mottling and granularity of the RPE, migration of pigment to form intraretinal clumps and bone spicules, attenuation of retinal vessels, and "waxy" optic nerve pallor from reactive gliosis (Fig. 119.3). Electroretinography demonstrates reduced or absent rod and cone amplitudes.

RP is associated with many syndromes and systemic conditions, such as Usher syndrome, Bardet–Biedl syndrome, Kearns–Sayer syndrome, and neuronal ceroid lipofuscinosis. The most common is Usher syndrome, which is characterized by sensorineural hearing loss and RP. Systemic evaluation is important to prevent life-threatening conditions such as heart block in Kearns-Sayer syndrome or to prevent further degeneration (such as with vitamin A and E supplementation in abetalipoproteinemia). Work-up includes serum phytanic and ornithine levels, EKG, and a lipid profile.

J. Diffuse granular pigment clumping can occur as a reactive response of the RPE to a variety of infectious insults, such as rubella, congenital syphilis, diffuse unilateral subacute neuroretinitis caused by intraocular helminthic infection, and toxoplasmosis.

K. Thioridazine is a phenothiazine antipsychotic medication that can cause widespread retinal pigmentary degeneration, which early on, can be confused with RP. Phenothiazines bind to melanin and presumably concentrate in the RPE. Toxicity occurs within months of initiation of thioridazine use and it can result in significant central and peripheral vision loss. The classic feature of advanced chloroquine or hydroxychloroquine toxicity is bull's eye maculopathy, though the appearance of end-stage disease can be indistinguishable from RP with peripheral pigmentary changes and bone spicule formation, vascular attenuation, and optic disc pallor.

BIBLIOGRAPHY

1. Arepalli S, Kaliki S, Shields JA, et al. Growth of congenital hypertrophy of the retinal pigment epithelium over 22 years. J Pediatr Ophthalmol Strabismus. 2012;49 Online:e73-5.

2. Berson EL, Rosner B, Sandberg MA, et al. Ocular findings in patients with autosomal dominant retinitis pigmentosa and a rhodopsin gene defect (Pro-23-His). Arch Ophthalmol. 1991;109:92-101.

3. Choi JY, Sandberg MA, Berson EL. Natural course of ocular function in pigmented paravenous retino-choroidal atrophy. Am J Ophthalmol. 2006;141:763-5.

4. Dutton JJ, Anderson RL, Schelper RL, et al. Orbital malignant melanoma and oculodermal melanocytosis: Report of two cases and review of the literature. Ophthalmology. 1984;91:497-507.

5. Gass JDM, Braunstein RA. Further observations concerning the diffuse unilateral subacute neuroretinitis syndrome. Arch Ophthalmol. 1983;101:1689-97.

6. Givens KT, Lee DA, Jones T, et al. Congenital rubella syndrome: Ophthalmic manifestations and associated systemic disorders. Br J Ophthalmol. 1993;77:358-63.

7. Hobbs HE, Sorsby A, Freedman A. Retinopathy following chloroquine therapy. Lancet. 1959;2:478-80.

8. Kiss S, Damico FM, Young LH. Ocular manifestations and treatment of syphilis. Semin Ophthalmol. 2005;20:161-7.

9. Klein A, Barak A, Habot-Wilner Z, et al. The appearance of congenital hypertrophy of retinal pigment epithelium by high-resolution optical coherence tomography. Retina. 2011;31:1740-1.

10. Marmor MF, Kellner U, Lai TY, et al. Revised recommendations on screening for chloroquine and hydroxychloroquine retinopathy. Ophthalmology. 2011;118:415-22.

11. Meredith TA, Aaberg TM, Willerson WD. Progressive chorioretinopathy after receiving thioridazine. Arch Ophthalmol. 1978;96:1172-6.

12. Murray AT, Kirkby GR. Pigmented paravenous retinochoroidal atrophy: A literature review supported by a unique case and insight. Eye (Lond). 2000;14(5):711-6.

13. Parsons MA, Rennie IG, Rundle PA, et al. Congenital hypertrophy of retinal pigment epithelium: A clinico-pathological case report. Br J Ophthalmol. 2005;89:920-1.

14. Sandberg MA, Rosner B, Weigel-DiFranco C, et al. Disease course in patients with autosomal recessive retinitis pigmentosa due to the *USH2A gene*. Invest Ophthalmol Vis Sci. 2008;49:5532-9.

15. Sandberg MA, Rosner B, Weigel-DiFranco C, et al. Disease course of patients with X-linked retinitis pigmentosa due to RPGR gene mutations. Invest Ophthalmol Vis Sci. 2007;48:1298-304.

16. Shields CL, Kaliki S, Livesey M, et al. Association of ocular and oculodermal melanocytosis with the rate of uveal melanoma metastasis: Analysis of 7872 consecutive eyes. JAMA Ophthalmol. 2013. [EPub. In press].

17. Tiret A, Parc C. Fundus lesions of adenomatous polyposis. Curr Opin Ophthalmol. 1999;10:168-72.

Intraocular Hemorrhages

Negin Agange, Gelareh Abedi

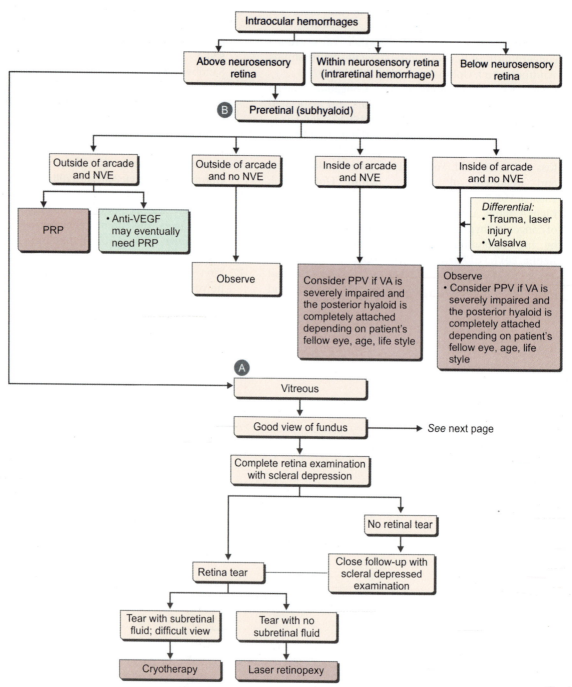

Contd...

Contd...

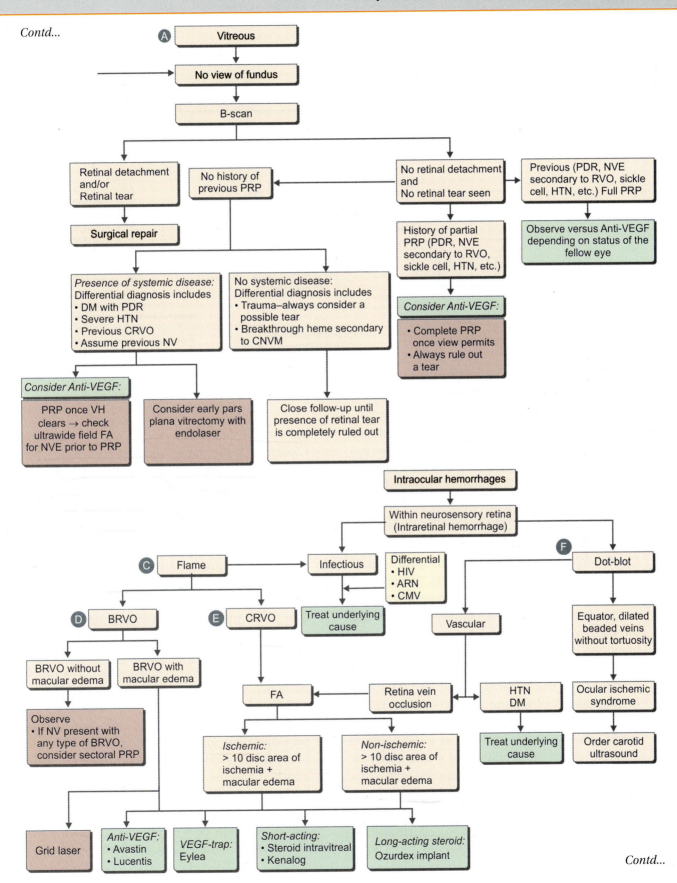

Contd...

Contd...

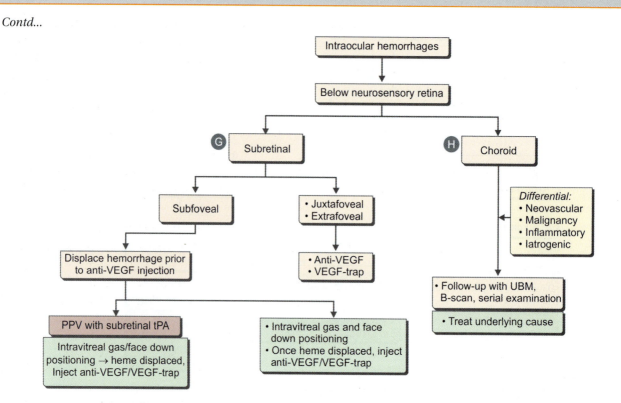

Intraocular hemorrhages have variable clinical appearances based on their location within the eye. The three main locations include: above the neurosensory retina (vitreous and preretinal hemorrhages), within the neurosensory retina (flame and dot blot hemorrhages), and underneath neurosensory retina (subretinal and suprachoroidal hemorrhages).

A. Excavation of blood into the vitreous space leads to decreased visual acuity, and floaters. Retinal break is a primary concern and must be completely ruled out by doing serial scleral depressed exams until the entire retina is completely viewed. If tears are identified, they need to be treated appropriately, as per the American Academy of Ophthalmology Preferred Practice Patterns guidelines.[1] If vitreous hemorrhage is obscuring the view of the retina, B-scan must be performed. Many times, postural modifications such as sleeping at a 45° angle or avoiding excessive bending and lifting can help the hemorrhage to settle inferiorly and allow for a proper view of the fundus. In patients with underlying diabetic retinopathy, severe chronic hypertension or retinal vascular events where there is a high rate of neovascularization (NV), early

pars plana vitrectomy (PPV) can be considered, especially if the patient does not have any prior panretinal photocoagulation (PRP). The decision to observe clinically with serial B-scans versus anti-vascular endothelial growth factor (anti-VEGF) injections versus early PPV is case dependent and all options must be discussed with the patient.

B. Preretinal (subhyaloid) hemorrhages are located between posterior vitreous face and internal-limiting membrane. Some preretinal hemorrhages arise from preretinal neovascular tissue and can form fluid levels secondary to gravity (boat-shaped hemorrhage). Others are secondary to change in pressure and rupture of capillaries such as valsalva retinopathy. Location of the hemorrhage (within or outside of the arcades) and the cause of hemorrhage (presence of NV versus change in capillary pressure) will influence the management plan. In a young patient, when the posterior hyaloids is attached and the hemorrhage causes a significant decline in visual acuity, early PPV can be discussed with the patient. Fluorescein angiography (FA) can aid in detection of NV. Hypofluorescence pattern of preretinal hemorrhage on FA is secondary to blockage and hyperfluorescence secondary to leakage is seen with NV. If the presence of NV is detected, PRP should be considered.

C. Flame-shaped hemorrhages are intraretinal bleeds. Flame hemorrhages are located within the nerve fiber layer (NFL). Their appearance is due to the blood running parallel to the surface of the retina within the NFL. Clinically, they are suggestive of ischemic leakage occurring in conditions such as hypertensive retinopathy, venous occlusion, and optic neuropathies. Management depends on the type and extent.

D. A common cause of flame hemorrhages is branch retinal vein occlusion (BRVO), which occurs in areas of arteriovenous crossing and is most common in the superotemporal quadrant of retina. Typical fundoscopic appearance is that of sectoral dilation of a venule with flame hemorrhage and cotton-wool spots. Based on BVOS, grid laser has been used in treating nonresolving macular edema secondary to BRVO, as well as treating areas of NV. More recently, the BRAVO trial demonstrated efficacy and safety of ranibizumab injection at the onset of BRVO in patients with macular edema.[2] In addition to anti-VEGF, intravitreal triamcinolone can also be used.[3]

E. Central retinal vein occlusion (CRVO) presents with dilated retinal venous hemorrhage in all four quadrants. Visual acuity is affected by macular involvement and secondary neovascular glaucoma. CRVO is subdivided into ischemic and nonischemic types. FA demonstrates prominent retinal capillary nonperfusion throughout the posterior fundus in the ischemic CRVO (>10 disc areas). Common complications of CRVO include vitreous hemorrhage and neovascular glaucoma. Close monitoring of intraocular pressure and evaluation of the iris and the angle is prudent. Options for treatment of macular edema secondary to CRVO include intravitreal corticosteroid (short versus long acting), as well as intravitreal anti-VEGF therapy.[4,5] Use of steroid may depend on factors such as lens status (phakic versus pseudophakic), history of ocular hypertension or glaucoma, and refractory macular edema. COPERNICUS

(Controlled Phase 3 Evaluation of Repeated intravitreal administration of VEGF Trap-Eye in CRVO: Utility and Safety) and GALILEO (General Assessment Limiting Infiltration of Exudates in CRVO with EYLEA) show some promise with VEGF-trap in treatment of CRVO.

F. Dot blot hemorrhages are present in the retina's inner nuclear and outer plexiform layers. They are deeper and can be associated with microvascular edema as commonly seen with diabetic and hypertensive retinopathies. Adequate treatment of underlying disease is the key.

G. Subretinal hemorrhages are of dark-red or maroon color and are located below the neurosensory retina. Choroidal neovascular membranes are a frequent cause. If the hemorrhage is subfoveal, one should attempt to displace the blood prior to anti-VEGF or VEGF-trap treatment. Techniques to displace the hemorrhage can vary from intravitreal gas injection with face down positioning to PPV and subretinal tPA injection. Failure to displace the hemorrhage will lead to poor visual outcome. An extensive subretinal hemorrhage can lead to breakthrough hemorrhage (vitreous hemorrhage).

H. Choroidal hemorrhages have a broad differential and should be treated based on the underlying cause. Suprachoroidal hemorrhage is a feared intraoperative or immediate postoperative complication. Elderly hypertensive men with history of glaucoma are at a great risk. Preoperative patient selection and appropriate treatment of underlying HTN and/or glaucoma, intraoperative precautions such as maintaining a normal blood pressure and being prepared to close the eye immediately in an event of hemorrhage and appropriate management of suprachoroidal hemorrhage such as drainage if indicated can improve the patient's final visual outcome.

REFERENCES

1. Posterior vitreous detachment, retinal breaks, and lattice degeneration preferred practice pattern guidelines. AAO, 2008.
2. Campochiaro PA, Heier JS, Feiner L, et al. Ranibizumab for macular edema following branch retinal vein

occlusion: Six-month primary end point results of a phase III study. Ophthalmology. 2010;117:1102-12.

3. Scott IU, Ip MS, Van Veldhuisen PC, et al. A randomized trial comparing the efficacy and safety of intravitreal triamcinolone with standard care to treat vision loss associated with macular edema secondary to branch retinal vein occlusion: The Standard Care vs Corticosteroid for Retinal Vein Occlusion (SCORE) study report 6. Arch Ophthalmol. 2009;127:1115-28.

4. Haller JA, Bandello F, Belfort R Jr, et al. Dexamethasone intravitreal implant in patients with macular edema related to branch or central retinal vein occlusion twelve-month study results. Ophthalmology. 2011;118:2453-60.

5. Brown DM, Campochiaro PA, Singh RP, et al. Ranibizumab for macular edema following central retinal vein occlusion: Six-month primary end point results of a phase III study. Ophthalmology. 2010;117:1124-33.

Cotton-Wool Spots in the Fundus 121

Gelareh Abedi

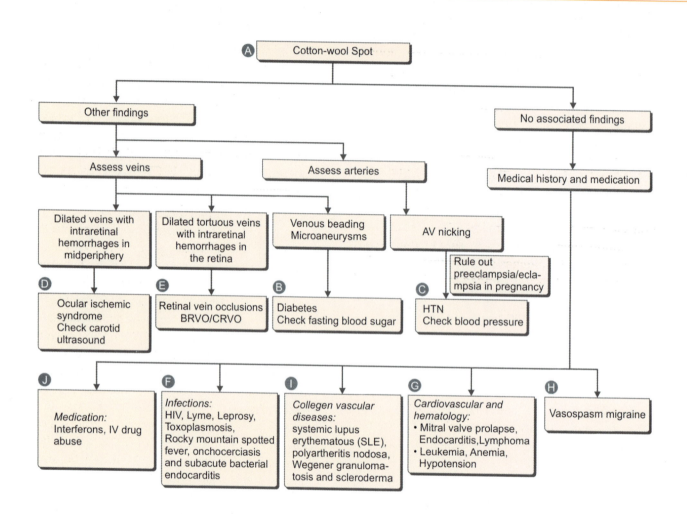

Cotton-wool spots (CWSs), also known as 'soft exudates,' are fluffy white patches seen typically near the optic nerve and around the arcades. Occlusion of a precapillary retinal arterioles leads to microinfarction of the nerve fiber layer (NFL). As a result, axoplasm builds up inside ganglion cells and the cells extrude their exoplasm debris in the NLF. Histological hallmark of a CWS is 'cystoid bodies' or end bulbs of Cajal. Cystoid bodies represent terminal swelling of ganglion cell axons with mitochondria and other materials. Any

vascular disease that causes occlusion of retinal arterioles such as diabetes, chronic or acute hypertension, or retinal vascular occlusions contributes to CWS formation. The presence of even a single CWS in a nondiabetic, nonhypertensive patient who does not have retinal vein occlusion requires a full systemic work up.

In approximately 95% of cases, a serious underlying systemic disorder can be found. In addition to the conditions discussed here, other disease entities associated with CWSs include papilledema, papillitis, radiation retinopathy, hypotension, acute blood loss, anemia, metastatic carcinoma, Purtscher, and pseudo-Purtscher retinopathy.

A. Using indirect biomicroscopy, CWSs are easily identified as superficial areas of white patches with variable sizes that are typically less than one-fourth of the disk diameter. Those associated with hypertension and diabetes last longer. They can cause decreased visual acuity and permanent relative scotomas depending on their size and location. Using microperimetry, these relative scotomas are denser in diabetic patients compared with hypertensive patients. CWSs are not associated with vitreous cells, inflammation, or vascular leakage. They appear within the NFL on optic coherence tomography (OCT). An acute CWS has a hyper-reflective pattern on OCT that continues to remain even after its resolution (hyper-reflective sign). On fluorescein angiography, the patches are hypofluorescent due to blockage and are surrounded by a rim of dilated capillaries, sometimes showing multiple beadlike microaneurysmal changes.

B. Diabetes mellitus is the most common cause of CWSs, with an overall incidence of 32–44%. CWSs tend to last longer in diabetic patients than in nondiabetic patients (half-life in patients < 40 years old is 8 months, > 40 years old, 1–7 months). The presence of more than eight CWSs has been correlated with a higher risk of proliferative diabetic retinopathy.

C. Multiple CWSs can be seen in at least 50% of patients with acute or chronic systemic hypertension (HTN). Optic disc swelling, hard exudates, intraretinal hemorrhages, and exudative retinal detachment can be seen with acute HTN. Chronic HTN on the other hand is associated with retinal arteriole narrowing and flame hemorrhages. In a pregnant patient, pre-eclampsia and eclampsia should be ruled out.

D. Ocular ischemic syndrome or venous stasis retinopathy is caused by severe carotid artery obstruction. Five percent of the patients usually have CWSs in the posterior pole. Flare in the anterior chamber, mild disc edema, dilated tortuous retinal venules, and intraretinal hemorrhages in mid-periphery are seen. The syndrome is associated with a significant risk of rubeosis of the iris and gonioscopy must be done. In addition, carotid ultrasound should be performed to determine whether there is an ipsilateral carotid stenosis of greater than 75%.

E. Multiple, unilateral intraocular hemorrhages associated with venous dilation and tortuosity are commonly seen in vein occlusions. In central retinal vein occlusion, intraretinal hemorrhages are spread throughout the fundus, whereas in branch retinal vein occlusion, the hemorrhages follow the distribution of the occluded vein, usually superotemporal. Multiple CWSs, usually six to 10, are associated with ischemic vein occlusions.

F. CWSs are the most common ocular sign in HIV seen in up to 64% of patients. Single or multiple CWSs can be a sole sign of HIV retinopathy. Increased plasma viscosity, immune-complex deposition, and a direct cytopathic effect of the virus on the retinal vascular endothelium are some of the causes of microvascular disease in HIV that ultimately lead to CWSs. They correlate with higher serum beta-2 microglobulin levels and lower CD4 T-cell counts and thus may be an important clinical sign of the severity of HIV-related disease. CWSs do not cause significant visual decline and are notably rare in children with HIV. Other infectious causes of CWSs include lyme disease, leprosy, toxoplasmosis, Rocky Mountain spotted fever, onchocerciasis, and subacute bacterial endocarditis. Appropriate work-up and management is indicated based on the final diagnosis.

G. Cardiac valvular diseases including mitral valve prolapse, rheumatic heart disease, and endocarditis may produce CWSs due to a microembolic phenomenon. CWSs associated with leukemia may be caused by local factors, such as an abnormally large cell or cluster of cells occluding retinal arterioles and may not be related to the overall peripheral blood composition. CWSs and retinal hemorrhages related to anemia or thrombocytopenia are also common in patients with non-Hodgkin's lymphoma.

H. Vasospasms are partially thought to be responsible for migraines and can result in CWSs. The visual defect seen in migraine patient is usually transient and due to central nervous system processes. If migraine is suspected, a referral to a migraine specialist is indicated.

I. Collagen vascular diseases including systemic lupus erythematous (SLE), polyartheritis nodosa, Wegener granulomatosis, and scleroderma are a host of diseases where the immune system plays a significant role. The most common retinal vascular manifestation in SLE includes CWSs with or without intraretinal hemorrhages. The retinal vascular changes occur independently of hypertension and are thought to be related to the underlying microangiopathy of SLE. If such diseases are expected, a referral to a rheumatologist is indicated with a close follow-up with the ophthalmologist. With the systemic control of underlying disease, majority of the CWS will disappear without causing a significant visual decrease.

J. Drugs, either for recreational use or medication such as interferon, can also be responsible for the appearance of CWSs. Therefore, it is important to take a good social and medication history. The spots disappear after discontinuation of the drug(s).

BIBLIOGRAPHY

1. Kestelyn P, Lepage P, Karita E, et al. Ocular manifestations of infection with the human immunodeficiency virus in an African pediatric population. Ocul Immunol Inflamm. 2000; 8:263-73.
2. Kim JS, Maheshwary AS, Bartsch DU, et al. The microperimetry of resolved cotton-wool spots in eyes of patients with hypertension and diabetes mellitus. Arch Ophthalmol. 2011; 129:879-84.
3. Kozak I, Bartsch DU, Cheng L, et al. Hyperreflective sign in resolved cotton wool spots using high-resolution optical coherence tomography and optical coherence tomography ophthalmoscopy. Ophthalmology. 2007; 114:537-43.

Retinal Vascular Anomalies

Ambar Faridi, Mark Pennesi

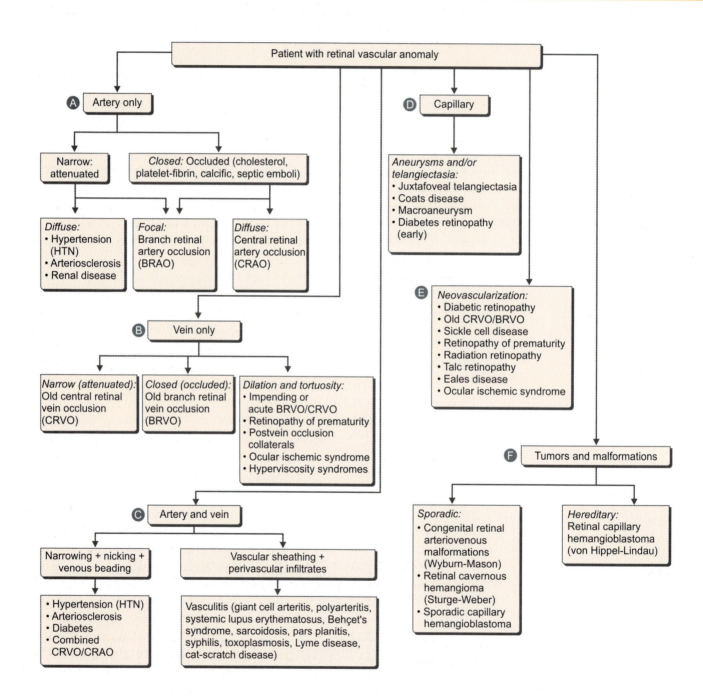

Retinal vascular anomalies encompass a wide variety of conditions that can be subdivided by the vessel system primarily affected: arterial, venous, arterio-venous (AV), capillary, neovascular, or vascular tumors and malformations.

A. Retinal arterial narrowing, or attenuation, should be estimated as a function of other landmarks in the fundus because the actual viewed size of a vessel varies with the refractive status. However, pathologic narrowing of retinal arteries is usually obvious when it is moderate or severe. Retinal arterial attenuation can be seen in patients with systemic vascular diseases, including hypertension, arteriosclerosis, diabetes, and renal diseases. Other retinal changes seen in these chronic diseases include microaneurysms, intraretinal microvas-cular abnormalities, blot hemorrhages, lipid exudates, nerve fiber layer infarcts, and venous beading (Figs. 122.1A and B). Retinal arteries generally cross superficial to the veins, and a common adventitia binds the artery and the vein together at the AV crossing. This predisposes the veins to occlusion with either sclerosis of the artery or congestion of the veins. In hypertension and arteriosclerosis, thickening of the arterial wall occurs, which can compress the vein and lead to branch retinal vein occlusion or central retinal vein occlusion. Retinal ischemia as a result of vein occlusions may lead to the formation of new blood vessels, or neovascularization of the retina. Retinal arterial occlusions are usually seen as a focal or diffuse whitening of the retina due to embolization or thrombosis of the affected artery supplying a given region of the retina. On optical coherence tomography scans, this pathology is seen as thickening of the inner retina. Carotid artery disease, arteriosclerosis, and cardiac valve disorders can lead to central or branch retinal artery occlusion. The different types of emboli include cholesterol (Hollenhorst plaques), platelet-fibrin, calcific, septic, and leukemic (Fig. 122.2).

B. Retinal veins are approximately one and a half to twice the size of corresponding arteries, resulting in a normal AV ratio of 3:2. With congestion, they may exceed this difference by several times. The corresponding blood column appears darker. Ancillary signs of venous congestion are tortuosity, accentuation of AV crossings, and superficial retinal hemorrhages (Fig. 122.3). These retinal findings can be seen in branch and central retinal vein occlusions, which most commonly occur at an arteriovenous crossing (Fig. 122.4). Acutely, the occluded vein is tortuous and dilated, but with time, it can become narrow and sheathed. Sheathing of veins is caused by the infiltration of their walls or cellular changes in the walls secondary to venous stasis. Extreme sheathing occurs with venous occlusion, producing a white, bloodless column. Another retinal manifestation of chronic vein occlusion is the development of collateral vessels (Fig. 122.5).

C. Inflammatory and infectious diseases can affect both retinal arteries and veins. In retinal vasculitis, vascular sheathing and perivascular infiltrates occur. Veins are usually involved early in the disease course. A variety of diseases can cause retinal vasculitis, including giant cell arteritis (GCA), systemic lupus erythematosus, Behçet syndrome, sarcoidosis, syphilis, and toxoplasmosis. In acute retinal necrosis, granulomatosis with polyangiitis (formerly known as Wegener granulomatosis), polyarteritis nododa, and GCA, retinal arteries are primarily affected. In contrast, veins tend to be the target of inflammation in sarcoid and Eales disease (Fig. 122.6). Behçets disease usually manifests as a nonspecific vasculitis.

D. Vascular dilatations, or retinal telangiectasia, are observed in Coats disease, juxtafoveal retinal telangiectasia (JFT), and retinal arterial macroaneurysms. Coats disease is characterized by "light bulb" microaneurysms, venous dilations, and ectatic arterioles, often with areas of capillary nonperfusion and exudative retinal detachment (Figs. 122.7 and 122.8). Telangiectasia confined to the juxtafoveal capillary bed is seen in JFT and leads to vision loss due to macular edema from incompetent, leaky capillaries. In contrast to Coats disease and JFT, retinal macroaneurysms are acquired ectasias, usually of second-order retinal arterioles. They are typically associated with systemic arterial hypertension and can follow a vascular occlusion. Retinal macroaneurysms

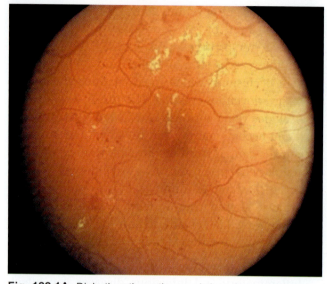

Fig. 122.1A: Diabetic retinopathy consisting of numerous micro-aneurysms, dot and blot hemorrhages, and lipid exudates in the macula. *Courtesy:* Dr Thomas Hwang at the Casey Eye Institute.

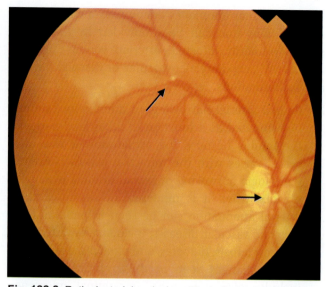

Fig. 122.2: Retinal arterial occlusion with cholesterol emboli called Hollenhorst plaques (arrows) and associated retinal whitening in the region of ischemic retina. *Courtesy:* Dr Christina Flaxel at the Casey Eye Institute.

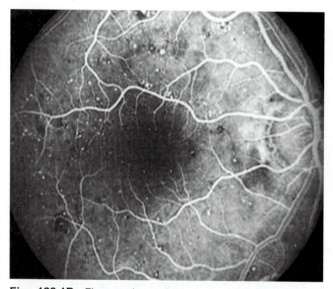

Fig. 122.1B: Fluorescein angiogram demonstrating areas of pinpoint hyperfluorescence corresponding to microaneurysms in a patient with diabetic retinopathy. *Courtesy:* Dr Thomas Hwang at the Casey Eye Institute.

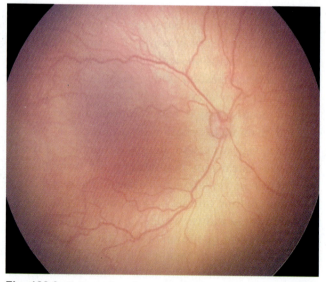

Fig. 122.3: Retinopathy of prematurity demonstrating engorged, tortuous retinal vessels. *Courtesy:* Dr Michael Chiang at the Casey Eye Institute.

may lead to hemorrhage in all the retinal layers: subretinal, intraretinal, and preretinal (Fig. 122.9).

E. The growth of new, abnormal blood vessels in the retina is referred to as neovascularization. Retinal ischemia from a variety of conditions leads to new blood vessel growth from the retina into the vitreous to lie on the surface of the retina. The new vessels have fragile walls and are permeable to

serum and fluorescein, creating a characteristic hyperfluorescence and leakage on fluorescein angiogram. These vessels are at risk of hemorrhage, vitreoretinal traction, and retinal detachment. Retinal neovascularization is observed in numerous retinal vascular diseases, such as proliferative diabetic retinopathy, old vein occlusion, sickle cell retinopathy, retinopathy of prematurity, radiation

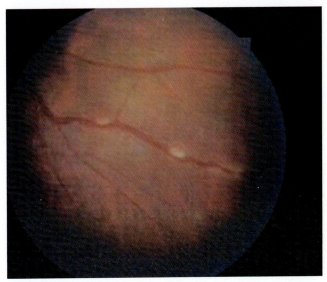

Fig. 122.4: Central retinal vein occlusion with diffuse retinal hemorrhages and macular edema. *Courtesy:* Dr Christina Flaxel at the Casey Eye Institute.

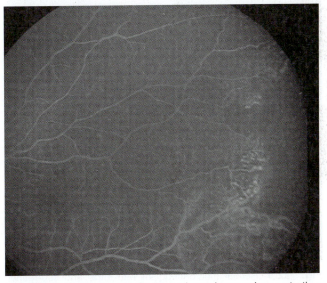

Fig. 122.6: Vasculitis (periphlebitis) in ocular sarcoidosis demonstrating segmental cuffing and perivenous exudates resembling candlewax drippings. *Courtesy:* Dr Seema Gupta at the Casey Eye Institute.

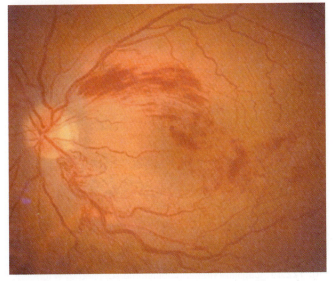

Fig. 122.5: Branch retinal vein occlusion with retinal hemorrhages and the development of collateral vessels adjacent to the optic nerve. *Courtesy:* The Casey Eye Institute collection.

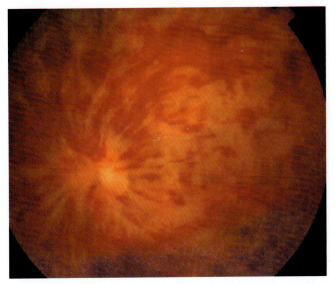

Fig. 122.7: Coats disease: Fluorescein angiogram demonstrating hyperfluorescence from "light bulb" microaneurysms. *Courtesy:* Dr Timothy Stout at the Casey Eye Institute.

retinopathy, and talc retinopathy. In sickle cell retinopathy, characteristic peripheral "sea fan" neovascularization is seen (Fig. 122.10).

F. Vascular tumors and malformations in the retina have a very distinctive appearance in a number of syndromes referred to as the phakomatoses. Most of these syndromes are hereditary but can

occur sporadically. Retinal angiomatosis, or von Hippel-Lindau disease (VHL), is inherited in an autosomal-dominant fashion. In VHL disease, capillary hemangioblastomas develop in the retina and the optic nerve head. A developed hemangioblastoma is a spherical, orange-red lesion supplied by a dilated, tortuous retinal artery and

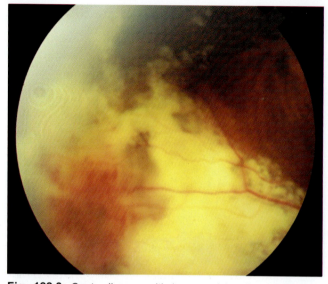

Fig. 122.8: Coats disease with large peripheral exudates and ectatic retinal vessels. *Courtesy:* Dr Christina Flaxel at the Casey Eye Institute.

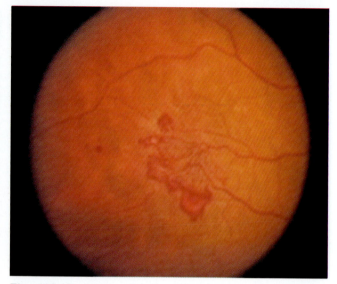

Fig. 122.10: Sickle cell retinopathy demonstrating peripheral "sea fan" neovascularization. *Courtesy:* Dr Christina Flaxel at the Casey Eye Institute.

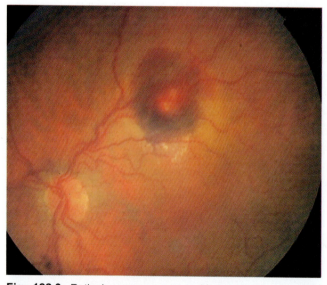

Fig. 122.9: Retinal macroaneurysm with intra- and sub-retinal hemorrhage and small amount of lipid exudation. *Courtesy:* Dr Christina Flaxel at the Casey Eye Institute.

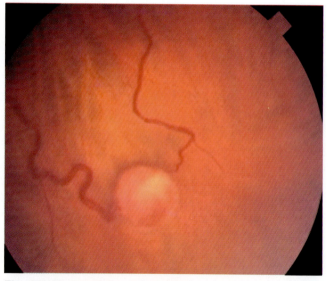

Fig. 122.11: Capillary hemangioblastoma supplied by a tortuous retinal artery and drained by an engorged retinal vein. *Courtesy:* The Casey Eye Institute collection.

drained by an engorged vein (Fig. 122.11). Multiple tumors can occur in the same eye. Extravasation from the tumors may lead to retinal edema, vitreous hemorrhage, and exudative retinal detachment. Patients with VHL disease also have central nervous system tumors and renal cell carcinoma. Capillary hemangiomas can also occur sporadically. Genetic testing can be a useful tool to differentiate sporadic from hereditary capillary hemangioblastomas as in VHL. Racemose angioma is defined by the presence of congenital retinal arteriovenous malformations in which no intervening capillary plexus exists. It is usually an incidental finding in young adults without visual complaints. The fundus appearance may range from a solitary arteriovenous communication

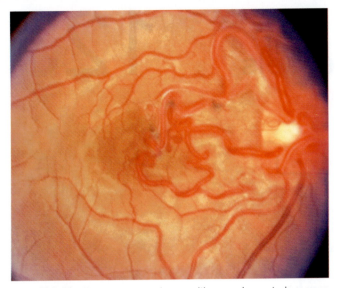

Fig. 122.12: Racemose angioma with complex arteriovenous anastomosis and a "bag of worms" appearance. *Courtesy:* The Casey Eye Institute collection.

to a very complex AV anastomoses with a "bag of worms" appearance (Fig. 122.12). Racemose angioma is nonhereditary and usually unilateral. The condition is termed Wyburn-Mason syndrome if associated with ipsilateral vascular malformations in the brain, face, or orbit. Encephalotrigeminal angiomatosis, or Sturge-Weber syndrome, occurs sporadically and is characterized by peripheral retinal arteriovenous malformations and diffuse cavernous choroidal hemangiomas, resulting in the classic "tomato ketchup fundus". Systemic findings in Sturge-Weber syndrome include nevus flemmeus (port-wine stain), leptomeningeal vascular malformations, and intracranial calcifications.

BIBLIOGRAPHY

1. Agarwal A. Gass' Atlas of Macular Diseases, 5th Edition. Elsevier Inc: Vanderbilt Eye Institute at the Vanderbilt University in Nashville, TN; 12.
2. Archer DB, Deutman A, Ernest T, et al. Arteriovenous communications of the retina. Am J Ophthalmol. 1973;75:224-41.
3. Cohen SB, Goldberg MF, Fletcher ME, et al. Diagnosis and management of ocular complications of sickle hemoglobinopathies, part I. Ophthalmic Surg. 1986;17:57-9.
4. Committee for the Classification of Retinopathy of Prematurity. An International Classification of Retinopathy of Prematurity. Arch Ophthalmol. 1984;102:1130-4.
5. Egerer I, Tasman W, Tomer TL. Coats' disease. Arch Ophthalmol. 1974;92:109-12.
6. Ehlers N, Lenses VA. Hereditary central retinal angiopathy. Acta Ophthalmol. 1973;51:171-8.
7. Grennan OM, Forrester J. Involvement of the eye in SLE and scleroderma. Ann Rheum Dis. 1977;36:152-6.
8. Hayreh SS. Classification of central retinal vein occlusion. Ophthalmology. 1983;90:458-74.
9. Lavin MJ, Marsh RJ, Peart S, et al. Retinal arterial macroaneurysms: A retrospective study of 40 patients. Br J Ophthalmol. 1987;71:817-25.
10. Merimee TJ. Diabetic retinopathy: A synthesis of perspectives. N Engl J Med. 1990;322:978-83.
11. Orth DH, Patz A. Retinal branch vein occlusion. Surv Ophthalmol. 1978;22:357-76.
12. Ryan SJ, Hinton DR, Schachat AP, et al. Retina, 4th edition. Elsevier Inc. 2006.
13. Tso MOM, Jampol LM. Pathophysiology of hypertensive retinopathy. Ophthalmology. 1982;89:1132-45.

Lina Marouf, Lanny S Odin, Juan E Rubio Jr, Timothy P Cleland

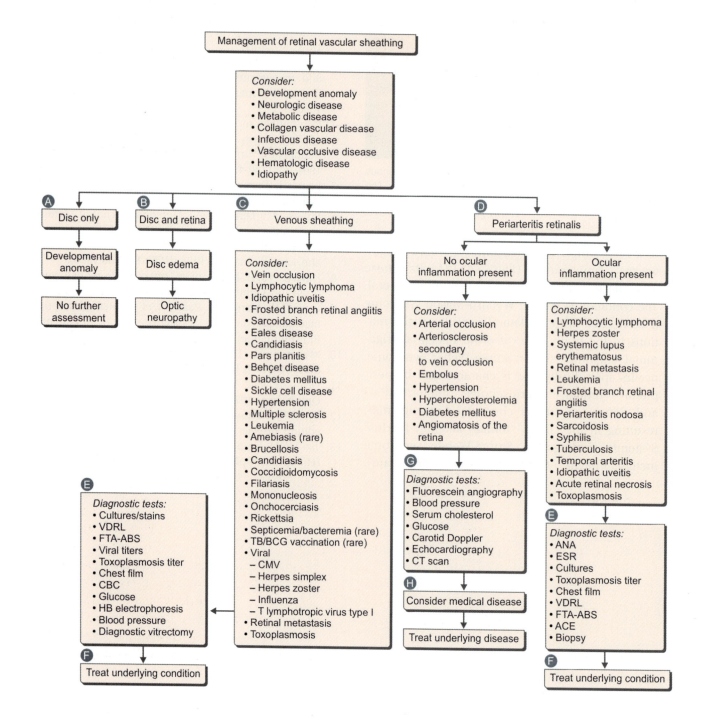

The retinal vascular walls are usually transparent and invisible. What one sees clinically is the blood column within the vascular lumen. *Vascular sheathing* is a general term used to describe clinically visible whitening of the vessel wall. Complete occlusion of a retinal vessel, resulting in obliteration of the funduscopically visible blood column, results in a ghost vessel, rather than vascular sheathing. Sheathing comprises several pathologic changes that can involve the arteries and/or veins. It may be primarily occlusive, with secondary exudation of the vascular elements, or it may be inflammatory in origin, with or without altered blood flow in the affected vessel. Infiltration of a retinal vessel (vein) with lymphocytes, as seen in leukemia, is an example of occlusive vascular sheathing. Sheathing secondary to retinal phlebitis or arteritis, as seen in sarcoidosis and syphilis, presents as white, fuzzy, irregular cuffing of the retinal vasculature associated with other signs of anterior uveitis, vitreitis, or chorioretinitis and is an example of inflammatory sheathing. Aging, retinal vascular occlusive disease, hypertension, and diabetes can also result in thickening of the retinal vascular wall and obscuration of the blood column, giving the vessel wall a whitish sheathed appearance.

Patients with retinal vascular sheathing may be asymptomatic or present with decreased visual acuity, visual field defects, pain, floaters, photophobia, and redness. A thorough systemic history is important. Ocular examination helps in determining the site and extent of the vascular sheathing. Many disorders associated with retinal vascular sheathing are likely to affect other ocular structures, and uveitis is also commonly seen. General medical history and examination often help in narrowing the differential diagnosis. Neurologic involvement (multiple sclerosis, sarcoidosis, Behçet, and optic neuropathies), metabolic abnormalities (diabetes mellitus and hypercholesterolemia), immunosuppressive therapy (acute retinal necrosis and CMV[*] retinitis), collagen vascular disease (SLE[*] and periarteritis nodosa), shortness of breath (TB and Wagner granulomatosis), diarrhea (Whipples, infectious diseases, helminthic, mycobacterial, mycotic, protozoan, rickettsial, spirochetal, and viral), vascular occlusive disease (embolic and arteriosclerotic), hematologic problems (sickle cell and leukemia), and idiopathic disease (idiopathic uveitis, Behçet disease, Eales disease, and sarcoidosis) are all signs and symptoms of disease entities that may display retinal vascular sheathing.

A. White sheathing of disc vessels and immediate peri-papillary venules or arterioles is a developmental anomaly. The sheathing is smooth and is densest over the disc. It is most easily diagnosed when associated with papillary membranes or Bergmeister papilla.

B. Sheathing of disc and retinal vessels may also occur after papillitis and optic disc edema. Unlike congenital vascular sheathing, the vascular whitening is less uniform and is often associated with abnormalities of the optic nerve and retina (e.g. pallor, atrophy, filled-in physiologic cup, retinal folds, and loss of nerve fiber layer).

C,D. It is important to categorize the sheathing as venous or arterial. Sarcoidosis, Behçet disease, and multiple sclerosis, present primarily with venous sheathing. TB, syphilis, and various connective tissue diseases present with primarily arterial sheathing. Frosted branch angiitis is an example of both. Associated systemic findings are helpful in establishing a diagnosis. Skin rash/lesions may be present in Lyme disease, sarcoidosis, Behçet, syphilis, and herpes. Genital ulcers may be present in sexually transmitted diseases and Behçet. Aphtous ulcers are seen in Behçet.

E. When either retinal arterial or venous sheathing is present in association with ocular or systemic inflammation, a medical work-up directed by the medical history and systemic findings should be initiated. A basic screen includes CBC[*], ESR[*], VDRL[*], serum angiotensin-converting enzyme, toxoplasma titers, tuberculin skin test, interferon-gamma release assays, and chest X-ray. Retinal biopsy and diagnostic anterior chamber and vitreous taps/vitrectomy for serology, PCR[*], stains, and cultures may be necessary in some patients to determine the etiology of the disease (infectious, autoimmune, or malignant).

---

[*]*Abbreviations:* CMV: Cytomegalovirus; SLE: Systemic lupus erythematosus; CBC: Complete blood count; ESR: Erythrocyte sedimentation rate; VDRL: Venereal disease research laboratory test; PCR: Polymerase chain reaction

F. When inflammation is present, once the underlying cause of the vascular sheathing is established it is of utmost importance to promptly initiate the treatment. Infectious diseases are treated with specific antimicrobial agents with or without systemic corticosteroids. Ocular syphilis is treated like neurosyphilis with intravenous penicillin 4M units every 4 hours for 3 weeks.

Acute retinal necrosis is treated with intravenous acyclovir for 10 days (15 mg/kg three times per day) followed by oral acyclovir 800 mg five times per day for 6 weeks plus oral corticosteroids.

Steroid therapy, immunosuppressive therapy, and immunomodulatory therapy may be necessary in the treatment of some autoimmune, malignant, and idiopathic ocular inflammatory disease (Behçet disease, Wegener granulomatosis). Long-term use of oral corticosteroids (>7.5 mg per day) should be avoided. Immunosuppressive therapy should be administered in conjunction with a trained specialist. Vitrectomy may be needed to clear vitreous hemorrhage, vitreous opacities, or reattach the retina.

G. In the absence of ocular inflammatory disease, fluorescein angiography may demonstrate vascular occlusion. Retinal emboli should alert one to look for a source (i.e. carotid or cardiac). Blood pressure, blood sugar, and serum cholesterol determination may lead to the cause of vascular sheathing. Retinal angiomas can represent isolated ocular abnormalities or can be associated with systemic abnormalities; therefore, CT scanning of the head, upper cervical spine, and abdomen may be indicated.

H. Specific medications may be indicated to treat the underlying disorder (i.e. antihypertensives, hypoglycemic agents, cholesterol-lowering drugs, and antiplatelet medications). More invasive intervention could be indicated in carotid artery disease and angiomatosis of the retina.

BIBLIOGRAPHY

1. Gass JDM. Stereoscopic Atlas of Macular Diseases Diagnosis and Treatment, 4th Edition. St Louis, MO: Mosby, 1997.
2. Nussenblatt RB, Whitcup S. Uveitis, 3rd Edition. St Louis, MO: Mosby, 2004.
3. Roy FH. Ocular Differential Diagnosis. Baltimore, MD: Williams and Wilkins, 1997.
4. Ryan SJ, (Ed). Retina, 2nd Edition (Vol. 2). St Louis, MO: Mosby, 1994.

Retinal Arterial Occlusive Disease

124

Timothy P Cleland, Lina Marouf

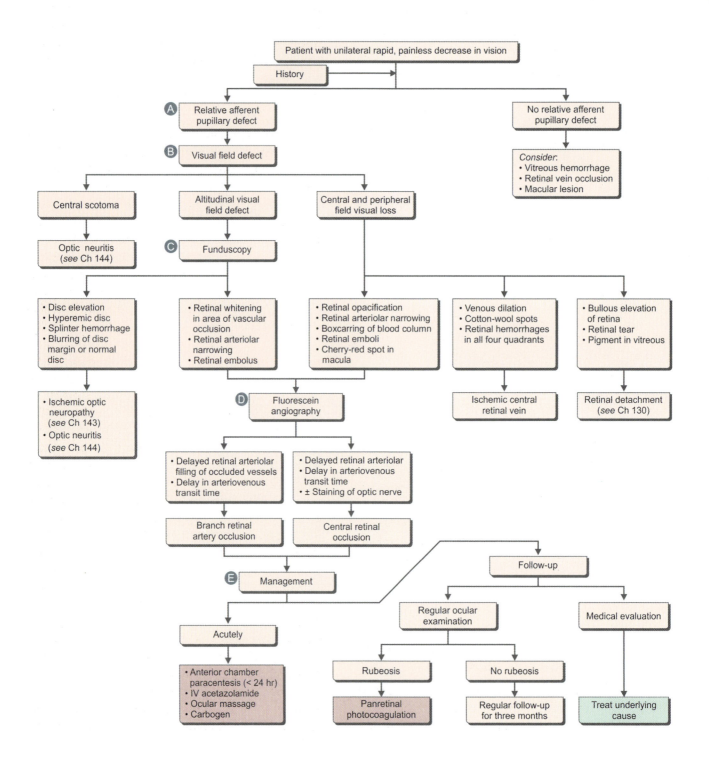

Central retinal artery occlusion (CRAO) has been reported to occur in one in 10,000 outpatient visits. It involves men and women >60 years of age with an equal frequency. Unilateral involvement is the rule in 98% of the patients. Bilateral involvement should alert the physician to consider cardiac valvular disease and inflammatory vasculopathies including giant cell arteritis.

A. Ninety percent of the patients present with painless, sudden onset of decreased vision to the finger counting to light perception range. The absence of the light perception should raise the suspicion of ophthalmic artery occlusion or optic nerve disease. The presence of a cilioretinal artery in 25% of the population accounts for sparing of central vision in the remaining 10% of the patients. An afferent pupillary defect can be detected within seconds of visual symptom onset.

B. The site of vascular occlusion determines the type of visual field defect produced. An altitudinal or nerve fiber bundle field defect occurs in branch retinal artery occlusion (BRAO), and complete loss of the central and peripheral visual fields occurs in CRAO.

C. Funduscopic examination reveals retinal opacification in the area of vascular occlusion. Emboli have been detected in 20–60% of eyes. "Boxcarring" of the blood column may be present in both retinal arterioles and venules. A cherry-red spot is present in the macula.

D. Although ancillary studies such as fluorescein angiography and electroretinography may be helpful in confirming the diagnosis, careful funduscopic examination alone should establish the diagnosis of a retinal arterial occlusion. On fluorescein angiography, there is delayed perfusion of the involved artery (normal retinal arterial filling time is approximately 12 seconds). There may be retrograde filling of the obstructed branch by neighboring collateral vessels in a BRAO. In a CRAO, filling of the optic nerve capillaries by way of the central retinal artery and vein. As a result of inner retinal ischemia, the electroretinogram reveals decreased B-wave amplitude.

E. Although studies in primates have suggested that irreversible damage occurs to the retina after 90 minutes in a complete CRAO, it is still considered an ocular emergency in patients who present within 24 hours of the onset of symptoms. As soon as the diagnosis is established, an attempt should be made to dislodge the embolus to a more distal arteriole in cases that are caused by embolic phenomena. Dislodgement may be accomplished by inducing retinal vasodilation. Intermittent ocular massage and inspiration of a mixture of 95% oxygen and 5% carbon dioxide can result in increased retinal vascular caliber. The intraocular pressure should be reduced by performing an anterior chamber paracentesis and instituting intravenous acetazolamide.

Patients with retinal embolic phenomena have a 10% risk of stroke during the first year and an additional 6% risk per year subsequently. Patients with retinal artery occlusive disease have a higher risk of death because of cardiac or cerebrovascular disease and therefore should undergo a thorough medical evaluation. Of patients with retinal arterial occlusive disease, 90% have associated medical abnormalities, the most common of which are hypertension (66%), carotid atherosclerosis (45%), diabetes mellitus (25%), cardiac valvular disease (25%), and giant cell arteritis (2%). Retinal vascular occlusive disease in the young may occur secondary to migraine, coagulation abnormalities, ocular anomalies, trauma, IV drug abuse, pregnancy, use of oral contraceptives, disseminated intravascular coagulopathy (DIC), and the antiphospholipid antibody syndrome. Tests should include completed blood count (CBC), platelets, erythrocyte sedimentation rate (ESR), C-reactive protein, lipid profile, coagulation profile, lupus anticoagulant antibody, antinuclear antibody (ANA), serum complement, protein electrophoresis, echocardiography, and duplex carotid ultrasonography. Patients should be observed closely during the first 3 months for the development of rubeosis iridis and neovascular glaucoma, which have been reported to occur in 18.2% and 15.2% of patients, respectively, in one prospective study. A retrospective uncontrolled study by Duker and Brown have demonstrated the beneficial effects of panretinal photocoagulation in inducing regression of the rubeosis in 89% of patients and preventing the occurrence of neovascular glaucoma in all patients when performed early in the course of rubeosis iridis following CRAO. Additionally, intravitreal anti-VEGF agents may be considered as adjuvant therapy or if significant media opacity is present.

BIBLIOGRAPHY

1. Atebara NH, Brown GC, Cater J. Efficacy of anterior chamber paracentesis and carbogen in treating acute nonarteritic central retinal artery occlusion. Ophthalmology. 1995;102:2029-34.
2. Duker SJ, Brown GC. The efficacy of panretinal photocoagulation for neovascularization of the iris after central retinal artery obstruction. Ophthalmology. 1989;96:92-5.
3. Duker SJ, Sivalingam A, Brown GC, et al. A prospective study of acute central retinal artery obstruction. The incidence of secondary ocular neovascularization. Arch Ophthalmol. 1991; 10:339-42.
4. Hayreh SS, Kolder HE, Weingeist TA. Central retinal artery occlusion and retinal tolerance time. Ophthalmology. 1980; 87:75-8.
5. Wiznia A, Pearson WN. Use of transesophageal echo-cardiography for detection of a likely source of embolization to the central retinal artery. Am J Ophthalmol. 1991;111:104-5.

125

Retinal Vein Occlusion

Omar S Punjabi, Lina Marouf

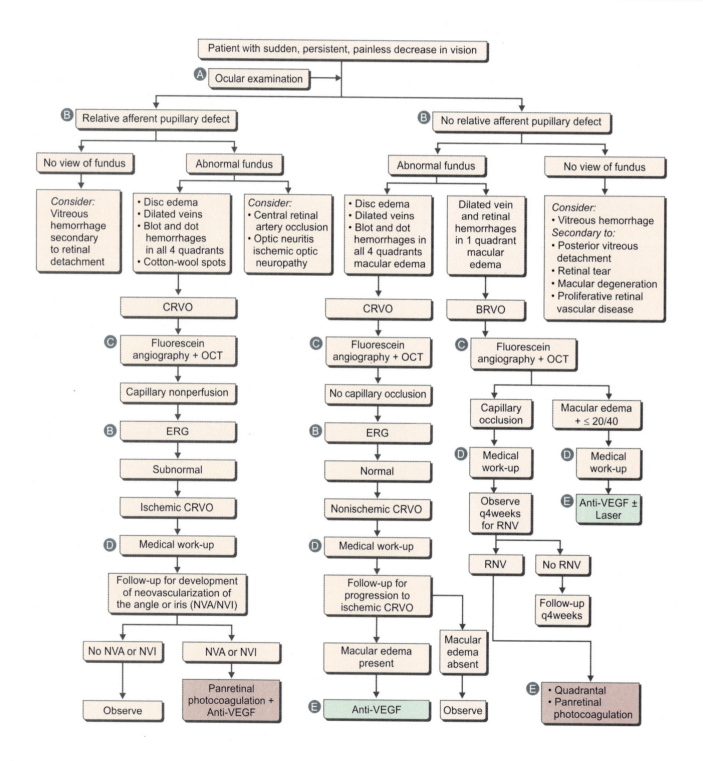

Branch and central retinal vein occlusions (CRVOs) are the second and third most common retinal vascular diseases, respectively. They occur in the 50- to 70-year-old age group. Ocular involvement is unilateral in 90% of cases. Diabetic retinopathy predisposes the patient to the development of bilateral disease. The histopathologic change in venous occlusive disease is a thrombus at the site of occlusion. In branch retinal vein occlusion (BRVO), there is usually sclerosis of the corresponding branch retinal artery. A mechanical factor is proposed in the development of the BRVO. Occlusion usually occurs at the site of an arteriovenous crossing. The artery has been reported to lie anterior to the vein at the site of crossing in more patients with vein occlusion as compared with controls. Atherosclerotic arteriolar changes plus the presence of a common perivascular adventitial sheath result in narrowing of the venular lumen, turbulent blood flow, intimal damage and initiation of the clotting mechanism. Patient usually present with painless decrease in vision associated with a visual field defect.

A. Patients with BRVO or CRVO should undergo a thorough ocular examination. Glaucoma or increased intraocular pressure, trauma and optic disc drusen may be present in 23–69%, 14% and 7% of patients with CRVO, respectively. Pupillary testing is helpful in differentiating optic nerve and widespread retinal disease from localized retinal abnormalities. This is particularly important in the presence of opaque media. Retinal findings in CRVO include disc edema, macular edema, dilated and tortuous retinal veins, and retinal hemorrhages with or without cotton-wool spots in all four quadrants of the retina. Funduscopic findings for BRVO in the acute phase of the disease include intraretinal hemorrhages, retinal edema, and retinal venous dilation and tortuosity in the involved quadrant. Later in the course of the disease collateral vessel formation, microaneurysms, retinal, iris and angle neovascularization may be observed.

B. Central retinal vein occlusion has two forms: (1) ischemic and (2) nonischemic, with each requiring different management and bearing different prognoses. Ocular neovascularization attributable to CRVO is the major complication of the ischemic CRVO. Earlier studies have shown that rubeosis developed in 60%, angle neovascularization in 47% and neovascular glaucoma in 33% of patients. The Central Vein Occlusion Study (CVOS) showed that 34% of nonischemic CRVO converted to ischemic CRVO. An abnormal electroretinogram (ERG) with subnormal B-wave amplitude, reduction of oscillatory potentials, B-A-wave amplitude ratio greater than 1, decrease in ERG sensitivity, and delay in ERG implicit time are indicative of an ischemic CRVO. Poor visual acuity, a relative afferent pupillary defect 0.7 log units, and retinal nonperfusion greater than 10 disc areas by fluorescein angiogram are also indicative of ischemic CRVO. BRVO is said to be ischemic, if there is greater than 5 disc areas of neovascularization.

C. Fluorescein angiogram may not be helpful initially in differentiating ischemic from nonischemic retinal vein occlusion due to the presence of retinal hemorrhages. As the hemorrhage clears angiography of the posterior pole and periphery can help quantitate the extent of retinal ischemia in the macula and periphery and assess the presence of macular edema. Patients with CRVO and BRVO can experience decrease in vision as the result of hemorrhage in the fovea, macular edema, vitreous hemorrhage or macular ischemia. Optical coherence tomography (OCT) is another useful tool in evaluating the presence of macular edema on initial examination and a guide in following-up the patient to assess treatment with antivascular endothelial growth factor (VEGF) therapy. OCT also can help quantitate the amount of retina atrophy from chronic macular ischemia.

D. Several medical conditions have been reported in association with CRVO—cardiovascular disease (70%), platelet function abnormalities (73%), elevation of serum lipids (30–60%), hyperviscosity (53%), elevated blood glucose (15–34%) and chronic obstructive pulmonary disease (20%). Hypertension and arteriosclerosis are the most common medical problems associated with BRVO. A medical work-up is usually limited to patients less than 55 years of age.

E. Several studies have shown the benefit of panretinal photocoagulation in preventing neovascular glaucoma and rubeosis iridis in ischemic CRVO. The central retinal vein occlusion study (CVOS) showed that prophylactic panretinal photocoagulation did not prevent neovascularization of the iris (NVI) or neovascularization of the angle (NVA) in ischemic CRVO and one could wait for the development of NVI or NVA before proceeding with panretinal photocoagulation. The CVOS also showed the lack of benefit of macular grid photocoagulation for macular edema in patients with CRVO. The CRUISE study showed a significant improvement in macular edema and visual acuity at 6 months after 6 monthly intravitreal injections of ranibizumab in patients with CRVO and best corrected visual acuity (BCVA) of 20/40 to 20/320. Improved visual acuity occurred in 48% eyes in the treatment group and 17% eyes gained 15 or more letters. BRVO trial showed that patients with decreased vision less than 20/40 secondary to macular edema should undergo macular grid laser photocoagulation and patients with retinal nonperfusion defined as 5 disc diameters or more should be observed every 4 months for the development of retinal neovascularization (RNV), at which time they should receive scatter laser photocoagulation to the involved quadrant. The BRAVO study showed a significant improvement in macular edema and visual acuity at 6 months after 6 monthly intravitreal injections of ranibizumab in patients with BRVO and BCVA between 20/40 and 20/400.

Intravitreal bevacizumab (Avastin), an anti-VEGF agent, is widely used off label for the treatment of macular edema and retinal and iris neovascularization in patients with BRVO and CRVO.

The Standard Care versus Corticosteroid for Retinal Vein Occlusion Study showed the benefit of corticosteroids compared to observation in patients with symptomatic macular edema from BRVO and CRVO. The study compared the observation, laser and 1 mg and 4 mg doses of intravitreal triamcinolone acetonide. In addition, an intravitreal dexamethasone implant (Ozurdex™) has been approved for macular edema in retinal vein occlusions. Recently, intravitreal aflibercept (Eylea™) has received approval for the treatment of macular edema for both CRVO and BRVO.

BIBLIOGRAPHY

1. Campochiaro PA, Heier JS, Feiner L, et al. Ranibizumab for macular edema following branch retinal vein occlusion: six-month primary end point results of a phase III study. Ophthalmology. 2010;117:1102-12.
2. Haller JA, Bandello F, Belfort R, et al. Randomized, sham-controlled trial of dexamethasone intravitreal implant in patients with macular edema due to retinal vein occlusion. Ophthalmology. 2010;117:1134-46.
3. Hayreh SS, Klugman MR, Podhajsky P, et al. Electroretinography in central retinal vein occlusion. Correlation of the electroretinographic changes with pupillary abnormalities. Graefe's Arch Clin Exp Ophthalmol. 1989;227:549-61.
4. Hayreh SS, Rojas P, Podhajsky P, et al. Ocular neovascularization with retinal vascular occlusion-Ill. Incidence of ocular neovascularization with retinal vein occlusion. Ophthalmology. 1983;90:488-506.
5. McAllister IL, Constable IJ. Laser-induced chorioretinal venous anastomosis for treatment of nonischemic central retina vein occlusion. Arch Ophthalmol. 1995;113:456-62.
6. Scott IU, Ip MS, VanVeldhuisen PC, et al. A randomized trial comparing the efficacy and safety of intravitreal triamcinolone with standard care to treat vision loss associated with macular edema secondary to branch retinal vein occlusion: the Standard Care vs Corticosteroid for Retinal Vein Occlusion (SCORE) study report 6. Arch Ophthalmol. 2009;127:1115-28.
7. The Branch Vein Occlusion Study Group. Argon laser photocoagulation for macular edema in branch vein occlusion. Am J Ophthalmol. 1984;98:271-82.
8. The Branch Vein Occlusion Study Group. Argon laser scatter photocoagulation for prevention of neovascularization and vitreous hemorrhage in branch vein occlusion. A randomized clinical trial. Arch Ophthalmol. 1986;104:34-41.
9. The Central Vein Occlusion Study Group M Report. Evaluation of grid pattern photocoagulation for macular edema in central vein occlusion. Ophthalmology. 1995;102:1425-33.
10. The Central Vein Occlusion Study Group N Report. A randomized clinical trial of early panretinal photocoagulation for ischemic central vein occlusion. Ophthalmology. 1995;102:1434-44.
11. Varma R, Bressler NM, Suñer I, et al. Improved vision-related function after ranibizumab for macular edema after retinal vein occlusion: results from the BRAVO and CRUISE trials. Ophthalmology. 2012;119:2108-18.

126

Retinal Elevation

Steven Ness

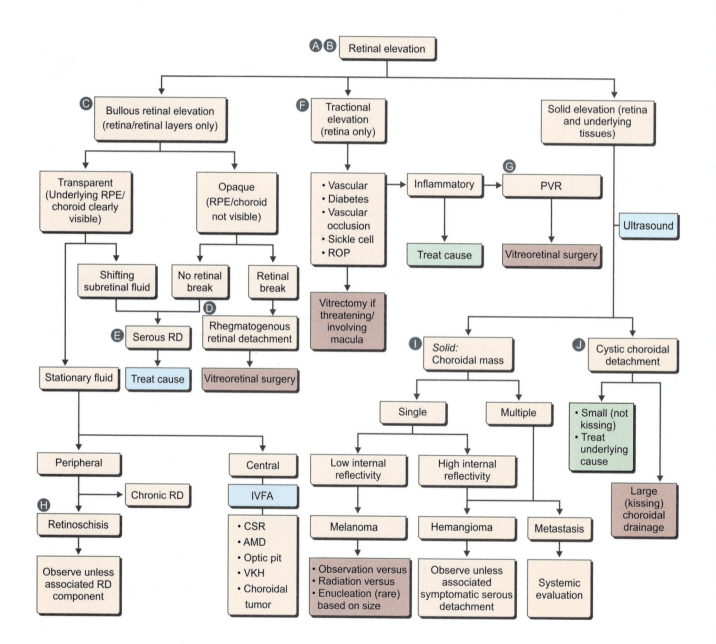

A. Peripheral retinal elevation may be asymptomatic, but when symptoms are present, their character provides clues as to the diagnosis. Acute vitreoretinal traction most commonly presents with photopsias and floaters. Peripheral field loss associated with retinal detachment progresses more rapidly than that associated with slowly growing tumors, but in both cases, central acuity is spared until posterior progression involves the macula. Highly myopic patients or patients with a family or fellow eye history of retinal detachment are at higher risk for retinal detachment. A history of systemic inflammatory disease raises suspicion for serous retinal or choroidal detachment, and systemic conditions often result in bilateral disease.

B. A dilated funduscopic examination is required for accurate diagnosis of the cause of retinal elevation. Slit-lamp examination with ancillary lenses provides a detailed view of the posterior pole and mid-periphery, whereas indirect ophthalmoscopy, in conjunction with scleral depression, allows complete examination of the retinal periphery. Fluorescein angiography is indicated when a vascular or inflammatory etiology is suspected, and ultrasonography is valuable in cases of choroidal elevation or when media clarity hinders examination of the posterior segment. Ocular coherence tomography, while indispensable for macular lesions, is of limited use for the examination of the far periphery.

C. The healthy retina is transparent, with the underlying retinal pigment epithelium (RPE) and choroidal circulation imparting the red-orange coloration seen on normal funduscopic examination. The retina has a dual blood supply, with the inner retina supplied by the retinal circulation. When bullous subretinal fluid separates the outer retina from its underlying choroidal circulation, resulting retinal edema and opacification obscure the normal red reflex (Fig. 126.1).

D. By definition, rhegmatogenous retinal detachments (RRD) are caused by retinal breaks, predominantly acute horseshoe tears. The passage of liquefied vitreous through the retinal break and into the subretinal space results in an elevated, opacified retina with a corrugated surface.

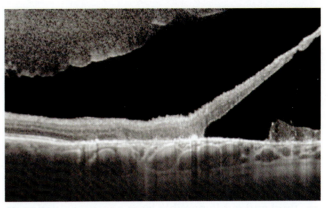

Fig. 126.1: Spectral domain (SDOCT) of retinoschisis with outer retinal hole. In retinoschisis, the inner retina is elevated while the outer retina remains opposed to the retinal pigment epithelium.

Posterior vitreous detachment is the usual source of vitreoretinal traction and acute retinal breaks, although retinal dialysis can also occur in association with blunt ocular trauma.

The treatment of acute RRD is surgical, with macula-sparing RRD representing a surgical emergency. Surgical options include pneumatic retinopexy, scleral buckle, and vitrectomy with intraocular tamponade. Factors influencing the choice of surgical technique include the number, size, and location of retinal tears, media clarity, the lens status, and the presence and degree of proliferative vitreoretinopathy (PVR). In all cases, however, the surgical goals are to locate and remove vitreous traction from all retinal breaks and to create a chorioretinal irritation to permanently reattach the retina.

E. Serous or exudative retinal detachment occurs when a breakdown of the blood retinal barrier overwhelms the RPE's ability to dehydrate the subretinal space. Commonly associated ocular conditions include severe intraocular inflammation, retinal vasculopathy (i.e. Coats Disease), and choroidal tumors. Non-inflammatory serous macular detachments can be seen in central serous retinopathy or in association with optic nerve pits. Systemic conditions, including severe hypertension, eclampsia, or chronic renal failure should also be considered, especially in cases of bilateral serous RD.

Serous retinal detachments tend to have a smooth, transparent surface. Due to its exudative nature, underlying subretinal fluid is often opaque and gravity dependent, shifting with patient positioning. The retina is intact, without breaks, and lacks preretinal traction. Treatment of serous retinal detachment requires identification and treatment of the underlying cause, and surgery is generally not indicated. In cases of abnormal retinal vascular permeability, fluorescein angiography can be helpful to establish the source of subretinal fluid and guide possible laser photocoagulation or cryotherapy.

F. Traction retinal detachment most commonly results when fibrovascular tissue proliferating from the retinal surface to the posterior hyaloid pulls the retina away from the underlying RPE. While proliferative diabetic retinopathy is the most common vascular cause, any condition resulting in retinal ischemia, including vascular occlusions, sickle cell retinopathy, retinopathy of prematurity, or severe intraocular inflammation can result in traction retinal detachment. As opposed to the convex appearance of rhegmatogenous and serous retinal detachments, traction retinal detachments are generally concave and tend to be localized. Clinical examination reveals preretinal fibrovascular proliferation. Retinal breaks are not necessary for the development of traction retinal detachment, but severe traction can cause breaks and result in combined traction-rhegmatogenous detachment. Localized or peripheral traction detachments may progress only slowly and can be observed often. When the macula is threatened, however, vitrectomy surgery with membrane peeling is indicated.

G. Proliferative vitreoretinopathy (PVR) occurs when RPE, glial, and inflammatory cells proliferate on both the anterior and posterior retinal surfaces resulting in severe traction and often causing retinal breaks. PVR is the most common cause of failed retinal detachment repair, but can also occur in cases of penetrating ocular trauma or chronic retinal detachment without prior surgical repair. Clinical findings in cases of PVR include pigment in the vitreous, epiretinal proliferation resulting in fixed retinal folds, and subretinal fibrosis.

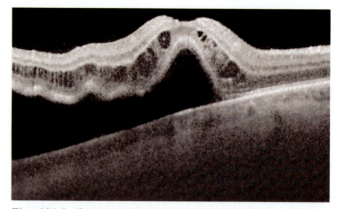

Fig. 126.2: Spectral domain optical coherence tomography (OCT) of fovea involving retinal detachment. In acute rhegmatogenous detachment, retinal edema results in an opacified retina, obscuring the normal red reflex.

Findings are usually most severe in the inferior retina, where liberated RPE and glial cells settle in a gravity-dependent manner. When PVR results in or threatens to cause retinal detachment, surgical intervention is necessary, often requiring both vitrectomy and scleral buckling techniques and long-term intraocular tamponade.

H. It is important to distinguish retinal detachment, involving the full-thickness retina, from retinoschisis in which only the inner retinal layers are elevated. Senile retinoschisis typically involves the inferotemporal retinal periphery and is often bilateral, although asymmetric. The inner retinal elevation has a smooth, transparent surface, and underlying pigmentary changes are absent. Whitish opacities are frequently seen on the retinal surface or in the schisis cavity. Uncomplicated retinoschisis is generally asymptomatic but can cause peripheral field defects. It progresses only slowly and almost never extends to the posterior pole. Due to its low risk of progression, laser demarcation of uncomplicated retinoschisis is probably unnecessary. When outer retinal holes occur (Fig. 126.2), fluid in the schisis cavity can enter the subretinal space resulting in localized, slowly progressive retinal detachment. In such cases, laser retinopexy is often adequate to prevent progression, although more aggressive surgical methods may be necessary when detachment threatens the posterior pole. Schisis complicated by both inner and outer layer breaks can result in rhegmatogenous detachment and may require surgical intervention.

I. Ocular ultrasound is helpful in the differentiation of retinal elevation caused by mass or fluid in the underlying choroid. Elevation due to a solid mass is most commonly associated with neoplasm, including choroidal nevus and melanoma, choroidal hemangioma, and metastatic choroidal tumors. A-scan of elevated choroidal masses can differentiate choroidal melanoma (low internal reflectivity) from hemangioma (high internal reflectivity). Metastatic choroidal lesions tend to be hypopigmented and multifocal with lung (males) and breast (females) representing the most common sources.

J. Cystic choroidal elevation can be either serous or hemorrhagic. Serous choroidal detachments are associated with ocular hypotony (often following glaucoma filtering surgery) or severe intraocular inflammation. Rare causes of serous choroidal detachments include nanophthalmos and uveal effusion syndrome. The rupture of choroidal vessels, either intra- or postoperatively, in association with blunt or penetrating trauma, or rarely spontaneously (especially in patients on systemic anticoagulation), causes hemorrhagic choroidal detachment. Large hemorrhagic detachments often have associated subretinal or vitreous hemorrhage. The size of choroidal detachments varies, but even in cases of large choroidals, their extent will be limited by the vortex veins. Small choroidal detachments can often be observed, with efforts made to address the causative factors, but surgical evacuation may be necessary in cases of large (kissing) detachments. When possible, drainage of hemorrhagic detachment is delayed 10–14 days to allow liquefaction of choroidal clots.

BIBLIOGRAPHY

1. Aylward GW. Proliferative vitreoretinopathy. In Yanoff M, Duker JS (Eds). Ophthalmology, 2nd Edn. St Louis, MO: Mosby. pp. 1002-6.
2. Bird, A. Pathogenesis of serous detachment of the retina and pigment epithelium. In Ryan SJ (Ed). Retina, 4th Edn. Philadelphia, PA: Elsevier. 2006. pp. 971-8.
3. Collaborative Ocular Melanoma Study Group: comparison of clinical, echographic, and histologic measurements from eyes with medium-sized choroidal melanoma in the Collaborative Ocular Melanoma Study. COMS Report No. 21. Arch Ophthalmol. 2003;121: 1163-71.
4. Kanski J. Clinical Ophthalmology: A Systematic Approach, 5th Edn. Philadelphia, PA: Elsevier. 2003. pp. 348-88.

Malignant Melanoma of the Choroid

127

Thanos D Papakostas, Vasiliki Poulaki

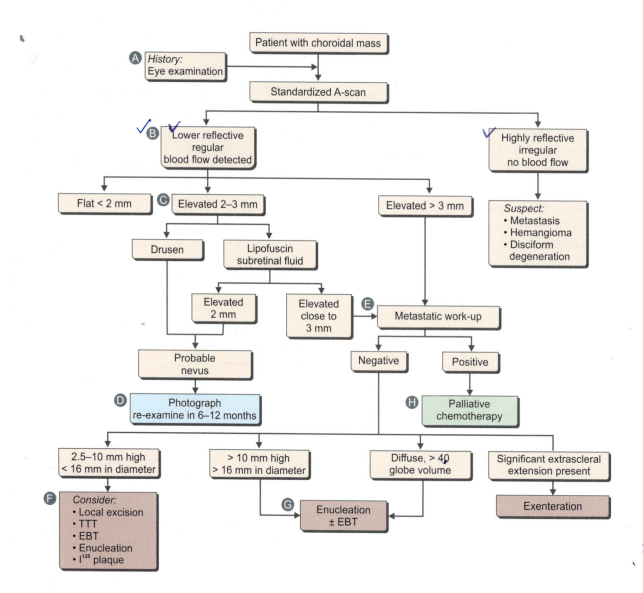

Choroidal melanoma is the most common primary intraocular tumor, but it is nevertheless infrequent with an incidence of about six cases per one million people in the USA. It most commonly affects Caucasians of Northern European descent and it is extremely rare among blacks. The median age at diagnosis is about 55 years and is usually discovered during routine indirect ophthalmoscopy.

A. The majority of melanomas are diagnosed on asymptomatic patients during routine ophthalmoscopy. Patients present with decreased vision only if their macula is involved either by direct involvement by the tumor or through secondary exudative retinal detachment, or if their lens has cataractous changes from contact with the tumor. They are usually painless unless

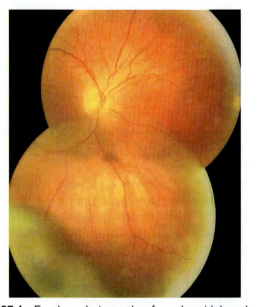

Fig. 127.1: Fundus photograph of a choroidal melanoma showing an inferotemporal-pigmented collar button-shaped mass with associated shallow retinal detachment the borders of which show mild pigmentation (melanophagocytes).

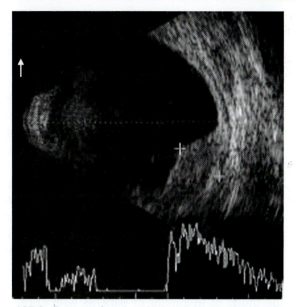

Fig. 127.2: B-scan of a choroidal melanoma showing low to medium reflectivity of the tumor.

they cause severe inflammation, neovascular glaucoma, or extrascleral extension. The classical presentation is a pigmented dome-shaped or collar button-shaped mass with associated characteristic orange pigment (lipofuscin) and overlying or adjacent retinal detachment that is evident in indirect ophthalmoscopy in 95% of cases (Fig. 127.1). Melanomas can have variable degree of pigmentation and in some cases can be completely amelanotic. Tumors with light pigmentation can be associated with abnormal vasculature that is evident in ophthalmoscopy. Anterior melanomas can show sentinel vessels that are dilated episcleral vessels that directly feed the tumor. In rare cases of extrascleral extension, brown areas of pigmentation can be seen subconjunctivally.

B. According to the Collaborative Ocular Melanoma Study (COMS), the accuracy of clinical diagnosis of ocular melanoma is 99.7%. Combined A-mode and B-mode ultrasonography is the most important test in the evaluation of patients with melanoma. By B-scan ultrasonography, the classic features of choroidal melanoma are: (1) low to medium reflectivity within the melanoma (Fig. 127.2), (2) choroidal excavation, (3) shadowing in the orbit, (4) internal vascularity, and (5) an acoustic quiet zone at the tumor base called acoustic hollowing. For very anterior (ciliary body melanomas),

ultrasound biomicroscopy (UBM) can define the anterior tumor borders better than B-scan and it is preferentially used. On A-scan ultrasonography, choroidal melanoma shows medium to low internal echoes (Fig. 127.2). For tumors greater than 3 mm in thickness, a combination of A-scan and B-scan ultrasonography can diagnose choroidal melanomas with greater than 95% accuracy. Other tests include fluorescein angiography that can show a dual circulation pattern due to the intrinsic tumor circulation as well as late staining of the lesion with multiple pinpoint leaks and optical coherence tomography that can highlight small amounts of subretinal fluid or subretinal deposits corresponding to orange pigment that can be missed in clinical examination. On autofluorescence, melanomas demonstrate slightly increased autofluorescence with brightness corresponding to the amount of pigment, RPE atrophy, and lipofuscin accumulation. Although choroidal biopsy of the tumor is usually not necessary, it is done in diagnostic challenging cases, and frequently it is done at the time of plaque implantation for cytogenetics to assess chromosome 3 and 1 deletion or chromosome 8 amplification or classification of the tumors into type I or II with gene arrays that carry prognostic significance. Tumors with chromosome 3 and 1p deletion or type II tumors tend to metastasize earlier than the rest.

C. According to J and C Shields, the factors in the clinical examination that differentiate a choroidal melanoma from a nevus can be found in the mnemonic (T)o (F)ind (S)mall (O)cular (M)elanoma; (T)hickness > 2 mm, subretinal (F)luid, (O)range pigment, (M)argin touching the optic disk. Tumors that display one factor have a 38% chance of growth within the next 5 years; tumors that have two or more factors have a 50% chance of growth.

D. The liver is the most common site of metastasis (~90%) and screening is performed with liver function tests. If any abnormalities are found, abdominal imaging is recommended and these patients should be also followed by a medical oncologist.

E. Several factors are taken into account to decide the mode of treatment in patients with choroidal melanoma, such as the dimensions and location of the tumor, the presence of metastasis and the overall health of the patient. Choroidal melanomas are classified as either small (<10 mm in diameter and < 3 mm in height), medium (10–15 mm in diameter and 3–5 mm in height), or large (>15 mm in diameter and > 5 mm in height). Small tumors, in which the diagnosis of choroidal melanoma is not established, can be observed every 4–6 months until growth is documented. For tumors < 10 mm high or 16 mm across, no specific therapy has proven to be superior, although it is generally accepted that treatment is better than none. Therefore, small tumors with documented growth, medium, and large tumors are generally treated. Although the traditional mode of treatment used to be enucleation, it is currently only used in cases of large tumors with poor vision or pain. Vision-sparing treatment such as brachytherapy with I-125 plaques or proton beam therapy are currently implemented, especially after the COMS found that the cumulative all cause 10-year mortality of each treatment is comparable in medium and large tumors. COMS also found that enucleation alone does not increase the incidence of metastasis and does not affect the overall survival in patients with malignant melanoma when compared with enucleation with preoperative irradiation tests that, if abnormal, should prompt abdominal imaging. An examination by an oncologist is recommended, with special attention to subcutaneous tissues.

F. External beam (charged particle), either helium ions or protons, may have several theoretical advantages over plaque therapy including optimal irradiation delivery to the entire tumor, with a theoretical reduction of radiation damage to surrounding normal tissue, and has been performed since 1975. Proponents praise the treatment's accuracy and ability to treat larger tumors, up to 30% of the ocular volume. Access to a cyclotron limits the widespread availability of the procedure, and there is no proof that it is any better than plaque irradiation.

G. Other treatments like local excision, transpupillary thermotherapy, stereotactic photon beam irradiation, and photodynamic therapy have been employed but their safety and efficacy has not been demonstrated in prospective comparative trials.

H. If the metastatic work-up is positive, the prognosis for survival is generally < 18 months. Palliative and systemic chemotherapy can be used.

BIBLIOGRAPHY

1. Byron SF, Green RL. Ultrasound of the Eye and Orbit. St. Louis, MO: Mosby, 1992. p 134-87.
2. COMS Group. Radiation treatment for eye cancer does not change patients' five year survival. Am J Ophthalmol. 1998; 125:779-96.
3. Finger PT. Radiation therapy for choroidal melanoma. Surv Ophthalmol. 1997;42:215-32.
4. Gass IDM. Problems in the differential diagnosis of choroidal nevi and malignant melanomas: The XXXIII Edward Jackson Memorial Lecture. Am J Ophthalmol. 1997;83:299-323.
5. Grin JM, Grant-Kels JM, Grin CM, et al. Ocular melanomas and melanocytic lesions of the eye. J Am Acad Dermatol. 1998; 38:716-30.
6. Shields CL, Shields JA, Cater J, et al. Transpupillary thermotherapy for choroidal melanoma: Tumor control and visual results in 100 consecutive cases. Ophthalmology. 1998; 105:581-90.
7. Zimmerman LE, Mclean IW. An evaluation of enucleation in the management of uveal melanomas. Am J Ophthalmol. 1979; 87:4741-60.
8. Hawkins BS. Collaborative Ocular Melanoma Study Group. The Collaborative Ocular Melanoma Study (COMS) randomized trial of pre-enucleation radiation of large choroidal melanoma: IV. Ten-year mortality findings and prognostic factors. COMS report number 24. Am J Ophthalmol. 2004;138(6):936-51.
9. Collaborative Ocular Melanoma Study Group. The COMS randomized trial of iodine 125 brachytherapy for choroidal melanoma: V. Twelve-year mortality rates and prognostic factors: COMS report No. 28. Arch Ophthalmol. 2006;124:1684-93.
10. Gragoudas ES. Proton beam irradiation of uveal melanomas: The first 30 years. The Weisenfeld lecture. Invest Ophthalmol Vis Sci. 2006;47:4666-73.

Vitreous Opacities

128

Lina Marouf, Lanny S Odin, Bailey L Lee

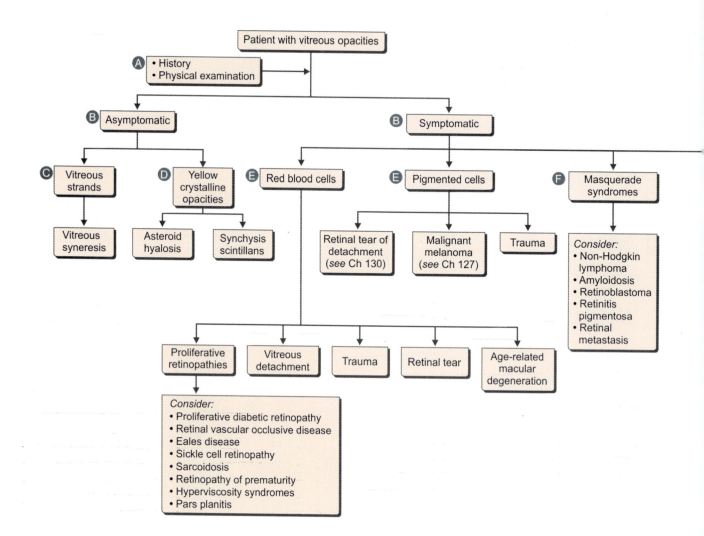

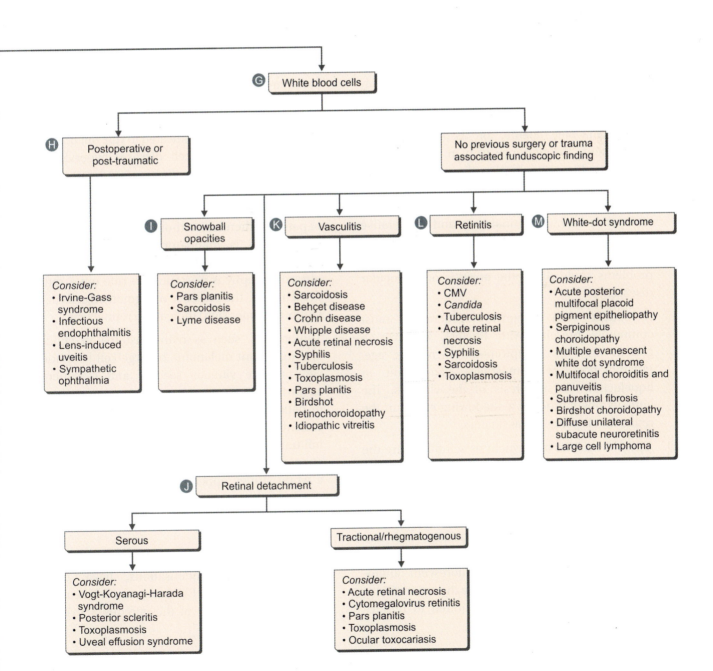

G White blood cells

H Postoperative or post-traumatic

No previous surgery or trauma associated funduscopic finding

I Snowball opacities

K Vasculitis

L Retinitis

M White-dot syndrome

Consider:
• Irvine-Gass syndrome
• Infectious endophthalmitis
• Lens-induced uveitis
• Sympathetic ophthalmia

Consider:
• Pars planitis
• Sarcoidosis
• Lyme disease

Consider:
• Sarcoidosis
• Behçet disease
• Crohn disease
• Whipple disease
• Acute retinal necrosis
• Syphilis
• Tuberculosis
• Toxoplasmosis
• Pars planitis
• Birdshot retinochoroidopathy
• Idiopathic vitreitis

Consider:
• CMV
• *Candida*
• Tuberculosis
• Acute retinal necrosis
• Syphilis
• Sarcoidosis
• Toxoplasmosis

Consider:
• Acute posterior multifocal placoid pigment epitheliopathy
• Serpiginous choroidopathy
• Multiple evanescent white dot syndrome
• Multifocal choroiditis and panuveitis
• Subretinal fibrosis
• Birdshot choroidopathy
• Diffuse unilateral subacute neuroretinitis
• Large cell lymphoma

J Retinal detachment

Serous

Tractional/rhegmatogenous

Consider:
• Vogt-Koyanagi-Harada syndrome
• Posterior scleritis
• Toxoplasmosis
• Uveal effusion syndrome

Consider:
• Acute retinal necrosis
• Cytomegalovirus retinitis
• Pars planitis
• Toxoplasmosis
• Ocular toxocariasis

A. Examination of the vitreous should be done using the slit lamp with the pupil dilated. This allows evaluation of the anterior third of the vitreous. High-power magnification provides information about the size, shape, and intensity of the vitreous cells when present. Use indirect biomicroscopy using 90-D or 78-D lenses, or contact lens biomicroscopy to visualize the posterior vitreous and retina. In cases of vitritis, the location of the cells in the vitrous is important in classifying the type of inflammation. The vitritis may be primary in origin, or it could be a sign of spillover from the anterior chamber or retina. Indirect ophthalmoscopy with scleral depression should also be performed to assess the peripheral retina and pars plana.

B. Patients with vitreous opacities may be asymptomatic, may complain of floaters, or may present with decreased vision. The change in vision may be secondary to dense vitreous opacities, cystoid macular edema, or associated retinal detachment. The presence of pain, photophobia, and eye redness should alert the physician to an inflammatory process. Floaters accompanied by photopsia indicate vitreoretinal traction, as seen in vitreous detachment, retinal tears, and proliferative retinal diseases. A thorough ocular and medical history of trauma, surgery, or active medical problems could direct the analysis of the ocular disease.

C. A patient with vitreous degeneration most commonly presents with floaters. However, a patient may be asymptomatic. Increasing age, inflammation, or hemorrhage can result in liquefaction and syneresis of the vitreous. The vitreous fibers produce a shadowing effect on the retina that is perceived as floaters.

D. Asteroid hyalosis and synchysis scintillans are the two main entities associated with yellow crystalline opacities in the vitreous. Asteroid hyalosis are opacities composed of calcium-containing phospholipids and are found to be unilateral in 75% of patients. There has been an association with diabetes mellitus. When the retina detail is limited by dense asteroid hyalosis, fluorescein angiography may allow one to visualize the retina. Occasionally, vitrectomy may be required to remove incapacitating vitreous opacities or to facilitate the treatment of an underlying retinal pathologic condition. Synchysis scintillans or cholesterolosis occurs in eyes that have had repeated vitreous hemorrhages and is composed of cholesterol crystals. The opacities tend to settle inferiorly because these eyes often have a posterior vitreous detachment, in contrast to the eyes with asteroid hyalosis.

E. Pigmented cells in the vitreous can be seen in conditions associated with the release of retinal pigment epithelium (RPE) cells into the vitreous or with vitreous hemorrhage, as seen in posterior vitreous detachment, retinal, tears, and proliferative retinopathies. Proliferative retinal disease tends to be bilateral (except in retinal vascular occlusive disease). Examination of the fellow eye may help in establishing the diagnosis. In the absence of a known medical illness, a medical evaluation is indicated to rule out diabetes, hypertension, sickle cell disease, hyperviscosity syndrome, retinal embolization, and sarcoidosis. Posterior vitreous detachment resulting in vitreous hemorrhage is associated with a retinal tear in 80% of patients; therefore, a thorough peripheral retinal examination is mandatory. When the vitreous hemorrhage precludes retinal visualization, ocular ultrasonography is warranted to rule out a retinal detachment. The presence of pigmented cells in the vitreous (Shafer sign) indicates a retinal tear.

F. Tumor cells, such as retinoblastoma in children and malignant melanoma or large cell lymphoma, can produce vitreous seeding and masquerade as vitritis. Intraocular large cell lymphoma occurs in patients in their sixties. It is bilateral in 80% of patients. The retina and choroid may also be infiltrated by tumor cells, which have a yellow-white appearance. Amyloidosis of the vitreous produces a white stringy appearance of the vitreous fibrils that resembles a string of pearls. The diagnosis is established by the presence of the associated ocular findings.

G. Inflammation of the vitreous can present as vitreous cells, opacities, condensations, haze, cystoid macular edema (CME), or areas of vitreoretinal traction. The severity of the vitreous activity can be graded by assessing the amount of vitreous haze, the clarity of the optic nerve, retinal vessels, and nerve fiber layer reflex using a 20-D lens and indirect ophthalmoscopy.

H. Prior trauma or surgery to the eye can result in infectious endophthalmitis, lens-induced uveitis, or Irvine-Gass syndrome in the involved eye. The presence of bilateral iritis, vitritis, and a yellow subretinal nodule after trauma is diagnostic of sympathetic ophthalmia. The clinical presentation, ocular findings, and course of the vitritis should help in establishing the diagnosis.

I. Snowball opacities over the peripheral retina and pars plana occur in pars planitis, sarcoidosis, and Lyme disease. The medical history (e.g. tick bites, Lyme disease) and associated systemic findings such as erythema chronicum migrans (Lyme), erythema nodosum, and restrictive lung disease (sarcoidosis); laboratory tests such as VDRL, FTA-ABS, and Lyme titers; and chest film can help narrow the difference.

J. Vitritis caused by posterior uveitis, as seen in Vogt-Koyanagi-Harada syndrome, or posterior scleritis can result in serous retinal detachment in the acute stage secondary to disruption of the outer blood retinal barrier. Chronic vitritis and uveitis can lead to vitreous condensation, proliferative changes, and vitreous detachment, resulting in tractional or rhegmatogenous retinal detachment, as seen in acute retinal necrosis, CMV retinitis, and pars planitis.

K. The diagnosis of several disorders associated with vasculitis is facilitated by multisystem evaluation (e.g. Behçet disease, Crohn disease, Whipple disease, and sarcoidosis). Ocular involvement in sarcoidosis occurs in about 40% of patients. Usually, posterior segment disease is accompanied by granulomatous iridocyclitis. Posterior segment involvement includes snowball vitreous opacities, retinal vasculitis (termed candlewax dripping), and optic nerve and choroidal granulomas. Toxoplasmosis presents as an area of focal retinitis seen as a 'satellite' next to an old atrophic lesion. Consider syphilis in any patient with vitritis because the clinical presentation may vary. Acute retinal necrosis syndrome classically presents with the triad of vasculitis, peripheral necrotizing retinitis, and vitritis. Tuberculosis typically produces choroidal granulomas or iridocyclitis that is unresponsive to anti-inflammatory therapy. Pars planitis is characterized by bilateral ocular involvement, vitritis, and snowball vitreous opacities with or without periphlebitis, peripheral neovascularization, and CME. It occurs in teenagers or young adults. Birdshot choroidopathy occurs in middle-aged patients, is bilateral, and clinically presents as multiple white spots in the choroid, vitritis, CME, arteritis, and late optic atrophy. Color vision, electro-oculographic, and electroretinographic abnormalities have been noted. Other laboratory tests that may confirm the diagnosis in some of the disease entities include chest X-ray (sarcoid and tuberculosis); purified protein derivative (PPD) skin testing (tuberculosis); angiotensin converting enzyme (ACE) and serum lysozyme (sarcoidosis); microhemagglutination assay-treponema pallidum (MHA-TP), fluorescent treponemal antibody-absorption (FTA-ABS), and venereal disease research laboratory (VDRL) (syphilis); serologic tests (toxoplasmosis); barium enema (Crohn and Whipple diseases); HLA typing (B5, Behçet, A29 birdshot choroidopathy).

L. Retinitis presents as an indistinct area of retinal thickening and whitening with overlying vitritis. The most common cause in healthy individuals is toxoplasmic retinochoroiditis. Evidence points to members of the herpesvirus family in the etiology of acute retinal necrosis (ARN syndrome). In immunocompromised individuals, candida retinitis, cytomegalovirus (CMV), and septic retinitis should be considered. CMV retinitis produces a confluent hemorrhagic retinitis. Candida retinochoroiditis lesions are multiple, fluffy white, and may break into the vitreous to produce 'fluff balls'. Syphilis and tuberculosis can occur in both groups of patients. The medical work-up should include blood, urine, and catheter cultures.

M. Several entities have been found to present with vitritis associated with white outer retinal or sub-retinal lesions. The white-yellow lesions in serpi-ginous choroidopathy involve the RPE-choroid complex. They begin in the peripapillary region, have a geographic appearance, and progress in a centripetal fashion. Serpiginous choroidopathy is a bilateral disease that can affect both sexes in the age group of 10–60 years. Multiple evanescent white-dot syndrome is a self-limited ocular disease that affects young women, is unilateral, and is characterized by small discrete white dots occurring at the RPE level in the perifoveal region. The dots resolve, leaving RPE window defects. Accompanying vitritis and periphlebitis may be present. Fluorescein angiography reveals early hyperfluorescence with late staining of the lesions. Posterior multifocal placoid pigment epitheliopathy is a bilateral disease characterized by large creamy-colored placoid lesions at the level of the RPE. Vitritis and occasionally papillitis are present. The disease affects young people with good visual prognosis. Fluorescein angiography reveals early blockage and late staining of the lesions. Multifocal choroiditis, also called pseudopresumed ocular histoplasmosis, is a bilateral disease that usually affects women and is characterized by the presence of histoplasmosis-like 'punched-out' lesions in the peripheral fundus. However, unlike in presumed ocular histoplasmosis syndrome, these patients present with significant iritis and vitritis. In subretinal fibrosis and uveitis syndrome, a bilateral disease that affects young African-American women, irregular whitish lesions are seen in the subretinal space with accompanying vitritis and iritis. Diffuse unilateral subacute neuroretinitis occurs in healthy individuals and is thought to result from a wandering nematode in the subretinal space. It is characterized by vitritis, multiple evanescent gray-white outer retinal lesions, vasculitis, and papillitis. Several other parasitic infestations have also been reported to result in vitritis with various ocular manifestations.

BIBLIOGRAPHY

1. Bergren RL, Brown GC, Duker JS. Prevalence and association of asteroid hyalosis with systemic diseases. Am J Ophthalmol. 1991;111:289-93.
2. Hampton GR, Nelsen PT, Hay PB. Viewing through the asteroids. Ophthalmology. 1981;88:669-72.
3. Nussenblatt RB, Palestine AG, Chan CC, et al. Standardization of vitreal inflammatory activity in intermediate and posterior uveitis. Ophthalmology. 1985;92:467-71.
4. Nussenblatt RB, Whitcup SM, Palestine AG. Uveitis: Fundamentals and Clinical Practice, 2nd Edition. St Louis, MO: Mosby, 1996.
5. Roy FH. Ocular Differential Diagnosis. Baltimore, MD: Williams & Wilkins, 1997.

129

Retinal Holes and Tears

Maria Stephanie R Jardeleza, WAJ van Heuven

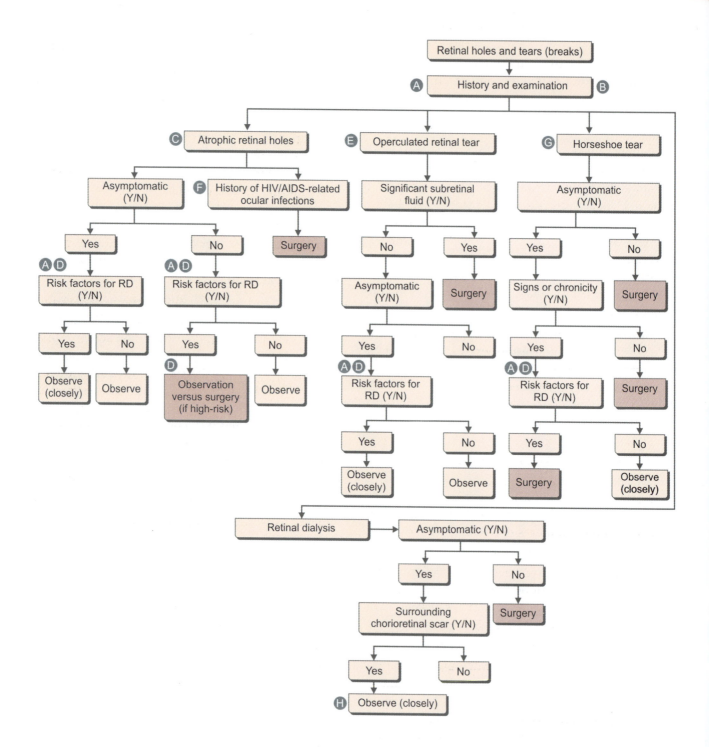

Retinal holes and/or tears (retinal breaks) are noted incidentally on routine eye examination or urgently for symptomatic vitreous traction. Partial or full thickness retinal holes or tears are rarely congenital; instead, they develop secondary to traction from age-related vitreous liquefaction or secondary to ocular trauma. Symptoms of active vitreous traction or a posterior vitreous detachment include new-onset floaters and flashes or a change in the number or size of pre-existing floaters. Certain vitreoretinal conditions (congenital, inflammation, vasculopathy, and/or trauma) can predispose to posterior vitreous detachment. Not all cases of posterior vitreous detachment cause retinal breaks.

Retinal break formation secondary to active vitreous traction may present with persistent flashes or numerous simultaneous floaters (described as a 'shower of red or black dots'—typically describing a vitreous hemorrhage). In general, if the patient sees <10–12 floaters, one can assume a benign vitreous detachment and the eye examination can be scheduled during regular office hours. However, >12 floaters often indicate hemorrhage from a retinal tear and demands prompt attention.

A. Not all retinal holes or tears require treatment. Obtaining a thorough history for risk factors of retinal detachment* or symptomatic vitreous traction is important. Asymptomatic retinal holes are noted during routine eye examination. Questioning yields no contributing factors.

B. Examination using the slit-lamp and fundus lens determines the presence of the posterior vitreous detachment, syneresis, or pigmented cells (Schaffer sign). Examination using the binocular indirect ophthalmoscope and wide field lens with scleral depression of both eyes determines type, size, and location of the retinal defects.

C. Atrophic round retinal holes are caused by retinal atrophy and may not be associated with a vitreous or choroidal component. Most, especially those which are asymptomatic, rarely progress to retinal detachment and do not require treatment.

D. Retinal holes associated with high/pathologic myopia or lattice degeneration do not always require treatment. Prophylactic treatment should be considered in patients with a strong family history of retinal detachment or a retinal detachment in the contralateral eye. Additionally, retinal breaks located at the edge of lattice lesions should be considered equivalent to horseshoe tears and treated with laser or cryotherapy (surgery).

E. An operculated tear is caused by active vitreous traction and is characterized by a retinal defect associated with retinal fragment within the immediate vicinity of the break without any active vitreous traction on the break itself. The retinal fragment or operculum, is now completely suspended within the vitreous cavity. If asymptomatic, these rarely lead to retinal detachment and may be observed. However, if significant subretinal fluid is present or other predisposing factors for retinal detachment exist, treatment should be considered. Clinically, significant subretinal fluid is defined as a rim of retinal detachment around a retinal break greater than the diameter of the break itself.

F. Atrophic and/or operculated holes in association with ocular complications of HIV/AIDS, such as cytomegalovirus (CMV) retinitis, acute retinal necrosis (ARN) or progressive outer retinal necrosis (PORN), merit special treatment considerations. These are often found in severe necrotic retina and due to the challenge of retinal detachment repair in such cases, prophylactic cryotherapy or laser is often recommended. Treatment should be carried out to involve areas of nondiseased retina to effect adequate formation of chorioretinal adhesions.

G. Horseshoe-shaped retinal tears (HSTs) have active vitreoretinal traction at the attached base (flap) of the tear. Three criteria must be met for most rhegmatogenous (retinal tear associated) retinal detachments to occur: a retinal break, active vitreous traction on the break, and vitreous liquefaction overlying the break. As a consequence, HSTs carry a higher risk for retinal detachments and are treated by most retina surgeons. HST that are asymptomatic or demonstrate signs of chronicity such as demarcation lines or surrounding

---

Risk factors for retinal detachment: Myopia, lattice degeneration, pseudophakia, trauma, retinal detachment in fellow eye, retinopathy of prematurity (ROP), hereditary vitreoretinopathies.

pigment may be observed; exceptions are those found in patients with limited access to ocular care or professions that carry a high-risk of trauma. Overall, a low threshold for treatment should be observed, especially in light of those with persistent symptoms of vitreoretinal traction or risk factors for retinal detachment (Section A).

H. Retinal dialysis is disinsertion of the retina at the ora serrata and usually occurs in the inferotemporal quadrant secondary to blunt trauma. If the dialysis is surrounded by a chorioretinal scar, observation may be a safe option. Although retinal detachments associated with dialysis can be slowly progressive and occur years after the initial insult, most retinal surgeons will treat symptomatic and asymptomatic dialysis with prophylactic cryotherapy or if associated with retinal detachment, scleral buckle placement.

▌BIBLIOGRAPHY

1. American Academy of Ophthalmology Retina/Vitreous Panel. Preferred Practice Patterns: Posterior vitreous detachment, retinal breaks and lattice degeneration. 2008.
2. Byer NE. Long-term natural history of lattice degeneration of the retina. Ophthalmology. 1989;9:1396-401.
3. Byer NE. The natural history of asymptomatic retinal breaks. Ophthalmology. 1982;89:1033-9.
4 Davis JL, Hummer J, Feuer WJ. Laser photocoagulation for retinal detachments and retinal tears in cytomegalovirus retinitis. Ophthalmology. 1997;104:2053-60.
5. Folk JC, Bennett SR, Klugman MR, et al. Prophylactic treatment to the fellow eye of patients with phakic lattice retinal detachment. Retina. 1990;10:165-9.
6. Ross WH. Traumatic retinal dialysis. Arch Ophthalmol. 1981;99:1371-4.
7. Wilkinson CP, Rice TA. Michel's Retinal Detachment, 2nd Edition. St. Louis, MO: Mosby, 1997.

Retinal Detachment

130

Mitchell J Goff, James E Bell

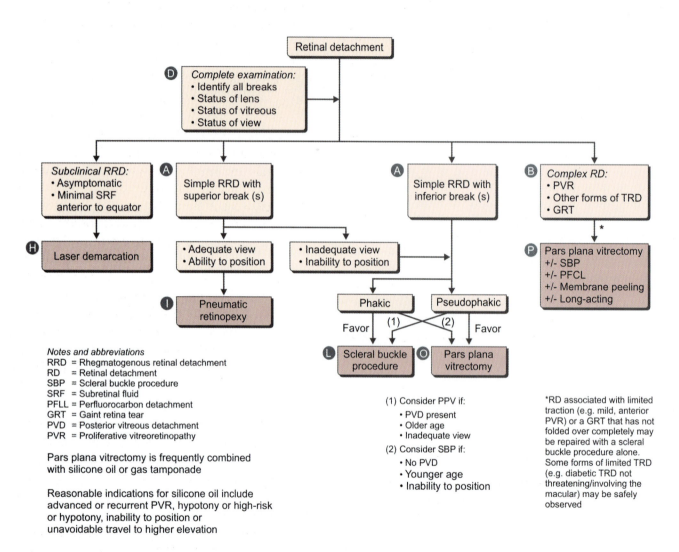

Retinal detachment

D *Complete examination:*
- Identify all breaks
- Status of lens
- Status of vitreous
- Status of view

Subclinical RRD:
- Asymptomatic
- Minimal SRF anterior to equator

A Simple RRD with superior break (s)

A Simple RRD with inferior break (s)

B *Complex RD:*
- PVR
- Other forms of TRD
- GRT

H Laser demarcation

- Adequate view
- Ability to position

- Inadequate view
- Inability to position

P Pars plana vitrectomy
+/- SBP
+/- PFCL
+/- Membrane peeling
+/- Long-acting

I Pneumatic retinopexy

Phakic

Pseudophakic

Favor (1) (2) Favor

L Scleral buckle procedure

O Pars plana vitrectomy

(1) Consider PPV if:
- PVD present
- Older age
- Inadequate view

(2) Consider SBP if:
- No PVD
- Younger age
- Inability to position

*RD associated with limited traction (e.g. mild, anterior PVR) or a GRT that has not folded over completely may be repaired with a scleral buckle procedure alone. Some forms of limited TRD (e.g. diabetic TRD not threatening/involving the macular) may be safely observed

Notes and abbreviations
RRD = Rhegmatogenous retinal detachment
RD = Retinal detachment
SBP = Scleral buckle procedure
SRF = Subretinal fluid
PFLL = Perfluorocarbon detachment
GRT = Gaint retina tear
PVD = Posterior vitreous detachment
PVR = Proliferative vitreoretinopathy

Pars plana vitrectomy is frequently combined with silicone oil or gas tamponade

Reasonable indications for silicone oil include advanced or recurrent PVR, hypotony or high-risk or hypotony, inability to position or unavoidable travel to higher elevation

OVERVIEW

Retinal detachment (Fig. 130.1) may be defined as a separation of the neurosensory retina from the retinal pigment epithelium (RPE). It is typically categorized as rhegmatogenous, tractional or exudative, and each has different causes and characteristic features. All forms of retinal detachment can cause significant and permanent visual loss; therefore, prompt recognition and appropriate treatment is of paramount importance.

The primary symptom of retinal detachment is a relative loss of peripheral vision. This will not be an absolute loss of vision in the affected area because the photoreceptors and associated neural connections to the ganglion cells are intact. The area of the visual field loss depends on the extent and location of the retinal detachment. If the retinal detachment involves the fovea, presenting visual acuity will be poor, generally 20/100 or less. Preceding symptoms are often present and may include photopsias and floaters due to the

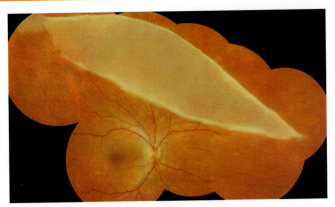

Fig. 130.1: Retinal detachment due to giant retinal tear.

presence of vitreous traction and posterior vitreous detachment, respectively.

A. Rhegmatogenous retinal detachment (RRD) is the most common form of detachment and has an estimated annual incidence of approximately 10.5 per 100,000.[1] For a RRD to occur, three predisposing factors must be present: (1) a tear or hole in the retina, (2) traction on the retina in the vicinity of the tear or hole, and (3) liquefied vitreous to pass into the subretinal space. The tear in the retina is typically but not always, a flap tear, also referred to as a horseshoe tear because of its U-shaped appearance. Vitreous traction is usually present and accounts for the appearance of these tears (vitreous traction elevates the flap anteriorly, toward the peripheral retina). Without associated vitreous traction, the edges of the retinal tear or hole are likely to remain apposed to the RPE and liquefied vitreous cannot pass into the subretinal space. This is the reason that some retinal tears and most round or atrophic retinal holes do not lead to retinal detachment. Likewise, in very young people with minimal liquefied vitreous, retinal detachment may not occur, or will progress much more slowly, even in the setting of retinal breaks and vitreous traction.

B. Tractional retinal detachment occurs when there are proliferative membranes on the surface of the retina, often involving the posterior hyaloid face, which contract leading to separation of the retina from the RPE. Common examples of proliferative membranes include fibrovascular tissue from proliferative diabetic retinopathy or fibrous

membranes from proliferative vitreoretinopathy. Vitreous traction is often present but not required. Often, proliferative membranes grow into the posterior hyaloid and progression of posterior vitreous detachment accelerates or worsens the vector forces leading to retinal detachment. Tractional retinal detachment is less common as it frequently represents the advanced stages of proliferative disease or a secondary outcome of RRD.

C. Exudative retinal detachment is a separation of the neurosensory retina from the RPE due to the accumulation of fluid in the subretinal space from underlying structures. By definition, there is no tear or hole in the retina. Many underlying conditions can cause exudation of fluid from the choroid including vascular disease such as hypertensive choroidopathy, eclampsia, or central serous chorioretinopathy, inflammatory diseases such as Vogt-Koyanagi-Harada syndrome, choroidal tumors such as malignant melanoma, hemorrhagic conditions such as advanced macular degeneration with massive subretinal hemorrhage, and many more. It is critical to distinguish exudative retinal detachment from rhegmatogenous or tractional retinal detachment as the treatment is not surgical in most cases and is directed at the underlying cause of exudation.

D. A complete ocular examination with scleral depression is required in patients with retinal detachment. It is imperative to find all breaks and holes to ensure success with any procedure used to repair retinal detachment. Many examination findings are important to determine the optimal procedure for repair.

E. The RRD has a characteristic appearance with a corrugated, mobile, elevated retina with a variably convex configuration and associated retinal tears or holes. Tractional retinal detachment is characterized by the presence of proliferative membranes, relatively immobile retina, and sometimes areas with a concave configuration representing traction. Full thickness retinal folds, sometimes in a star pattern can be seen. If tears or holes are present, they may have an oval or stretched appearance due to traction by proliferative membranes.

Exudative retinal detachment generally demonstrates a smooth, relatively immobile surface and a convex configuration with no associated retinal tears or holes. The subretinal fluid may shift with changes in position.

F. The location and configuration of the detachment can aid in localization of retinal tears and holes as they tend to be present in the most superior part of the detachment. Exceptions occur such as an inferior detachment that extends symmetrically temporally and nasally, in which case the retinal tear or hole is likely to be directly inferior.

G. Treatment options for the repair of retinal detachment include laser demarcation, pneumatic retinopexy, scleral buckle procedure, and pars plana vitrectomy techniques. There is a considerable variation in the treatment approach among surgeons, and frequently surgeon preference, experience, and training will influence the chosen procedure. Procedures to repair retinal detachment have similar outcomes if used in the appropriate setting, with most series reporting anatomic success rates of 90% or higher with one or multiple procedures. Flow chart 1 is an algorithm for the surgical treatment of retinal detachment based on key examination findings and results of clinical trials. This algorithm applies to rhegmatogenous and tractional retinal detachments only as exudative retinal detachments are usually treated medically.

H. Laser demarcation involves creating a continuous chorioretinal adhesion around the retinal detachment to prevent further posterior progression. Two to three near-confluent rows of easily visible laser spots should be delivered just posterior to the entire border of the retinal detachment, extending anteriorly to the ora serrata. This is performed either at the slit lamp with a wide-field viewing lens or using laser indirect ophthalmoscopy. Generally, topical anesthesia is sufficient. The existing retinal detachment will not resolve as nothing has been done to relieve the vitreous traction or to remove the subretinal fluid. The purpose of the procedure, instead, is to prevent progression of the detachment. This procedure should be reserved for subclinical retinal detachments extending posteriorly no

further than the equator. Due to their limited extent, these are typically asymptomatic. Attempting to repair more extensive retinal detachments with laser demarcation may result in a permanent and noticeable visual field defect or other secondary complications such as chronic macular edema or hypotony.

I. Pneumatic retinopexy (Fig. 130.2) involves creating a chorioretinal adhesion around the retinal tears or holes and injecting an intravitreal gas bubble into the eye to aid in resolution of subretinal fluid. The gas bubble will occlude the retinal tear or hole, preventing additional liquefied vitreous from passing into the subretinal space, and allowing the RPE to maintain a net outward transport of fluid from the subretinal space. The buoyant force of the bubble may also aid in displacing subretinal fluid through the retinal tear or hole and further promote retinal reattachment.

J. Pneumatic retinopexy requires an adequate view to visualize the retinal tear or hole and the patient must be able to position appropriately for the gas bubble to occlude the tear or hole. Ideally, the tears or holes should be in the upper two-thirds of the peripheral retina, and there should only be a single

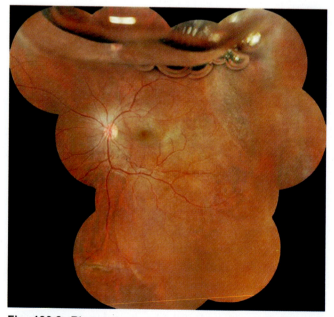

Fig. 130.2: Rhegmatogenous retinal detachment with repair by pneumatic retinopexy.

tear or hole or a small cluster of tears or holes. Inferiorly located, or numerous tears and holes in different locations render appropriate positioning difficult and success rates may be lower.

K. Complications of pneumatic retinopexy include subretinal injection of gas, missed or new retinal tears or macular hole, proliferative vitreoretino-pathy, and macular detachment due to displacement of subretinal fluid into the macula.

L. A scleral buckle procedure involves the placement of an external band or sponge beneath Tenon's capsule, underneath the rectus muscles to indent the sclera and relieve traction. A segmental or radial scleral buckle indents the sclera in the area of retinal tears or holes and relieves vitreous traction associated with the tears or holes. An encircling scleral buckle reduces the entire circumference of the eye and minimizes tractional forces pulling the retina toward the center of the eye leading to retinal detachment. A chorioretinal adhesion is created around all retinal breaks and holes using cryotherapy or laser photocoagulation. Scleral buckle procedures are often combined with external drainage of subretinal fluid, either using a needle passed through the sclera and choroid into the subretinal space, or by creating a small radial scleral incision with a puncture through the choroid to allow subretinal fluid to exit the eye.

M. Scleral buckle techniques, such as pneumatic retinopexy, require adequate visualization to treat all retinal tears and holes appropriately. Specific positioning requirements are not necessary. Because the scleral buckle indents the eye, it may affect the axial length and can cause a myopic shift.

N. Additional complications of scleral buckle procedures include extrusion or infection of the scleral buckle element, motility disturbances, choroidal detachment or angle-closure glaucoma, cystoid macular edema, and anterior segment ischemia. Complications associated with external drainage of subretinal fluid include retinal incarceration and choroidal hemorrhage.

O. Pars plana virectomy for the repair of retinal detachment involves the removal of all the vitreous via an approach through the pars plana, thereby relieving vitreous traction. Proliferative membranes may be removed at the time of vitrectomy as well. A chorioretinal adhesion is created using laser photocoagulation or cryotherapy. Tamponade can be applied using intravitreal air, gas [typically sulfur hexafluoride (SF6), perfluoroethane (C2F6), or perfluoropropane (C3F8)], or silicone oil.

P. Vitrectomy is sometimes necessary to clear media opacity such as vitreous hemorrhage to visualize all peripheral pathology. Induction of a posterior vitreous detachment during vitrectomy surgery can be difficult, particularly in younger patients because the posterior hyaloid is firmly adherent, and this can lead to iatrogenic retinal breaks. Therefore, the presence or absence of a posterior vitreous detachment and the age of the patient are important considerations when deciding upon vitrectomy surgery. Additionally, pars plana vitrectomy may cause formation or progression of cataract, requiring subsequent surgery for optimal vision.

Q. Additional complications of pars plana vitrectomy for retinal detachment include endophthalmitis, iatrogenic retinal breaks, intraocular hemorrhage, elevated intraocular pressure, visual field defects, intraocular lens subluxation or dislocation, cystoid macular edema, epiretinal membrane, and proliferative vitreoretinopathy.

R. Surgical adjuncts for the repair of retinal detachment include perfluorocarbon liquids (PFCL) and silicone oil. PFCL are optically clear, heavy liquids that may be used intraoperatively to aid in flattening the retina by compressing subretinal fluid and forcing it through peripheral tears or holes or by unfolding the retina in the case of giant retinal tears. It has a low viscosity allowing it to be easily passed through small-gauge cannulas, a high-specific gravity making it heavy, and a refractive index of approximately 1.3, making it visible among saline or silicone oil due to their different refractive indices. It is most often used intraoperatively and not as long-term tamponade and care should be taken to remove it completely from the eye at the time of surgery. Subretinal migration or anterior chamber migration of PFCL may lead to RPE atrophy or glaucoma, respectively.

S. Silicone oil is another optically clear vitreous substitute used for long-term tamponade. It has a low-specific gravity making it lighter than saline or PFCL. It has a high viscosity requiring special instrumentation to inject and remove it from the eye. It has a refractive index of 1.4, making it visible among other clear liquids with different refractive indices. The use of silicone oil in aphakic eyes requires a peripheral iridotomy to prevent angle-closure glaucoma. Silicone oil may emulsify over time and migration of tiny silicone oil bubbles into the anterior chamber may cause a psuedohypopyon appearance and cause secondary open-angle glaucoma. Long-term silicone oil contact with the corneal endothelium may cause dysfunction and result in corneal opacification. A second surgery is required for removal of silicone oil. Reasonable indications for the use of silicone oil include complex retinal detachments, inability to position, and hypotony.

T. The pneumatic retinopexy study was a prospective, randomized clinical trial comparing pneumatic retinopexy to scleral buckle for patients with a single or small cluster of tears and absence of proliferative vitreoretinopathy. With regard to retinal reattachment, there was no statistical difference between the two treatments with pneumatic retinopexy successful in 73% of eyes and scleral buckle successful in 82% of eyes. Final anatomic success was similar between the two groups for patients who required additional surgery (99% for the pneumatic retinopexy group versus 98% for the scleral buckle group). Interestingly, among patients who had macula-off retinal detachments, visual acuity results were better in patients who underwent pneumatic retinopexy with 80% achieving 20/50 or better versus 56% in the scleral buckle group.[2]

U. The scleral buckling versus primary vitrectomy in RRD study was a large multicenter study comparing techniques with 1 year of follow-up. Treatment groups were separated into phakic eyes ($n = 416$) and pseudophakic eyes ($n = 265$). In the phakic group, better visual acuity outcomes were achieved with scleral buckle procedures (improvement of 0.71 log MAR versus 0.56 log MAR for the pars plana vitrectomy group) and similar anatomic outcomes were observed with both procedures. The trend of better visual acuity outcomes in the sclera buckle procedure group remained after removal of patients with significant cataracts. Conversely, in the pseudophakic group, better anatomic outcomes, defined as retinal reattachment without any secondary retina-affecting surgery, were achieved with pars plana vitrectomy techniques (72% versus 53% in the scleral buckle group) and similar visual acuity outcomes were achieved with both procedure. This study suggests a benefit of scleral buckle procedures for phakic eyes and a benefit of pars plana vitrectomy in pseudophakic eyes.[3] A meta-analysis of randomized controlled clinical trials supports this notion.[4]

V. The silicone oil study compared short-acting gas tamponade (SF6) with long-acting tamponade (C3F8 or silicone oil) for complex retinal detachment with proliferative vitreoretinopathy and found that long-acting tamponade with either C3F8 gas or silicone oil was superior to short-acting tamponade. There was noted to be a higher rate of hypotony in patients treated with C3F8 compared with those treated with silicone oil.[5,6]

W. The timing of retinal detachment repair is extremely important to maximize visual outcomes, and generally speaking new retinal detachments should be treated promptly. Macula-on retinal detachments, particularly recent onset, superior retinal detachments should be repaired as soon as possible to prevent the retinal detachment from extending posteriorly and involving the macula. In the case of macula-off retinal detachments, longer duration of macular detachment negatively impacts final visual acuity. Waiting for 4 or more days from the beginning of symptoms has been correlated with worse visual acuity outcomes, whereas waiting up to 3 days was found to have no impact on final visual acuity.[7] After 6 weeks of macular detachment, final visual acuity outcomes are poor.[8]

X. Reasonable guidelines for the timing of the repair of new RRDs include: (1) macula threatening or recent macula-off retinal detachments should be repaired urgently (within 1 to 2 days). The goal is to avoid more than 3 days of macular detachment. (2) Macula-off retinal detachments of 4 or more days should be repaired as soon as possible, though not urgent. The goal is still to minimize the number of days of macular detachment. (3) Macula-off retinal detachments of more than 6 weeks can be repaired on a routine basis.

REFERENCES

1. Mitry D, Charteris DG, Fleck BW, et al. The epidemiology of rhegmatogenous retinal detachment: Geographical variation and clinical associations. Br J Ophthalmol. 2010;94:678-84.
2. Tornambe PE, Hilton GF. Pneumatic retinopexy: A multicenter randomized controlled clinical trial comparing pneumatic retinopexy with scleral buckling. The Retinal Detachment Study Group. Ophthalmol. 1989;96:772-83.
3. Heimann H, Bartz-Schmidt KU, Bornfeld N, et al. Scleral buckling versus primary vitrectomy in rhegmatogenous retinal detachment: A prospective randomized multicenter clinical study. Ophthalmol. 2007;114: 2142-54.
4. Sun Q, Sun T, Xu Y, et al. Primary vitrectomy versus scleral buckling for the treatment of rhegmatogenous retinal detachment: A meta-analysis of randomized controlled clinical trials. Curr Eye Res. 2012;37:492-99.
5. Vitrectomy with silicone oil or sulfur hexafluoride gas in eyes with severe proliferative vitreoretinopathy: Results of a randomized clinical trial. Silicone Study report 1. Arch Ophthalmol. 1992;110:770-9.
6. Vitrectomy with silicone oil or perfluoropropane gas in eyes with severe proliferative vitreoretinopathy: Results of a randomized clinical trial. Silicone Study report 2. Arch Ophthalmol. 1992;110:780-92.
7. Henrich PB, Priglinger S, Klaessen D, et al. Macula-off retinal detachment—a matter of time? Klin Monbl Augenheilkd. 2009; 226:289-93.
8. Mowatt L, Shun-Shin GA, Arora S, et al. Macula-off retinal detachments. How long can they wait before it is too late? Eur J Ophthalmol. 2005;15:109-117.

Diabetic Retinopathy

131

Maria Stephanie R Jardeleza, WAJ van Heuven

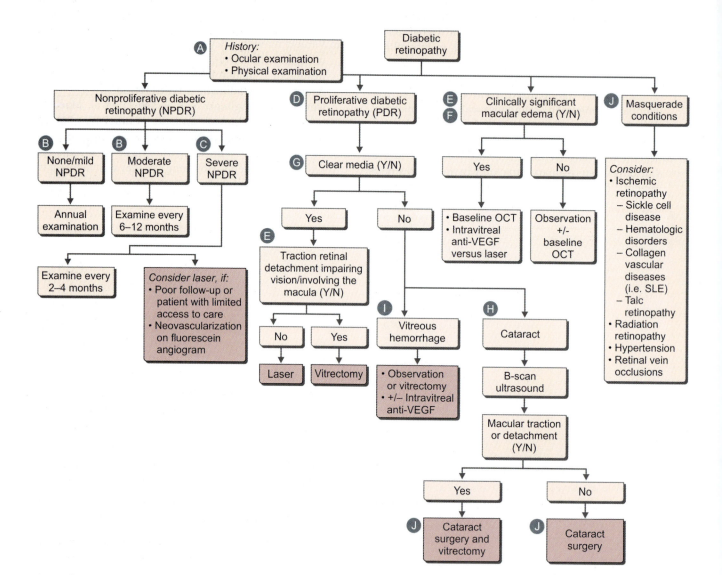

Diabetes is now the leading cause of newly diagnosed blindness among adults of the age between 20 and 74 years. Generally, all of the changes of diabetic retinopathy are seen in both type 1* (5-10% of diabetes) and type 2† diabetes (90-95% of diabetes). However, type 1 diabetes usually develops retinopathy several years after diagnosis, whereas type 2 diabetes often has retinopathy present at the time of diagnosis. Duration of diabetes is a risk factor for the development of diabetic retinopathy. Therefore, approximately 25% of type 1 diabetes patients have some retinopathy after 5 years of having diabetes and 80% have

*Previously known as insulin dependent/juvenile onset diabetes
†Previously known as noninsulin dependent diabetes

retinopathy after 15 years of having diabetes. In type 2 diabetes, 84% of patients on insulin and 53% of patients not on insulin presented with retinopathy at 19 years after diagnosis.

Duration of diabetes and severity of hyperglycemia are major risk factors for development of retinopathy. Once retinopathy is present, however, severity of hyperglycemia appears to be the key alterable risk factor associated with the progression of diabetic retinopathy. Hypertension and elevated serum lipids contribute to the progression of diabetic retinopathy. Therefore, intensive management of hypertension is recommended. Patients with severe proliferative diabetic retinopathy (PDR) are at a higher risk of stroke, myocardial infarction, and nephropathy.

Largely responsible for prevention of blindness secondary to diabetes have been the three national collaborative studies supported by the National Institutes of Health (NIH)—the Diabetic Retinopathy Study (DRS), which demonstrated the value of laser treatment for PDR; the Early Treatment Diabetic Retinopathy Study (ETDRS), which proved the value of earlier intervention with laser as well as the value of laser treatment for macular edema; and the Diabetic Retinopathy Vitrectomy Study (DRVS), which showed the value of early vitrectomy in some patients with severe retinopathy.

With the advent of intravitreal antivascular endothelial growth factor (anti-VEGF) treatment, however, management of diabetic retinopathy has undergone a paradigm shift. More recent data from The Diabetic Retinopathy Clinical Research Network (DRCR.net) and other studies demonstrate that anti-VEGF agents are effective treatments for CSME. Although studies suggest that intravitreal corticosteroids may play an important role in the treatment of CSME, long-term results failed to demonstrate superiority over macular focal/grid laser treatment.

A. Any patient recently diagnosed with diabetes and/or has retinal vascular changes suggestive of diabetic retinopathy should undergo a thorough eye examination. The eye examination should obtain a thorough ocular history and complete ocular examination. Pertinent medical history details include: duration of diabetes, past-glycemic control (hemoglobin A_{1c}), medications (especially use of insulin), comorbid systemic conditions (e.g. obesity, renal disease, systemic hypertension, serum lipid levels, pregnancy), and ocular history (e.g. trauma, ocular injections, surgery, including laser treatment and refractive surgery). Ocular examination should document visual acuity, slit-lamp biomicroscopy (looking for rubeosis), intraocular pressure, gonioscopy when indicated [to look for angle neovascularization (NV)], dilated funduscopy including stereoscopic examination of the posterior pole, and examination of the peripheral retina and vitreous. Depending on the severity of the retinopathy, fluorescein angiography may be useful in detecting macular and peripheral ischemia and proliferative changes. Physical examination of patients with retinal findings suspicious for diabetic retinopathy is best performed by an internist or endocrinologist to evaluate for end organ damage secondary to diabetes and/or investigate other comorbid systemic conditions. Communication between the ophthalmologist and the internist/endocrinologist should be facilitated.

B. Nonproliferative diabetic retinopathy (NPDR) consists of microaneurysms (MA), small round hemorrhages (blots and dots), and hard exudates. It is classified as mild, moderate or severe, depending on the number of intraretinal hemorrhages and extent of microvascular abnormalities. If a patient has good vision even with systemic diabetes and has no retinopathy, the patient should be re-examined annually. Five to ten percent of patients with no retinopathy will develop some retinopathy within 1 year. Re-examination of patients with mild and moderate NPDR should be in 6-12 months. In addition, if any severe systemic disease develops or the patient becomes pregnant during that year, it is wise for the ophthalmologist to be consulted again.

C. *Severe NPDR is characterized by any one of the following (4:2:1 rule):* Severe intraretinal hemorrhages and microaneurysms in each of the four quadrants, venous beading in two or more quadrants, or intraretinal microvascular abnormalities (IRMA) and no retinal vascular proliferation. Fifty percent of patients with severe NPDR will progress to PDR in 1 year. Thus, identification of severe NPDR became a useful clinical tool for recommending the frequency of patient visits and for preparing the patient for future laser treatment. Because some IRMAs are difficult to differentiate from retinal NV, fluorescein angiography is recommended to detect occult NV. If patients are deemed reliable and can be expected to keep appointments, severe NPDR can simply be documented and observed every 2–4 months until high-risk characteristics develop. However, in an unreliable patient or remote population, it may be wise to treat at least one eye with severe NPDR with panretinal photocoagulation.

D. PDR is, by definition, preretinal proliferation of NV at the disc (NVD) or elsewhere in the fundus (NVE). The DRS demonstrated that laser photocoagulation is beneficial at this stage. The DRS also identified high-risk characteristics for profound visual loss, which include NVD greater than one quarter of the disc area and vitreous or preretinal hemorrhage associated with NVD or with NVE. When these criteria are present, there is an urgency in doing laser treatment soon, before further vitreous hemorrhage develops.

E. In a diabetic patient with decreased vision and clear media, the probable cause of vision loss is diabetic macular edema. Extensive preretinal fibrosis and macular traction due to regressed or active PDR can also be the causes. Not all cases of traction retinal detachment due to diabetes require surgery; those not involving or threatening the macula can be observed safely. Slit-lamp biomicroscopy with examination of the posterior pole with a macular lens can determine the etiology for vision loss. Some ophthalmologists will obtain a macular optical coherence tomography image to confirm the presence of diabetic macular edema and serve as a baseline prior to onset of treatment. Angiography is also useful in determining the presence of macular ischemia, which can contribute to decreased vision.

F. The determination of whether macular edema is clinically significant, which was defined by the ETDRS, is important in deciding whether to institute treatment or observe. The definition of clinically significant macular edema is as follows:

1. Thickening of the retina within 500 μ of the center of the macula

2. Hard exudates within 500 μ of the center of the macula, if associated with thickening of adjacent retina

3. A zone of retinal thickening one disc area or larger, a part of which is within one disc diameter of the center of the macula.

The ETDRS demonstrated that laser treatment, according to its protocol, significantly reduced the risk of visual loss in clinically significant macular edema. The first line of treatment for CSME, however, is rapidly becoming intravitreal anti-VEGF injections, especially for cases of fovea-involving CSME.

G. In eyes with opaque media due to dense vitreous hemorrhage and/or cataract, B-scan is useful to determine the nature of vitreoretinal abnormalities in the posterior half of the eye. B-scan ultrasonography can provide good topographic information about the complex vitreoretinal adhesions and the presence of a retinal detachment. Quantitative A-scan ultrasonography is helpful to differentiate retinal detachment from vitreous membranes. If the ultrasonography indicates vitreous traction on the macula or macular detachment, vitrectomy may be indicated.

H. If a cataract is present and the lens opacities are sufficient to explain significantly decreased vision, cataract surgery is indicated. If significant lens opacification is coexisting with a nonclearing vitreous hemorrhage or macular detachment/traction on ultrasonography, concomitant pars plana vitrectomy may need to be performed. Both vitrectomy and cataract surgery tend to remove barriers between the posterior and anterior segments of the eye. Presumably, this permits endovascular factors produced by the ischemic retina to enter the anterior segment and produce NV of the iris and angle, resulting in glaucoma. This scenario is especially likely if panretinal photocoagulation has not been previously done. Thus, if a combined cataract extraction and vitrectomy are planned for an eye that has not had laser treatment, panretinal photocoagulation should be done at the same time.

I. The DRVS demonstrated that early vitrectomy was better than vitrectomy after 1 year of vitreous hemorrhage in juvenile-onset diabetes. This benefit was not found in adult-onset diabetic vitreous hemorrhage. Thus, if more than trace vitreous hemorrhage occurs in a juvenile diabetic patient, vitrectomy is indicated unless it can be clearly demonstrated that the entire vitreous gel is detached from the posterior retinal surface. If vitreous hemorrhage occurs in a patient with adult-onset diabetes, biomicroscopy can be used to gauge the amount, mobility, and color of the hemorrhage. If the amount of hemorrhage is little and the fundus can be seen through the hemorrhage, if the mobility of the blood is great, if the vitreous is detached from the posterior retina, and if the color is reddish, the vitreous hemorrhage can be observed and will probably be clear spontaneously. However, if the vitreous hemorrhage is severe, relatively immobile, and yellow ochre in color or is associated with multiple vitreoretinal traction points, vitrectomy should be considered. Some vitreoretinal specialists use anti-VEGF treatment as an adjuvant to panretinal photocoagulation or vitrectomy in the management of vitreous hemorrhage.

J. Many retinal ischemic conditions have features similar to those of diabetic retinopathy. These conditions include sickle cell disease and other hemoglobinopathies, hematologic diseases that cause small vessel occlusions, collagen vascular diseases, that is, systemic lupus erythematosus that cause arteriolar occlusions, and talc retinopathy (which causes embolic phenomena in drug addicts). Many of these conditions show peripheral retinal occlusive phenomena with peripheral NV, unlike the more central NV of diabetes. Radiation retinopathy can mimic diabetic retinopathy precisely. The history indicates this as a possibility. Systemic hypertension and increased coagulability of the blood are common with diabetes. Thus, patients may have a combination of hypertensive and diabetic retinopathy and may also have central or branch retinal vein occlusions together with diabetic retinopathy. Hypertensive retinopathy has many of the same features as diabetic retinopathy, except that the hemorrhages are in the nerve fiber layer and therefore are streaked rather than round, and microaneurysms occur only late in the disease. Vein occlusions also show many of the same features of diabetic retinopathy but are more prominently hemorrhagic, often with streak hemorrhages; are always associated with edema in the occluded areas; and have significant venous dilation, which is uniform, unlike the beading or sausage-like dilations in diabetic retinopathy.

BIBLIOGRAPHY

1. American Academy of Ophthalmology Preferred Practice Patterns: Diabetic Retinopathy, October 2012.
2. Diabetic Retinopathy Study Research Group. Indications for photocoagulation treatment of diabetic retinopathy, DRS Report No. 14. Int Ophthalmol Clin. 1987;27:239-53.
3. Diabetic Retinopathy Study Research Group. Photocoagulation treatment of proliferative diabetic retinopathy: the second report of DRS findings. Ophthalmology. 1978;85:82-106.
4. Diabetic Retinopathy Vitrectomy Study Research Group. Early vitrectomy for severe proliferative diabetic retinopathy in eyes with useful vision results of a randomized trial. DRVS Report No. 3. Ophthalmology. 1988;95:1307-20.
5. Early Treatment Diabetic Retinopathy Study Research Group: case reports to accompany ETDRS reports 3 and 4. Int Ophthalmol Clin. 1987;27:254-64.
6. Early Treatment Diabetic Retinopathy Study Research Group. Photocoagulation for diabetic macular edema: ETDRS Report No 1 Arch Ophthalmology. 1985;103:1796-806.
7. Elman MJ, Aiello LP, Beck RW, et al. Diabetic Retinopathy Clinical Research Network. Randomized trial evaluating ranibizumab plus prompt or deferred laser or triamcinolone plus prompt laser for diabetic macular edema. Ophthalmology. 2010;117:1064-77.
8. Zhao LQ, Zhu H, Zhao PQ, et al. A systematic review and meta-analysis of clinical outcomes of vitrectomy with or without intravitreal bevacizumab pretreatment for severe diabetic retinopathy. Br J Ophthalmol. 2011; 95:1216-22.

132

Retinal Drug Toxicity

Bailey L Lee

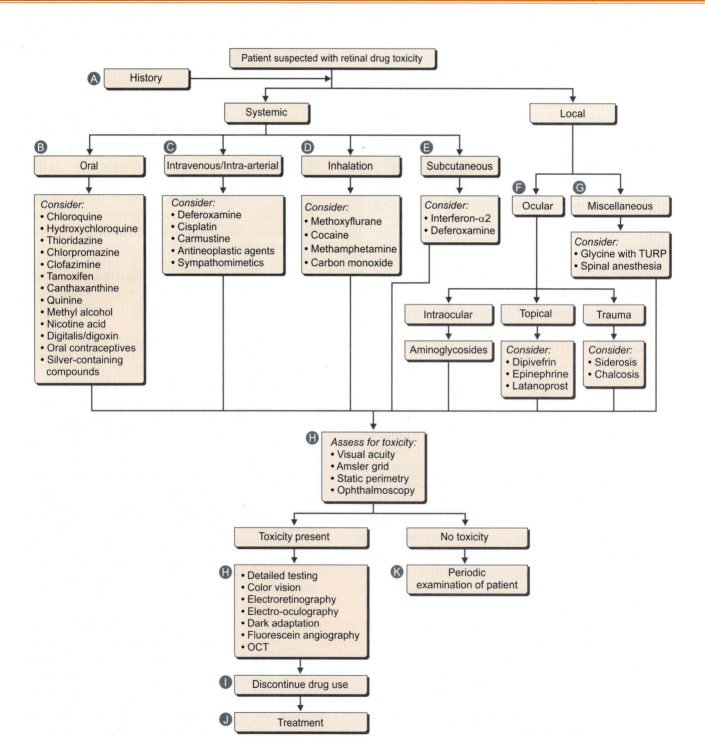

A. A careful drug history must be taken in patients with suspected retinal drug toxicity, especially in patients whose medical history is incomplete or vague. Of course, there will be those patients with an obvious history of drug use who are referred or evaluated, but even in those patients, the dosage and duration of the drug still needs to be documented.

B. Certain oral medications are well known for potential retinal toxicity. Chloroquine and hydroxychloroquine are used at higher dosages for the treatment of rheumatoid arthritis and systemic lupus erythematosus than for the treatment of malaria, and it is the patients taking these higher dosages who are at risk for toxicity. For chloroquine, toxicity rarely occurs at a total cumulative dose of <300 g, but maintaining a daily dose of <250 mg may be more important. For hydroxychloroquine, toxicity rarely appears at dosages of greater than 400 mg/day, but patients with many years of cumulative use may be at risk. These patients can develop macular pigmentary changes, often seen in a bull's eye pattern, thus this retinal toxicity is in the differential for bull's eye maculopathy. The phenothiazines, such as thioridazine and chlorpromazine, are believed to be concentrated within the melanin granules of the uvea and retinal pigment epithelium. Pigmentary retinopathy from chlorpromazine use is rare, whereas with thioridazine severe retinopathy can develop within weeks of taking dosages >800 mg/day. Clofazimine, used to treat *Mycobacterium avium* complex infections in AIDS patients, can also cause a bull's eye pattern of maculopathy. The antiestrogen drug tamoxifen, widely used for breast carcinoma, can lead to loss of central vision, macular edema, and superficial white refractile deposits in the inner layers of the retina with cumulative doses >90 g and also in cumulative doses as low as 15 g. Canthaxanthine is a carotinoid dye used as a tanning agent that can lead to deposits of golden-yellow crystal in the macular region, which usually does not affect the vision. Quinine toxicity typically occurs with doses >4 g and leads to atrophy of the inner layers of the retina. Used in the treatment of hypercholesterolemia, nicotinic acid can lead to cystoid macular edema without inflammation or leakage on fluorescein angiography. Digitalis and digoxin may cause blurred vision, color defects, and xanthopsia ("yellow vision") with normal-appearing fundus. Chronic ingestion of silver-containing compounds can lead to argyrosis, which can manifest itself as loss of normal choroidal markings, leopard-spot mottling, and a "dark" choroid on fluorescein angiography as a result of deposition of silver in Bruch's membrane. Oral contraceptives can predispose patients to vascular occlusions.

C. Deferoxamine, whether administered intravenously or subcutaneously, can lead to a maculopathy with decreased vision, color vision abnormalities, nyctalopia, and ring scotoma. Vision may return after cessation of the drug. Intracarotid injection of cisplatinum and/or carmustine for the treatment of malignant gliomas of the brain can lead to either a clinical picture of retinal infarction or pigmentary retinopathy. Patients who have received chemotherapy intravenously for bone marrow transplantation have developed retinopathy even without radiation to the orbit or brain. A clinical picture similar to acute macular neuroretinopathy has developed after IV injections of sympathomimetics and iodine-contrast dye.

D. The anesthetic inhalation agent methoxyflurane, when administered to patients with renal dysfunction over a prolonged period, can lead to oxalosis or the deposition of oxalate crystals throughout the posterior pole. Inhalation of methamphetamine and cocaine may be associated with amaurosis fugax, retinal vasculitis, retinal hemorrhages, cotton-wool patches, and retinal artery occlusion. These manifestations are presumably caused by the rapid increase in systemic blood pressure. Carbon monoxide retinopathy presents as superficial retinal hemorrhages, disc edema, or retinal venous engorgement and tortuosity. This may represent hypoxic damage to the vascular endothelium.

E. Patients receiving subcutaneous interferon-α2 for the treatment of systemic disorders (e.g. metastatic renal cell carcinoma, skin melanoma, Kaposi sarcoma), as well as for subretinal neovascular membranes can develop multiple cotton-wool patches and retinal hemorrhages. Deferoxamine administered subcutaneously can lead to a maculopathy with decreased vision, color vision abnormalities, nyctalopia, and ring scotoma.

F. Retinal toxicity can result from ocular medications or retained intraocular foreign bodies. Inadvertent injection of large doses of aminoglycosides into the anterior chamber after cataract surgery or even a previously considered safe dose of 200 micrograms for intravitreal injection of either amikacin or gentamicin in the treatment of endophthalmitis can lead to macular toxicity. Topical medications such as epinephrine, dipivefrin, and latanoprost used in the treatment of glaucoma have been noted to cause cystoid macular edema. After penetrating ocular injury, retained iron and copper can lead to siderosis and chalcosis, respectively.

G. Other local treatments away from the eye can also lead to retinal changes. Glycine is a substance used in irrigating fluid during transurethral resection of the prostate (TURP). Excessive systemic absorption can lead to transient visual loss lasting several hours with associated electroretinographic changes and a normal appearing fundus. This may be because of glycine's role as an inhibitory neurotransmitter. A hemorrhagic maculopathy has been noted after subarachnoid and epidural injections, with the presumed mechanism being the sudden increase of the retinal venous pressure transmitted from elevated CSF pressure.

H. Routine testing includes visual acuity, Amsler grid testing, and ophthalmoscopy on any patient taking or exposed to a drug that may cause retinal toxicity. Detailed studies, including color vision testing, electroretinography, electro-oculography, dark adaptation, IV fluorescein angiography and OCT may be helpful in some cases. Relative paracentral scotomas can be detected with a high degree of sensitivity using a red test object with static perimetry. Unfortunately, no single test is uniquely sensitive in detecting early retinal toxicity.

I. Visual function may improve with cessation of the drug at the earliest sign of retinopathy in the case of chloroquine or hydroxychloroquine. But even if these or other sight-threatening drugs are discontinued, visual defects may persist indefinitely or may progress.

J. Besides cessation of the suspected drug, there is no proven benefit of any therapy except the removal of the intraocular foreign body in the cases of siderosis and chalcosis.

K. Periodically examine the patients who take high dosages of chloroquine, hydroxychloroquine, thioridazine, or other medication for a long term for the development of retinal toxicity.

BIBLIOGRAPHY

1. Fraunfelder FT. Drug-induced Ocular Side Effects and Drug Interaction, 3rd Edition. Philadelphia, PA: Lea and Febiger. 1989.
2. Gass JDM. Stereoscopic Atlas of Macular Diseases Diagnosis and Treatment, 4th Edition. St Louis, MO: Mosby; 1997. pp. 775-808.
3. Grant WM. Toxicology of the Eye: Effects on the Eyes and Visual System from Chemicals, Drugs, Metals and Minerals, Plants, Toxins and Venoms: Also, Systemic Side Effects from Eye Medications, 3rd Edition. Springfield, IL: Thomas, 1986.
4. Swartz M. Other diseases: Drug toxicity and metabolic and nutritional conditions. In: Ryan SJ (Ed). Retina, 2nd Edition (Vol. 2). St Louis, MO: Mosby; 1994. pp. 1755-66.
5. Weinberg DV, D'Amico OJ. Retinal toxicity of systemic drugs. In: Albert OM, Jakobiec FA (Eds). Principles and Practice of Ophthalmology. Philadelphia, PA: WB Saunders; 1994. pp. 1042-50.

SECTION 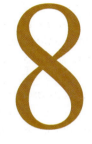 8

Uveitis

External Ocular Inflammation

133

Olga A Shif, Daniel A Johnson

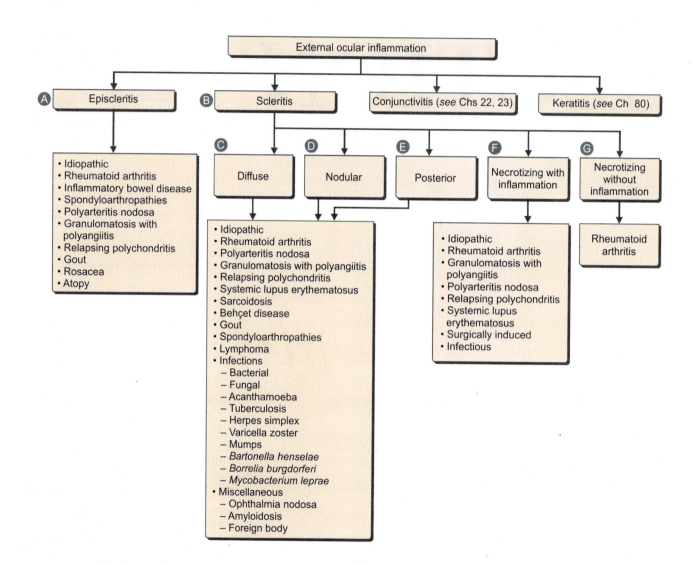

External ocular inflammation

A. Episcleritis
B. Scleritis
Conjunctivitis (*see* Chs 22, 23)
Keratitis (*see* Ch 80)

A. Episcleritis
- Idiopathic
- Rheumatoid arthritis
- Inflammatory bowel disease
- Spondyloarthropathies
- Polyarteritis nodosa
- Granulomatosis with polyangiitis
- Relapsing polychondritis
- Gout
- Rosacea
- Atopy

C. Diffuse / D. Nodular
- Idiopathic
- Rheumatoid arthritis
- Polyarteritis nodosa
- Granulomatosis with polyangiitis
- Relapsing polychondritis
- Systemic lupus erythematosus
- Sarcoidosis
- Behçet disease
- Gout
- Spondyloarthropathies
- Lymphoma
- Infections
  – Bacterial
  – Fungal
  – Acanthamoeba
  – Tuberculosis
  – Herpes simplex
  – Varicella zoster
  – Mumps
  – *Bartonella henselae*
  – *Borrelia burgdorferi*
  – *Mycobacterium leprae*
- Miscellaneous
  – Ophthalmia nodosa
  – Amyloidosis
  – Foreign body

E. Posterior

F. Necrotizing with inflammation
- Idiopathic
- Rheumatoid arthritis
- Granulomatosis with polyangiitis
- Polyarteritis nodosa
- Relapsing polychondritis
- Systemic lupus erythematosus
- Surgically induced
- Infectious

G. Necrotizing without inflammation
- Rheumatoid arthritis

Patients with external ocular inflammation often present with a red eye and symptoms that may include pain, itching, tearing, and photosensitivity. The inflammation may involve the cornea, conjunctiva, episclera, and/or sclera. Corneal and conjunctival inflammatory conditions are discussed elsewhere in this text.

The episclera is composed of connective tissue, which includes Tenon capsule and a superficial vascular plexus. The sclera consists of thick collagenous tissue, which is supplied by a deep vascular plexus. Either or both vascular plexuses may become engorged when inflamed. Recognizing the key features of scleritis and episcleritis allows the clinician to distinguish these processes from one another and from the superficial inflammatory response of the conjunctiva and cornea. An accurate diagnosis is important to identify potentially lethal systemic associations, to initiate therapy, and to provide meaningful prognostic information.

A. Episcleritis is typically a self-limited, painless inflammatory condition affecting the radial superficial episcleral vessels. Visual acuity is usually preserved. The inflammation may be diffuse (simple) or nodular. Episcleritis may be associated with systemic diseases in up to 30% of the cases. Topical 10% phenylephrine will blanch the inflamed episcleral vessels but not the deeper vessels, and is useful to distinguish episcleritis from scleritis. The coloration of episcleritis is usually bright red, whereas that of scleritis is more violaceous. A laboratory evaluation is recommended in patients with episcleritis if the patient's review of systems is suggestive of a systemic disease, if the inflammation does not improve with treatment, or if it recurs. Episcleritis may resolve spontaneously. Since ocular complications are rare, treatment is often not necessary. Chilled artificial tears, topical corticosteroids, and topical nonsteroidal anti-inflammatory drops may be effective. Systemic therapy with nonsteroidal anti-inflammatory drugs (NSAIDs) and systemic corticosteroids, while effective, generally is not necessary.

B. Deeper and potentially more destructive inflammation is a feature of scleritis. Edema of episcleral and scleral tissues as well as injection of the superficial and deep episcleral vessels is usually present. Blanching of the deep vessels is typically not seen with 10% phenylephrine drops and, as noted, can help to differentiate scleritis from episcleritis. Scleritis is often accompanied by severe boring or piercing pain that may awaken the patient at night. Tenderness is common and gentle pressure on the eyelid during an examination will often elicit pain with scleritis but not with episcleritis. Scleritis often results from immune-mediated vasculitis and without proper treatment can lead to scleral thinning and even perforation. Ocular complications including glaucoma, keratitis, and uveitis are common. A correct systemic diagnosis is necessary to reduce long-term morbidity. As a result, a full physical examination and directed laboratory evaluation are recommended. A grading system for scleritis has been described in which the degree of ocular surface inflammation is graded following the application of 10% phenylephrine. The inflammation is recorded as "0" (complete blanching), "+0.5" (localized, minimally dilated, deep episcleral vessels), "+1" (diffuse, mildly dilated episcleral vessels), "+2" (moderate, significantly tortuous, and engorged deep episcleral vessels), "+3" (severe, diffuse redness with indistinguishable details of superficial and deep vessels), or "+4" (necrotizing, diffuse redness with scleral thinning).

Initial treatment includes systemic NSAIDs such as indomethacin or flurbiprofen, then, if control is inadequate, oral corticosteroids. The use of subtenon injections of triamcinolone in patients with non-necrotizing, noninfectious anterior scleritis has been reported, but has not gained widespread acceptance due to the historic concerns of scleral perforation. Immunomodulatory therapy may be required for recalcitrant diseases or to allow reduction in the dose of oral corticosteroids. Immunomodulatory therapy is usually recommended for noninfectious, necrotizing scleritis.

C. Anterior scleritis (Fig. 133.1) can present with either diffuse or focal involvement, is most common in women, and in patients in the fifth decade of their life. With resolution, the affected sclera can take on a slate gray or brown appearance due to scleral thinning, which allows visualization of the underlying pigmented choroid (Fig. 133.2).

D. Nodular anterior scleritis presents as an immobile area of focal scleral thickening that has the appearance of a nodule. Multiple nodules may be present and may coalesce into one larger lesion. An association between nodular scleritis and a history of herpes zoster ophthalmicus has been identified. More than 10% of patients with nodular scleritis progress to necrotizing scleritis. Systemic therapy with oral NSAIDs is often effective in the management of nodular scleritis.

E. Often considered a variant of idiopathic orbital inflammatory syndrome, posterior scleritis can present with pain, photophobia, redness, proptosis, and lower eyelid retraction on upgaze. Involvement of the anterior segment may occur. Exudative retinal

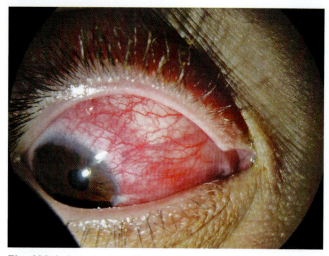

Fig. 133.1: Anterior scleritis. Note deep vascular engorgement.

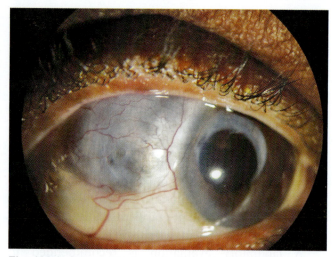

Fig. 133.2: Scleral thinning following anterior scleritis.

detachment, myositis, uveal effusion, choroidal folds, and disc edema are features. Early diagnosis is critical to prevent vision loss. Ultrasonography reveals a characteristic "T sign" formed by a collection of fluid in the subtenon space. Posterior scleral thickening and proptosis seen on computed tomography (CT) scanning further support the diagnosis.

F. Necrotizing scleritis with inflammation is often associated with severe pain. It can begin as nodular scleritis with deep vascular congestion. In later stages of the disease, an avascular edematous region of sclera is seen surrounded by an area of inflammation. Without treatment, areas of scleral thinning develop a blue-gray or brownish appearance due to progressive scleral thinning that may ultimately perforate. Ocular complications are common and may result in partial or total loss of vision. Marginal keratitis and anterior uveitis suggest aggressive disease. Extraocular morbidity of necrotizing scleritis demonstrates a strong correlation with rheumatoid arthritis (RA), granulomatosis with polyangiitis (formerly Wegener granulomatosis), and other vasculitides. A complete physical examination of the skin, joints, heart, and lungs can provide clues to systemic associations. Rheumatologic laboratory

workup should be obtained. Necrotizing scleritis frequently requires a more aggressive approach to treatment, which includes systemic corticosteroids and immunomodulatory therapy. Areas of scleral thinning may require surgical reinforcement.

G. Necrotizing scleritis without inflammation, also known as scleromalacia perforans, is most often associated with RA. The typical signs and symptoms of inflammation such as redness, pain, and swelling are usually not present. Areas of scleral thinning with exposure of uveal tissue are often identified. Scleral rupture can result from minimal trauma to the globe.

BIBLIOGRAPHY

1. Akpek EK, Thorne JE, Qazi FA, et al. Evaluation of patients with scleritis for systemic disease. Ophthalmology. 2004;111:501-6.
2. Jabs DA, Mudun A, Dunn JP, et al. Episcleritis and scleritis: Clinical features and treatment results. Am J Ophthalmol. 2000; 130:469-76.
3. Sen NH, Sangave AA, Goldstein DA, et al. A standardized grading system for scleritis. Ophthalmology. 2011; 118:768-71.
4. Sohn EH, Wang R, Read R, et al. Long-term, multicenter evaluation of subconjunctival injection of triamcinolone for non-necrotizing, noninfectious anterior scleritis. Ophthalmology. 2011;118:1932-37.

134

Anterior Uveitis

Daniel A Johnson

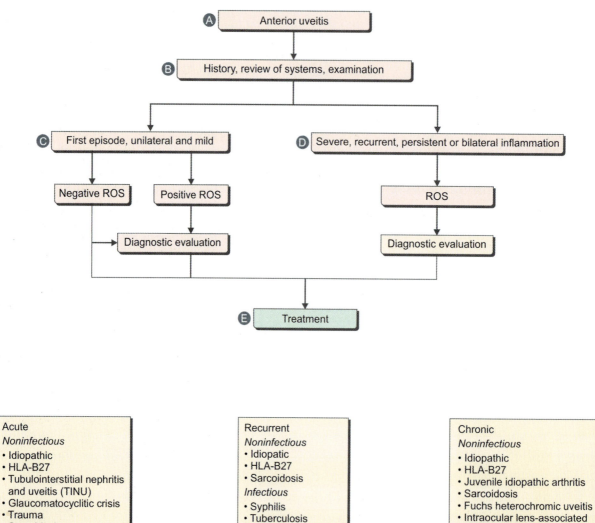

Acute
Noninfectious
- Idiopathic
- HLA-B27
- Tubulointerstitial nephritis and uveitis (TINU)
- Glaucomatocyclitic crisis
- Trauma
- Sarcoidosis
Infectious
- Syphilis
- Tuberculosis
- Brucellosis
- Viral (CMV, HSV, VZV)
Masquerade
- Leukemia
- Retinoblastoma
- Drug-related

Recurrent
Noninfectious
- Idiopatic
- HLA-B27
- Sarcoidosis
Infectious
- Syphilis
- Tuberculosis
- Brucellosis
- Viral (CMV, HSV, VZV)
Masquerade
- Leukemia

Chronic
Noninfectious
- Idiopathic
- HLA-B27
- Juvenile idiopathic arthritis
- Sarcoidosis
- Fuchs heterochromic uveitis
- Intraocular lens-associated
- Vogt-Koyanagi-Harada
Infectious
- Syphilis
- Tuberculosis
- Brucellosis
- Viral (CMV, HSV, VZV)
Masquerade
- Ocular ischemia
- Leukemia
- Retinoblastoma

A. Anterior uveitis (Table 134.1) is defined as inflammation in which the primary site of inflammation is in the anterior chamber, and accounts for approximately 60% of cases of uveitis. Symptoms often include pain, decreased vision, and photophobia; however, the process may be asymptomatic. Signs include anterior chamber cell with or without perilimbal redness, pupillary constriction (miosis), posterior synechiae, band keratopathy, and inflammatory deposits on the corneal endothelium (keratic precipitates) or in the anterior chamber (nodules). Keratic precipitates can be small and fine, medium, or large and greasy (also known as "mutton fat" keratic precipitates).

Table 134.1: Anterior Uveitis. Onset—sudden (S), insidious (I); Course—acute (A), recurrent (R), chronic (C); Keratic precipitates (KP)—granulomatous (G), non-granulomatous (NG); Intraocular pressure (IOP)—low (L), high (H); Laterality—unilateral (U), bilateral (B). Polymerase chain reaction (PCR)

Etiology	Onset (S,I)	Course (A,R,C)	Hypopyon	KP	Intraocular pressure	Laterality	Evaluation	Notes
NONINFECTIOUS								
HLA-B27	S	A,R	Y, N	NG	L	U	HLA-B27	Episodes unilateral but can affect both eyes at different times. Low back stiffness, plantar fasciitis, Achilles tendinitis.
Juvenile idiopathic arthritis (JIA)	I	C	N	NG	Variable	B	Clinical diagnosis, anti-nuclear antibody (ANA), rheumatology consultation	Often asymptomatic. Band keratopathy, posterior synechiae.
Tubulointerstitial nephritis and uveitis (TINU)	S	A	N	NG	Variable	B	Urinalysis, blood urea nitrogen (BUN), creatinine	Systemic symptoms (fever, myalgias, arthralgias, fatigue) may precede uveitis. Hematuria, proteinuria.
Traumatic	S	A	N	NG	L	U	Clinical diagnosis	History of trauma.
Sarcoidosis	S,I	A,R,C	Usually N	G, NG	L	U, B	Tissue diagnosis, chest imaging, gallium scan, angiotensin converting enzyme (ACE), lysozyme, anergy, liver function tests	Shortness or breath, cutaneous nodules, lacrimal gland enlargement.
Behçet disease	S	A,R,C	Y, N	NG	L	U, B	Clinical diagnosis, HLA-B5	Oral, genital ulcers.
Fuchs Heterochromic Iridocyclitis	I	C	N	NG, stellate	H	U	Clinical diagnosis, aqueous PCR	Rubella implicated. Iris heterochromia, posterior subcapsular cataract, secondary open angle glaucoma. Posterior synechiae uncommon.
Glaucomatocyclitic crisis/ Posner-Schlossman Syndrome	S	R	N	N	H	U	Clinical diagnosis	Low grade inflammation, elevated IOP (40–70 mm Hg), iris heterochromia.

Contd...

Contd...

Etiology	Onset (S,I)	Course (A,R,C)	Hypopyon	KP	Intraocular pressure	Laterality	Evaluation	Notes
INFECTIOUS								
Syphilis	S, I	A	Usually N	G, NG	L	U, B	Treponemal or Non-treponemal serology, Lumbar puncture	Intravenous penicillin as for neurosyphilis.
Herpes simplex virus (HSV)	S, I	A,R,C	Y, N	G, NG, stellate	Variable	U	Clinical diagnosis, aqueous PCR	Sector iris atrophy, keratitis, secondary glaucoma, hyphema.
Varicella-zoster virus (VZV)	S, I	A,R,C	Usually N	G, NG, stellate	Variable	U	Clinical diagnosis, aqueous PCR	Herpes zoster ophthalmicus (HZO), sector iris atrophy, keratitis, secondary glaucoma, hyphema.
Cytomegalovirus (CMV)	S, I	A,R,C	Usually N	G, NG, fine	Variable	U	Clinical diagnosis, aqueous PCR	Sector iris atrophy and posterior synechiae uncommon.
Tuberculosis	S, I	A,C	N	G, NG	Variable	U, B	Interferon gamma release assay, purified protein derivative (PPD), chest imaging	Rare cause of uveitis in the USA.

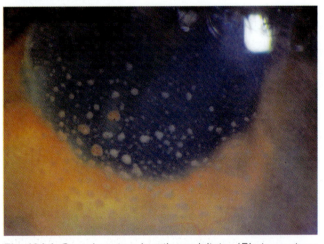

Fig. 134.1: Granulomatous keratic precipitates (*Photo courtesy:* Carrie Cooke).

Granulomatous keratic precipitates (Fig. 134.1) can be seen in lens-induced uveitis, sarcoidosis, syphilis, and tuberculosis. Anterior chamber nodules are named "Koeppe" if at the pupillary margin, "Busacca" if on the iris surface, and "Berlin" if in the anterior chamber angle.

The Standardization of Uveitis Nomenclature Working Group clarified the terminology used to describe uveitis. Anterior uveitis onset is defined as "sudden" or "insidious." Its duration is described as "limited" if it lasts equal to or less than 3 months, or "persistent" if it lasts more than 3 months. Its course is defined as "acute" if it is of sudden onset and limited duration, "recurrent" if it returns in 3 or more months *without* therapy, and "chronic" if it returns in less than 3 months *without* therapy. The grading of anterior chamber cell is based on the number of cells in an average 1×1 mm^2 slit-lamp beam as follows: 0 (<1 cell), 0.5+ (1–5 cells), 1+ (6–15 cells), 2+ (16–25 cells), 3+ (26–50 cells), and 4+ (>50 cells). Anterior chamber flare is graded as 0 (none), 1+ (faint), 2+ (moderate; iris and lens details clear), 3+ (marked; iris and lens details hazy), and 4+ (intense; fibrin).

B. Evaluation of patients with anterior uveitis starts with a thorough history and review of systems, with emphasis on symptoms suggestive of autoimmune diseases. Low back pain or stiffness, plantar fasciitis, and Achilles tendinitis raise the suspicion for a spondyloarthropathy. Oral or genital ulcers and arthritis raise the suspicion for Behçet disease. Other important review items include shortness of breath for sarcoidosis and a history of sexually transmitted diseases for syphilis. A list of the patient's medications should be reviewed since certain medications have been associated with anterior uveitis such as brimonidine, cidofovir, etanercept, metipranolol, and rifabutin.

C. Mild, first episodes of anterior uveitis of limited duration with preserved visual acuity and a negative review of symptoms do not necessarily require additional diagnostic testing.

D. More severe, bilateral, persistent or recurrent disease, or in patients with symptoms suggestive of a systemic disorder should undergo additional diagnostic studies. At a minimum, a chest X-ray and syphilis serology should be obtained. Additional studies based on the history may include HLA-B27, interferon-gamma release assay, urinalysis, and serology for bartonellosis and brucellosis. Angiotensin-converting enzyme and lysozyme are obtained by many to evaluate for sarcoidosis; however, definitive diagnosis of this condition requires biopsy. Although tuberculosis is considered a rare cause of uveitis, evaluation for this condition is recommended in the event that systemic immunosuppressive therapy is required to control the uveitis. Analysis of aqueous fluid (polymerase chain reaction/PCR or antibody assays) may be considered to assess for viral uveitis (cytomegalovirus, varicella-zoster virus, herpes simplex virus, rubella).

E. The therapy for noninfectious anterior uveitis generally consists of topical steroids to control the inflammation, and a cycloplegic agent to reduce the risk of synechiae (Fig. 134.2) forming between the iris and lens. Severe cases that are not responsive to topical steroids may require periocular steroid injections and/or oral steroids. Due to the risks associated with the use of chronic systemic corticosteroids, steroid-sparing immunomodulatory therapy should be considered for patients requiring chronic systemic immunosuppression.

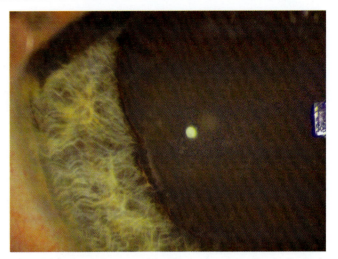

Fig. 134.2: Posterior synechia (*Photo courtesy:* Carrie Cooke).

Children should not be maintained on chronic oral steroids due to the risk of growth retardation. Therapy for infectious uveitis is dependent upon the infection identified.

BIBLIOGRAPHY

1. Amaratunge BC, Camuglia JE. Syphilitic uveitis: A review of clinical manifestations and treatment outcomes of syphilitic uveitis in human immunodeficiency virus-positive and negative patients. Clin Exp Ophthalmol. 2010;38:68-74.
2. Barisani-Asenbauer T, Maca SM, Mejdoubi L, et al. Uveitis—a rare disease often associated with systemic diseases and infections—a systematic review of 2619 patients. Orphanet J Rare Dis. 2012;7:1-7.
3. Baughman RP, Lowder EE, Kaufman AH. Ocular sarcoidosis. Sem Resp Crit Care Med. 2010;31:452-62.
4. Cunningham ET. The expanding spectrum of viral anterior uveitis. Ophthalmology. 2011;118:1903-4.
5. El-Asrar AM, Abouammoh M, Al-Mezaine HS. Tuberculous uveitis. Int Ophthalmol Clin. 2010;50: 19-39.
6. Jabs DA, Nussenblatt RB, Rosenbaum JT, et al. Standardization of uveitis nomenclature for reporting clinical data. Results of the First International Workshop. Am J Ophthalmol. 2005; 140:509-16.
7. Qian Y, Acharya NR. Juvenile idiopathic arthritis-associated uveitis. Curr Opin Ophthalmol. 2010;2: 468-72.
8. Siddique SS, Suelves AM, Baheti U, et al. Glaucoma and uveitis. Surv Ophthalmol. 2013;58:1-10.
9. Wendling D. Uveitis in seronegative arthritis. Curr Rheumatol Rep. 2012;14:402-8.

Intermediate Uveitis

135

Daniel A Johnson

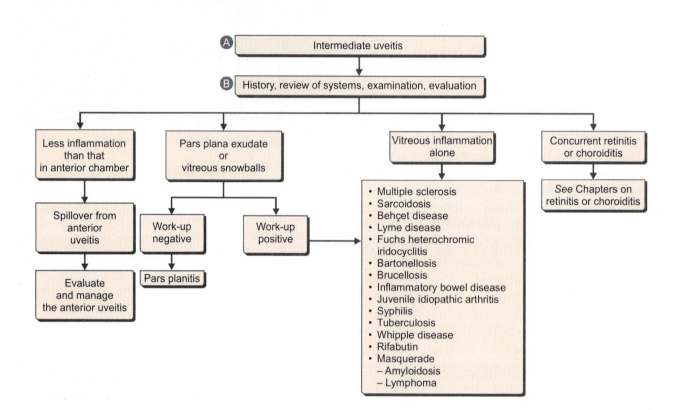

A. Intermediate uveitis is defined as inflammation in which the primary site of inflammation is in the vitreous cavity, and accounts for approximately 15% of the cases of uveitis. Peripheral vascular sheathing may or may not be present and is not required for the diagnosis. Idiopathic intermediated uveitis, in which there is a snowbank or vitreous snowballs (Fig. 135.1), is termed *pars planitis*.

Symptoms include decreased vision and floaters. Pain is not usually present. Signs include anterior chamber cell with or without perilimbal redness, vitreous cell, and vitreous debris. Peripheral retinal vascular sheathing, a snowbank, and vitreous snowballs may or may not be present. There is no consensus regarding the standardization of the vitreous cell; however, the Standardization of Uveitis Nomenclature Group accepted the vitreous haze grading of Nussenblatt et al., with the modification

of changing the "trace" to "0.5+." Vitreous haze (Fig. 135.2) is graded on a scale of "0" to "4+" as viewed with a 20 diopter lens and an indirect ophthalmoscope on mid power as follows: 0 (no haze), 0.5+ (slight blurring of optic nerve margin and retina), 1+ (optic nerve and retinal blood vessels visible but hazy), 2+ (optic nerve and retinal blood vessels visible but poorly defined), 3+ (optic nerve visible but poorly defined, retinal vessels poorly visualized), and 4+ (optic nerve and retinal blood vessels not visualized). Terminology related to uveitis onset, duration, and course, as defined by the Standardization of Uveitis Nomenclature Working Group, is described in the chapter on Anterior Uveitis.

B. Evaluation of patients with intermediate uveitis starts with a thorough history and review of systems. The history of a tick bite in endemic areas

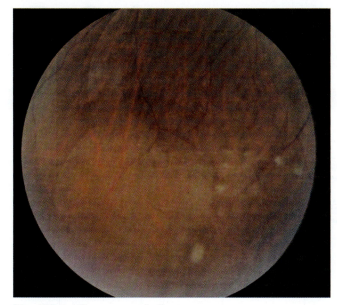

Fig. 135.1: Vitreous snowballs.

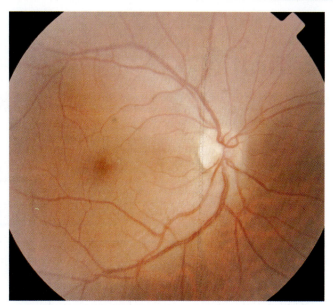

Fig. 135.2: Vitreous haze.

for Lyme disease should be sought, as well as episodes of neurologic dysfunction, which could indicate multiple sclerosis. Other important review items include shortness of breath for sarcoidosis and a history of sexually transmitted diseases for syphilis. Oral or genital ulcers and arthritis raise the suspicion for Behçet disease.

Diagnostic evaluation of patients with intermediate uveitis should include, at a minimum, a chest X-ray and syphilis serology. Additional studies based on the history may include HLA-B5, interferon-gamma release assay, serology for Lyme disease, bartonellosis, and brucellosis, and neuroimaging. Angiotensin-converting enzyme and lysozyme are obtained by many to evaluate for sarcoidosis; however, definitive diagnosis of this condition requires biopsy. Although tuberculosis is considered a rare cause of uveitis, evaluation for this condition is recommended in the event that systemic immunosuppressive therapy is required to control the uveitis.

The therapy for noninfectious intermediate uveitis generally consists of systemic, intraocular or periocular steroids, and/or immunomodulatory therapy. Administration of a cycloplegic agent to reduce the risk of synechiae forming between the iris and lens is recommended. Due to the risks associated with the use of chronic systemic corticosteroids, steroid sparing immunomodulatory

therapy should be considered for patients with chronic disease. Children should not be maintained on chronic oral steroids due to the risk of growth retardation. Therapy for infectious uveitis is dependent upon the infection identified.

BIBLIOGRAPHY

1. Amaratunge BC, Camuglia JE. Syphilitic uveitis: A review of clinical manifestations and treatment outcomes of syphilitic uveitis in human immunodeficiency virus-positive and negative patients. Clin Exp Ophthalmol. 2010;38:68-74.
2. Barisani-Asenbauer T, Maca SM, Mejdoubi L, et al. Uveitis–a rare disease often associated with systemic diseases and infections–a systematic review of 2619 patients. Orphanet J Rare Dis. 2012;7:1-7.
3. Baughman RP, Lowder EE, Kaufman AH. Ocular sarcoidosis. Sem Resp Crit Care Med. 2010;31:452-62.
4. El-Asrar AM, Abouammoh M, Al-Mezaine HS. Tuberculous uveitis. Int Ophthalmol Clin. 2010;50:19-39.
5. Jabs DA, Nussenblatt RB, Rosenbaum JT, et al. Standardization of uveitis nomenclature for reporting clinical data. Results of the First International Workshop. Am J Ophthalmol. 2005; 140:509-16.
6. Nussenblatt RB, Palestine AG, Chan CC, et al. Standardization of vitreal inflammatory activity in intermediate and posterior uveitis. Ophthalmology. 1985;92:467-71.
7. Qian Y, Acharya NR. Juvenile idiopathic arthritis-associated uveitis. Curr Opin Ophthalmol. 2010;2:468-72.
8. Sauberan DP. Pediatric uveitis. Int Ophthalmol Clin. 2010; 50:73-85.

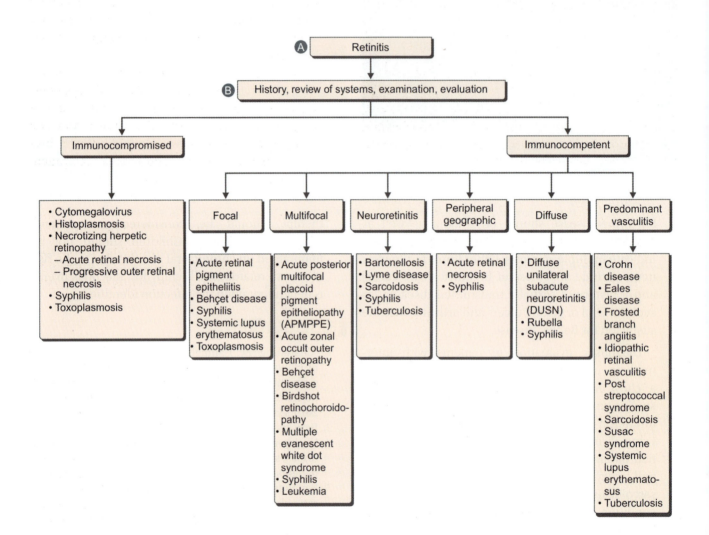

Figure:

- **A** Retinitis
- **B** History, review of systems, examination, evaluation

Immunocompromised
- Cytomegalovirus
- Histoplasmosis
- Necrotizing herpetic retinopathy
  - Acute retinal necrosis
  - Progressive outer retinal necrosis
- Syphilis
- Toxoplasmosis

Immunocompetent

Focal
- Acute retinal pigment epitheliitis
- Behçet disease
- Syphilis
- Systemic lupus erythematosus
- Toxoplasmosis

Multifocal
- Acute posterior multifocal placoid pigment epitheliopathy (APMPPE)
- Acute zonal occult outer retinopathy
- Behçet disease
- Birdshot retinochoroidopathy
- Multiple evanescent white dot syndrome
- Syphilis
- Leukemia

Neuroretinitis
- Bartonellosis
- Lyme disease
- Sarcoidosis
- Syphilis
- Tuberculosis

Peripheral geographic
- Acute retinal necrosis
- Syphilis

Diffuse
- Diffuse unilateral subacute neuroretinitis (DUSN)
- Rubella
- Syphilis

Predominant vasculitis
- Crohn disease
- Eales disease
- Frosted branch angiitis
- Idiopathic retinal vasculitis
- Post streptococcal syndrome
- Sarcoidosis
- Susac syndrome
- Systemic lupus erythematosus
- Tuberculosis

A. Retinitis (Fig. 136.1) is defined as inflammation in which the primary site of inflammation is the retina. Symptoms may include decreased vision, floaters, photopsia, and scotomata. Signs include anterior chamber cell, vitreous cell, vitreous debris, retinal infiltrates, arteritis or periphlebitis. The grading of any associated vitreous haze is described in the chapter on Intermediate Uveitis. Terminology related to uveitis onset, duration, and course, as defined by the Standardization of Uveitis Nomenclature Working Group, is described in the chapter on anterior uveitis.

B. Evaluation of patients with retinitis starts with a thorough history, review of systems, and ocular examination. Many causes of retinitis are diagnosed by clinical examination. A history of prior varicella-zoster virus infection and a tick bite in endemic areas for Lyme disease should be sought.

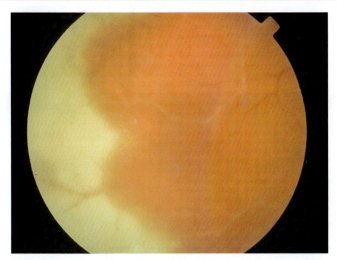

Fig. 136.1: Acute retinal necrosis. Note necrotizing retinitis, retinal vasculitis, and vitreous inflammation.

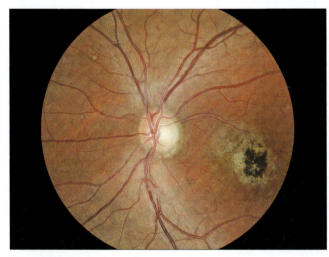

Fig. 136.2: Retinal scar from toxoplasmosis.

Other important review items include shortness of breath for sarcoidosis and a history of sexually transmitted diseases for syphilis.

Diagnostic evaluation of patients with retinitis should include, at a minimum, a chest X-ray and syphilis serology. Additional studies based on the history may include HLA-B5, interferon-gamma release assay, and serology for Lyme disease, bartonellosis, and brucellosis. Angiotensin-converting enzyme and lysozyme are obtained by many to evaluate for sarcoidosis; however, definitive diagnosis of this condition requires biopsy. Although tuberculosis is considered a rare cause of uveitis, evaluation for this condition is recommended in the event that systemic immunosuppressive therapy is required to control the uveitis. Analysis of aqueous or vitreous fluid (polymerase chain reaction/PCR or antibody assays) may be considered to assess for certain causes of infectious retinitis (cytomegalovirus, varicella-zoster virus, herpes simplex virus, toxoplasmosis).

The therapy for noninfectious retinitis (Fig. 136.2) generally consists of systemic, intraocular or periocular steroids, and/or immunomodulatory therapy. Administration of a cycloplegic agent to reduce the risk of synechiae forming between the iris and lens is recommended. Due to the risks associated with the use of chronic systemic corticosteroids, steroid-sparing immunomodulatory therapy should be considered for patients with chronic disease. Children should not be maintained on chronic oral steroids due to the risk of growth retardation. Therapy for infectious retinitis is dependent upon the infection identified.

BIBLIOGRAPHY

1. Amaratunge BC, Camuglia JE. Syphilitic uveitis: A review of clinical manifestations and treatment outcomes of syphilitic uveitis in human immunodeficiency virus-positive and negative patients. Clin Exp Ophthalmol. 2010;38:68-74.
2. Baughman RP, Lowder EE, Kaufman AH. Ocular sarcoidosis. Sem Resp Crit Care Med. 2010;31:452-62.
3. Bhaleeya SD, Davis J. Imaging retinal vascular changes in uveitis. Int Ophthalmol Clin. 2012;52:83-96.
4. El-Asrar AM, Abouammoh M, Al-Mezaine HS. Tuberculous uveitis. Int Ophthalmol Clin. 2010;50: 19-39.
5. Jabs DA, Nussenblatt RB, Rosenbaum JT, et al. Standardization of uveitis nomenclature for reporting clinical data. Results of the First International Workshop. Am J Ophthalmol. 2005; 140:509-16.
6. Nussenblatt RB, Palestine AG, Chan CC, et al. Standardization of vitreal inflammatory activity in intermediate and posterior uveitis. Ophthalmology. 1985;92:467-71.
7. Sauberan DP. Pediatric uveitis. Int Ophthalmol Clin. 2010; 50:73-85.

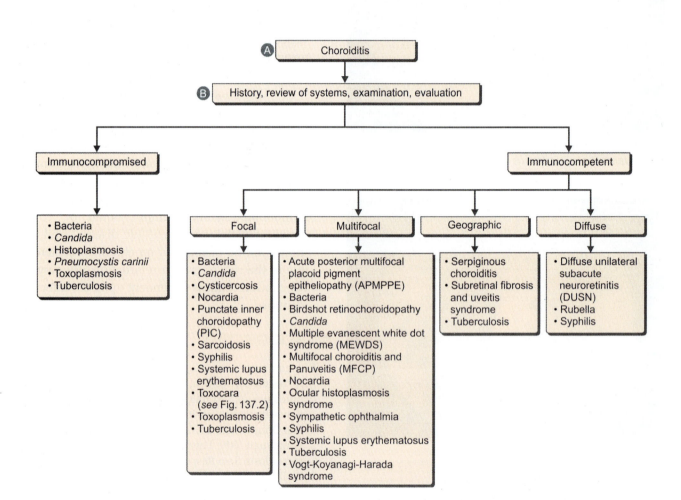

A. Choroiditis is defined as inflammation in which the primary site of inflammation is the choroid. *Symptoms* may include decreased vision, floaters, photopsia, metamorphopsia, and scotomata. *Signs* include anterior chamber cell, vitreous cell, vitreous debris, retinal infiltrates, choroidal infiltrates (Fig. 137.1), arteritis, or periphlebitis. The grading of any associated vitreous haze is described in the chapter on intermediate uveitis. Terminology related to uveitis onset, duration, and course, as defined by the Standardization of Uveitis

Nomenclature Working Group, is described in the chapter on Anterior Uveitis.

B. Evaluation of patients with choroiditis starts with a thorough history, review of systems, and ocular examination. Many causes of choroiditis are diagnosed by clinical examination. Since metastatic infection or neoplasia can present with choroidal involvement, an assessment of the patient's overall health is necessary. Other important review items include shortness of breath for sarcoidosis and a history of sexually transmitted diseases for syphilis.

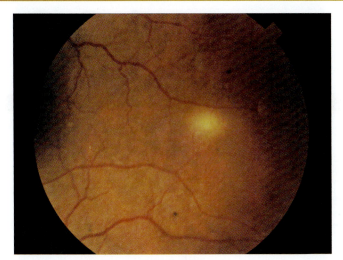

Fig. 137.1: Staphylococcal choroiditis.

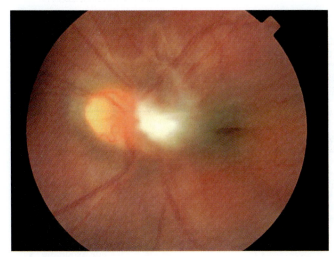

Fig. 137.2: Toxocara choroiditis.

Diagnostic evaluation of patients with choroiditis should include, at a minimum, a chest X-ray and syphilis serology. Additional studies based on the history may include HLA-B5, interferon-gamma release assay, blood cultures, and serology for Lyme disease, bartonellosis, and brucellosis. Angiotensin-converting enzyme and lysozyme are obtained by many to evaluate for sarcoidosis; however,

definitive diagnosis of this condition requires biopsy. Although tuberculosis is considered a rare cause of uveitis, evaluation for this condition is recommended in the event when systemic immunosuppressive therapy is required to control the uveitis.

The therapy for noninfectious choroiditis generally consists of systemic, intraocular or periocular steroids, and/or immunomodulatory therapy. Administration of a cycloplegic agent to reduce the risk of synechiae forming between the iris and lens is recommended. Due to the risks associated with the use of chronic systemic corticosteroids, steroid-sparing immunomodulatory therapy should be considered for patients with chronic disease. Children should not be maintained on chronic oral steroids due to the risk of growth retardation. Therapy for infectious choroiditis is dependent upon the infection identified.

BIBLIOGRAPHY

1. Amaratunge BC, Camuglia JE. Syphilitic uveitis: a review of clinical manifestations and treatment outcomes of syphilitic uveitis in human immunodeficiency virus-positive and negative patients. Clin Exp Ophthalmol. 2010;38:68-74.
2. Baughman RP, Lowder EE, Kaufman AH. Ocular sarcoidosis. Sem Resp Crit Care Med. 2010;31:452-62.
3. El-Asrar AM, Abouammoh M, Al-Mezaine HS. Tuberculous uveitis. Int Ophthalmol Clin. 2010;50: 19-39.
4. Jabs DA, Nussenblatt RB, Rosenbaum JT, et al. Standardization of uveitis nomenclature for reporting clinical data. Results of the First International Workshop. Am J Ophthalmol. 2005;140:509-16.
5. Mrejen S, Spaide RF. Imaging the choroid in uveitis. Int Ophthalmol Clin. 2012;52:67-81.
6. Nussenblatt RB, Palestine AG, Chan CC, et al. Standardization of vitreal inflammatory activity in intermediate and posterior uveitis. Ophthalmol. 1985; 92:467-71.
7. Sauberan DP. Pediatric uveitis. Int Ophthalmol Clin. 2010;50:73-85.

Panuveitis

138

Daniel A Johnson

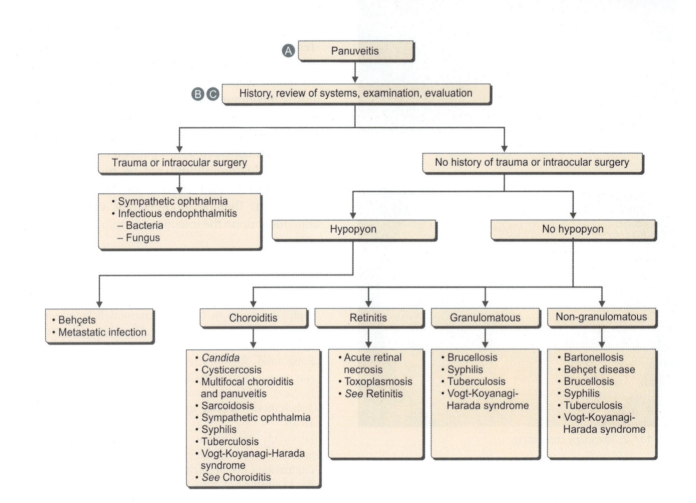

A. Panuveitis is defined as inflammation in which all segments of the eye are affected similarly, including the anterior chamber, vitreous, and the retina and/or choroid, and accounts for approximately 7% of cases of uveitis. *Symptoms* may include pain, photophobia, conjunctival injection, decreased vision, floaters, and photopsia. *Signs* include anterior chamber cell, vitreous cell, vitreous debris, and evidence of retinitis and/or choroiditis. The grading of any associated vitreous haze is described in the chapter on Intermediate Uveitis.

Terminology related to uveitis onset, duration, and course, as defined by the Standardization of Uveitis Nomenclature Working Group, is described in the chapter on Anterior Uveitis.

B. Evaluation of patients with panuveitis starts with a thorough history, review of systems, and ocular examination. Oral or genital ulcers and arthritis raise the suspicion for Behçet disease. Other important review items include shortness of breath for sarcoidosis (Fig. 138.1) and a history of sexually transmitted diseases for syphilis. Bilateral

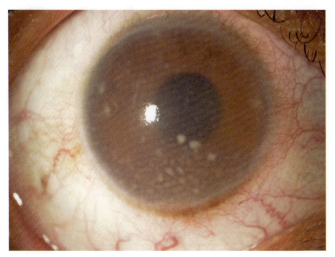

Fig. 138.1: Granulomatous panuveitis in a patient with sarcoidosis.

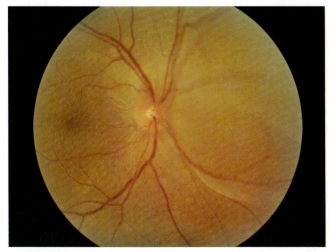

Fig. 138.2: Vogt–Koyanagi–Harada—serous retinal detachment.

serous retinal detachments are suggestive of Vogt-Koyanagi-Harada syndrome (Fig. 138.2).

C. Diagnostic evaluation of patients with panuveitis should include, at a minimum, a chest X-ray and syphilis serology. Additional studies based on the history may include blood cultures, HLA-B5, interferon-gamma release assay, and serology for Lyme disease, bartonellosis, and brucellosis. Angiotensin-converting enzyme and lysozyme are obtained by many to evaluate for sarcoidosis; however, definitive diagnosis of this condition requires biopsy. Although tuberculosis is considered a rare cause of uveitis, evaluation for this condition is recommended in the event that systemic immunosuppressive therapy is required to control the uveitis.

The therapy for noninfectious panuveitis generally consists of systemic or intraocular steroids. Administration of a cycloplegic agent to reduce the risk of synechiae forming between the iris and lens is recommended. Due to the risks associated with the use of chronic systemic corticosteroids, steroid-sparing immunomodulatory therapy should be considered for patients with chronic disease. Children should not be maintained on chronic oral steroids due to the risk of growth retardation. Therapy for infectious panuveitis is dependent upon the infection identified.

BIBLIOGRAPHY

1. Amaratunge BC, Camuglia JE. Syphilitic uveitis: a review of clinical manifestations and treatment outcomes of syphilitic uveitis in human immunodeficiency virus-positive and negative patients. Clin Exp Ophthalmol. 2010;38:68-74.
2. Barisani-Asenbauer T, Maca SM, Mejdoubi L, et al. Uveitis: a rare disease often associated with systemic diseases and infections: a systematic review of 2619 patients. Orphanet J Rare Dis. 2012;7:1-7.
3. Baughman RP, Lowder EE, Kaufman AH. Ocular sarcoidosis. Sem Resp Crit Care Med. 2010;31:452-62.
4. El-Asrar AM, Abouammoh M, Al-Mezaine HS. Tuberculous uveitis. Int Ophthalmol Clin. 2010;50: 19-39.
5. Jabs DA, Nussenblatt RB, Rosenbaum JT, et al. Standardization of uveitis nomenclature for reporting clinical data: results of the First International Workshop. Am J Ophthalmol. 2005; 140:509-16.
6. Nussenblatt RB, Palestine AG, Chan CC, et al. Standardization of vitreal inflammatory activity in intermediate and posterior uveitis. Ophthalmol. 1985; 92:467-71.
7. Sauberan DP. Pediatric uveitis. Int Ophthalmol Clin. 2010; 50:73-85.

Local Ocular Therapy

139

Steven R Cohen, Daniel A Johnson

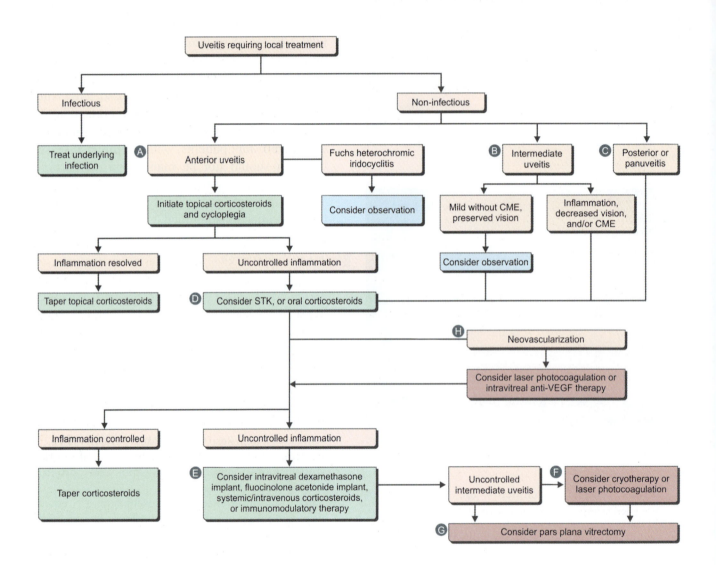

The broad-spectrum of disease processes associated with uveitis results in a variety of treatment options ranging from observation to surgical intervention to systemic immunosuppression. In all cases of uveitis, infection must be excluded. Any underlying infection that is identified should be treated. Treatment of infectious uveitis with corticosteroids alone can result in significant ocular morbidity. The most common therapy for noninfectious uveitis is corticosteroids, whether administered topically, periocularly, intra-vitreally, or systemically. Local therapy is not without side effects and patients must be monitored closely for cataract formation and elevated intraocular pressure (IOP).

A. Treatment of anterior uveitis usually consists of a topical corticosteroid to control the inflammation, and a cycloplegic agent to reduce the formation of posterior synechiae and relieve photophobia. Different cycloplegic drops can be used depending upon the desired duration of action, and include tropicamide, cyclopentolate, atropine, and others.

The topical steroid should be dosed frequently initially (generally hourly), and tapered once inflammation resolves. Choices for topical steroids vary and can be chosen based on potency or side-effect profiles. For initial control of inflammation, a more potent agent should be used such as prednisolone acetate or difluprednate; however, these agents may have a higher risk of elevated IOP than other topical corticosteroids. Once this initial medication has been tapered, some patients may require prolonged treatment with a milder topical steroid to suppress inflammation and minimize IOP response. These options include fluorometholone, rimexolone, loteprednol etabonate, and others. Once inflammation has resolved, the patient should be tapered off of the corticosteroid drop with monitoring to identify any recurrence of inflammation.

If inflammation cannot be controlled with topical therapy, additional therapy should be considered. One exception in which inflammation in the anterior chamber is often observed is with Fuchs heterochromic iridocyclitis.

B. Some clinicians do not treat mild cases of intermediate uveitis without vision loss or cystoid macular edema (CME). If the patient has decreased visual acuity or CME, treatment should be considered, such as with systemic or periocular corticosteroids.

C. Active posterior uveitis or panuveitis generally requires treatment to prevent vision loss. The initial control may be attempted with periocular or systemic corticosteroids. If inflammation remains uncontrolled or if the patient requires more prolonged therapy, intravitreal steroid implants or immunomodulatory therapy may be considered. Once again, one must be certain to rule out an infectious etiology before initiating these treatments.

D. If inflammation is uncontrolled, periocular corti-costeroids may be considered. Triamcinolone acetonide or methylprednisolone acetate may be administered either by a sub-Tenon or by a trans-septal route. These agents have a more prolonged duration of effect when compared with topical steroids, and may be repeated after four weeks, if needed. Potential complications include periorbital hemorrhage, prolonged IOP elevation, cataract formation, globe perforation, infection, ptosis, and skin discoloration (depending on approach). They should not be used in infectious uveitis or in necrotizing scleritis as there is a risk of scleral thinning and perforation. They are also not recommended for long-term control of chronic inflammation since each recurrence of inflamma-tion between injections produces cumulative ocular damage. The use of immunomodulatory agents for the management of chronic diseases is described in Chapter 140 of this text.

E. If inflammation remains uncontrolled, or if the patient requires more prolonged local treatment, intravitreal corticosteroids are available in several delivery modalities. They all carry the risk of retinal detachment, endophthalmitis, vitreous hemorrhage, cataract formation, and glaucoma. Intravitreal triamcinolone acetonide has been used for many years to manage CME in uveitis, but the

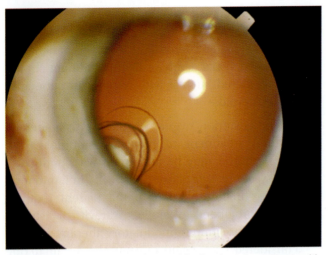

Fig. 139.1: Fluocinolone acetonide implant in patient with Behçet disease.

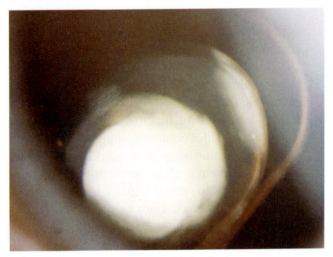

Fig. 139.2: Fluocinolone acetonide implant.

duration of the effect is limited, and injection often needs to be repeated. Sustained-release intravitreal implants have longer durations of action as compared with intravitreal injections and include the fluocinolone and dexamethasone implants (Figs. 139.1 and 139.2). The fluocinolone implant is approved by the US-Food and Drug Administration (FDA) for the treatment of chronic noninfectious posterior uveitis, and can control inflammation for up to 3 years. Studies have shown the implant to be useful in controlling intermediate uveitis and panuveitis as well, while decreasing the need for other local or systemic therapy. The intravitreal dexamethasone implant is also approved by the US FDA for the treatment of noninfectious uveitis

affecting the posterior segment. This implant is bioerodible and delivers dexamethasone for approximately 6 months.

F. Destruction of the pars plana snowbank with cryotherapy or treatment of the peripheral retina with laser photocoagulation may be considered in patients with intermediate uveitis in whom other treatment modalities have failed. Laser therapy to the snowbank has been associated with retinal tears and should be avoided.

G. If cryotherapy or laser photocoagulation fail, pars plana vitrectomy may be considered to control inflammation. Additionally, vitrectomy may be considered for the treatment of dense vitritis/vitreous debris, retinal detachment, vitreous hemorrhage, persistent CME, or for diagnostic purposes.

H. Neovascularization may occur in eyes with long-standing inflammation. Control of the inflammation alone may resolve the stimulus for neovascularization. Inflammatory choroidal neovascularization (CNV) can be a significant cause of vision loss. Several small studies have shown that the therapy directed against vascular endothelial growth factor may be effective in managing CNV secondary to uveitis.

BIBLIOGRAPHY

1. Gallego-Pinazo R, Dolz-Marco R, Martínez-Castillo S, et al. Update on the principles and novel local and systemic therapies for the treatment of non-infectious uveitis. Inflamm Allergy Drug Targets. 2013;12:38-45.
2. Lowder C, Belfort R Jr, Lightman S, et al. Dexamethasone intravitreal implant for noninfectious intermediate or posterior uveitis. Arch Ophthalmol. 2011;129:545-53.
3. Multicenter Uveitis Steroid Treatment (MUST) Trial Research Group. Kempen JH, Altaweel MM, et al. Randomized comparison of systemic anti-inflammatory therapy versus fluocinolone acetonide implant for intermediate, posterior, and panuveitis: The multicenter uveitis steroid treatment trial. Ophthalmology. 2011;118:1916-26.
4. Rouvas A, Petrou P, Douvali M, et al. Intravitreal ranibizumab for the treatment of inflammatory choroidal neovascularization. Retina. 2011;31:871-9.
5. Tran TH, Fardeau C, Terrada C, et al. Intravitreal bevacizumab for refractory choroidal neovascularization (CNV) secondary to uveitis. Graefes Arch Clin Exp Ophthalmol. 2008;246:1685-92.

Systemic Therapy

140

Steven R Cohen, Daniel A Johnson

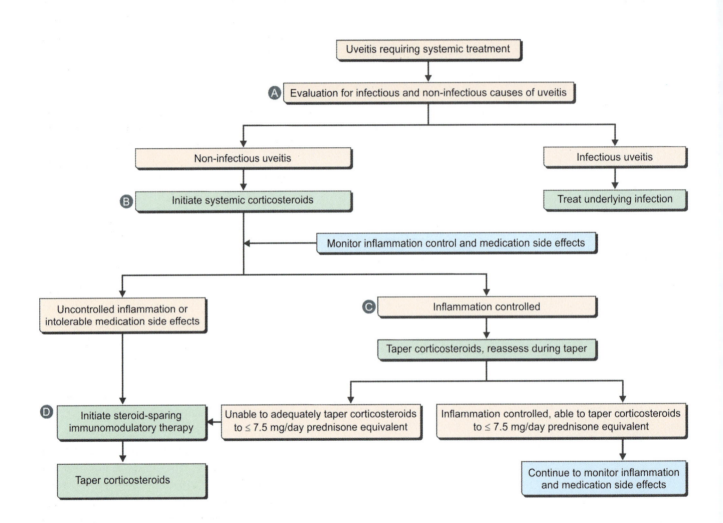

The incidence of uveitis in the United States is estimated to be up to 17 cases per 100,000 population. Untreated or undertreated ocular inflammation may lead to profound ocular morbidity. Topical therapy alone may control many cases of anterior uveitis. Systemic therapy may be indicated when there is inadequate control of inflammation with local therapy, for severe bilateral disease, for posterior segment disease, and when there is a need for nonocular immunosuppression.

A. A thorough evaluation including a detailed history, as well as laboratory and radiographic studies, is important to determine any potential underlying cause of inflammation. Failure to diagnose an infectious cause of uveitis may result in significant harm if inappropriately treated with immunosuppressive therapy.

B. Systemic corticosteroids have been the mainstay of therapy for inflammatory diseases for decades, and if used appropriately, can be extremely effective. Prednisone is the most commonly prescribed oral corticosteroid, with a typical starting dose of 1 mg/kg/day. Patients should be counseled on the potential serious side effects of oral corticosteroids including weight gain, hypertension, hyperglycemia, elevated lipids, osteoporosis, aseptic necrosis, and gastrointestinal bleeding. They should also be counseled on the risks of suddenly stopping the medication, due to the suppression of the hypothalamic-pituitary-adrenal axis. Calcium and vitamin D supplementation is recommended, as is gastrointestinal prophylaxis. Children should not be maintained on long-term systemic corticosteroids due to the risk of growth retardation.

Oral corticosteroids should be continued until the inflammation has resolved, but generally should not be continued at high doses for longer than one month. If the inflammation has not been controlled by one month, corticosteroids alone are unlikely to control the disease, and consideration should be given to the use of immunomodulatory therapy.

C. If the inflammation is well-controlled, oral corticosteroids should be tapered slowly over a period of weeks to months. The goal is to taper off the oral corticosteroids completely. If the patient requires chronic corticosteroid therapy, the dose should be tapered to ≤7.5 mg/day prednisone equivalent to minimize the long-term side effects. If this cannot be achieved, additional or alternative immunosuppressive therapies must be considered.

D. If the patient's inflammation cannot be controlled with oral corticosteroids, the patient cannot tolerate the side effects of oral corticosteroids, or if the corticosteroids cannot be tapered adequately, immunomodulatory therapy should be considered. Although no immunomodulatory agents are approved by United States-Food and Drug Administration (US-FDA) for the treatment of uveitis, many have proven to be safe and effective for the treatment of many ocular inflammatory diseases. In fact, they are the recommended monotherapy for many autoimmune conditions. Immunomodulatory therapy is often continued for 1–2 years. These agents are categorized according to their mechanism of action:

- **Antimetabolites**
  i. *Methotrexate:* Methotrexate is a folic acid analog that inhibits dihydrofolate reductase, producing several effects that inhibit rapidly dividing cells. It is used commonly in rheumatoid arthritis and juvenile idiopathic arthritis. It is often used in children due to its long track record and safety profile. Hepatotoxicity is a potential serious side effect and liver enzymes must be monitored. Other side effects include mucositis, pneumonitis, and secondary infections.
  ii. *Azathioprine:* Azathioprine is a prodrug that is converted to a purine analog that inhibits DNA and RNA production. It is utilized for several systemic autoimmune diseases. Gastrointestinal upset is the most common side effect limiting its use. Other side effects include bone marrow suppression, specifically leukopenia and thrombocytopenia, and secondary infections.
  iii. *Leflunomide:* Leflunomide is a prodrug that functions as a tyrosine kinase inhibitor, inhibiting T-cell and B-cell responses to interleukin-2. Side effects include diarrhea, weight loss, alopecia, neurologic effects, and upper respiratory infections.
  iv. *Mycophenolate mofetil:* Mycophenolate mofetil is an inosine monophosphate dehydrogenase inhibitor that disrupts the *de novo* purine synthesis pathway. It is used commonly for scleritis and other forms of uveitis. Gastrointestinal upset is its most common side effect. Other side effects include leukopenia, lymphocytopenia, and abnormal liver function tests.

- **Alkylating agents**
  i. *Cyclophosphamide:* Cyclophosphamide alkylates DNA bases leading to DNA crosslinking and cell death. For ocular inflammation, it is used most commonly in treating granulomatosis with polyangiitis (formerly Wegener granulomatosis), polyarteritis nodosa, necrotizing scleritis (Fig. 140.2) and peripheral ulcerative keratitis in rheumatoid arthritis, relapsing polychondritis, ocular

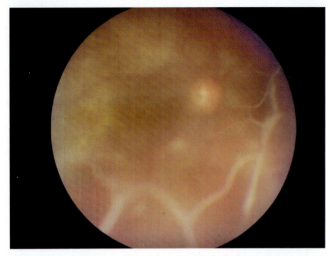

Fig. 140.1: Retinitis, vitritis in patient with Behçet disease.

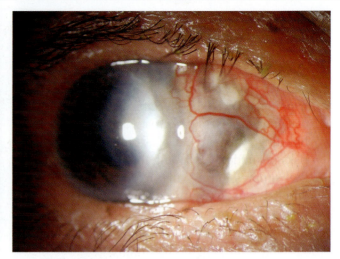

Fig. 140.2: Necrotizing scleritis.

cicatricial/mucous membrane pemphigoid, and in severe Behçet disease (Fig. 140.1). Potential side effects include hemorrhagic cystitis, sterility, leukopenia, opportunistic infections (often requiring prophylaxis for *Pneumocystis carinii*), and secondary malignancy.

ii. *Chlorambucil:* The mechanism of action of chlorambucil is similar to that of cyclophosphamide. It has been found to be especially effective in uveitis associated with Behçet disease. One of the most severe side effects is potentially irreversible bone marrow suppression. Other side effects include sterility and amenorrhea, reactivation of varicella-zoster virus, opportunistic infections (often requiring prophylaxis for *P. carinii*), and possibly increased risk of secondary malignancy.

- **Antibiotics**

i. *Cyclosporine:* Cyclosporine is a calcineurin inhibitor that decreases the activation of T-cells and has been used extensively in the treatment of uveitis. The main side effect is hypertension. Other side effects include renal toxicity, immunosuppression, gingival hyperplasia, myalgias, hirsutism, hypomagnesemia, cutaneous neoplasia, and tremor.

ii. *Tacrolimus:* Tacrolimus is a macrolide antibiotic that inhibits calcineurin. Major side effects include hypertension and nephrotoxicity. Other side effects include gastrointestinal upset, hyperglycemia, hypomagnesemia, and tremor.

iii. *Sirolimus:* Sirolimus is a macrolide antibiotic that functions similarly to cyclosporine and tacrolimus. Limited data exist regarding its use in the treatment of ocular inflammatory diseases. Side effects include infection, edema, gastrointestinal upset, erythema nodosum, myalgias, and dermatologic issues.

iv. *Dapsone:* Dapsone is a synthetic sulfone that has anti-inflammatory properties. Its ophthalmic use is predominantly for patients with ocular cicatricial or mucous membrane pemphigoid. Methemoglobinemia is the most frequent side effect and is especially severe in patients with glucose-6-phosphate dehydrogenase deficiency. Other side effects include aplastic anemia, peripheral neuropathy, hepatitis, and jaundice, among others.

- **Microtubule inhibitors**

i. *Colchicine:* Colchicine binds to tubulin dimers and prevents the formation of the mitotic spindle that stops cell division. It is used for prophylaxis against the recurrences of anterior uveitis in patients with Behçet disease. Gastrointestinal upset is a common side effect.

- **Antibodies**

  i. *Tumor necrosis factor inhibitors*

     1. *Etanercept:* Etanercept is a dimeric protein formed by the fusion of two human tumor necrosis factor (TNF) receptors and one human IgG1 Fc fragment. It binds to and inactivates circulating TNF, which results in decreased leukocyte migration and cytokine production. The most common side effect is a reaction at the site of injection. Other side effects include anaphylaxis, immunosuppression, sepsis, and demyelinating disease. Latent or active tuberculosis must be ruled out prior to beginning therapy.

     2. *Infliximab:* Infliximab is an IgG monoclonal antibody that binds to and inhibits circulating and membrane bound TNF-α. It has been used in treating the inflammatory diseases resistant to other treatments. Serious infections have been reported with its use. Side effects include headache, diarrhea, rash, and autoantibodies. Latent or active tuberculosis must be excluded prior to beginning therapy.

     3. *Adalimumab:* Adalimumab is a human IgG1 TNF-α antibody. It has been used successfully in uveitis secondary to juvenile idiopathic arthritis, ankylosing spondylitis, Vogt-Koyanagi-Harada, birdshot retinochoroidopathy, and scleritis. Side effects include reactivation of tuberculosis, fungal infections, and opportunistic infections.

  ii. *Anti-interleukin-2 (IL-2) receptor antibodies*

     1. *Daclizumab:* Daclizumab is a humanized IgG1 monoclonal antibody that binds to CD25, inhibiting the IL-2 response. Its production has been discontinued due to low demand, but it is still being studied in trials.

  iii. *Other antibodies:* Intravenous immune globulin, anakinra, rituximab, toclizumab.

BIBLIOGRAPHY

1. Durrani K, Zakka FR, Ahmed M, et al. Systemic therapy with conventional and novel immunomodulatory agents for ocular inflammatory disease. Surv Ophthalmol. 2011;56:474-510.
2. Jabs DA, Rosenbaum JT, Foster CS, et al. Guidelines for the use of immunosuppressive drugs in patients with ocular inflammatory disorders: recommendations of an expert panel. Am J Ophthalmol. 2000;130:492-513.
3. Nguyen QD, Hatef E, Kayen B, et al. A cross-sectional study of the current treatment patterns in noninfectious uveitis among specialists in the United States. Ophthalmology. 2011;118:184-90.
4. Suttorp-Schulten MS, Rothova A. The possible impact of uveitis in blindness: a literature survey. Br J Ophthalmol. 1996;80:884-8.

SECTION  9

Neuro-Ophthalmic Disorders

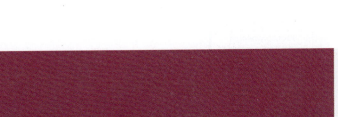

The Abnormal Pupil

141

Angela M Herro, Martha P Schatz, John E Carter

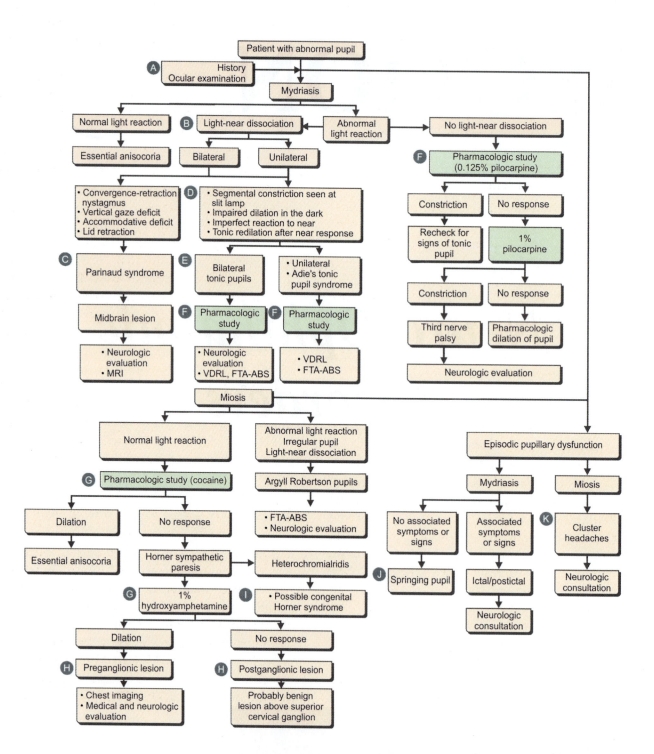

This chapter gives the diagnostic pathway for the etiology of the abnormal pupil in an awake and alert patient. This does not include evaluation of the comatose patient nor does it incorporate the relative afferent pupillary defect into diagnostic criteria.

A. A thorough history and ocular examination of the eye will lead to the determination of the abnormal pupil as either mydriatic or miotic. The examination of the iris should exclude previous surgery of the iris or trauma producing traumatic mydriasis or pupillary irregularity. The pupil should be observed in bright and dim environments. Anisocoria that is accentuated in dim light implicates the smaller pupil as abnormal, whereas anisocoria greater in bright light indicates the larger pupil is abnormal. A unilateral tonic pupil may be smaller in dim light but larger in bright light.

B. Light-near dissociation indicates a stronger constriction to a near stimulus than to light. This can be a unilateral or bilateral phenomenon.

C. If bilateral, light-near dissociation likely represents a central source, such as the midbrain, as seen in dorsal midbrain syndrome (Parinaud syndrome). This can be caused by an intrinsic process such as a neoplasm, infarct, vascular malformation, or demyelinating plaque or from an extrinsic lesion causing compression, such as a pinealoma.

D. In the case of unilateral light-near dissociation, or a tonic pupil, there will be a slow, "tonic" contraction and dilation, segmental constriction, or spontaneous "vermiform movements" of the iris best evaluated at the slit lamp.

E. A tonic pupil can also be bilateral or unilateral, however, most commonly presents as a unilateral phenomenon. Each year, about 4% of patients with an Adie tonic pupil develop a tonic pupil in the fellow eye. Sequential onset of the tonic pupils, either by history or observation, is typical of Adie tonic pupil syndrome. There is an extensive list of causative processes including infection that result in a peripheral neuropathy and cholinergic denervation hypersensitivity.

F. Pharmacologic testing of the mydriatic pupil helps confirm a tonic pupil when 0.125% pilocarpine induces pupillary constriction. This should be done before any manipulation of the eye, including tonometry or instillation of anesthetic drops. Approximately 80% of tonic pupils react to dilute pilocarpine, thus a negative result does not rule out the diagnosis. If unclear, instill 1% pilocarpine. Failure to respond to 1% indicates a pharmacologically dilated pupil, usually caused by accidental exposure to a mydriatic. This may be caused by organophosphate or cocaine exposure. A mydriatic pupil due to injury to the third nerve will react to pilocarpine 1%, but there may also be a small response to dilute pilocarpine, thus emphasizing the importance of clinical history and slit-lamp examination.

G. Pharmacologic testing of the miotic eye, on the other hand, uses other agents. As mentioned earlier, these studies should be done before manipulating the cornea or instilling other drops. To confirm the presence of a Horner syndrome, or deficiency of sympathetic activity, a drop of either cocaine (4% or 10%) or apraclonidine should be instilled into the eye (Of note, do not use apraclonidine in children because of respiratory depression and lethargy). Keep in mind that 10% cocaine is the gold standard but 4% is widely available and sufficient for diagnostic testing. Cocaine blocks the reuptake of norepinephrine resulting in the dilation of a normal pupil, but would leave a Horner pupil unaffected. Apraclonidine is a α_1- and α_2-adrenergic agonist that may cause slight dilation in a normal iris. However, because of denervation hypersensitivity, the Horner pupil dilates to a greater degree, thus producing reversal of anisocoria. Testing with hydroxyamphetamine should not be done until 24 to 48 hours after cocaine testing.

H. Hydroxyamphetamine can be used to localize the lesion. Hydroxyamphetamine causes a release of norepinephrine from intact adrenergic nerve endings causing pupillary dilation. Therefore, if there is dilation 1 hour after the instillation of the eyedrops, this would indicate a first- or second-order lesion. If the pupil fails to dilate, this indicates a lesion of the third-order neuron. Malignancy is responsible for up to 50% of first- or second-order lesions (between C8-T1 and superior cervical ganglion), but is rarely the cause of the third-order order lesions. Associated CNS symptoms or signs may identify the lesions; however, the apex of the chest, mediastinum, or neck account for most cases of Horner syndrome (Customary evaluation for Horner depends on the age of the patient and clinical circumstances).

I. If the cocaine and/or apraclonidine test shows a Horner syndrome in the setting of heterochromia iridis, this suggests a congenital cause, but has also been documented in a few cases of acquired Horner. The authors recommend all children with Horner should be considered for the evaluation of neuroblastoma.

J. When the pupil is not consistently affected, but shows episodic dysfunction, the history again becomes more important. A mydriatic springing pupil is a benign syndrome with episodic mydriasis, usually in young women, associated with nonspecific headache or sensations in the eye, and defective accommodation. Episodic mydriasis can also be produced by migraine.

K. Episodic miosis, on the other hand, is characteristic of cluster headaches, as this can produce sympathetic paresis during the headache.

BIBLIOGRAPHY

1. Bradley WG, Daroff RB, Fenichel GM. Neurology in Clinical Practice, 3rd Edition. Butterworth-Heinemann, 2000. pp. 223-6.
2. Miller NR, Newman NJ. Walsh and Hoyt's Clinical Neuro-ophthalmology, 6th Edition. Baltimore, MD: Williams & Wilkins, 2005.

Nystagmus

142

Jorge A Montes, Martha P Schatz, John E Carter, Susan M Berry

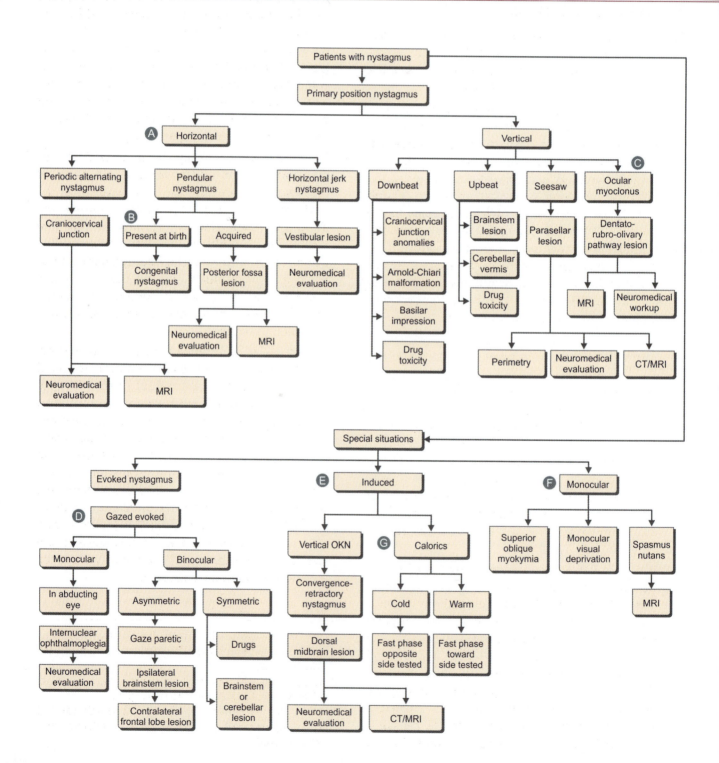

Acquired nystagmus is most helpful diagnostically when it is present in the primary position. Any type of nystagmus discussed here may be caused by lesions in a variety of locations or may be congenital. In addition, drugs, especially anticonvulsants and psychoactive medications, may cause nystagmus in the primary position resulting in oscillopsia.

A. Three types of horizontal nystagmus maintain their horizontal character when the patient moves the eyes vertically: vestibular, periodic alternating nystagmus, and congenital nystagmus.

B. Congenital nystagmus has been described with delayed onset for several years after birth but typically presents by 6 months of age. Congenital nystagmus can take many forms to include pendular with jerk component, usually horizontal but very occasionally vertical or rotary. A null point is often present. Pendular nystagmus in the primary position, which maintains its horizontal direction in vertical gaze, does not produce oscillopsia, and dampens with convergence in a patient without other neurologic symptoms or signs, may still be congenital nystagmus, even though it was not present for several years after birth.

C. Despite its name, ocular myoclonus is a nystagmus, in that it is a steady, rhythmic oscillation of the eyes. It is a slow, coarse, vertical nystagmus, and accompanies palatal myoclonus in which the palate or pharyngeal musculature exhibits the same rhythmic movement. Small lesions in the dentatorubro-olivary pathway may produce only the palatal movements, whereas larger or bilateral lesions produce oculopalatal myoclonus. This is a delayed effect that may not develop for several months after the neurologic injury and does not necessarily mean that there is a new or progressive lesion.

D. Gaze-evoked nystagmus in the extremes of eccentric gaze is common. It is usually not sustained. Many drugs amplify gaze-evoked nystagmus. Gaze-evoked nystagmus to one side suggests a recovering gaze palsy from a lesion of the brainstem on the same side or contralateral hemispheric lesion in the frontal lobe. However, significantly asymmetric gaze-evoked nystagmus may also be seen with ipsilateral brainstem lesions, especially cerebellopontine mass lesions. If eccentric gaze produces nystagmus in the abducting eye, there may have been an internuclear ophthalmoplegia that has recovered; slowing of adducting saccades in the fellow eye or saccadic dysmetria in the same eye confirms the diagnosis.

E. Upward saccades, whether a single large amplitude movement or repetitive saccades induced by optokinetic stimulation, may produce co-contraction of all third nerve muscles and consequent convergence and retraction of the globe into the orbits. The repetitive phenomenon is convergence-retractory nystagmus when induced with optokinetic stimulation. This is one element of Parinaud syndrome (lid retraction, light-near dissociation, and upward gaze palsy).

F. Superior oblique myokymia is identifiable by a history of intermittent vertical and torsional movement of one of the two images of the environment. It may be induced during the slit-lamp examination by various vertical eye movements. Spasmus nutans has a characteristic clinic profile of early onset, fine nystagmus, head bobbing, and resolution by the age of 3 years. Although it is usually benign, consideration should be given to intracranial mass lesions, especially if atypical features exist.

G. Testing of the VOR can be done by caloric testing. The VOR aims to produce an eye movement equal and opposite to head movement so that the gaze is stabilized during head rotation. Cold water in the right ear elicits a clockwise current in the semicircular canal and movement of the stereocilia to the right (similar effect as turning head to the left). Therefore, there will be slow pursuit to the right and a fast saccade to the left. Similarly, warm water in the right ear produces a counter clockwise current and movement of the stereocilia to the left (similar effect as turning head to the right). Therefore, there will be a slow saccade to the left and a fast saccade to the right.

BIBLIOGRAPHY

1. Burde RM, Savino PF, Trobe JD. Clinical Decisions in Neuro-ophthalmology, 2nd Edition. St Louis, MO: Mosby, 1992.
2. Glaser JS. Neuro-ophthalmology, 2nd Edition. Hagerstown, MD: Harper and Row, 1989.
3. Miller NR, Newman NJ. Walsh and Hoyt's Clinical Neuro-ophthalmology, 6th Edition. Williams and Wilkins, 2005.

143

Swollen Disc

Martha P Schatz, Angela M Herro

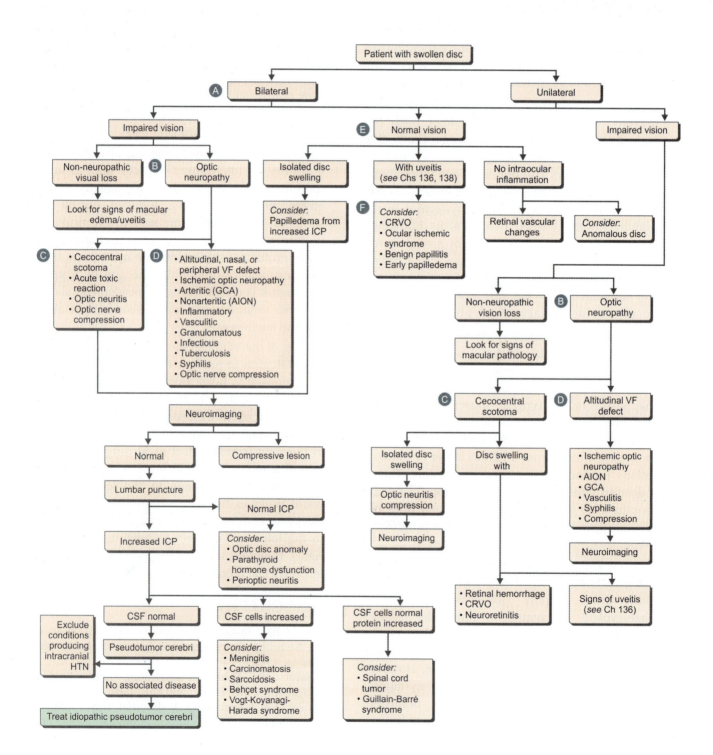

Optic disc swelling can be caused by many processes, either by direct invasion or indirectly from a secondary intracranial process. There are also many terms used to describe swelling of the optic nerve head. In general, many use the term *disc swelling* descriptively and reserve the term *papilledema* for disc swelling caused by intracranial hypertension. Others use *papilledema* for any disc swelling but indicate passive disc swelling by the term *choked disc*. However, whatever the term used, the most important question is whether the vision is affected. Impaired vision often indicates an active process affecting the nerve versus passive swelling. The pattern of the visual field (VF) defect and the laterality is most helpful in determining the nature of the process.

A. In any patient with bilateral disc swelling, one must consider increased intracranial pressure unless the clinical examination indicates otherwise (e.g. uveitis).

B. In a patient with bilateral disc swelling, the next question is whether or not there is vision impairment. If there is decreased vision, the etiology is either the optic nerve or retina. An optic neuropathy is diagnosed by the presence of an afferent pupillary defect, color vision deficit, and a characteristic neuropathic VF defect (i.e. altitudinal, arcuate, cecocentral, or constrictive). Nonneuropathic VF loss is that which does not have these features (i.e. macular or central).

C. The presence of a bilateral swollen disc with impaired vision and cecocentral scotoma leads to a broad differential including methanol poisoning, optic neuritis, chronic infectious processes, and infiltrative processes, and warrants neuroimaging. Bilateral optic neuritis is common in children but uncommon in adults. The differential should include syphilis, tuberculosis, and fungus, whereas inflammation can be the consequence of sarcoidosis or collagen vascular diseases, or infiltrative as in leukemia and lymphoma.

D. Disc swelling in the presence of an altitudinal VF defect is highly suggestive of ischemia of the optic disc. The differential should include those in step "C" as well as ischemic optic neuropathy of the arteritic or non-arteritic form, as well as the infectious, inflammatory, or compressive etiologies outlined above. Bilateral, simultaneous ischemic optic neuropathy is more often caused by temporal arteritis.

E. Monocular disc swelling with preserved vision may be seen with uveitis, which is often accompanied by white blood cells in the vitreous and anterior chamber. If there is intraocular inflammation, the appearance of the retinal vasculature should be examined. If normal, an anomalous disc or disc drusen should be considered. In the presence of vascular congestion or venous inflammation, one must consider diabetic papillopathy, diabetic or HTN retinopathy, CRVO or *venous stasis retinopathy* in older patients; or venous inflammation or papillophlebitis in children.

F. A patient with isolated unilateral disc edema with normal vision can be seen in intracranial hypertension; however, this usually becomes bilateral over weeks to months. Other symptoms and clinical signs may be used to determine the need to proceed with additional studies.

BIBLIOGRAPHY

1. Burde RM, Savino PJ, Trobe JD. Clinical Decisions in Neuroophthalmology, 2nd Edition. St Louis, MO: Mosby; 1992.
2. Glaser JS. Neuro-ophthalmology, 2nd Edition. Philadelphia, PA: JB Lippincott; 1989.
3. Miller NR, Newman NJ. Walsh and Hoyt's Clinical Neuro-ophthalmology, 6th Edition (Vol. 1). Baltimore, MD: William & Wilkins; 2005.

144

Optic Neuropathy

John E Carter, Susan M Berry, Martha P Schatz, David K Scales

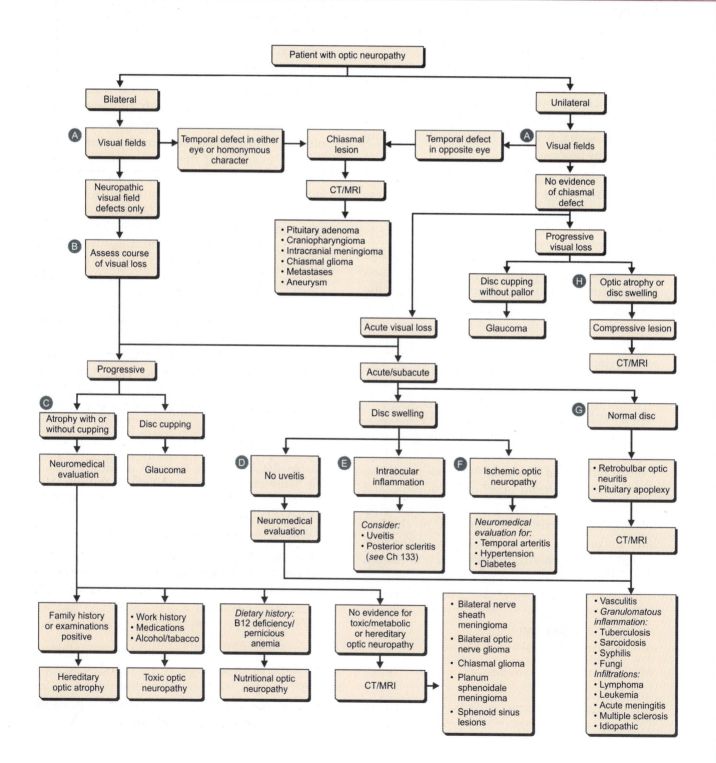

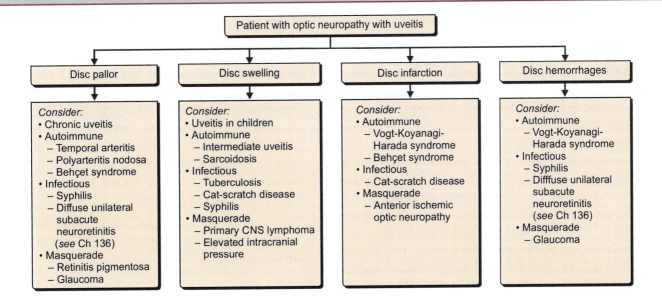

Patient with optic neuropathy with uveitis

Disc pallor

Consider:
• Chronic uveitis
• Autoimmune
  – Temporal arteritis
  – Polyarteritis nodosa
  – Behçet syndrome
• Infectious
  – Syphilis
  – Diffuse unilateral subacute neuroretinitis (*see* Ch 136)
• Masquerade
  – Retinitis pigmentosa
  – Glaucoma

Disc swelling

Consider:
• Uveitis in children
• Autoimmune
  – Intermediate uveitis
  – Sarcoidosis
• Infectious
  – Tuberculosis
  – Cat-scratch disease
  – Syphilis
• Masquerade
  – Primary CNS lymphoma
  – Elevated intracranial pressure

Disc infarction

Consider:
• Autoimmune
  – Vogt-Koyanagi-Harada syndrome
  – Behçet syndrome
• Infectious
  – Cat-scratch disease
• Masquerade
  – Anterior ischemic optic neuropathy

Disc hemorrhages

Consider:
• Autoimmune
  – Vogt-Koyanagi-Harada syndrome
• Infectious
  – Syphilis
  – Difffuse unilateral subacute neuroretinitis (*see* Ch 136)
• Masquerade
  – Glaucoma

Optic neuropathy is diagnosed when complaints of decreased vision are accompanied by impaired color vision, afferent pupillary defect, and a visual field defect (or a combination thereof). Subjective abnormalities also include decreased color saturation and brightness in the involved eye. The appearance of the optic disc varies according to the duration of the process. Acute disease anteriorly produces disc swelling, but acute disease in the retrobulbar optic nerve may not change the appearance of the optic disc. Disease of the optic nerve of a more chronic nature usually produces atrophy, although compressive lesions may produce disc swelling for many months before atrophy develops.

A. Visual field testing in both eyes should be performed. Any defect that respects the vertical meridian indicates that the disease process is intracranial at the anterior chiasm and optic nerve junctions. Because most chiasmal lesions are caused by mass lesions, this distinction is critical in directing the diagnostic work-up.

B. The temporal profile of the visual loss is the most reliable indicator of the cause and permits tailoring of the examination and diagnostic studies toward the most likely diagnosis.

C. Bilateral, chronic, progressive optic atrophy is usually attributable to a hereditary optic neuropathy, a nutritional or deficiency state, or toxic exposure (environmental or medicinal).

Visual field defects in these conditions are usually cecocentral. Examination of family members may be helpful. However, neuroimaging is recommended to exclude mass lesions that simultaneously involve both optic nerves in most cases.

D. Young patients with acute or subacute visual loss and disc swelling most commonly have an inflammatory process involving the optic disc and/or anterior optic nerve. Idiopathic optic neuritis is the most common, but history and laboratory studies should be used to exclude other more specific and more treatable inflammatory and infiltrative conditions (Patients with Leber hereditary optic neuropathy may appear to have segmental disc swelling; however, there is no leakage on fluorescein angiography, and genetic testing should be done).

E. The optic nerve head may be swollen with uveitis involving the posterior globe or with posterior episcleritis. Visual loss may or may not be present when the nerve is swollen in association with uveitis; when present, visual loss may be caused by inflammation of the nerve or by effects of the uveitis on the macula.

Note: When neuroimaging is indicated, magnetic resonance imaging (MRI) with contrast (brain and/or orbits) is recommended. If a contraindication exists for MRI, then CT scan should be performed.

F. Visual loss with a very sudden onset is usually vascular in nature and in older patients indicates retinal vascular occlusion or, if disc swelling is present, ischemic optic neuropathy. Most ischemic optic neuropathy is related to either atherosclerosis of small arterioles, mechanical factors associated with small cup/disc, or a combination of these. However, temporal arteritis (TA) also causes ischemic optic neuropathy, and early treatment is important to prevent further visual loss. Symptoms that suggest TA are progressive headache of recent onset, jaw claudication, nocturnal fevers or a recurrent fever of unknown origin, and polymyalgia rheumatica. Immediate lab oratory work-up to include erythrocyte sedimentation rate (ESR), C reactive protein (CRP), and complete blood count should be obtained. A combination of thrombocytosis and elevated ESR or CRP is highly suggestive of TA in the right clinical setting. A strong clinical suspicion with appropriate labs is usually sufficient to make the diagnosis and begin treatment immediately without a temporal artery biopsy. The biopsy can be performed after treatment has been started.

G. Acute optic neuropathy with a normal optic disc indicates abnormality in the retrobulbar optic nerve. The diagnostic considerations are similar to those of patients with optic neuritis. Pituitary apoplexy (hemorrhage into a pituitary tumor) may cause acute visual loss bilaterally and is usually associated with severe headache and eye movement disturbances. An older patient with a history of cancer may have meningeal carcinomatosis, which involves the optic nerves bilaterally in a large percentage of patients.

H. A progressive optic atrophy in one eye is likely to indicate a compressive lesion, either neoplastic or aneurysmal.

▌BIBLIOGRAPHY

1. Burde RM, Savino PJ, Trobe JD. Clinical Decisions in Neuro-ophthalmology, 2nd Edition. St. Louis, MO: Mosby; 1992.
2. Glaser JS. Neuro-ophthalmology, 2nd Edition. Philadelphia, PA: JB Lippincott; 1989.
3. Miller NR, Newman NJ. Walsh and Hoyt's Clinical Neuro-ophthalmology, 6th Edition (Vol 1). Baltimore, MD: Williams & Wilkins; 2005.

Angela M Herro, Johan Zwaan

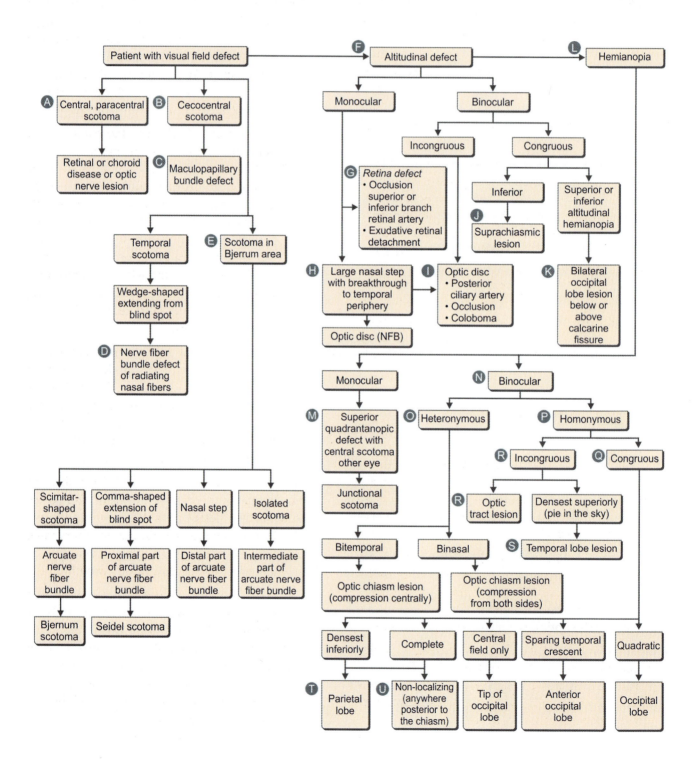

The interpretation of the loss of visual field (VF) is based on the anatomic organization of the retina throughout the visual pathway to the occipital lobe. Because lesions of different parts of the visual system can cause similar VF defects, interpretation of the VF alone is not always sufficient to localize a lesion. This test should be used in conjunction with tests such as pupillary reaction, color vision, ocular motility, ophthalmoscopy, perception of brightness, and light-stress recovery time to further refine the location of the lesion. Often, MRI, CT scanning, or electrophysiologic testing are also necessary. The initial branch in the flow chart starts with classification of the VF defect as central, cecocentral, temporal, Bjerrum scotoma, altitudinal, or a hemianopia.

A. A central or paracentral VF defect can result from retinal, macular, or choroidal disease or from a lesion of the optic nerve. Careful inspection of the defect with respect to the vertical or horizontal meridian is often helpful. Retinal lesions generally do not respect either meridian, whereas optic nerve lesions respect the nasal horizontal but not the vertical meridian. Ophthalmoscopy will aid in differentiating between the two. If the VF is bilateral and similar between both eyes, suspect optic neuropathies of hereditary (Leber optic neuropathy, Kjer dominant optic atrophy), nutritional {vitamin B_{12} or folate deficiency, tobacco or alcohol}, or toxic {methanol, medications, heavy metals} causes.

B. A cecocentral scotoma is a nerve fiber bundle (NFB) defect of the papillomacular bundle. It is, by definition, an extension of the blind spot. These can be caused by optic neuritis, hereditary conditions, toxic insults, and nutritional deficits, or less commonly, retinal diseases affecting these fibers such as serous exudate from an optic nerve pit (often unilateral).

C. The maculopapillary bundle consists of nerve fibers from the macula that enter the optic disc on the temporal side. Thus, they represent the fibers that represent the VF temporal from fixation and leading to the optic disc, or a cecocentral scotoma.

D. A temporal scotoma that appears as a wedge emanating from the blind spot peripherally is likely from a process on the nasal side of the retina as they enter the nerve radially. This type of defect does not always respect the horizontal meridian.

E. A scotoma in the Bjerrum area, or an arcuate scotoma, comes from nerve fibers from the temporal peripheral retina as they arch around the maculopapillary bundle and the fovea on their way to the optic disc. This part of the VF is about 15 degrees away from the fixation point and is called *Bjerrum area*. Defects within this area, often are an early indication of glaucomatous damage, as the superior and inferior temporal parts of the optic nerve are more susceptible to glaucoma. This scotoma can range from a full scimitar shape to only portions of the arch involved, depending on which segment of the arcuate NFB is damaged.

F. An altitudinal defect is larger than those from a NFB defect alone. Those respecting the nasal horizontal meridian but not the temporal, are most likely caused by optic nerve or NFB defects. If the entire horizontal meridian is respected in both eyes, this points to a lesion of the calcarine cortex. Occipital cortex and retinal or optic disc lesions may also cause such defects, as can contusions of the optic nerves or the chiasm, although less commonly. The first diagnostic division when encountering a patient with an altitudinal defect is whether it involves one or both eyes.

G. A monocular altitudinal defect is most commonly caused by embolism of the superior or inferior branch of the retinal artery. It is possible for an embolus to affect both eyes but unusual for the defect to be congruous. Bilateral retinal detachments, rhegmatogenous or exudative, may also cause incongruous altitudinal defects.

H. A large monocular nasal step with breakthrough to the temporal periphery may give rise to an altitudinal field defect. This defect would respect the horizontal meridian nasally but not temporally, and most likely indicates an optic nerve lesion as from glaucoma or ischemic optic neuropathy.

I. A binocular altitudinal VF defect can be classified as congruous or incongruous. One example of an incongruous VF defect is described in "K" as a retinal artery occlusion. Another cause may be occlusion of the vascular supply to the optic disc due to damage to the posterior ciliary arteries. Other causes include bilateral optic disc colobomas and advanced glaucoma in both eyes.

J. Bilateral congruous inferior altitudinal VF defects are generally caused by suprachiasmatic lesions. A meningioma originating from the olfactory groove may grow backward onto the planum sphenoidale and compress the chiasm from above.

K. Bilateral and congruous altitudinal VF defects, respecting both nasal and temporal horizontal raphe, are caused by lesions of the occipital lobe. This can be caused by infarction of the brain tissue superior or inferior to the calcarine fissure caused by occlusion of branches of both posterior cerebral arteries. Similarly, inhibited circulation through the middle cerebral arteries may lead of infarction of the superior lips of the calcarine fissure. A VF defect such as this could also be caused by trauma from above, as trauma from below most likely involves laceration of the dural sinuses, which would likely result in death of the patient.

L. Hemianopic VF defects split the point of fixation (macula) and respect the vertical meridian. In contrast, NFB defects originate from the blind spot (optic disc) and do not respect the vertical meridian.

M. A junctional scotoma results when an optic nerve lesion of one eye impinges on the chiasm at the same side. Depending on its extent, the optic nerve lesion may cause a central or complete scotoma and the contralateral VF shows a superior temporal defect or a hemianopic temporal defect due to compression of the crossed fibers in the chiasm.

N. A binocular hemianopia can be further classified as either heteronymous or homonymous depending on the laterality within each eye. Any lesion of the optic pathway behind the chiasm will affect the VF of both eyes.

O. A heteronymous hemianopia involves either both nasal or both temporal halves of the VF. Pituitary tumors will first affect the inferior part of the center portion of the chiasm, leading to bitemporal superior quadrantanopia that may progress to complete bitemporal hemianopia. Binasal hemianopia is rare. It is caused by compression of both lateral sides of the chiasm, usually secondary to aneurysmal or arteriosclerotic enlargement of both internal carotid arteries.

P. VF defects on the same side in both eyes (nasal hemianopia in one eye and temporal in the contralateral eye) are called *homonymous*. They are caused by lesions behind the chiasm and can be incongruous or congruous.

Q. Congruity is determined by performing central VF tests. If the hemianopia affects the entire half of the central field, congruity cannot be determined. It can be tested only when the VF defect is incomplete. In general, the more congruous the hemianopia, the further posterior the causative lesion is located. The exception to this is the lateral geniculate body where nerve fibers of corresponding areas are organized.

R. An incongruous homonymous hemianopia points to the optic tract because of the loose association of corresponding areas.

S. An incongruous VF defect that is densest superiorly localizes to the temporal lobe. These lesions usually produce incongruous defects as the fibers in the optic radiation tend to be wider apart. Furthermore, it is the inferior fibers that swing anteriorly into the temporal lobe, forming Meyer loop, which accounts for the superior VF defect. Superior fibers run back directly toward the optic radiation within the parietal lobe and thus would cause an inferiorly denser VF defect.

T. A congruous homonymous hemianopia generally localizes to the parietal lobe or occipital lobe. The nerve fibers of the optic radiation become closer together and more homologously arranged in the parietal lobe and farther posterior, still separated anatomically into superior and inferior fibers. Therefore, a lesion of the parietal lobe would tend to affect the superior fibers first, resulting in a congruous inferior quadrantanopia, or a hemianopia denser inferiorly.

U. Occipital lobe lesions are the most congruous with one major exception. Each eye has a temporal crescent of VF for which there is no counterpart in the contralateral eye. This portion is represented in the occipital cortex along the most anterior part of the calcarine fissure. The macula is represented at the tip of the occipital lobe. Lesions that spare the anterior cortex will cause congruous homonymous hemianopias with sparing of the temporal crescent of the contralateral eye. Similarly, a lesion of the anterior lip of the calcarine fissure alone will cause a monocular VF defect that only involves the temporal crescent of the contralateral eye.

BIBLIOGRAPHY

1. Trobe JD, Glaser JS. The visual fields manual. Gainesville, FL: Triad, 1983.
2. Walker HK, Hall WD, Hurst JW, (Eds). Clinical methods: The history, physical, and laboratory examinations, 3rd edition. Boston: Butterworths; 1990. Available at: http://www.ncbi.nlm.nih.gov/books/NBK201/.

Index

Note: Page numbers followed by *f* and *t* denote for figures and tables respectively.